D0713007

Corpus Hippocraticum, the treatise ΠΕΡΙ ΑΡΘΡΩΝ, XXXII, 6 to XXXIII, 5:

If the teeth at the point of injury are displaced or loosened, when the bone is adjusted fasten them to one another, not merely the two which are loose, but several, preferably with gold wire, but, lacking that, with linen thread, till consolidation takes place. . . . If the jaw is broken right across, which rarely happens, one should adjust it in the manner described (one thumb inside the mouth; the fingers outside, for reduction). After adjustment [reduction] *one should fasten the teeth together as was described above* [*i.e., with gold wire or, lacking that, with linen thread*], *for this will contribute greatly to immobility, especially if one joins the teeth closely and fastens the ends of the wire, or thread, as they should be (fastened).*

(The work "On Joints" possibly may not have been written by Hippocrates, but might be an abridgment of an earlier work by another author, or even perhaps a collection of student's notes. It is, nonetheless, an important part of the Corpus Hippocraticum, the whole of which probably is only, after all, the remains of the library of the School of Medicine of Cos.)

The nonchalant way in which the Hippocratic author writes might lead one to suspect that the wiring of teeth in cases of fractures of the mandible was not an uncommon procedure.

G. Kasten Tallmadge

MORGAN L. LUCID, M. D.
2100 FOREST AVE. SUITE 107
SAN JOSE, CALIFORNIA 95128

SURGERY OF FACIAL FRACTURES

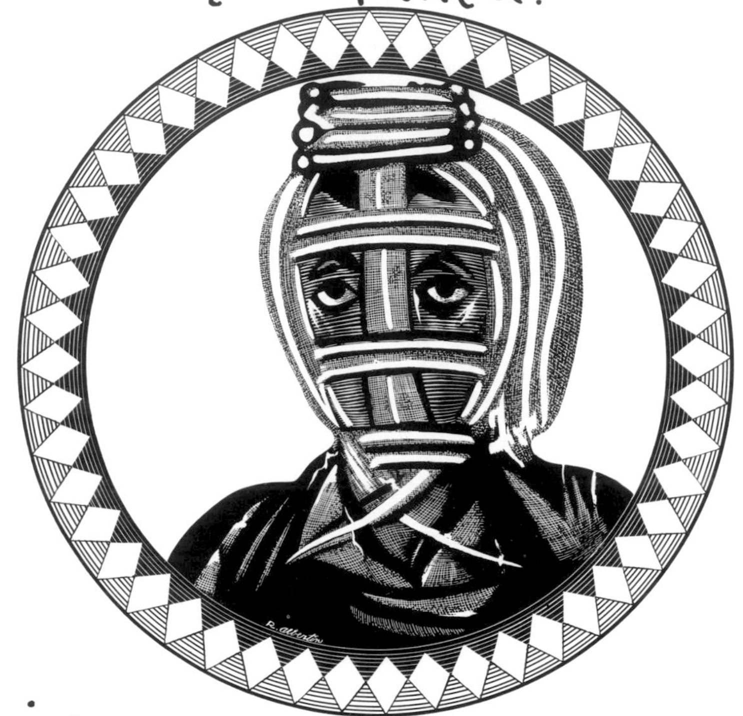

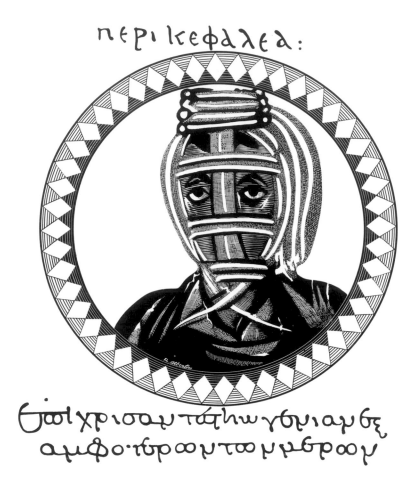

Redrawn by Robert H. Albertin

Laurentian MS, Plut. LXXIV, 7;
f. 232 verso.

PERIKEPHALEA

illustration from a medieval copy of a Greek scroll

Perikephalea (περικεφαλέα), a "casque," was the term used to describe bandages of the face and head. The illustration shows the position of a properly applied long bandage. The bandage was applied over an ointment and covered both the head and the face. From the chin the two ends were carried across opposite sides of the face, with several turns, to the back of the head and then to the top of the head, where many turns were made. Then the ends were carried downward across each cheek to be crossed beneath the chin, carried beneath the arm pits, and secured between the shoulder blades in back. It seems evident that this strikingly complex bandage was used in the treatment of fractures and injuries of the face and head. This beautiful illustration from a medieval copy of a Greek scroll has been attributed by Garrison to Niketas (ca. 900 A.D.); it could also have come from a manuscript of Soranus about 800 years earlier. The spiritual, melancholy appearance of the eyes, so familiar in countless Byzantine icons, and the graceful and delicate depiction of the folds of the garment suggest that the illustration was drawn by a Byzantine artist rather than by the compiler of the book. The text is generally Hippocratic. The excellent cursive (except in the superscription, which appears to have been done by another hand) confirms the tenth century dating of the manuscript.

G. KASTEN TALLMADGE, A.M., M.D., Ph.D.
Professor and Director of the Department of the History of Medicine, Marquette University School of Medicine, Milwaukee, Wisconsin.

FOREWORD BY

CHARLES G. CHILD, III, A.B., M.D.
Professor of Surgery and Chairman of the Department of Surgery, University of Michigan Medical School, Ann Arbor, Michigan.

ILLUSTRATIONS

ROBERT H. ALBERTIN, B.F.A., M.A.
Assistant Professor and Director, Division of Medical Illustration, Marquette University School of Medicine, Milwaukee, Wisconsin.

SURGERY OF FACIAL FRACTURES

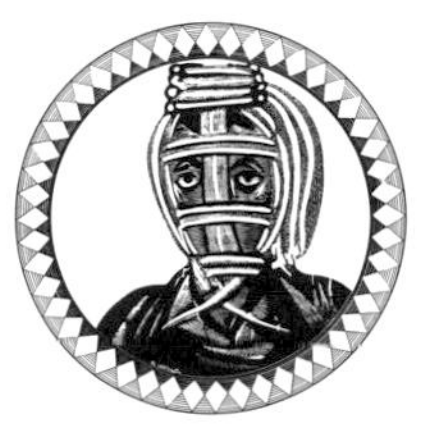

REED O. DINGMAN, A.B., D.D.S., M.S., M.D.
Assistant Professor of Surgery, University of Michigan Medical School. Associate Professor of Dentistry (Oral Surgery), University of Michigan School of Dentistry. Chief of the Department of Plastic Surgery, St. Joseph Mercy Hospital, and Staff Surgeon, University Hospital and Veterans Administration Hospital, Ann Arbor, Michigan.

PAUL NATVIG, B.A., D.D.S., M.D.
Assistant Clinical Professor of Plastic and Reconstructive Surgery, Marquette University School of Medicine. Staff Surgeon, Milwaukee Hospital, Milwaukee Children's Hospital, Milwaukee County General Hospital, and St. Mary's Hospital, Milwaukee, Wisconsin.

W. B. SAUNDERS COMPANY
Philadelphia and London
1964

Surgery of Facial Fractures

© 1964 by W. B. Saunders Company. Copyright under the International Copyright Union. All rights reserved. This book is protected by copyright. No part of it may be duplicated or reproduced in any manner without written permission from the publisher. Made in the United States of America. Press of W. B. Saunders Company. Library of Congress catalog card number 63-14507.

For

THELMA MUIR DINGMAN

and

ANNE CAMPBELL NATVIG

FOREWORD

In search of perfection, the science of surgery is certain to continue to reflect greater and greater specialization. The time has passed when one surgeon could pretend to master every competence of his craft. Today, as each surgeon pursues his special interests, he moves from the general to the specific, inevitably developing and thereby providing a whole new body of surgical knowledge. His work may be original, but often it represents a resynthesis of old facts and principles in new form and in new usefulness.

Two world wars, great advances in sciences basic to human health and disease, and rapid changes in the socioeconomic environment have stimulated surgery to incredible expansion. Today, achievements in support of human life which were unthought of not very many years ago, are commonplace. To display this new knowledge widely, books on special surgical subjects have appeared in great numbers. These, the oldest but still the newest and most reliable of teaching machines, mirror breadth and depth in surgery's contribution to alleviating an ever-increasing number of man's ills.

This text by Doctors Dingman and Natvig encompasses past and present knowledge of facial injuries. It clearly points the way toward a better understanding of one of surgery's most humanitarian accomplishments: the mending of fractured faces. The book is also a lively tribute to specialization in pursuit of progress and excellence.

In both these dimensions—progress and excellence—this volume has great significance for surgery and for surgeons. Even in periods of specialization there are beginners: medical students, interns, residents, practitioners, and specialists. As these learn, so must they teach and be taught. For them, the authors of this book on the surgery of facial fractures have captured the past with charm and the present with vigor. Guides are abundantly available for teaching and learning principles, for practicing applications, and for achieving competence.

Although men and women may be known by their deeds, they are recognized by their faces.

> The human features and countenance, although composed of but some ten parts or little more, are so fashioned that among so many thousands of men there are no two in existence who cannot be distinguished from one another.
>
> Pliny the Elder

The authors' enthusiasm for their science is infectious, and their skill in their art is unchallenged. Their ability to teach their skills by word and by picture is limited only by their students' capacity and motivation to learn. In these times of acceleration, deceleration, and dashboards, students, teachers, practitioners, and patients are greatly in their debt.

Professor of Surgery and
Chairman of the Department,
University of Michigan Medical School

PREFACE

In our time a torrent of technological advances has accelerated productivity, but this acceleration has proved to be not an unmixed blessing. Together with increases in the number of machines—automotive and otherwise—and in the rates at which they operate, it has brought new and different and difficult problems to Medicine. Far from the least of these is the alarmingly persistent increase in the incidence of injuries to the face. And this increase concerns a branch of medical practice which must be of high importance to all physicians and to some dentists, and of the highest importance to plastic surgeons, to otolaryngologists, to ophthalmologists, and to general and orthopedic surgeons.

Our book recognizes these important developments and is intended to provide for our colleagues a definitive illustrated work concerned with the contemporary management of fractures of the face. In the treatment of such fractures, this book is intended to fill the need for a concise and accurate description of the technique of internal fixation by wiring.

The technique of wiring, made popular about 1940 by Dr. William Milton Adams, lends itself admirably to the attainment of the accuracy required for its purpose: to return the patient swiftly to his normal functional state and to active participation in the life of his community.

But these purposes must be achieved with the fewest possible psychological complications. The face is the key to recognition, the center of attention, and no one's psyche is more severely injured as a result of trauma than is his whose face is disfigured. If the purpose of treatment is the restoration of normal anatomic relations and normal function—both of which include the restoration of functional dental occlusion—it is no less the restoration of the symmetry and intrinsic beauty of the features.

Our book, then, explains and demonstrates (as far as description and profuse illustration can explain and demonstrate) the manners in which these purposes can be achieved by combining internal fixation by wiring with intermaxillary fixation. This combination of procedures has proved to be eminently successful in our management of many cases.

Our colleagues will notice that we have not described or illustrated other methods of treatment: these—using multiple bandage-like splints, plaster head-caps, complex metallic frames, and other external appliances—are familiar to all. It would be of small consequence for us to elaborate new descriptions of these cumbersome methods.

We have divided several of the chapters in this book into two parts for the sake of clarity in presentation. In such chapters, part I is a discussion of the problems involved and part II is an illustrated, step-by-step description of the surgical procedure.

ACKNOWLEDGMENTS

We are happy to acknowledge our debt of gratitude to our friend, Dr. G. Kasten Tallmadge, who by his scholarship, wisdom, and judgment made such excellent additions to our volume. We are deeply appreciative of the many hours and days he contributed in preparation and reading of the manuscript.

In great measure the stimulation for preparation of this book was initiated by our learned colleague and teacher, Dr. Harry Sicher. His valuable suggestions, his constructive criticism, and the many hours devoted to the reading of the text have contributed much to this work.

We thank Mr. Robert H. Albertin and Miss Jean Moberg for the beautiful art renderings and illustrations.

We are grateful to the staff of the W. B. Saunders Company for their excellent advice and counsel concerning many technical problems of production.

Mr. Joseph Stodolo, Jr., has been patient and helpful in preparation and reading of the text.

The help and consideration of these others have done much to make this book possible: Dr. Donald P. Bobbitt, Miss Frances Beckwith, Mrs. Mary-Ann Brichta, Mr. C. Roland Burd, Mr. Ralph S. Cavan, Dr. Charles G. Child, III, Dr. J. C. Devine, Dr. Christopher R. Dix, Dr. Edwin H. Ellison, Dr. Sherwood W. Gorens, Dr. James R. Hayward, Mr. Gerald P. Hodge, Dr. Robert H. Ivy, Miss Ellen Johnson, Dr. Arthur C. Kissling, Jr., Mr. Anthony M. Kuzma, Dr. Richard H. Lillie, Dr. Jerome L. Marks, Dr. John K. Olinger, Dr. James A. Schelble, Mrs. Doris Schilling, Miss Ruth Schmidt, Mr. Robert H. Teevan, Mr. George J. Wing, and Dr. Walter Zeit.

Reed O. Dingman

Paul Natvig

CONTENTS

CHAPTER

1

PROFILING THE PIONEERS

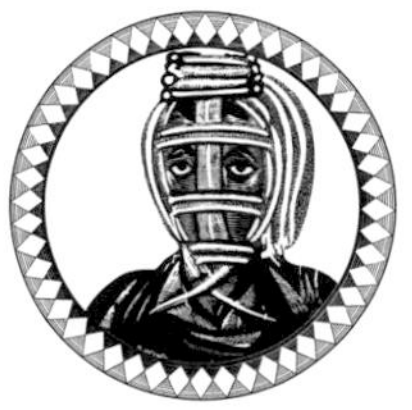

It is hoped that the biographical sketches in the following pages will interest all who concern themselves with the treatment of facial fractures. Here are sketched briefly the lives and careers of some of the pioneers who helped to lay the foundations of the modern surgical techniques that are the subjects of this work.

There is no doubt that many others contributed to the advances which we shall be describing. We acknowledge their work with gratitude and admiration. We wish it were possible to include biographies of all of them in this book.

Surveying the lives of these pioneers, we are impressed by an attitude they shared. None ever despaired of the ability of his profession to find, eventually, better methods of treating facial fractures. All had the critical judgment and the courage to recognize that any great progress is the result of many small gains.

In the search for a better way, no new way is necessarily final.

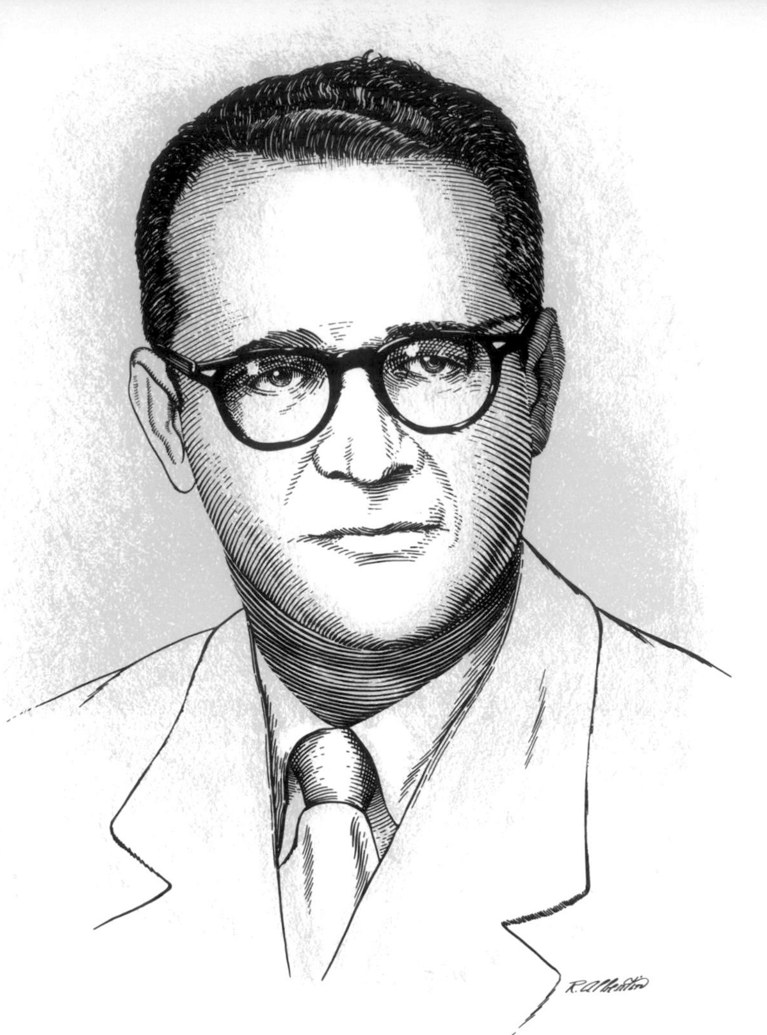

WILLIAM MILTON

ADAMS

(1905–1957)

"He is the greatest artist who has embodied, in the sum of his works, the greatest number of the greatest ideas."—John Ruskin

Nineteen hundred and thirty was the year William Milton Adams was graduated from the School of Medicine of Tulane University.

This was the year which initiated a career of concentration, a single dedication to a painstaking search for improved techniques of plastic and reconstructive surgery.

His was a brief career; he died at the age of 52. In the light of his excellent accomplishments, the brevity of his lifespan appears all the more tragic. Today we can only speculate on the achievements that might have come.

In terms of the essential subject of this work—the surgery of facial fractures—his accomplishments are as vital at this moment as they were in his own day.

He was the first to propose the modern technique of treating facial fractures by internal fixation by wire.

Milton Adams' original application of this technique is acknowledged as one of the truly great advances in the field of plastic surgery. Subsequent development by Adams helped popularize the technique, broadened its range of effectiveness, and multiplied its applications.

The accomplishments which have resulted from the great aims of William Milton Adams cannot be listed within the limited borders of a thumbnail biography.

The spirit that moved the man in his relentless search for a better way can best be expressed in the words of the man himself: *"A good surgeon should always be his own severest critic."*

The story of Greene Vardiman Black is the story of an American genius. One is reminded of Arnold's lines on Shakespeare:

But thou who didst the stars and sunbeams know,
Self-school'd, self-scann'd, self-honour'd, self-secure,
Didst walk on earth unguessed at . . .

For when he began his career, he was a self-taught practitioner of dentistry. When he completed his career, he was Dean of the School of Dentistry of Northwestern University and a man of science whose greatness was acknowledged everywhere.

At the beginning of this career, dentistry was hardly more than a crude trade. At its end, dentistry had become a respected scientific profession. To Greene Vardiman Black we owe gratitude for the largest share in the implementation of this evolution.

Not only was he an expert practitioner—we still refer to Black's lines of extension in operative dentistry—but he was also a proficient educator, as is proved by his ranking in Northwestern University.

Again, not only did he improve techniques and apparatus in dentistry, but he published many scientific articles concerned with the more technical problems of his specialty.

These accomplishments were stimulating to most of his students and to many of his colleagues. Thus Black brought to the profession of dentistry that excellence for which the state of Illinois long has been distinguished.

Greene Vardiman Black has been called the Father of Modern Dentistry. He advanced techniques and knowledge in a field which is peculiarly germane to the subjects that are discussed in our book.

Black was the first American to maintain reduction in fractures of the jaw by means of circumferential wiring.

"What's past is prologue."—Shakespeare

GREENE VARDIMAN

BLACK

(1836–1915)

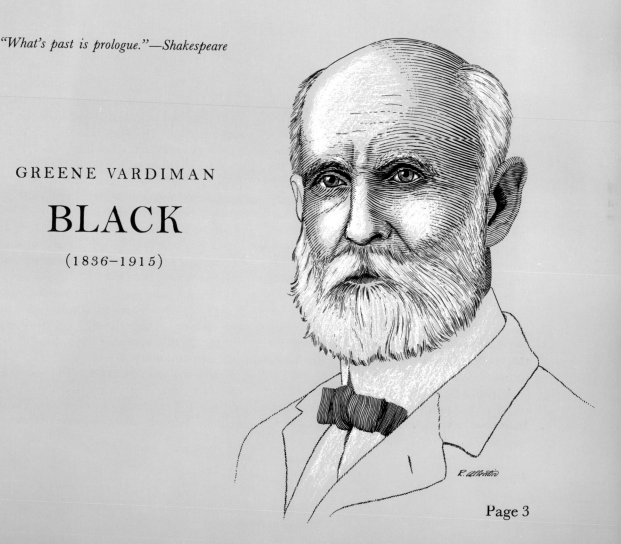

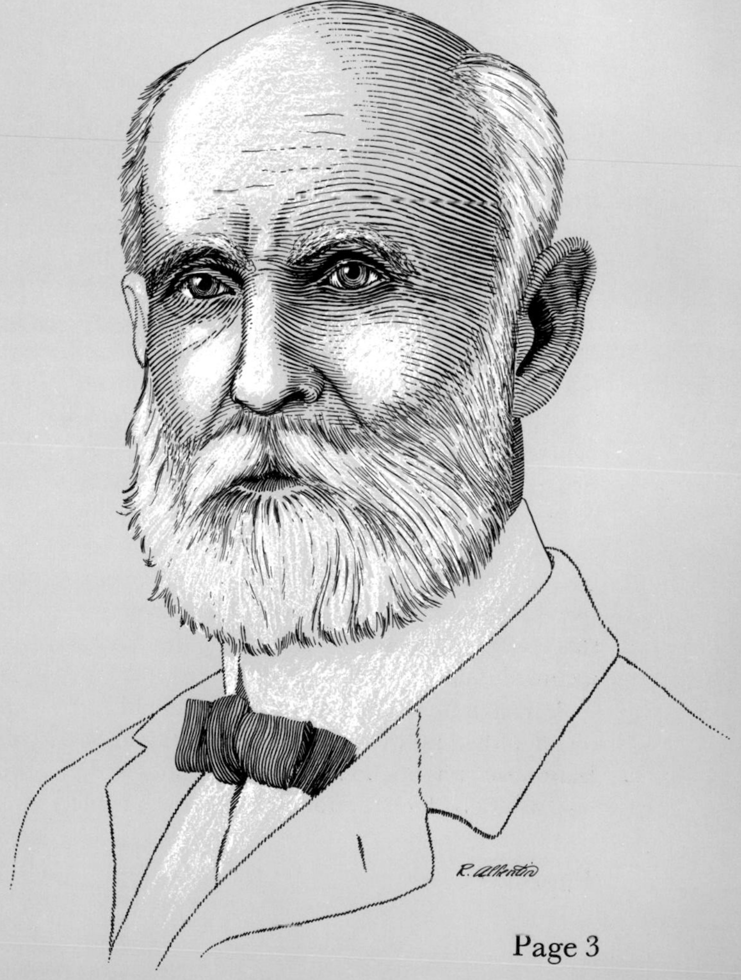

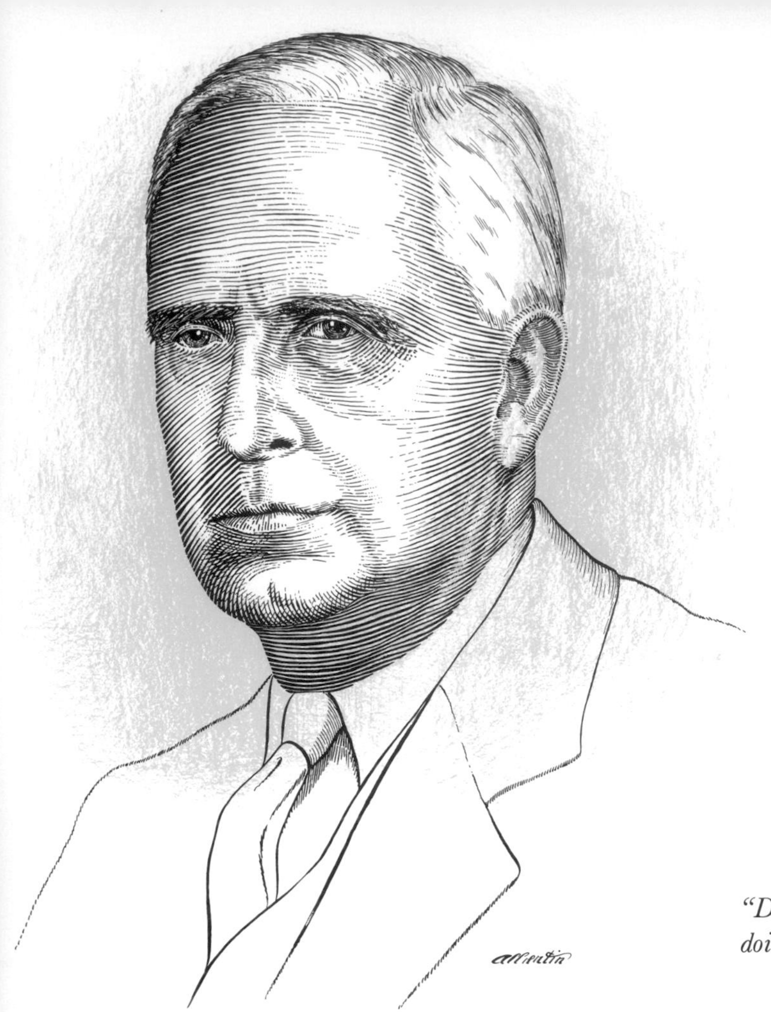

VILRAY PAPIN

BLAIR

(1871–1955)

"Doing easily what others find difficult is talent; doing what is impossible FOR TALENT *is genius."*
—Amiel

The medical profession is hardly given to the thoughtless encomium or exaggerated statement at any level. Thus, there can be little doubt about the true greatness of Vilray Papin Blair—hailed by his colleagues as the man most responsible for raising the standards of plastic surgery in the United States.

An inspired surgical innovator, a man of remarkable organizational genius, Blair was both the instigator and the prime moving force behind the establishment of the American Board of Plastic Surgery. And, having made major contributions toward establishing this specialty, his surgical accomplishments in the treatment of facial injuries, and in other operative procedures as well, helped make plastic surgery ever more valuable in the battle against human ills.

Although he was a descendant of an old and distinguished family of St. Louis, Vilray Papin Blair never was one to let traditions stand in the way of independent action. His approach to life or to science never was hidebound. He was imbued with the investigative spirit of the "Renaissance Man." In keeping with this spirit, he was immensely articulate and was a writer of unusual eloquence.

Vilray Blair was graduated in 1893 from the St. Louis Medical College, now extinct. His first teaching position was that of instructor in practical anatomy at Washington University, a position which supplied a valuable foundation for the highly creative surgical procedures that made him famous.

During World War I he was Head of the Section of Oral and Plastic Surgery in the United States Army and then Chief Consultant in Maxillofacial Surgery with the American Expeditionary Forces.

His subsequent career as a surgeon, teacher, and writer was consistently dynamic. The story of his life is epic in its proportions. The guide lines he left for his colleagues will stand for years to come.

An admiring colleague once described James Barrett Brown as "Mr. Plastic Surgery." While discounting its colloquial qualities, the appellation aptly defines the stature of this man and his work. On the basis of performance to date—and without considering the potentialities of his future—the work of Dr. Brown stands as a giant's mark upon the entire field of plastic surgery.

To the authors of this book, one of Dr. Brown's most impressive characteristics is an almost uncanny ability to simplify complex surgical problems. This ability was of infinite value to our nation during World War II, when Barrett Brown served the government's medical services as consultant-coordinator in plastic surgery. By introducing simplified procedures—techniques that made it easier for the clinician to perform effectively under tough wartime conditions—he became the man behind the scenes of thousands of surgical victories.

His war record also demonstrates the man's talent in the communication of ideas. His ability in the clear exposition of medical complexities is shown further in the wide-ranging, standard-setting contributions he has made to the literature of our profession.

Dr. Brown was born in Hannibal, Missouri—a fortuitous circumstance which led to a hobbyist's interest in the life and works of another prominent Hannibalian, Mark Twain. (Dr. Brown's collection of Twain memorabilia is reputed to be one of the finest in the country.)

A graduate of the Washington University School of Medicine in St. Louis, he continues to serve his alma mater as Professor of Clinical Surgery and as Professor of Maxillofacial Surgery at the university's School of Dentistry.

Although he makes Missouri his home, the scope of James Barrett Brown's contributions to medicine are of international significance.

"In science, the thing is to modify and change one's ideas as science advances."—Claude Bernard

JAMES BARRETT
BROWN
(1899-)

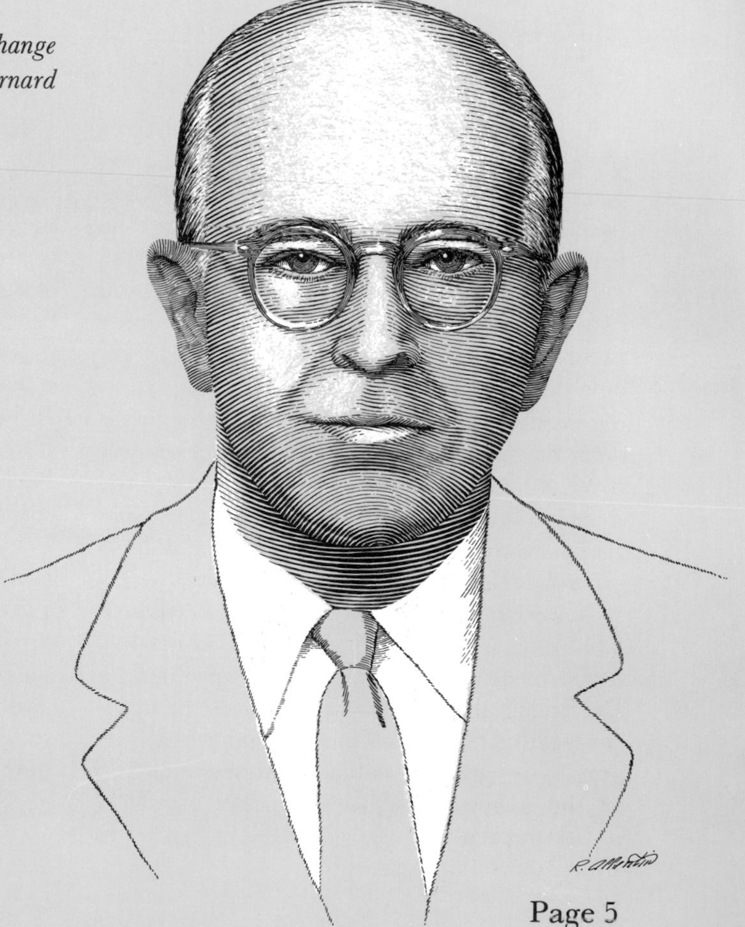

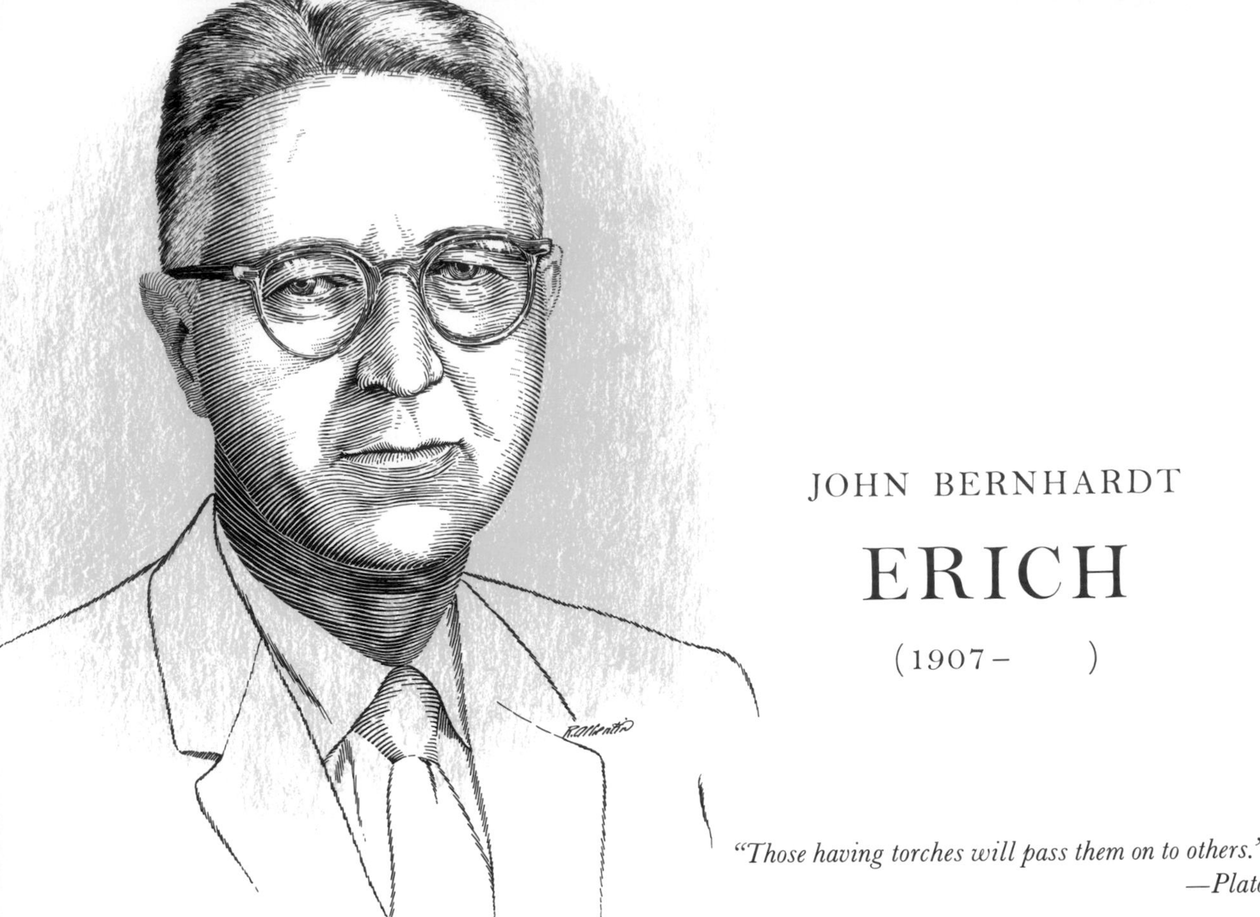

JOHN BERNHARDT
ERICH
(1907–)

"Those having torches will pass them on to others."
—Plato

Among the remarkable characteristics of America's medical profession is the capacity to rise to great heights in times of extreme stress—when both the facilities and the trained practitioners of a specialty are in sore danger of becoming overextended. One reason behind this unique capacity is the fortunate presence of men who are able to multiply their own skills . . . *to pass the torches on to others.*

During World War II and the Korean incident no medical specialty was under greater stress than was plastic surgery. To meet the shortage of trained clinicians, many great specialists worked tirelessly to teach their skills to physicians not trained in the specialty.

A leader in this work was John Bernhardt Erich. During the major conflict, some 200 naval medical and dental officers profited by Dr. Erich's ability to teach his skill in the surgical treatment of facial injuries and plastic surgery. They learned valuable lessons from him at the Mayo Clinic to which he, himself a naval medical officer, had been assigned to train others in his specialty.

In addition to these direct beneficiaries of Dr. Erich's teaching, many others gained through study of his book, *Traumatic Injuries of the Facial Bones,* a definitive volume in the writing of which he collaborated with Dr. Louis T. Austin, Director Emeritus of the Mayo Clinic's Section on Dentistry.

John Bernhardt Erich's own basic training started at the University of Illinois in Chicago. In just seven years of study at that institution, from 1926 to 1933, he received the degrees of Bachelor of Science, Doctor of Medicine, Doctor of Dental Surgery, and Master of Science.

In 1933, he entered the Mayo Foundation as a fellow in plastic surgery.

Today, after years of consistent accomplishment, he is head of the Mayo Clinic's Section on Plastic Surgery and also serves his specialty and the medical community as Professor of Plastic Surgery at the Mayo Foundation Graduate School of the University of Minnesota.

No roster of pioneers of our medical specialty would be complete unless it included the name of Harold Delf Gillies. Founder of the British Association of Plastic Surgeons, Harold Gillies was an inspirational leader on an international scale.

A native of New Zealand, Harold Gillies traveled to England to attend Cambridge University, after having been graduated from Wanganui College. He received his medical training at St. Bartholomew's Hospital, qualifying in medicine in 1908 and becoming a fellow of the Royal College of Surgeons in 1910.

As it did for many of his colleagues, World War I directed his career toward specialized treatment of facial injuries. As chief of the unit in plastic surgery of the Royal Medical Corps at Sidcup, in Kent, Gillies was responsible for the handling of more than 11,000 surgical cases in the final two years of the war.

In the years between the two great wars, the continuing achievements of Harold Gillies helped create the clinical standards of plastic surgery. In 1930, he was knighted in worthy recognition of his formidable achievements.

Gillies greeted the outbreak of World War II with strength and ingenuity. It was largely through his efforts that units in plastic surgery were organized in the British Isles. In the unit which he himself headed, hundreds of plastic surgeons were trained for service elsewhere. In 1941 he was sent to the United States, Canada, and South America to acquaint his colleagues of the West with the latest British methods of treating war casualties.

Among the enduring contributions made by Harold Gillies are two great books. The first, *Plastic Surgery of the Face,* published in 1920, summarized the lessons learned in the First World War. The second, *The Principles and Art of Plastic Surgery,* written in collaboration with Dr. D. Ralph Millard, Jr., was published in two volumes in 1957.

"Execute every act of thy life as though it were thy last."—Marcus Aurelius

HAROLD DELF

GILLIES

(1882–1960)

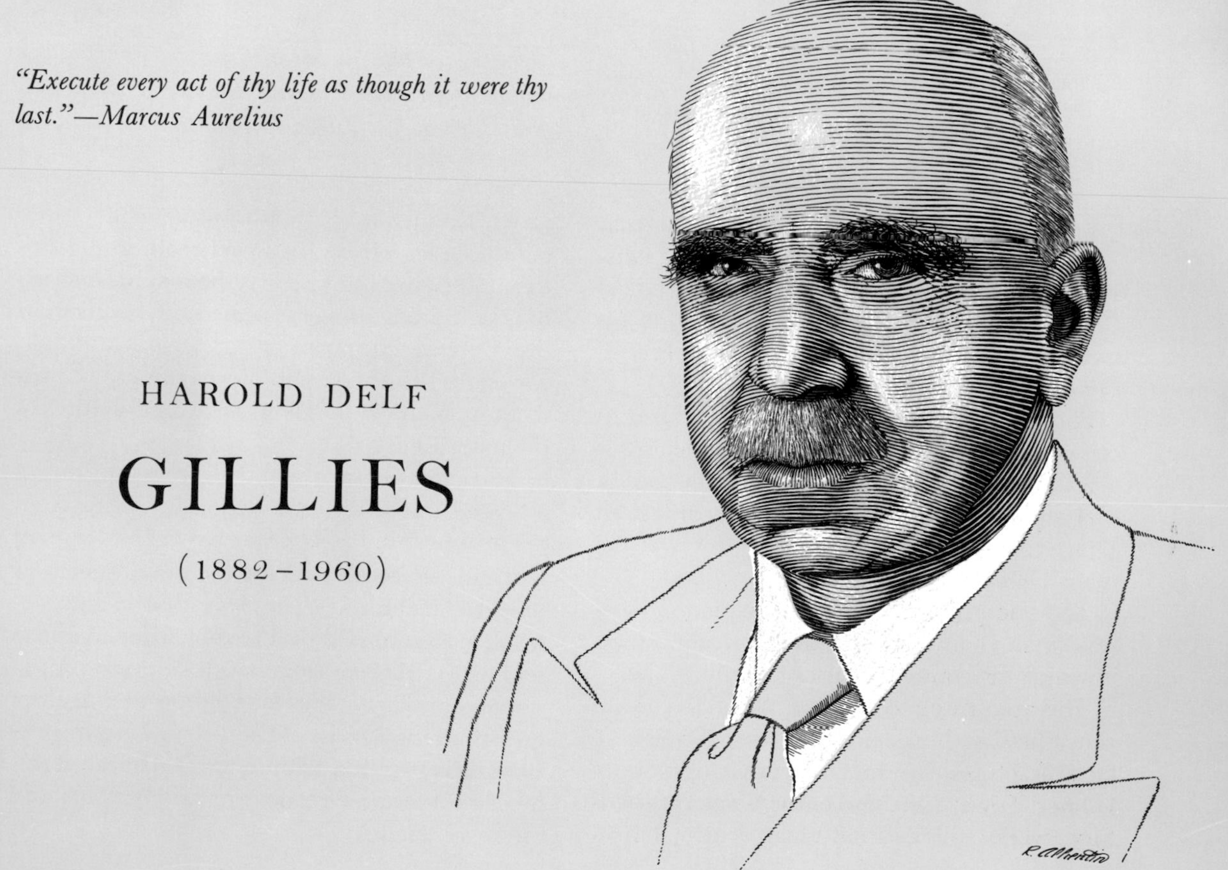

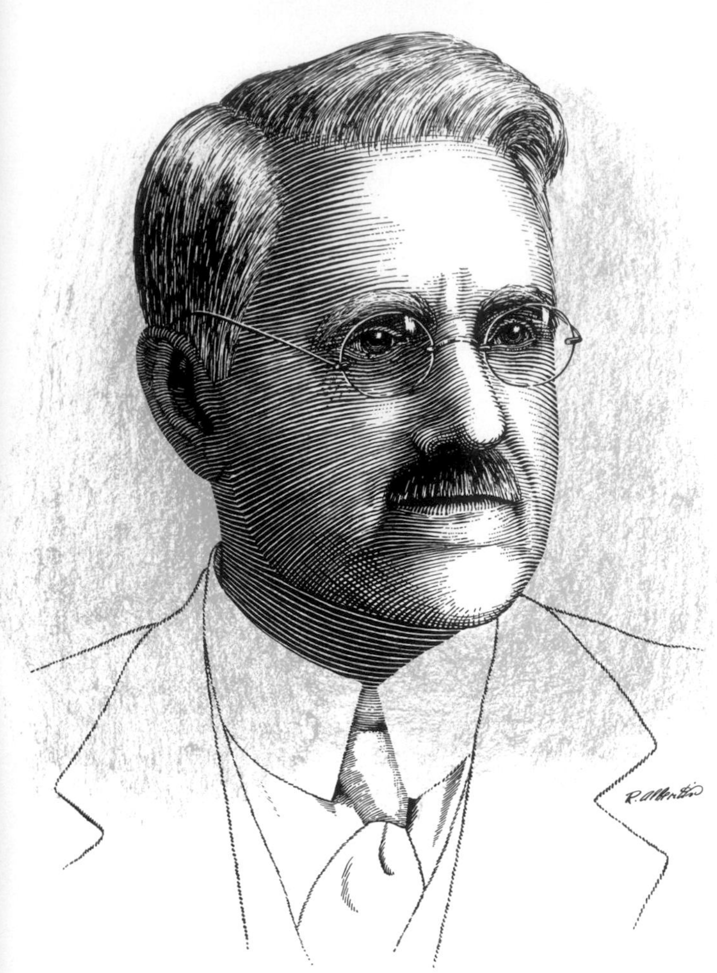

THOMAS LEWIS

GILMER

(1849–1931)

"You regard him as one of the great lights of the dental profession—I would claim him as a very great surgeon."—Vilray Papin Blair

Thomas Gilmer was born in Lincoln County, Missouri. He attended Missouri Dental College and St. Louis Medical College simultaneously—later completing his medical training at Quincy Medical College in Quincy, Illinois.

Son of a country physician, trained and licensed to practice medicine as well as dentistry, a leader in the development of techniques in oral surgery, a founder of the Northwestern University School of Dentistry—this was the man, Thomas Lewis Gilmer.

The quotation from his fellow-pioneer, Vilray Papin Blair, sums up the high admiration in which his contemporaries held him.

This admiration continues. All of us who are concerned with the modern management of facial fractures owe much to the good work of Gilmer. Toward the end of the nineteenth century, while still a small-town dentist, he revived the idea of treating fractures of the mandible by wiring the lower teeth to those of the upper jaw. Thus he was the first in America to take full advantage of a method described in the Corpus Hippocraticum, where attention was called to the suitability of the use of firm teeth as fixation points in treating fractures of the mandible.

The example mentioned above is only one of a host of important innovations to spring from the prolific mind of Thomas Lewis Gilmer. And with all his good work in the development of modern techniques, he was also a devoted teacher who passed on his knowledge to others and who worked tirelessly to elevate professional standards. The foundation and healthy growth of the School of Dentistry of Northwestern University is a tribute to his dedicated collaboration with Greene Vardiman Black and other colleagues.

In 1954, the plastic surgeons of Philadelphia and its environs decided to form a regional professional society which would enhance the reputation of their specialty. To find an appropriate name for the new organization was scarcely a problem. It seemed only natural that they should name it after the man who had given so much of his life to the progress of plastic surgery. They called it The Robert H. Ivy Society.

Born in England, Robert Henry Ivy came to the United States in 1898. Seventeen years of age, he promptly enrolled in the University of Pennsylvania's School of Dentistry. In 1901, when the nation's first dental internship was established at the Philadelphia General Hospital, Dr. Ivy became one of the first to serve. Subsequently, he entered the School of Medicine, was graduated in 1907, and completed his residency in 1910.

During the earlier years of his professional career, there was some question as to the specific direction his preferences might lead him. He was attracted strongly by the still unformulated specialty of plastic surgery; he was also deeply interested in urology. And to further broaden his horizon of experience, he spent five years as clinical pathologist and bacteriologist in the West Philadelphia Hospital for Women.

But World War I finally directed his career. Serving as an assistant to Vilray Papin Blair and later charged with direction of maxillofacial surgery at Walter Reed Hospital, he moved to the front of our specialty.

The scope of Dr. Ivy's competence as a teacher is indicated by the fact that he was the first American to hold the title of Professor of Plastic Surgery in any university—this at his alma mater, the University of Pennsylvania. The scholarly contributions of Professor Emeritus Ivy were fully recognized by the University in 1954, when he was awarded the degree of Doctor of Science.

Currently serving the specialty of plastic surgery as editor of its journal, Dr. Ivy ranks among the truly great contributors to our progress.

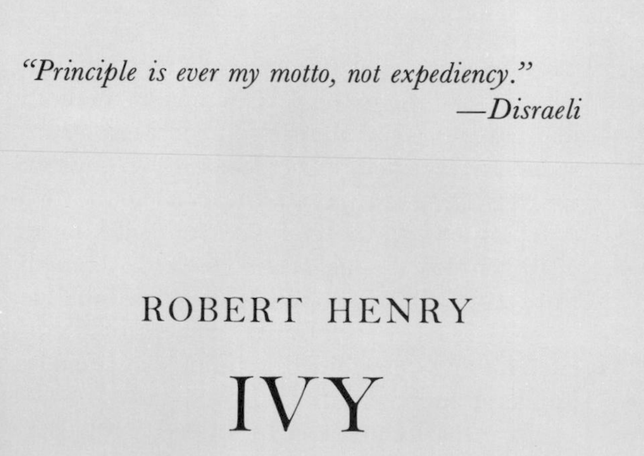

"Principle is ever my motto, not expediency."
—Disraeli

ROBERT HENRY

IVY

(1881–)

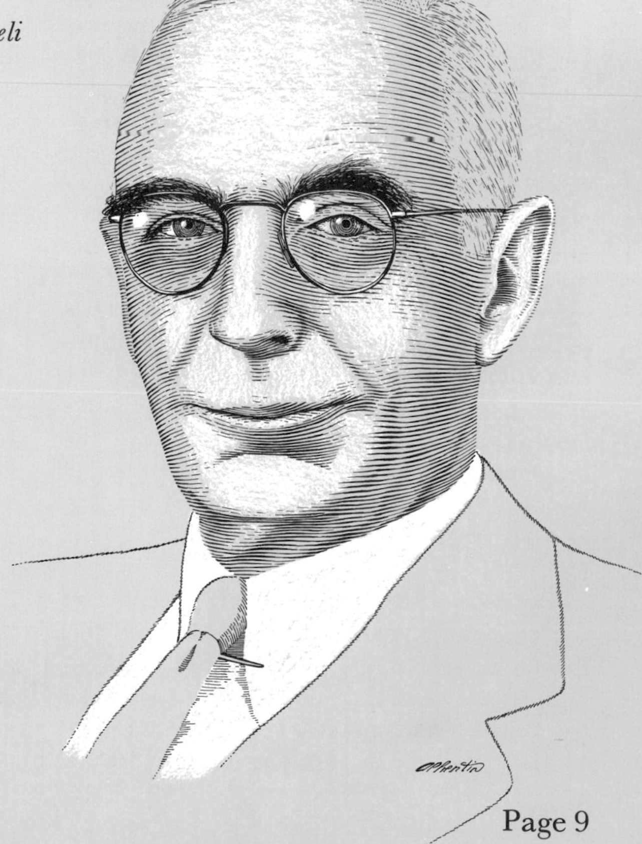

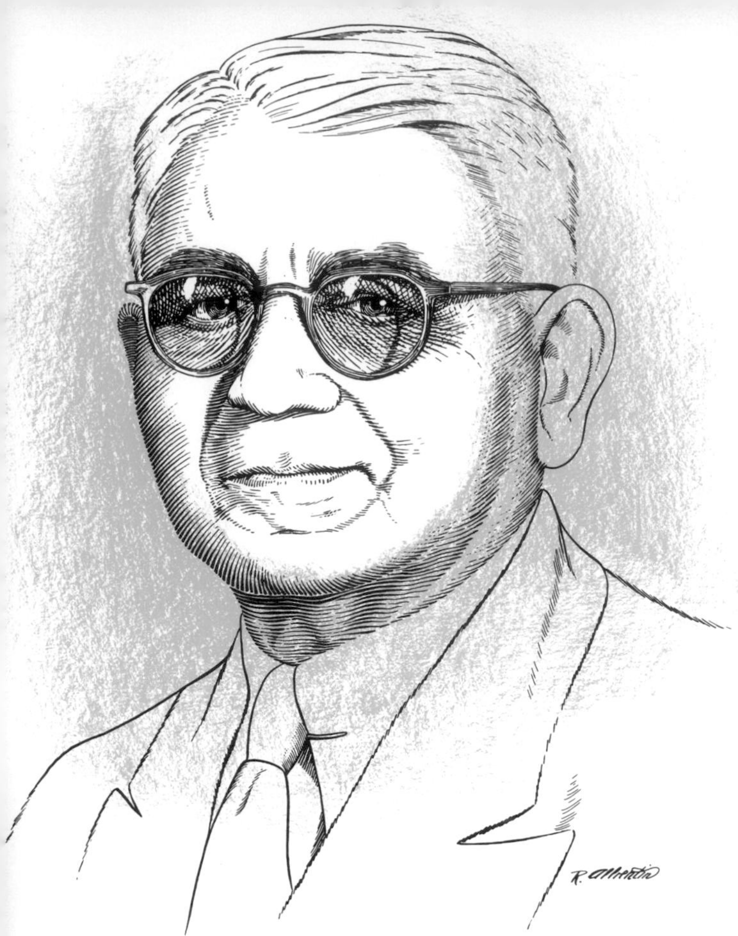

VARAZTAD HOVHANNES

KAZANJIAN

(1879–)

"Healing is a matter of time, but it is sometimes also a matter of opportunity."

—Hippocrates—Precepts

When he came to the United States from Turkish Armenia in 1895, Varaztad Hovhannes Kazanjian was only sixteen. Behind him lay the seemingly endless strife and turmoil that scarred his ancient homeland. Ahead of him lay the New World, exhibiting broad vistas of opportunity. The young newcomer viewed these vistas with enthusiasm and chose to devote his life to the healing arts.

In 1902 he entered Harvard University's School of Dentistry. The year after his graduation in 1906 he was retained by his alma mater as an instructor in prosthetic dentistry. His professional interests were concentrated upon the development of appliances for the correction of various abnormalities and defects of the jaw, and he treated many kinds of fractures of the jaw.

The year 1915 was exceedingly significant for Varaztad Kazanjian. He was named Chief Dental Surgeon in the Volunteer Surgical Unit organized by Harvard University to serve with the British Expeditionary Forces. He accepted this assignment, one of the great tests of his life, with strength and courage, applying all his talent and training to the development of methods for treating facial injuries and techniques for reducing the deformities caused by gunshot wounds.

Upon leaving the Harvard Surgical Unit in 1919, he took the logical step toward which all the events of his life had been leading him. He entered Harvard University School of Medicine, having determined to become a specialist in plastic surgery.

His remarkable capacities were swiftly recognized. Upon graduation from the Harvard University School of Medicine in 1921, Dr. Kazanjian was appointed Visiting Surgeon in Plastic Surgery at the Boston City Hospital, the Massachusetts General Hospital, and the Massachusetts Eye and Ear Infirmary. He is now Professor Emeritus of Plastic Surgery at Harvard University.

Dr. Kazanjian's brilliant career encompasses many valuable contributions to the treatment of facial fractures. Skilled clinician, dedicated teacher, prolific writer, he is honored as one of the valued pioneers in our specialty.

CHAPTER

2

THE MEN OF THE ELDER DAYS

Surely since the days of the cave dwellers, surely during the Old Stone Age, men (and doubtless women) have attempted to treat fractures of the face. We of course have no records of such attempts.

The earliest writings we possess occur in the Smith Papyrus, whose author (or authors) is thought to have written about twenty-five or thirty centuries before Christ. The only hieroglyphs which can be interpreted to indicate the use of bandages in the treatment of fractures are those which mention the use of lint (linen). In a part of the papyrus the author advised against any attempt to treat compound fractures of the mandible: "If thou examinest a man having a fracture of his mandible, thou shouldst place thy hand upon it. Shouldst thou find that fracture crepitating under thy fingers, thou shouldst say concerning him: 'One having a fracture in his mandible, over which a wound has been inflicted . . . (and) he has fever from it. An ailment not to be treated.'"[1]

The author, however, did advise treatment for dislocation of the mandible: "If thou examinest a man having a dislocation in his mandible, shouldst thou find his mouth open (and) his mouth cannot close for him, thou shouldst put thy thumb(s)

[1] Breasted tr.

upon the ends of the two rami of the mandible in the inside of his mouth, (and) thy two claws (meaning two groups of fingers) under his chin, (and) thou shouldst cause them to fall back so that they rest in their places. Thou shouldst say concerning him: 'One having a dislocation in his mandible. An ailment which I will treat.' Thou shouldst bind it with *ymrw,* (and) honey every day until he recovers."[2]

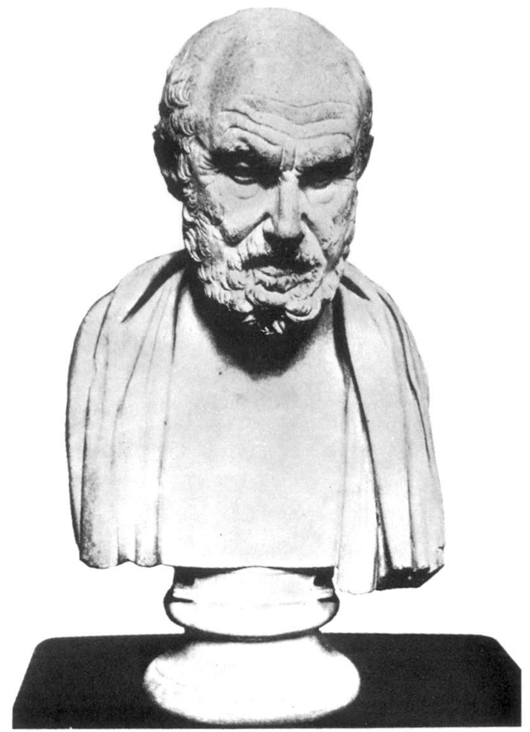

Figure 1. Hippocrates (460–375 B.C.). Greek marble bust in the British Museum.

THE MANDIBLE

Although no decipherable writings are extant, it is known that the Etruscans (ca. 600 B.C.) were expert in the use of gold and solder and had knowledge of the use of removable dental bridge appliances. These facts lead one to suspect that the Etruscans probably used monomaxillary gold wiring to treat fractures of the mandible.

"We have definite proof of the existence of the art . . . especially of dentistry among the Etruscans [600–500 B.C.]. In the tombs of Tarquinia, Capodimonte, and Civitá Castellana have been found teeth bound with gold wire (dentes auro juncti). These methods of treating the teeth passed from Etruria to Latium, whose dentures containing gold work have been found at Palestrina and Conca, and also at Rome, where a regulation of the Laws of the Twelve Tables forbade placing gold in tombs, except where it was in the teeth of the dead person."*

It is known, of course, that classical Greek science and culture influenced the Etruscans more profoundly in this period than did the Roman.

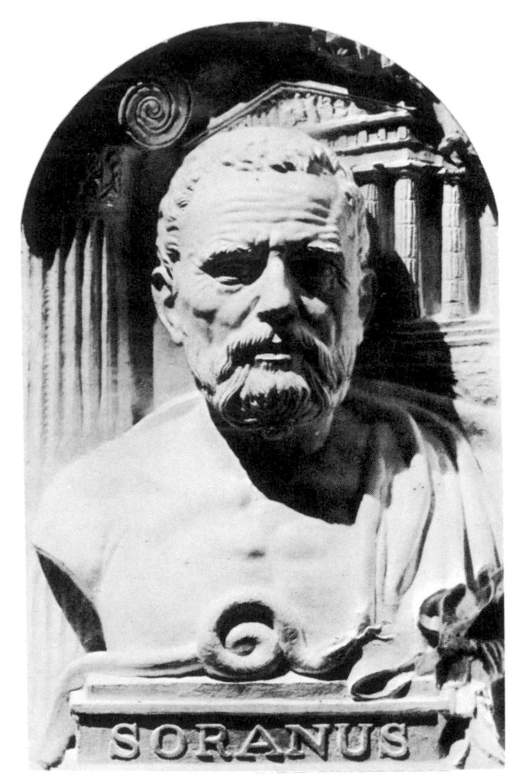

Figure 2. Soranus of Ephesus (98–138 A.D.). From the collection of the National Library of Medicine.

Bandages

Hippocrates (460–375 B.C.), as translated by Withington (1927), stated, "One should bear in mind that bandaging a fractured

[2] Breasted tr.

* Castiglioni, A.: *A History of Medicine* (Krumbhaar tr.). Ed. 2. New York, Knopf, 1947.

jaw will do little good when done well but would do great harm if done badly." Hippocrates (or the Hippocratic writer) recommended the use of leather straps for the chin, with a paste to cause them to adhere to the skin so that direct traction could be applied. He also mentioned the use of various bandages.

Apparently similar kinds of bandages were described by Galen of Pergamon and Soranus of Ephesus. An old calligraphic manuscript, with commentary, by Soranus of Ephesus (98–138 A.D.) contains illustrations of bandages used by the ancients for facial and head injuries (Figs. 3 and 4).

Figure 3 verso shows, at the upper left, the *polyrhomboid* bandage. At the upper right is the famous *perikephalea* (casque) bandage, while the lower right illustration shows a bandage apparently intended to maintain reduction of an outwardly displaced fragment of the mandible.

Figure 4, the left central illustration, shows the *geneiac* (chin) bandage, and the upper right illustration shows the *rhomboid* bandage, which derives its name perhaps

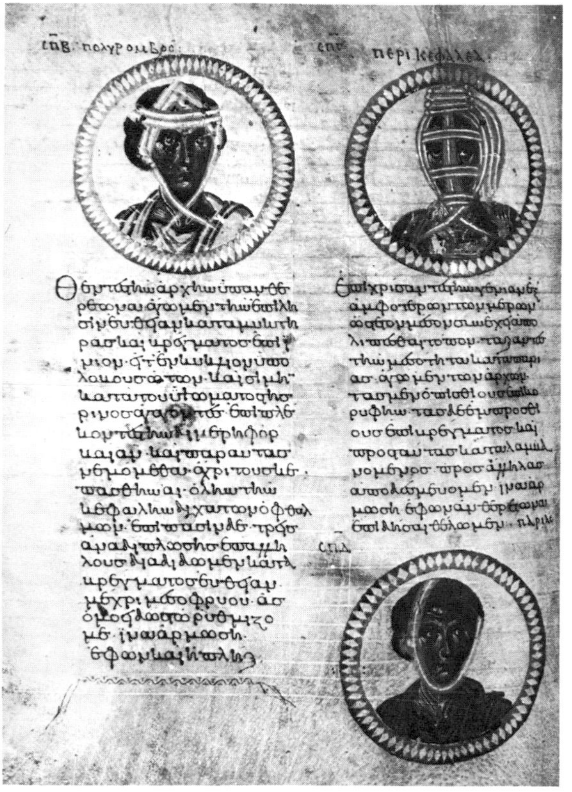

Figure 3

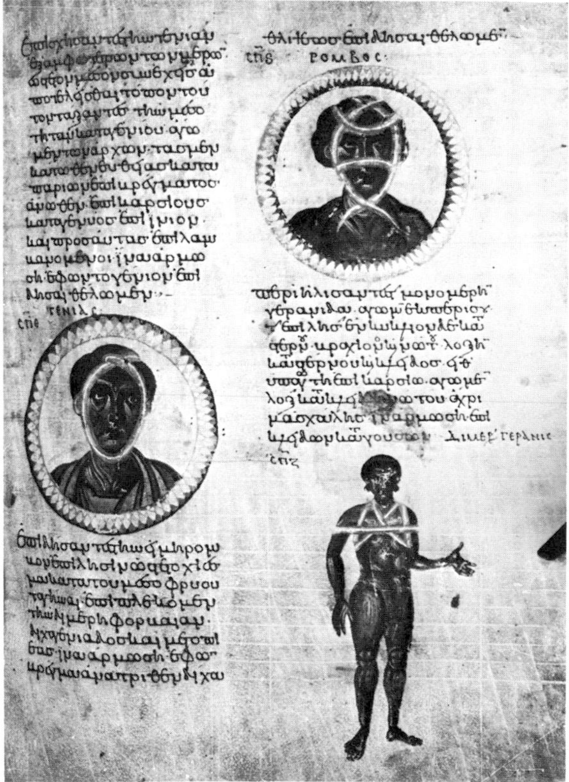

Figure 4

Figure 3. Illustrations from Laurentian MS LXXIV, 7; folio 232 verso. Upper left illustration shows the *polyrhomboid* bandage. Upper right shows the *perikephalea* bandage. The bandage at the lower right apparently was intended to maintain the reduction of a fragment of the mandible displaced outwardly. Faultiness of the illustrations is the result of damage to the manuscript. (Courtesy of the Laurentian Library, Florence, Italy.)

Figure 4. Illustrations from Laurentian MS LXXIV, 7; folio 233. The left central illustration shows the *geneiac* (chin) bandage. At the upper right is the rhomboid bandage. The lower right illustration does not pertain to injuries of the face; it shows the method of immobilizing the left shoulder, probably in the treatment of dislocation. (Courtesy of the Laurentian Library, Florence, Italy.)

from the appearance of the patient's face after the bandage had been applied. The illustration in the lower right does not pertain to injuries of the face; it shows the method of immobilizing the left shoulder, probably in the treatment of dislocation. The Laurentian MS LXXIV, 7, in Florence contains additional drawings of bandages of the face and head.[3]

From a translation of the Corpus Hippocraticum in the *Treatise on Joints* as interpreted by Tallmadge,[4] it is evident that fixation as a method of treating fractures was in vogue as far back as the fifth century B.C.

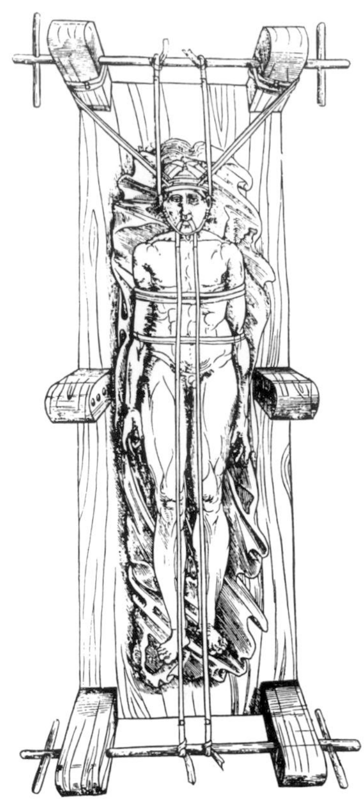

Figure 5. Copy of an illustration from the *Chirurgia* of Vidus Vidius, 1544. The illustration shows the manner of using the *scamnum*, probably of Hippocratic origin, for applying traction to correct displacement of a fractured mandible.

Monomaxillary and Intermaxillary Fixation

The following is direct quotation from the Corpus Hippocraticum (as translated by Tallmadge) (XXXII, 6 to XXXIII, 5): "If the teeth at the point of injury are displaced or loosened, when the bone is adjusted fasten them to one another, not merely the two, but several, preferably with gold wire, but, lacking that, with linen thread, till consolidation takes place.

"If the jaw is broken right across, which rarely happens, one should adjust it in the manner described (one thumb inside the mouth; the fingers outside, for reduction). After adjustment [reduction] one should fasten the teeth together as was described above [i.e., with gold wire or, lacking that, with linen thread], for this will contribute greatly to immobility, especially if one joins them properly and fastens the ends as they should be (fastened)." Tallmadge suggests that this method of wiring was not original with Hippocrates, but, because of the casual way in which the subject is presented, might have been a common procedure.

"These Greeks discovered the size of the earth, the distance of the moon from the earth; the fact that the earth revolves around the sun, the value of π. Should one not suspect that they practiced not only monomaxillary but intermaxillary wiring?"[5]

[3] We are indebted to Dr. Loren MacKinney, Kenan Distinguished Professor of Medieval History, and to the University of North Carolina, for their gracious help in supplying us with photographs and historical materials.

[4] Dr. G. Kasten Tallmadge, who has translated the French, German, Latin, and Greek texts used in this book, has remarked that his translations are not intended to be word for word or "interlinear," but are intended to express adequately to the contemporary reader the meanings of the authors whose writings have been translated from other languages.

[5] Tallmadge

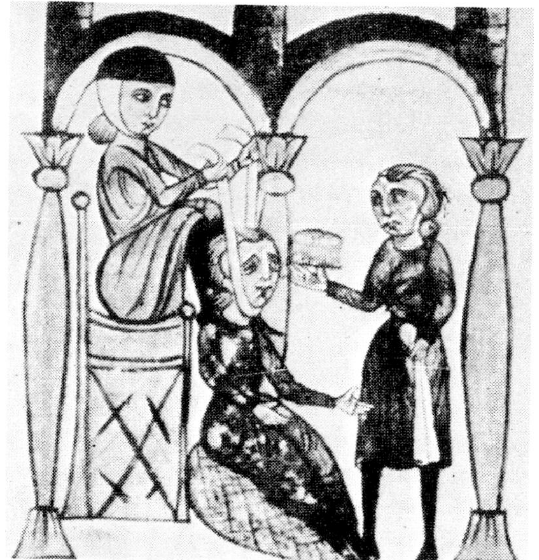

Figure 6. Illustration from the *Cirurgia Magistri Rolandi* (Codex 1382, in the Biblioteca Casanatense, Rome). Bettmann (*A Pictorial History of Medicine*) has described this as a method of treating fractures of the jaws. However, the accompanying text in the Codex describes this as a method of treating an injury to the neck.

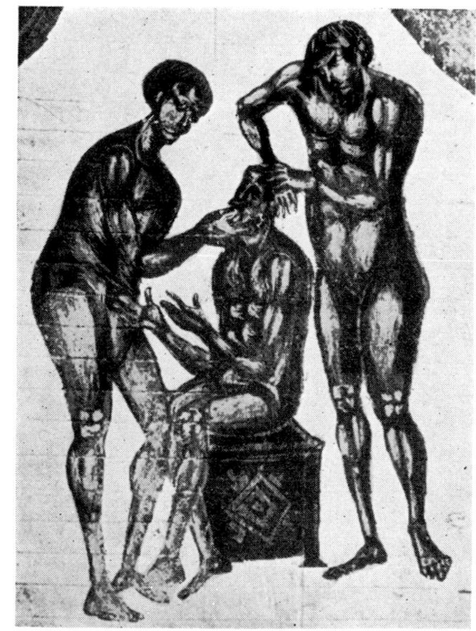

Figure 7. From Apollonius of Kitium, ΠΕΡΙ ΑΡΘΡΩΝ (Teubner, Leipzig, 1896). The plate shows the physician reducing a dislocated mandible by exerting pressure, with his thumbs inside the mouth, downward and backward against the mandibular molars. (We are indebted for the graciousness of the University of North Carolina for the loan of this volume, which is from the library of Charles Singer and bears his autograph.)

Many modern authors who mention the work of Hippocrates have said that he advocated the use of linen thread, if gold wire was not satisfactory or could not be obtained, for maintaining the position of the fragments. Linen was used, of course, in the wrapping of ancient Egyptian mummies.

Celsus in *De Medicina* VII, 12, wrote, "If some teeth are loosened by a blow, or by any cause, they should be ligated by means of gold [wire] to other teeth which still are firm in their sockets." In VIII, 7, he wrote: "[The fragments] of a fractured mandible always adhere, after reduction, to each other.

"Therefore, in the first place, with two fingers, one within the mouth, the other outside, all of the fragments should be reduced. Next, if the lower jaw has been fractured transversely [in which case one tooth will be higher than its neighbor], when the fragments have been reduced the two neighboring teeth should be tied together with a bristle [L. *seta*][6] or if these teeth are loose further teeth should be used in the ligature. Further treatment should be given: folded linen moistened in wine and oil should be placed on the buccal surface of the gum, with another such pad impregnated with myrrh placed on the lingual surface. Then a bandage of cloth or of soft leather should be applied. The bandage should be cut partially, lengthwise, so that the two ends may be passed beneath the chin and thence to the top of the head where they may be tied together . . . the treatment of fracture of any bone is approximately the same. But in respect of fracture of the mandible it should be added that only liquid nourishment should be taken for a long time. Later, the patient

[6] Translated by W. G. Spencer (1938) as "horsehair."

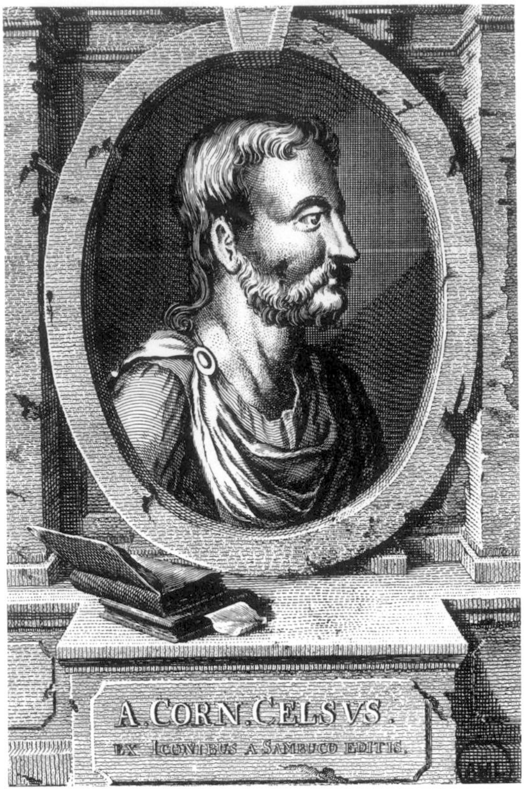

Figure 8. Aulus Cornelius Celsus (ca. 178 A.D.). From Sambucus' collection of illustrations. This engraving was made by T. M. Stock of Leipzig and is dated 1765.

should take gruel and similar things for an additional time, without solid foods, until the callus in the mandible has formed completely. Also the patient ought not to speak for a number of days."

Guglielmo Salicetti, or William of Saliceto, seems to have been one of the early surgeons who ligated the teeth of the lower jaw to the corresponding teeth of the upper jaw.

As noted by Rowe and Killey (1955), the first edition of Saliceto's *Cirurgia* was printed, in Italian, in Venice and was published on March 1, 1474. With a modification from a later edition printed at Lyons in 1492, the author wrote: "But if the bone of the upper or the lower jaw be fractured, put your hand into the mouth of the patient, the right if the upper jaw be fractured, the left if it be the lower. So reduce the parts, the hand outside helping the one inside in such a fashion that the fracture be leveled and the part perfectly restored. This done, bind the teeth in the parts of the injured jaw in this way: Take a linen thread and a silk thread and twist them together; then wax the twist with wax and bind the teeth with it as if you were weaving a hurdle, and continue this interlacing between the teeth of the uninjured part and those of the injured part, going from one tooth to another in such a way that the part be immobilized." The Lyons edition directed, "This done, tie the teeth of the uninjured jaw to the teeth of the injured jaw in the same way." Rowe and Killey have attributed this translation to F. N. L. Poynter, Librarian of the Wellcome Historical Medical Library.

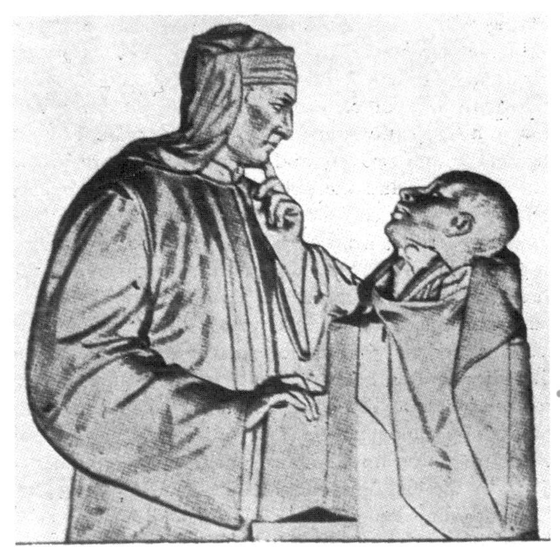

GUILLAUME DE SALICET
D'après le bas-relief de Ferrarini, à Plaisance
Et la photographie de Giuseppe Caldi.

Figure 9. William of Saliceto [1210(?)–1280(?)]. From *Chirurgie de Guillaume de Salicet* by Paul Pifteau, Toulouse, 1898.

Richard Wiseman in 1676 reported many facial injuries, including fractures of most of the facial bones.[7] He wrote:

At the Siege of *Taunton* one of Colonel *John Arundel's* men, in ftorming the Works, was fhot in the Face by Cafe-fhot. He fell down, and in the Retreat was carried off among the dead, and laid into an empty houfe by the way until the next day: when in the morning early, the Colonel marching by that houfe heard a knocking within againft the Door. Some of the Officers defiring to know what it was, lookt in, and faw this man ftanding by the Door without Eye, Face, Nofe, or Mouth. The Col. fent to me (my Quarters being neareft) to drefs the man. I went, but was fomewhat troubled where to begin. The Door confifted of two Hatches; the uppermoft was open, and the man ftood leaning upon the other part of the Door which was fhut. His Face, with his Eyes, Nofe, Mouth, and forepart of the Jaws, with the Chin, was fhot away, and the remaining parts of them driven in. One part of the Jaw hung down by his Throat, and the other part pafht into it. I faw the Brain working out underneath the lacerated Scalp on both fides between his Ears and Brows. I could not fee any advantage he could have by my Dreffing. To have cut away the lacerated Parts here had been to expofe the Brain to the Air. But I helpt him to clear his Throat, where was remaining the Root of his Tongue. He feemed to approve of my Endeavours, and implored my help by the Signs he made with his Hands. I askt him if he would drink, making a Sign by the holding up a Finger. He prefently did the like, and immediately after held up both his Hands, expreffing his Thirft. A Soldier fetcht fome Milk, and brought a little wooden Difh to pour fome of it down his Throat: but part of it running on both fides, he reacht out his Hands to take the Difh. They gave it him full of Milk. He held the Root of his Tongue down with the one Hand, and with the other poured it down his Throat, (carrying his Head backward,) and fo got down more than a quart. After that I bound his Wounds up. The dead were removed from thence to their Graves, and frefh Straw was fetcht for him to lie upon, with an old Blanket to cover him. It was in the Summer. There we left that deplorable creature to lodge, and while we continued there, which was about 6 or 7 days, he was dreft by fome of the Chirurgeons with a Fomentation made of Vulnerary Plants, with a little Brandy-wine in it, and with Stupes of Tow dipt in our common Digeftive. So we bound him up.

The absence of any reference in medical literature to the management of fractured facial bones over the period of the next several centuries seems to imply that the work of earlier authors was unknown or had become standard or that methods of fixation were found ineffective and so fell out of use.

The development of techniques of intermaxillary wiring was a definite advance over the use of monomaxillary wiring. These techniques permitted splinting of the fractured mandible and immobilizing it against the intact maxilla. Intermaxillary fixation provided not only a rapid method of dealing effectively with fresh fractures

[7] *Eight Chirurgical Treatises,* Third Edition, by Richard Wiseman, Serjeant-Chirurgeon to King Charles the Second. London, 1676.

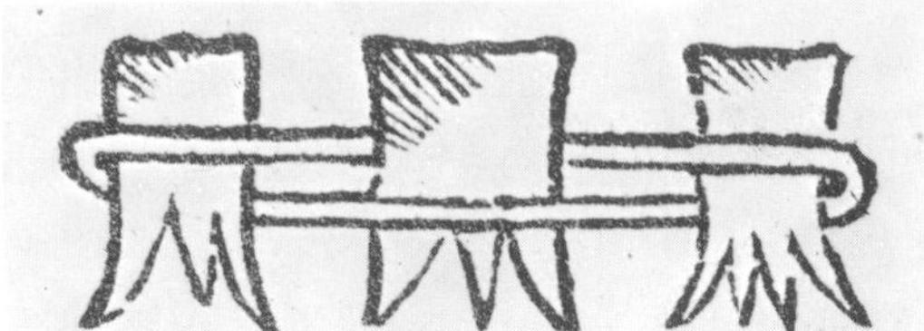

Figure 10. A method for treating fractured jaws, using silk thread or silver or brass wire. From Hieronymus Brunschwig: *Das Buch der Cirurgia.* Strassburg, Johann Grüninger, 1497, p. 195.

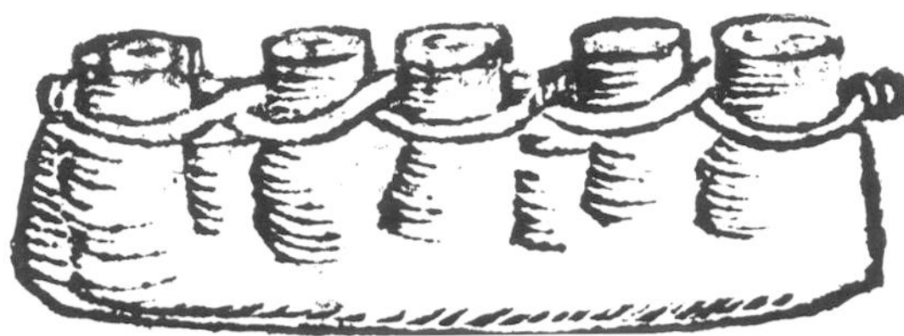

Figure 11. Old method of wattle-wiring of the teeth. From T. Priscianus: *Rerum medicarum lib. quatuor* . . . Albucasis. J. Schott, 1532, p. 177.

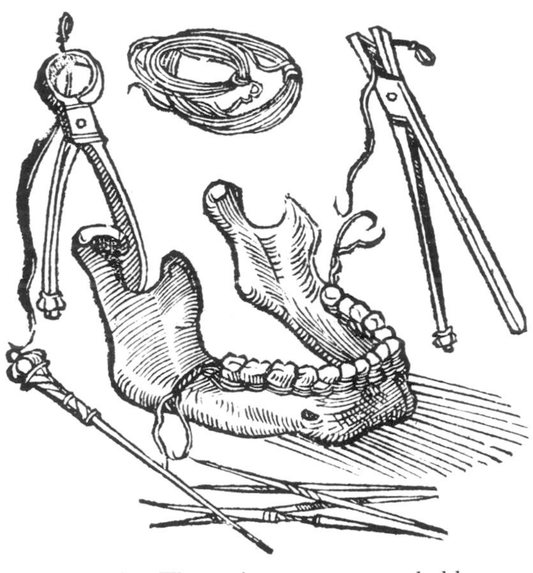

Figure 12. These instruments probably were used simply in the fixation of loosened teeth. However, they might also have been used in the fixation of fractures of the mandible. From W. H. Ryff: *Die grosz Chirurgei oder volkommene Wundartzenei.* Frankfurt am Main, Christian Egenolph, 1545, [6], p. 48v.

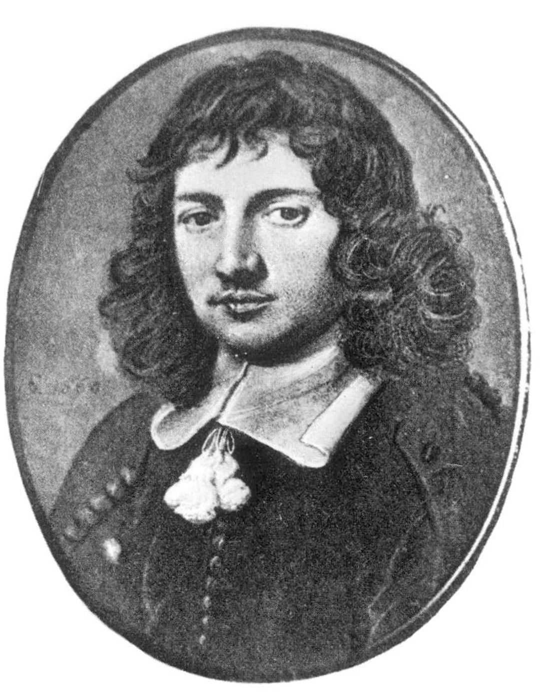

Figure 13. Richard Wiseman (1622–1676). "Carolo II Mag. Brit. Regi Archichirurgus," by S. Cooper, 1660, signed. From *The History of Portrait Minatures* by George C. Williamson. George Bell and Sons, 1904, plate XVI, number 4.

of the mandible but also an opportunity for early treatment. This was in contrast to the late treatment necessitated by the development of soreness and pain of the oral structures, which had made it impossible to take impressions for the fabrication of splints.

Credit for the development of intermaxillary fixation by wiring is due to an American, Thomas L. Gilmer, who used it in 1887. Gilmer's method of wiring consisted of twisting wires around the necks of the teeth of the upper and lower jaws, of adjusting the lower teeth to the occlusion of the upper jaw, and of twisting together the connecting upper and lower wires for stabilization.

Gilmer's method underwent many modifications, the most notable of which were made by Oliver, Winter, and Ivy. Ivy popularized several methods of intermaxillary fixation, and he is credited with having adopted the technique for dental practice. Darnall was one of the first to recommend the use of rubber bands for reduction and fixation of fractured segments.

Intermaxillary Splints

Early forms of intermaxillary splints were simple double gutters made of cork, wood, or metal. Later these gutters were filled with such materials as gutta-percha or modeling compound which allowed a firmer application to the teeth. Plaster of Paris or cement was used later in the gutters to provide still firmer fixation.

Späth, in his article, "Komplicirte Fraktur des Unterkiefers," published in 1836, wrote:

"Johannes Haug, farm laborer from Ziegelhutte, 22 years of age, of healthy and strong physique, was struck by the pole of a heavily loaded unyolked fruit wagon. While he pushed the wagon backward out of the barn, its left front wheel slipped in a rut and the pole crushed the left side of Haug's lower jaw between the first and second molar teeth. [At this time no distinction was made between premolars and molars.] A serious wound was inflicted; the mandible was exposed; the first molar was lost, and the second and third were dislocated. The lower jaw hung toward the right, and two fragments were so loosely attached that, in the absence of treatment, they would have been lost. The mouth was open and deformed; movement of the mandible was all but impossible; crepitation was easily perceived because of the looseness of the fragments. Hemorrhage from the inferior alveolar artery, which, of course, was severed, was profuse at first, but was easily controlled by the application of cold compresses. It was easy to move the fractured ends of the bone. The larger fragment was displaced downward by the traction of the muscles; the smaller was displaced upward and inward. The fragments could be reduced easily but could not be maintained in reduction. It was not possible to maintain reduction with either silver wire or silk because the teeth were loose in their phatnes. It was not possible to maintain reduction of the fragments with leather, pasteboard splints, wooden gutters held in place by means of bandages, or even with Boyer's single gutter of cork, because of the softness of the gutters, the accumulation of mucus, and the foulness of the odor which ensued. A cylinder of flax fixed by means of a bandage against the lingual surface of the mandible failed to maintain the freely movable fragments in reduction. I visited the patient several times every day only to discover that the reduction of the fragments had been lost. It would have taken too much time for me to obtain one of Rutenick's Mechanisms[8]

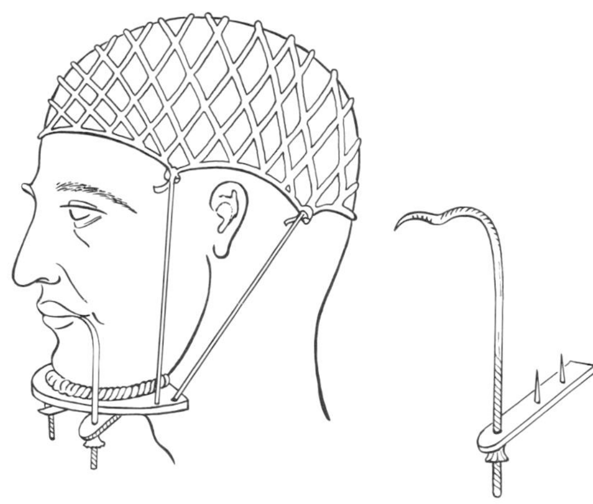

Figure 14. Our artist's copy of Rutenick's illustration of his apparatus for the treatment of fracture of the mandible. (*Dis. de fractura mandibulae,* Berol., 1823.)

[8] Rutenick's apparatus (1799) had connecting clamps of steel attached to the wooden chin piece by means of spikes. It was provided with variously curved silver pieces for the teeth, the shape of these pieces varying somewhat, according to the size of the fracture. Fabric bands ran from the chin piece to a light head cap. Rutenick's apparatus could be of value only in fractures within the alignment of the teeth.

(since perfected by Prof. Kluge): the lapse of time might have resulted in a deformation of the mandible.

"What could one do under such unfavorable circumstances? I summoned the skillful turner, Schilling, and showed him a skull whose maxilla and mandible were of a size and shape comparable to the patient's. I asked him to turn two double gutters of horn, which would correspond precisely to the teeth of the maxilla and the mandible. After I had reduced the fragments once more I adjusted both gutters—one on the intact side, the other on the injured, and bandaged the lower jaw. Thus the fragments were held reduced. The gutters stayed clean for a long time; they had to be removed only rarely for cleaning. A space was left between the incisor teeth and the forward edge of the gutters (a space which could be covered by the lips) so that meat-broth and other nourishing liquids could be fed to the patient easily and without disturbing the reduced fragments.

"The gutters were curved lengthwise to follow the natural curves of the jaws. Such

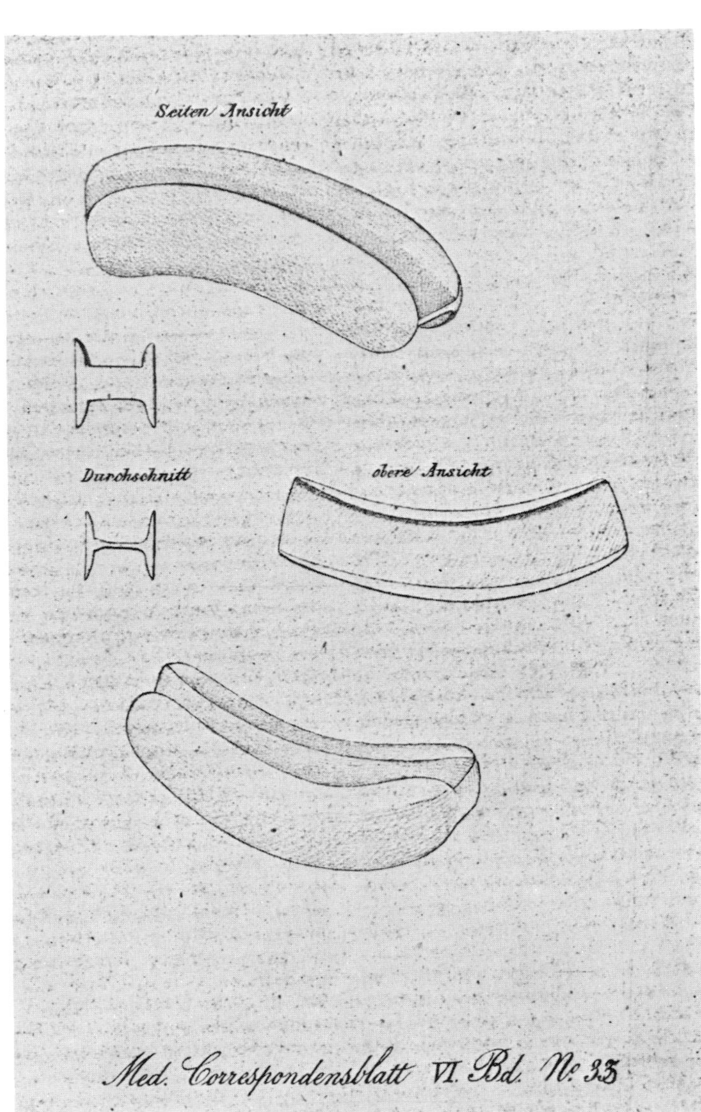

Figure 15. Two double gutters of horn designed by Späth and made by the turner, Schilling. From Späth's *Komplicirte Fraktur des Unterkiefers.* Med. Korbl Wurtemberg, *6*:1836, opp. p. 276.

gutters, with different curvatures, can be made to fit even edentulous fractured jaws. The gutters also may be varied to conform to the shape of any alveolar arch. Moreover when the jaw is fractured in the region of the incisors, a gutter can be turned to conform to the shapes of the teeth. In any case the free space between the incisors and the middle of the gutter should be left open to facilitate nourishment, and also irrigation of the mouth. These gutters are most useful also in cases of fractures occurring near the coronoid or condylar processes: they maintain the fragments in complete reduction, and the patient tolerates them without too much inconvenience. My patient suffered no complications and was completely healed in 45 days. I offer an illustration of the double gutter."[9]

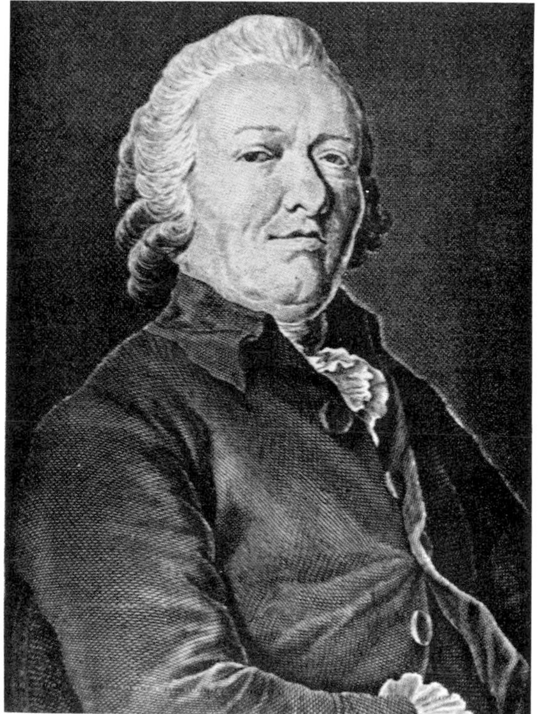

Figure 16. Pierre-Joseph Desault (1744–1795). From the collection of the National Library of Medicine.

Extra-intraoral Appliances

Before Rutenick published his monograph, the Chopart-Desault (1780) extra-intraoral appliance was described. Chopart either invented the appliance or made one, according to the record of a German method first published by him. The splint was made of a brace of metal, which was placed upon either side of the jaw and covered and fitted to the teeth by counterpressure made with screws against a plate of sheet-iron or other material under the chin. Chopart and Desault also used iron or steel hooks caught on the teeth on either side of the fracture and tightened by means of screws from a submental splint of sheet-iron or other material.

The reintroduction of bimaxillary (or intermaxillary) fixation, which occurred about 1836, was a great improvement in the management of fractures of the jaws, and led to the development of current methods of the treatment of facial fractures.

[9] Tallmadge tr.

Although monomaxillary splints do have a place in the management of fractures, in general they are inadequate, as most fractures of the mandible require the stability afforded by fixation to the intact maxilla.

Gutta-percha and vulcanized rubber made the use of intermaxillary splints even more popular. T. B. Gunning in New York appears to have been the first to use a vulcanite splint for fractured jaws; he made such a splint in 1861.

Kingsley reported that a simple and effective apparatus was constructed by Hayward of London in 1858. Hayward took casts of the jaw and made a metallic plate which fitted and covered the teeth on both sides of the fracture and, to some extent, the gingiva also. "From either side of this splint strong bent wires were soldered, which were curved in such a way that they passed out on each side of the mouth [Fig.

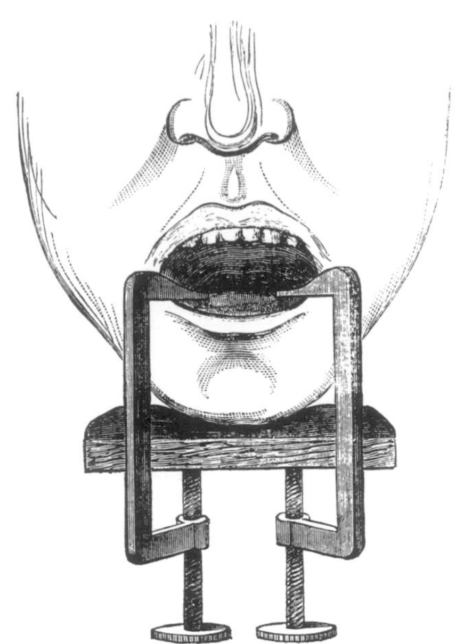

Figure 17. Apparatus of R. D. Stener of Grenoble, France, illustrating substantially the various extra-intraoral appliances in use. From "On the Treatment of Fractures of the Lower Maxilla," *British Journal of Dental Science,* vol. 20, page 660, 1877.

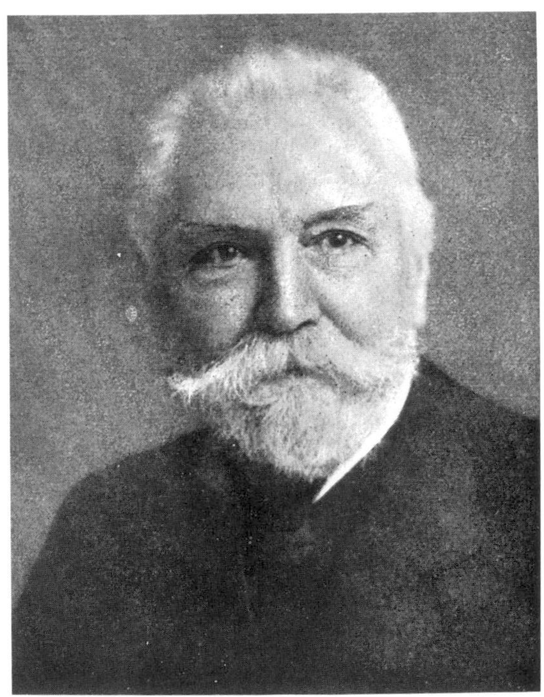

Figure 18. Norman W. Kingsley (1829–1913). From *Dental Chronology* by Hermann Prinz. Lea & Febiger, 1945, p. 90.

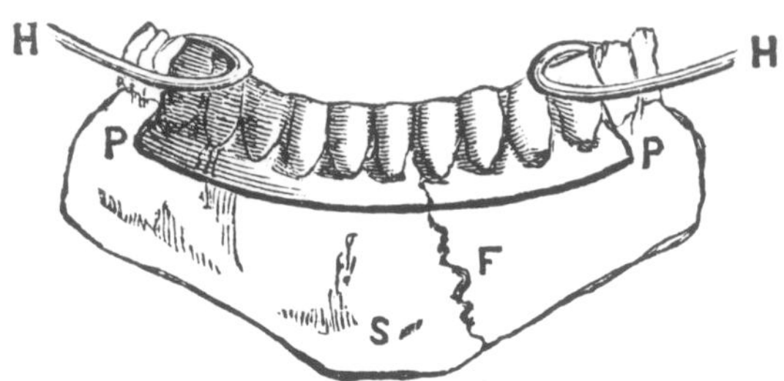

Figure 19. Splint of Hayward of London, 1858, as shown on page 397 of *A Treatise on Oral Deformities* by N. W. Kingsley. Appleton, 1880.

19]. To these arms, H H, a submental gutta-percha splint was fastened, and the whole secured by a four-tailed bandage—although just why a bandage was necessary is not patent." This was probably the first attempt at making a plate properly fitted to the teeth for fractures. Norman W. Kingsley, in his book *A Treatise on Oral Deformities,*[10] reported the following:

"For more than fifteen years I have made and used interdental splints in various forms, as the particular case seemed to require, and have experimented more or less successfully with splints made of silver, tin, vulcanite, and gutta-percha—the first three with and without gutta-percha lining.

"In cases of double or triple fracture, I have always found much displacement and much difficulty in replacing the fragments, the tendency to displace them being so strong that the pieces would fall away again immediately on the force which held them being relaxed; and this has been the case also sometimes with a single fracture. The effort to reduce the fracture has at times required much ingenuity in the management of pries or levers between the fragments or against the upper teeth, while at others pieces of stout cord have been tied around certain sound teeth, and one displaced fragment pulled in one direction and another in a different one.

[10] New York, Appleton, 1880, p. 398.

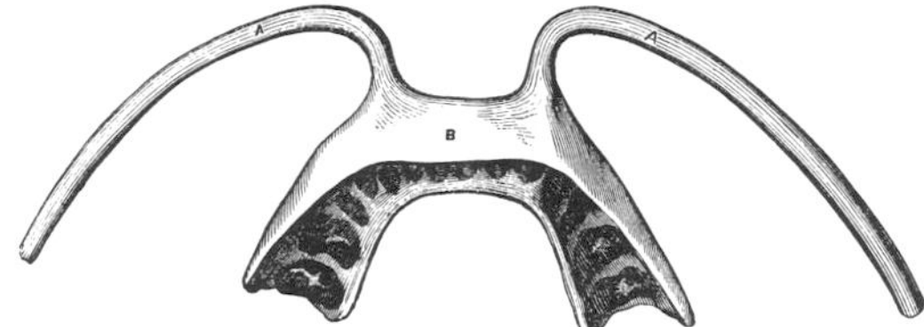

Figure 20. Kingsley splint. From *A Treatise on Oral Deformities* by N. W. Kingsley. Appleton, 1880, p. 399.

"The failure to always get the broken jaw into its original shape, so as to either fit a gutta-percha splint or to even get a correct impression, led me to abandon any attempt thereafter to reduce the fracture prior to making the splint, and instead thereof to take an impression of the parts as they were found, and restore the jaw in the model. The same want of success in bringing the parts into exact apposition made me devise the splint shown in Figure 20. This was entirely original with me, and its success was so great in a number of cases that it was with a shade of mortification that I afterward found that it was virtually a copy of Mr. Hayward's splint.

Figure 21 "shows the application of the splint to a reconstructed model, the same as it would be used in the mouth. It has been a favorite idea of mine that for all fractures of the body of the bone an interdental splint ought to be so nicely adjusted that the dental arch when placed in it would assume its exact original relation, *and that mastication might be performed upon the top of the splint.* In [Figure 21] are shown the indentations on the upper surface of the splint made to receive the cusps of the upper teeth; and, as such an appliance is used without binding the lower jaw against the upper, the patient is likely to use the splint to masticate upon as soon as he has the desire to."

The splint devised by Kingsley is shown being used by a patient (Fig. 22). Kingsley added: "The fragments resumed their natural position immediately upon the introduction of the splint and the application of the external bandage. This bandage was a simple, broad, elastic rubber band, such as are for sale by stationers; it covered a pad over the chin, made of gutta-percha, softened and modeled into proper form. The elasticity of the band was such as to force the

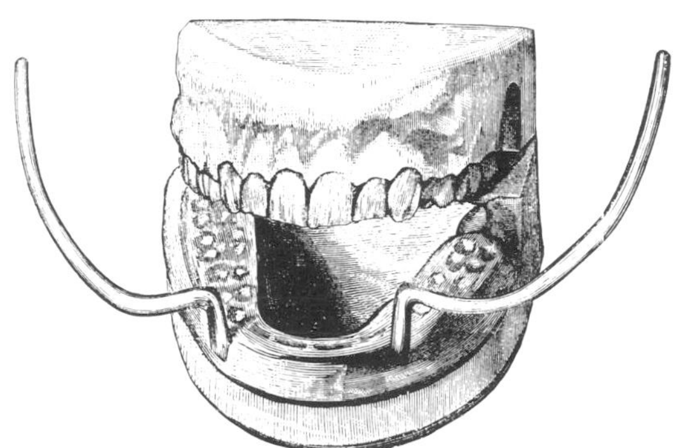

Figure 21. Kingsley splint applied to dental model. From *A Treatise on Oral Deformities* by N. W. Kingsley. Appleton, 1880, p. 401.

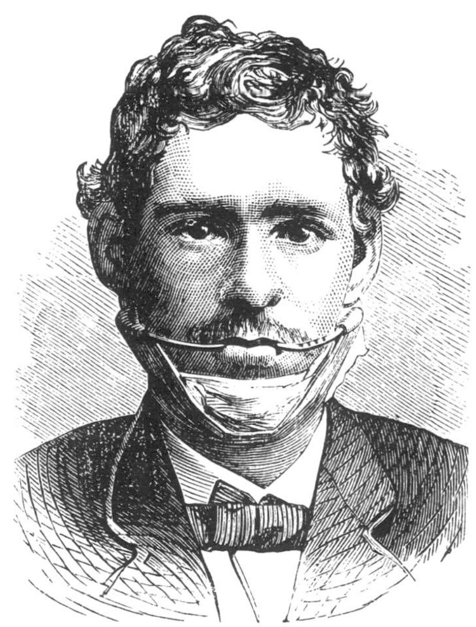

Figure 22. Sketch of Kingsley splint being worn by a patient. From *A Treatise on Oral Deformities* by N. W. Kingsley. Appleton, 1880, p. 404.

fragments into the splint and bind them firmly to it, thus allowing entire freedom to the jaw for reception of food. The superior surface of the splint was carefully articulated to the upper teeth, and a little experience enabled the patient to masticate without difficulty."

Numerous modifications of the Kingsley splint with head-cap attachments were made during the First World War. Kazanjian was one of the important Americans who used and developed extraskeletal appliances for the management of facial fractures. Federspiel (1927) demonstrated the use of wires attached to bone fragments (especially the zygoma) and held firm with support on a plaster head-cap.

Circumferential Wiring

A significant step leading to the development of modern methods of treating jaw fractures was the work of Jean-Baptiste Baudens (1840) (Fig. 23). His was the first reference in modern medical literature to circumferential wiring of the fractured mandible. Baudens had occasion to treat a soldier with an oblique fracture through the region of the angle of the mandible. He described severe displacement of the proximal fragment and stated that he was able to reduce the fracture and hold it securely in place by one circumferential wire around the mandible (passed with a needle). The two ends of the ligature were fixed over a posterior tooth. The following translation from the French gives a detailed description of the case as written by Baudens himself:

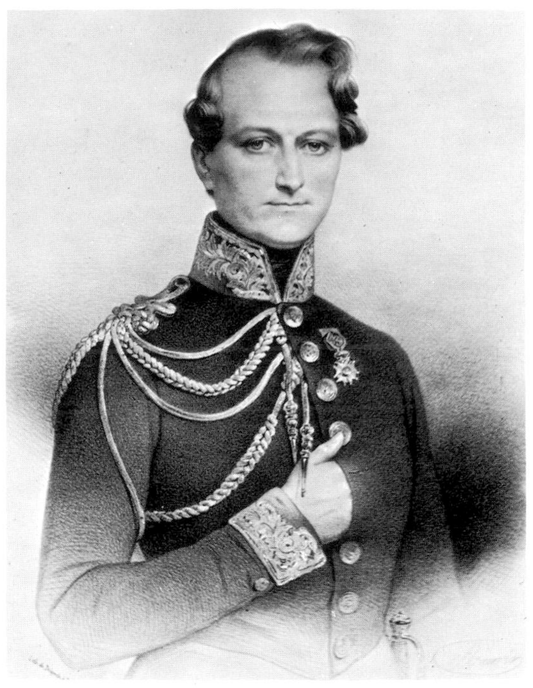

Figure 23. Jean-Baptiste Baudens (1804–1857). From the collection of the National Library of Medicine.

"I have just presented to the Academy, for the second time, the case of a soldier who, last May 4, suffered a fracture of the mandible; which case I had the honor to report to you after eight days of treatment.

"At that time I attempted to call attention to a new treatment which I used and which was original with me. The treatment consists in placing the fragments together immovable and in such a manner that they cannot become displaced. To obtain this result—and I cannot remember previous statements of its advantages—by means of a suture-needle I passed a strong ligature around the fragments. In a word, I made a bony suture such as one finds in the skull.

"The Academy has seen that there was a wide vertical hiatus in the soft cervico-facial structures, which complicated this fracture. This separation of the soft tissues was almost entirely healed by first intention thanks to the tightness of my ligature. Bony union was progressing satisfactorily and the best results were expected. Since then healing has progressed very rapidly because the fractured ends of the fragments were in complete apposition.

"Two criticisms were brought up by Professor Roux, who told me that, after the reduction of the oblique fragments from before and behind, and from above and below, no displacement should occur.

"I am compelled to answer that the displacement was very considerable and that surely the extensive injuries to the soft parts contributed much to the displacement of the fragments by failing to afford normal support to the fractured mandible. Furthermore, oblique fractures of the mandible always present a three-way displacement, each of which may be more or less pronounced.

"1. *Above-below,* caused by the elevation of the posterior fragment and the dropping of the anterior fragment; 2. *Longitudinally,* the anterior fragment is forward; 3. *According to thickness,* the posterior fragment is pulled backward. Now of all of these displacements, in our case the last is most remarkable because the fracture occurred through the entire thickness of the bone, and therefore I felt it necessary to treat this displacement by having recourse to a ligature around both fractured ends. By means of this treatment bony calluses were formed, without deformity, or without excessive callosity, and in a word, without any malformation, as all of you gentlemen may observe. You see the patient: his teeth are in perfect alignment; and one could deny that any fracture ever existed excepting that the posterior (or auricular) fragment is displaced inward almost imperceptibly. We think that we have answered Professor Roux's first criticism.

"Concerning his second criticism, which rests upon the supposition that the pressure of the ligature upon the bony tissue might alter the structure of the bone—this criticism is without foundation, as is shown by the fact that the ligature was in its place for 23 days.

"Moreover it should be noticed that, because of the mobility of the mandible, a ligature passed around it and attached to one of the molar teeth has only a partial and discontinuous action upon the bone.

"Since this soldier leaves Paris tomorrow I felt obliged to prove the fact of his complete cure, with no remaining deformity, to the Academy." [11]

César Alphonse Robert (1852) modified Bauden's method by passing his circumferential wiring over a small lead plate. Robert reported the following:

"Our most modern treatises on surgery, in describing fractures of the mandible, hardly mention fractures of the alveolar ridge of this bone. M. Malgaigne, in his learned treatise on fractures, limits himself to saying that such fractures are possible. In several works on dental surgery, and especially in the work by Gariot, it is stated that attempts made to extract impacted or embedded teeth sometimes have caused very extensive lesions, but he has not given any instructions concerning the treatment which these conditions require.

"Nevertheless, this aspect of practical surgery is interesting to study; because, aside from the bone lesion, of whose possible consequences one must be aware, one must understand the possible effect of the lesion upon the teeth. In fact, fracture of the alveolar ridge cannot occur without a separation of the vessels and nerves which supply the teeth in the fragment. Furthermore these teeth cannot live except through their connections with the alveolo-dental periosteum. It is difficult to say whether, under these new conditions, they might not sooner or later loosen and fall out. For this reason, as well as because of the new procedure which I have found it necessary to employ, the following case history seemed to me to be worth presenting to the surgical society.

"A 44 year old hack-driver, of sturdy frame, was knocked down in a brawl and received several kicks in the face. He was picked up unconscious and taken at once to the Beaujon Hospital. The next day, on my round, I observed a large swelling of the lower part of his face. There were two con-

[11] Tallmadge tr.

tused wounds above his chin, of which one, in the labiomental groove, could only have been caused by a blow from a man's bootheel. But what struck me most was a transverse fracture of the alveolar ridge of the mandible, about four finger-breadths long. The separated fragment of the bone was itself fractured into two parts; the larger one still held the four incisors and the left canine; the other, to the left of the former, held the first premolar and the first molar—the second premolar had been missing for many years. These two easily movable fragments were not attached to the body of the bone except by means of gingival mucous membrane, which itself was torn here and there. Thus there was a fracture of the alveolar ridge which involved a linear area corresponding to eight teeth, and whose fragments were so seriously separated that if they were left untreated they surely would have been lost by suppuration.

"In order to obtain union it was necessary to keep the two fragments completely immobile on the body of the bone. It seemed to me that enough blood vessels remained to nourish an adequate callus. But how could I perfect this immobilization? Some authors, and among others Gariot, whom I have named, thought it sufficient to attach the teeth of the fragment to unloosened teeth; but this method obviously is inadequate; indeed, it is even harmful in that it tends to destroy the connections which still unite the loose teeth to the fragments of the mandible. Boyer advised that one use a gutter of cork applied between the upper and lower teeth, and a bandage, which he uses in cases of fracture of the body of the mandible. But his method, like the other, was inapplicable because the bandage usually does not hold well, and in the case which I have been describing it was necessary, in order to obtain coaptation of the fracture, to work directly upon the fragments themselves.

"This is the procedure which I think one ought to follow. A lead plate, 1 mm. thick should be moulded to fit accurately the lingual ridge of the mandible, A, passing behind, B–C, the fragments [Fig. 24]. In order to keep this plate in place, a needle threaded with a silver thread should be passed along the internal surface of the mandible and through the floor of the mouth. The end of the silver thread should be left hanging. The other end of the silver thread should be passed in the same manner with a needle across the outer surface of the bone and directed through the same opening in the floor of the mouth. (In the illustration shown here the engraver has made an error: the anterior part of the silver loop ought to have been shown passing in front of the incisors.) The two ends of the silver thread, having been brought out beneath the chin, thus enclose the fragments in a loop of silver thread. The ends of the silver thread should be fixed over a small roller bandage impregnated with beeswax, D, and tightened by twisting until the lead plate be fixed firmly.

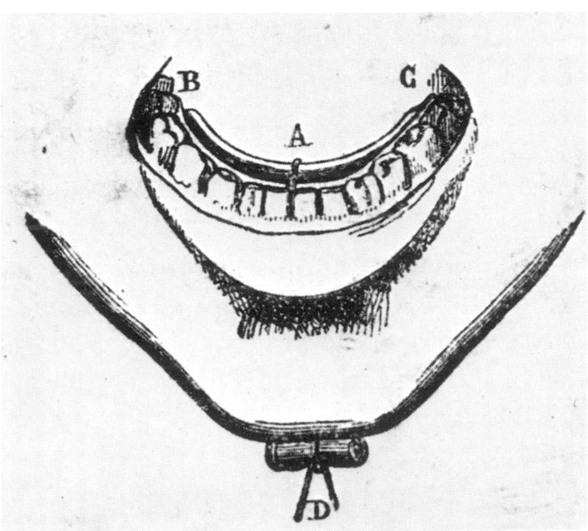

Figure 24. Copy of Robert's illustration shown on page 24 of "Nouveau procédé de traitement des fractures de la portion alvéolaire de la Machoire inférieure," *Bulletin général de thérapeutique médicale et chirurgicale,* Paris, 42, 1852.

"The complications produced by the manipulations of the fragments disappeared after some bleeding, and, remarkably, no sign of inflammation occurred in the line of the metallic suture during the entire duration of the treatment. In spite of the presence of silver thread the patient, after a few days, was able to eat without disturbing the reduction. On the 47th day the silver thread was removed from the lead plate.[12] Consolidation was perfect; all of the teeth were solidly fixed in their sockets, with the exception of the canine, which, lying in the line of fracture, was loose.

"And so, thanks to this method of treatment, this man was enabled to recover completely from an injury which otherwise would have resulted, without doubt, in the loss of eight teeth. It should be added that M. Baudens previously, in a case of a very oblique fracture most difficult to reduce, had the wisdom to bring the fragments together and to immobilize them by means of a metallic ligature. The success which he had, together with the success I have had in a similar case, should convince the surgeon that the excellence of this heroic method of treatment has been established."[13]

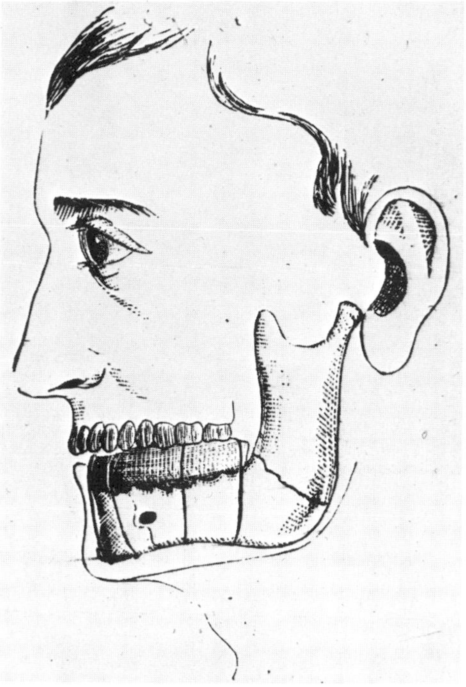

To G. V. Black of Jacksonville, Illinois, must go credit for the first use of circumferential wiring in the United States. In a paper entitled "Fractures of the Inferior Maxilla" by Thomas L. Gilmer of Quincy, Illinois, and illustrated by Black, Gilmer described many methods of fixation of fractures of the mandible including that of Black, who wired around the bone and over a splint in the mouth (Fig. 25). A gutta-percha or vulcanite splint was used by Black and retained by stout silver or platinum circumferential wire. Before inserting the wires, Black passed a double thread around the bone in two places by means of a doubly threaded needle. The double thread formed a loop, which was used to draw the wire around the bone. After reduction of the fragments, the wire was twisted tightly over the gutta-percha splint.

Figure 25. Copy of Gilmer's illustration shown on page 91 of "Fractures of the Inferior Maxilla," *Illinois State Dental Society Transactions*, 1881. Gilmer wrote that this method of wiring around the bone was first suggested and successfully used by G. V. Black of Jacksonville, Illinois.

Interosseous Wiring

Our studies suggest that the earliest report of direct wiring of bony fragments in a mandibular fracture was made by Gurdon Buck,

[12] "The length of time during which the lead plate must remain in the mouth reminds us that we ought to choose another metal rather than lead, in order to protect the wounded man from possible lead poisoning. Our last number records the case of a patient who contracted lead colic because he had been chewing thin pieces of lead. Laminated zinc is as easy as lead to obtain, and in its metallic state produces no signs of poisoning. A sheet of silver would be even more preferable. (Editor's remark.)"

[13] Tallmadge tr.

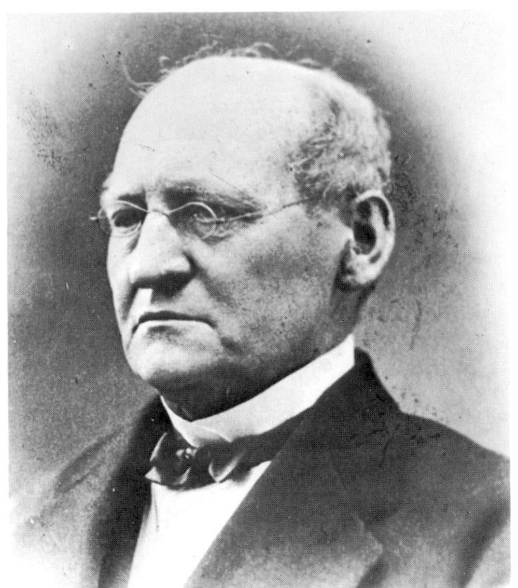

Figure 26. Gurdon Buck, Jr. (1807–1877). From the collection of the National Library of Medicine.

Jr. (1846–1847). He performed an open reduction of the mandible using malleable iron wire for fixation of the fragments. His report in *The Annalist* (New York) follows:

"Jeremiah Fredmore, æt. 19, New Jersey, boatman, admitted September 26, with fracture of the lower jaw between the first and second incisor teeth of the left side, that happened at sea two and a half weeks previous, from a block striking him on the left side of the face. The left fragment was driven towards the opposite side, and is firmly interlocked behind the right fragment of the jaw; the ends passing and overlapping each other, so that the second incisor tooth of the left side stands in a line posterior to the first incisor tooth of the right side, with a space of one finger's breadth between them. The fraenum of the lower lip remains attached to the left fragment, and passes round the first incisor tooth of the left side, which remains implanted in the right fragment. The relations of the dental arches on the right side are not disturbed, while on the left side, there is no contact of the upper and lower teeth. The fracture, instead of passing perpendicularly through the jaw, appears to have taken an oblique direction to the left before reaching the lower edge, so that the overlapping extremity of the right fragment presents a pointed prominence nearly in a line below the left angle of the mouth. Over the prominence just noted a small abscess has formed, and near it is a recent cicatrix, three-quarters of an inch in length—the remains of the wound caused by the block—depressed and firmly adherent to the bone. A slight degree of motion with grating of bony surfaces can be effected, though the parts seem firmly interlocked. All swelling and induration have for the most part disappeared, and the tissues have regained their natural suppleness. The speech is very much affected by the displacement. The symmetry of the face is less disturbed than might be supposed. In opening the mouth the lower lip is drawn to the right, and the upper to the left side. Chewing on the right side is embarrassed by the mobility of the jaw. Patient healthy, and of good constitution.

"Sept. 29. Operation. The patient being seated in a chair and his head supported, the lower lip was dissected up from the jaw, as low as the inferior margin of the chin, so as to expose the fracture and ascertain accurately the manner in which the ends of the bone were overlapped. After dividing all the soft tissues that bound the fragments together, it was still found impracticable to effect their reduction without excising the overlapping angle. To accomplish this, the lower lip was divided along the median line to the chin, and the flaps dissected up so as sufficiently to expose the ends of the bones—the remaining adhesions were divided, and a narrow chisel insinuated behind the fragment to be excised in order to protect the soft parts, while with a metacarpal saw a perpendicular section was effected. The left middle incisor tooth being loose in the right fragment, it was removed. The ends of the bone now admitted of accurate adjustment, so as to bring the teeth of both sides on the proper level. To maintain them in this position, a hole was drilled near the lower angle in each bone, and a piece of malleable iron wire passed through, with the ends drawn forward and twisted, so as to secure the desired object. The twisted ends were bent down and brought out at the lower angle of the wound, the edges of which were accurately brought into apposition by 5 or 6 sutures, supported by adhesive straps. The right fragment being inclined to fall below the left, owing to the depressing muscles of the jaw being alone connected with it, a thick compress was placed along the lower margin of the jaw on the right side, to give increased effect to the bandage which was next applied, so as to act from below upwards, as well as from before backwards, upon the chin.

"Oct. 5.—Union by first intention has taken place throughout the wound, except where the wire passes out.

"Oct. 23.—Union is quite firm. The wire being loose and moveable, was drawn out without much difficulty after untwisting the ends.

"Nov. 13.—The opening through which the wire passed has healed up. Union solid. Discharged cured."

Another early case of direct wiring of bony fragments in a mandibular fracture was that of R. A. Kinloch of Charleston, South Carolina, in 1858. By this method he treated successfully a compound oblique fracture of the mandible, the details of which fracture and treatment he reported in the *American Journal of the Medical Sciences* in July 1859. Kinloch states: "A stout silver wire was then passed through the perforations in the bone, from without inwards through the posterior fragment, and in the contrary direction through the anterior one; the ends of the suture were tightly twisted together, so as to bring the fragments into secure apposition; and, lastly, the wound of the soft parts was closed by silver wire sutures, the extremities of the large suture that passed through the bone being brought out at one of the corners, and the compress and bandage once more adjusted. Patient went to bed and took an anodyne." Kinloch most likely was unaware of the report by Buck, for Kinloch stated: "I know of no case except my own in which the lower jaw has been treated in this way."

He further stated, "M. Malgaigne says 'Duverney avait songé au cas où la Mâchoire fracturée serait tout à fait édentée. Ce cas ne parait pas s'être encore presents.' [Duverney considered also the cases in which the fractured mandible was completely edentulous. No such cases have been reported as such.] The report of my case, then, furnishes the learned Frenchman with a *reality*, and I am pleased to say that it also enables him to realize the sanguine hope he so long ago expressed, that 'la suture des fragments offriait une dernière ressource' [suture of the fragments would be the last resort]."

Kinloch suggested wiring the lower to the upper teeth to fix a fracture of the lower jaw but did not say that he had used this method. The method, nevertheless, was known at that time.

THE MAXILLA

There is little doubt that one of the very earliest references to fractures of the bones of the middle third of the face is in the Edwin Smith Papyrus given in the following case report:

"Case XIII: If thou examinest a man having a smash in his nostril, thou shouldst place thy hand upon his nose at the point of this smash. Should it crepitate under thy fingers, while at the same time he discharges

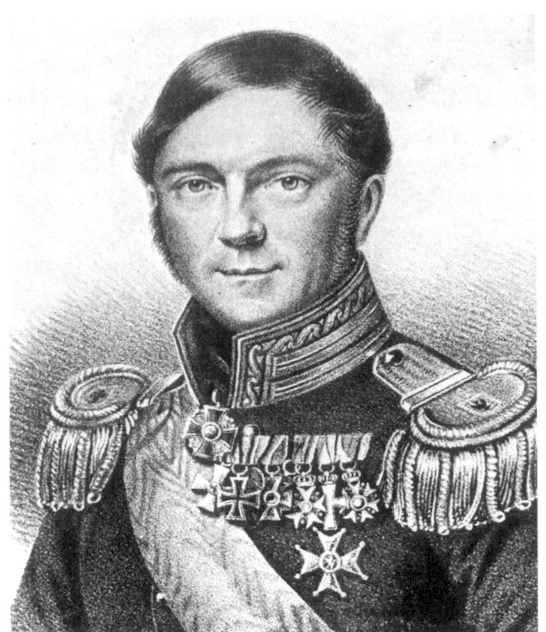

Figure 27. Carl Ferdinand von Graefe (1787–1840). From the collection of the National Library of Medicine.

blood from his nostril (and) from his ear, on the side of him having that smash; it is painful when he opens his mouth because of it; (and) he is speechless, thou shouldst say concerning him: 'One having a smash in his nostril. An ailment not to be treated.'"[14]

One of the earliest references to extraskeletal fixation was that of von Graefe (1823), who was one of the first to devise a special splint for fractures of the maxillary bone. His apparatus consisted of a horizontal fronto-occipital band of metal to which was attached an adjustable leather strap and buckle. Two vertical supports were fitted to this head band through cylindrical apertures. This arrangement permitted the supports to be fixed in any desired position by means of thumb screws, which made possible fixation of the supports. These vertical supports anchored suitably massive, curved hooks designed to fit over the teeth, and the appliance was used for the treatment of transverse fractures of the maxilla. This initial crude appliance became the basis for the development of more effective external appliances that could be used for the treatment of fractures of the upper jaw.

Graefe reported the following case: "A 42 year old hackney-coachman fell under his horse when the animal became frightened. He received several strong kicks from the heavily shoed animal and was brought into his house. He was thought to be dead. His left upper arm was fractured and his head was transformed into an almost unrecognizable bloody mass, as a strong kick had hit him directly in the face. The forehead was gaping widely and deeply depressed; the upper part of the right eye was severely injured; the nose was broken at its base and could be moved back and forth.

"Both upper jaw bones were loosened from their connections so completely that they, together with their sets of teeth, could be removed completely. In complete unconsciousness and absence of pulse, the only signs of life were the heartbeat and the infrequent, deep, stertorous breathing of a dying man.

"We cleaned the mouth and nostrils of the blood clots, but bleeding from both sinuses [antra] persisted, caused by the fractures of the upper jaw bones. Because of threatened suffocation, elastic tubes were put into the nose. The nose was reset into the normal position and stabilized by means of lateral padding. Both upper jaw bones were held fast and pressed against each other at a high level by means of a quickly assembled apparatus. Moreover, I ordered the necessary dressings for the remaining injuries: cold poultices on the head and an effective anti-inflammatory treatment.

"After a few days the patient resumed consciousness. After four weeks the nose and the upper jaw bones recovered their stability so that the patient was able to take ordinary

[14] Breasted tr.

food by mouth. Gradually, several bone pieces from the forehead fell away, the fracture of the arm was healed, and the patient who had been injured so severely recovered so well that he was able to return to his work.

"The apparatus to which the patient owes most for his recovery was described in detail and illustrated [Fig. 28] by Dr. Reiche in his inaugural dissertation, *De maxillae superioris fractura*."[15, 16]

In 1900 René Le Fort experimented on cadavers in his studies of fractures of the maxilla. Le Fort's monograph of 1900 follows:

"I have undertaken a series of experiments upon the cadaver for the purpose of studying fractures of the maxilla.

"The objects of these studies were limited to extensive fractures which reach frequently the bones of the face; partial or limited fractures were not considered.

"Most of the experiments were performed upon whole cadavers, and under differing conditions, varying the point of application, and also its direction, sometimes applying the force on a head supported against a resisting board, sometimes upon the unsupported head.

"If one generalizes upon local fractures produced by very violent blows within a limited area, one will see that there is close relation between the cause of the lesions and their natures. Lesions produced under analogous conditions on various heads are closely comparable and permit the description of a series of types of fractures.

[15] Charles Frederick William Reiche wrote, "That very simple appliance invented by the illustrious Graefe is most suitable to the treatment of fractures of the maxilla."

Tallmadge has noticed that von Graefe's publication is dated 1823, and that it gives credit to Reiche for the first description of the maxillary apparatus. On the other hand, Reiche's publication, dated 1822, gives credit to Graefe for the invention of the apparatus.

[16] Tallmadge tr.

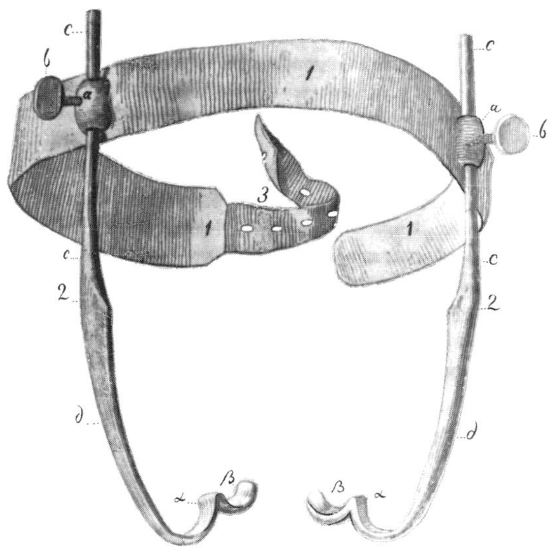

Figure 28. Graefe's apparatus for the treatment of fractures of the maxilla. From C. F. W. Reiche: *De maxillae superioris fractura*, Berol., 1822, p. 28. Legend printed in Latin: "Explicatio tabulae. 1. Arcus. 2. Trabeculae. 3. Lorum. a. Vaginae annulares. b. Trochleae. c. Extremitates superiores trabecularum. d. Extremitates inferiores trabecularum. α. Curvatura maior ad recipiendum labium. β. Curvatura minor ad recipiendum marginem alveolarem."

"Variations in the structure of the bone and in the degree of ossification of the sutures will cause variations in the extent or intensity of the lesion, as also will variations in the weight of the injuring tool, the swiftness of the blow and the duration of the action of the injuring agent; but these differences do not modify the general type of the fractures.

"My experiments (which numbered about 40) have been reported previously.[17] In this paper I limit myself to the formulation of some propositions which have been derived from my experiments and from the study of earlier papers on the same problem:

"1. Blows upon the face from before-backward at the level of the superior lip caused the production of a great transverse fracture which involves both maxilla and mandible. Such a blow detaches from the

[17] We have been unable to locate an earlier report on this subject by Le Fort.

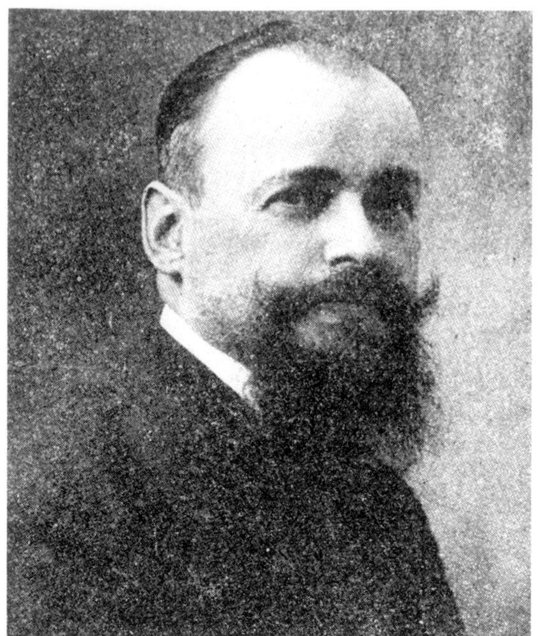

Figure 29. René Le Fort (1869–1951). From "Orthopédique et reparatrice de l'appareil moteur," *Revue de Chirurgie, 37:* 117, 1951.

maxilla, as a fragment, the whole palatine vault, the alveolar border, and the two pterygoid apophyses. This is the fracture of Guérin.

"Usually the fragment is separated into two parts by an antero-posterior fissure which passes at some distance from the median line.

"2. Blows delivered from the side at the level of the inferior part of the maxilla have a different effect depending upon whether the blow was directed horizontally or obliquely. Horizontally the blow produces a great double fracture, as has been described in the preceding case. Perhaps neither pterygoid apophysis may have been injured.

"If the blow is delivered obliquely, the fragment includes only the inferior part of the broken maxilla, which is separated from its fellow by a fracture or a subluxation of the sutures.

"If the blow is directed a little lower, the alveolar ridge will give way.

"3. Following a violent blow from below upward upon the superior alveolar ridge, if the mouth is open, the whole middle part of the face is knocked in, from the dental arch completely up to the nose, but the malar bones are uninjured. The large fragment, furthermore, is separated into two parts near the midline and a large horizontal fracture will have occurred as in the preceding cases, which may include one-half of one or both maxillary bones.

"4. Blows upon the front and middle part of the face produce analogous effects. The middle part of the face is detached and divided into two parts, as in the preceding case and it is evident that these injuries are about the same as those produced by a horizontal fracture.

"5. Wounds inflicted upon the root of the nose from above downward, grazing the face, may crush the maxilla between the wounding body and the mandible, which then will be resting against the sternum.

"M. Walther has shown that in such a case there may be a fracture of the maxilla with four fragments.

"6. Blows upon the chin may produce fractures of the maxilla by transmission of the force of the blow from the chin, or by the force of the blow meeting the inertia of the head. In such a case, the mandible may not be fractured. The resulting fractures should be compared with those which obtain by inflicting a direct blow upon the maxilla from below upward.

"7. Blows applied to the region of the malar bones are the most frequent of facial injuries; the resulting injuries are different depending upon whether the head is fixed against a resisting surface or whether it is unsupported.

"a) When the head is not supported the dominating lesion is a depression of the malar bone into the sinus because of the breaking of the pyramid. If the blow is somewhat higher, there will almost always be a comminuted fracture because of the great force required to produce more serious injury on a head which is not supported.

"b) When the head is not completely fixed or when, voluntary or by reflex action, one tries to avoid the striking body, there is a tendency toward complete separation of the bones of the face from the cranium and a division of the facial skeleton into two parts near the medial line, and a division, further, of these two fragments into secondary fragments.

"c) If the head is solidly supported against an immovable body, the malar bone is separated from its neighboring bones; the zygomatico-maxillary process constitutes a second fragment; and the whole arch of the palate, together with its alveolar ridge, separated by a large, transverse fracture from the rest of the face, constitutes a third fragment.

"8. When the blow is struck transversely across the whole anterior part of the face, including the malar, nasal, and maxillary bones, there is a complete separation of the face from the cranium. Furthermore the facial skeleton is divided from before backward, and laterally fragmented.

"9. Finally, when the blow is applied to the posterior part of the malar bone and the head is supported from the side, there is a great vertical separation of the face from the cranium, which divides the face transversely from the cranium as far back as the anterior cranial fossa.

"And so in general I draw the following conclusions from my work:

"Fractures of the face, although they are not frequent nevertheless are much less rare than we have thought and most of them are not discovered by the physician. Clinically, almost all reports have dealt with fractures where there is displacement of the bone; experimentally, there may be little or no displacement. No ordinary examination reveals externally the presence of even an extended fracture if there is little displacement, minor lesions of the soft parts, and small disturbance of mobility. Guérin, who was the first to describe fractures of the face without deformity, suspected that such fractures were more frequent than had been thought previously. We may add that usually they are not very extensive.

"Quite rarely, nevertheless, the base of the cranium is involved in these fractures. This hardly ever occurs except by bilateral compression of the head, that is, by pressure applied not only to the cranium but also to the face. In such cases the cranium may be fractured. One almost always notices the independence of the cranium from the face and also the complete separation of the cranium from the face at the pterygoid apophyses and the lateral plates of the ethmoid which, anatomically, belong rather to the face than to the cranium, and which adhere to the maxilla.

"The separation of the face from the cranium occurs in two manners. Usually the whole of the face is removed from the cranium, sometimes only in its middle part, sometimes from the root of the nose down to the teeth, with the malar bones still adhering to the cranium. In the first case there has been a blow at the level of the eyes, from the side or from before backward; in the second case the violence of the blow has been received only in the middle of the face, either from before backward or from above downward on the root of the nose or from below upward on the alveolar ridge, or even beneath the chin.

"Whether or not the face has been separated from the cranium, the facial skeleton tends to be broken into fragments and these fragments present constant characters whatever may be the means by which the fracture was produced.

"The most frequent fracture which we have obtained in our experiments corresponds to the great transverse fracture of Guérin. It includes the roof of the palate, the alveolar ridge, and the pterygoid apophyses.

"Sometimes the alveolar ridge is divided by an antero-posterior fissure which is usually at some distance from the midline.

"Frequently the malar bone forms a second fragment. This bone generally is intact, or nearly so, and has attached to it the tip of the pyramidal apophysis of the maxillary bone, or, more rarely, the whole apophysis.

"The ascending process of the maxilla, with part of the unguis and sometimes with the nasal bone, forms a third fragment.

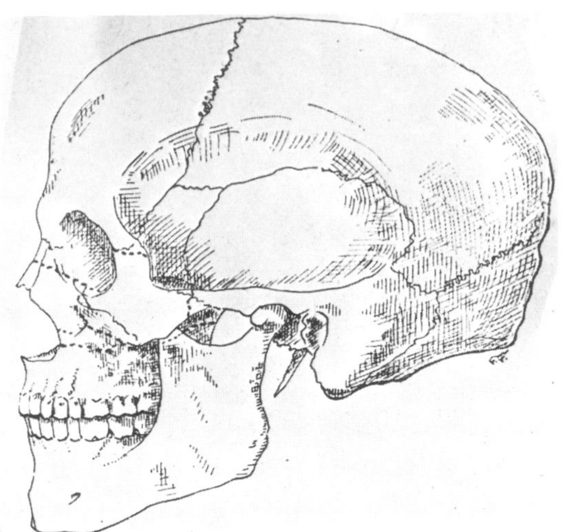

Figure 31. Copy of Le Fort's illustration shown on page 500 of "Etude expérimentale sur les fractures de la machoire supérieure," *Revue de Chirurgie,* Paris, 23, 1901. ("Fig. 10—Lines of greatest weakness in the face and fragments, seen from the side.")

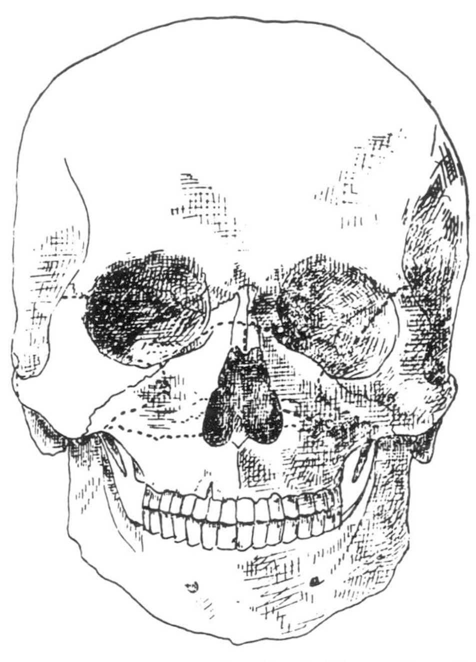

Figure 30. Copy of Le Fort's illustration shown on page 499 of "Etude expérimentale sur les fractures de la machoire supérieure," *Revue de Chirurgie,* Paris, 23, 1901. ("Fig. 9—The lines of greatest weakness in the skeleton of the face, and also the fragments which may be included in the areas which they bound. This anterior view shows, in dots, the lines where fracture is more frequent.")

"Splinters of the anterior wall of the maxillary antrum, the lateral plates of the ethmoid, the inferior part of the nasal bone, and others, may be included with those which constitute the bony mass of the maxilla.

"M. Le Fort has made photographs of these different kinds of fractures."[18]

In 1901 Le Fort continued his experiments on cadavers, and in his publications showed illustrations of sites of fractures which now have become known as Le Fort's classification of maxillary fractures.

Concerning such experiments performed upon cadavers, one is reminded of the similar tries of Sherlock Holmes in his efforts to determine whether a bruise could be produced after death, or what degree of strength would be required to transfix a dead sow with a whaler's harpoon.

Countless numbers of external appliances have been designed for the treatment of maxillary fractures. The definitive treat-

[18] Tallmadge tr.

ment waited upon the Adams method of suspension by wiring. In contemporary treatment, only rarely is some form of external appliance required.

THE ZYGOMA

Possibly the oldest reports of fractures of the zygoma are reported in the Smith Papyrus:

"Case XV: If thou examinest a man having a perforation in his cheek, shouldst thou find there is a swelling, protruding and black, (and) diseased tissue upon his cheek, thou shouldst say concerning him: 'One having a perforation in his cheek. An ailment which I will treat.' Thou shouldst bind it with *ymrw* and treat it afterward [with] grease (and) honey every day until he recovers.[19]

"Case XVI: If thou examinest a man having a split in his cheek, shouldst thou find that there is a swelling, protruding and red, on the outside of that split, thou shouldst say concerning him: 'One having a split in his cheek. An ailment which [I] will treat.' Thou shouldst bind it with fresh meat the first day. [Even today a "black eye" is treated by the application of a raw steak.]

"His treatment is sitting until its swelling is reduced (lit., drawn out). Thou shalt treat it afterward [with] grease, honey, (and) lint every day until he recovers.[20]

"Case XVII: If thou examinest a man having a smash in his cheek, thou shouldst place thy hand on his cheek at the point of that smash. Should it crepitate under thy fingers, while he discharges blood from his nostril, (and) from his ear on the side of him having that injury: (and) at the same time he discharges blood from his mouth, while it is painful when he opens his mouth because of it, thou shouldst say concerning him: 'One having a smash in his cheek, while he discharges blood from his nostril, from his ear, (and) from his mouth, (and) he is speechless. An ailment not to be treated': Thou shouldst bind with fresh meat the first day. His 'relief' is sitting until its swelling is reduced (lit., drawn out). Thou shalt treat it afterward [with] grease, honey (and) lint every day, until he recovers."[21]

[19] Breasted tr.

[20] Breasted tr.

Even though the hieroglyphs of the Edwin Smith Papyrus reported fractures of the zygoma or zygomatic region, as far as we have been able to determine, the zygomatic bone was not looked upon as a separate entity but was considered a part of the maxilla or the temporal or frontal bone.

The Corpus Hippocraticum does not give a description of fractures of the zygoma. Celsus in *De Medicina* does not mention fractures of the zygoma. Centuries elapsed before du Verney in 1751 gave a commentary on fractures of this bone along with two case reports:

"Article II: The zygomatic apophysis is part of the temporal bone. It arises slightly above the bony external auditory meatus and, passing horizontally from behind forward, articulates with the posterior angle of the zygoma. Thus it forms an arch beneath which is the point of the coronoid process of the mandible, and it covers the tendon of the temporal muscle, which is attached to the coronoid process. This arch has a connection with the temporal muscle by a strong aponeurosis as well as by muscular tissue.

"Fracture of the apophysis of the zygoma occurs from the same cause as does any other fracture. And, as in the case of any fracture, it may be either simple or comminuted. Usually the fragments are depressed inward. However it may happen that a frag-

[21] Breasted tr.

ment may be pushed outward, while the rest of the bone remains in its normal place.

"Such a fracture is characterized by these signs: firstly, the patient cannot move his mandible except with great difficulty; secondly, the patient has acute pain in the region of the fracture upon contraction of the temporal muscle; and thirdly, he has muscular fibrillations caused by pressure upon the small nerves about the bone.

"Complications are rare and the prognosis is good; the only thing necessary is reduction of the bone. Since I know of virtually no author who has mentioned the method of reduction let me describe what I have done in such cases."

Case History I

"A soldier of the French Guards was injured by a blow from the end of a log. This caused swelling of the entire cheek. The patient had great difficulty in moving his mandible. I examined the zygomatic apophysis and, by palpation, found a displacement. I placed my left index finger into his mouth, passing it above the first two or three molar teeth as far as I could and making pressure with the finger from within outward. By this manner of palpation I discovered that the apophysis had been fractured and depressed. Since there were no means of reducing the fragments from the outside with my fingers or with any instruments, I asked the patient to place between his last molar teeth a piece of wood, flattened, and about the thickness of a finger, and to occlude as strongly as he possibly could. After having maintained the occlusion for a few hours he felt considerable alleviation of his pain. Treatment was continued with a gradual increase in the size of the piece of wood, and by this means the fragments replaced themselves by the force of the temporal muscle, which exerted pressure upon the apophysis from within outward. The soft-tissue injury was treated by applying a compress soaked in brandy, which was held in place by a bandage passing beneath the chin, around the face, and fixed finally at the top of the head."

Case History II

"A child of three or four years was playing with a pea-shooter. The toy had a wooden mouthpiece made in the shape of an olive. While he had his toy in his mouth he fell down a flight of stairs headfirst. The wooden mouthpiece was driven into the mucous membrane of the cheek as far as the zygomatic apophysis, which was fractured from within outward. When the pea-shooter was withdrawn, the wooden mouthpiece remained concealed in the wound. However, no one noticed this. As time passed the child suffered from severe inflammation and pressure in the jaw. Those who noticed this paid little attention to it at first, and treated it unsuccessfully for about one month with compresses. Meanwhile the child could take nothing but fluid nourishment. The wound did not heal; its edges became thickened and from time to time a serosanguineous fluid exuded. I was summoned and was given the history of the case. I noticed that the injured child could not open his mouth. I inserted my finger into his mouth and palpated the wound. But as I passed my finger along the zygomatic apophysis I noticed the presence of a buried foreign body. I used a little pressure, and by placing my other hand against the cheek I discovered that the foreign body was within the wound. I advised the child's parents to apply to his cheek a cataplasm of bread soaked in milk and mixed with eggs and saffron. For the next three or four days I washed the small ulcer which was present with wine mixed with honey, and healing began. When the swelling had subsided to the point at which I could locate the foreign body more accurately I laid the child across a man's knees, belly down, and with the child's head held firmly. I introduced a curved forceps into the wound where the wooden tip of the peashooter lay, and removed the tip. The removal having been accomplished I laid the palm of my hand on the cheek, making some slight pressure, and in this manner reduced the fracture of the zygomatic apophysis. For a few days I treated the patient with suitable lavages, and he recovered completely."[22]

Monographs appeared more frequently after 1751. Lang (1889) probably was the first to describe the so-called "blow-out" fracture of the floor of the orbit. This fracture is usually classified in the zygomatico-maxillary complex of fractures. Matas (1896) treated depressed zygomatic fractures with silver wire wound around the bone with strong traction. In 1906 Lothrop used an antrostomy approach through Highmore's antrum, below the inferior turbinate. He passed a trocar into the maxillary sinus, contacted the lateral superior wall, and rotated the fractured zygoma upward and outward for proper repositioning. Keen, in 1909, described an intraoral approach: he passed a sharp elevator through the buccal vestibule behind the tuberosity of the maxilla. Pressure then could be exerted in an upward, forward, and outward direction. Manwaring (1913) advocated the "cow-horn" dental forceps for releasing impacted zygomas. The temporal approach was described by Gillies, Kilner, and Stone in 1927. The temporal approach is a popular and effective approach for the reduction of a fractured zygoma. Adams, in 1940, was probably the first to demonstrate internal wire fixation of the zygoma.

THE NOSE

The Edwin Smith Papyrus, from the age of the building of the pyramids, describes cases of fractures of the nose.

[22] Tallmadge tr.

"Case XI: If thou examinest a man having a break in the column of his nose, his nose being disfigured, and a 'depression' being in it, while the swelling that is on it protrudes, (and) he has discharged blood from both his nostrils, thou shouldst say concerning him: 'One having a break in the column of his nose. An ailment which I will treat.' Thou shouldst cleanse (it) for him [with] two plugs of linen. Thou shouldst place two (other) plugs of linen saturated with grease in the inside of his two nostrils. Thou shouldst put [him] at his mooring stakes until the swelling is reduced (lit., drawn out). Thou shouldst apply for him stiff rolls of linen by which his nose is held fast. Thou shouldst treat him afterward [with] grease, honey (and) lint, every day until he recovers. As for: 'The column of his nose,' it means the outer edge of his nose as far as its side(s) on the top of his nose, being the inside of his nose in the middle of his two nostrils. As for: 'His two nostrils,' [it means] the two sides of his nose extending to his [two] cheek[s], as far as the back of his nose; the top of his nose is loosened.

"Case XII: If thou examinest a man having a break in the chamber of his nose, (and) thou findest his nose bent, while his face is disfigured, (and) the swelling which is over it is protruding, Thou shouldst say concerning him: 'One having a break in the chamber of his nose. An ailment which I will treat.' Thou shouldst force it to fall in, so that it is lying in its place, (and) clean out for him the interior of both his nostrils with two swabs of linen until every worm of blood which coagulates in the inside of his two nostrils comes forth. Now afterward thou shouldst place two plugs of linen saturated with grease and put into his two nostrils. Thou shouldst place for him two stiff rolls of linen, bound on. Thou shouldst treat him afterward with grease, honey, (and) lint every day until he recovers. As for: 'A break in the chamber of his nose,' it means the middle of his nose as far as the back, extending to the region between his two eyebrows. As for: 'His nose bent, while his face is disfigured,' it means his nose is crooked and greatly swollen throughout; his two cheeks likewise, so that his face is disfigured by it, not being in its customary form, because all the depressions are clothed with swellings, so that his face looks disfigured by it. As for: 'every worm of blood which coagulates in the inside of his two nostrils,' it then means the clotting of blood in the inside of his two nostrils, likened to the 'n'r·t-worm, which subsists in the water."[23]

From the Corpus Hippocraticum ΠΕΡΙ ΑΡΘΡΩΝ, we quote, concerning fractures of the nose:

"XXXV. There are several kinds of fractures of the nose. Those who, without judgment, delight in fine bandagings may do more harm than good. For the nasal is the most complex of all bandages, having most of the turns of the bandage leaving rhomboidal intervals and uncovered spaces of the skin. As has been said, those who, without judgment, pretend to possess skill, are happy to encounter a case of fractured nose, for then they may apply this showy bandage. For a day or two thereafter the physician glories in his performance, and the patient who has been bandaged is well pleased, but soon the patient complains of the encumbrance of the bandage. Nevertheless, the physician is satisfied because he has had an opportunity to show his skill in applying this complex nasal bandage. Such bandaging, however, does everything the very reverse of what is proper; for, in the first place, those who have their nose flattened by the fracture clearly will have the part rendered still more flat if pressure from outside be applied to it; and, again, those cases in which the nose is displaced to either side, whether at the cartilage or higher up, clearly will derive no benefit from the bandage, but rather will be injured by it, for it will not admit of having pads properly arranged on either side of the nose, and indeed, persons applying this bandage do not even try to employ such pads. A nasal bandage appears to me to be most useful when the soft parts are bruised against the bone near the middle of the nose, or when the bone itself has sustained some slight injury. In such cases a superficial callus is formed and the nose becomes a little too prominent or misshapen. And yet even in these cases there is no need of a troublesome bandage; if, indeed, any bandage at all be required. It is enough if one lay a waxed compress across the contusion, keeping the compress in place with one turn of a two-tailed bandage. The best treatment for such lesions is the application of a small cataplasm of flour worked up with water into a viscid mass. If the flour be made from good wheat, and if it be glutinous, it should be used alone for all such cases, but if it be not very glutinous, a little frankincense, well pulverized in water, should be mixed with it, or a very little gum may be mixed in the same way.

"XXXVII. In those cases in which the fractured portions are depressed and flattened, if the depression is above the cartilage, something may be introduced into the nostrils to reduce the parts. If not, all such deformities may be reduced by introducing the fingers into the nostrils, if this can be managed; if not, a thick spatula may be introduced, directing it with the fingers, not to the fore part of the nose, but to the depressed portion. Then the physician should hold the nose externally on both sides, and at the same time elevate it. And if the fracture be mostly in the lower part, one may introduce into the nostrils, as already stated, either lint scraped from linen, or something of the kind, wrapped in a piece of cloth or, better, stitched in Carthaginian leather, and moulded into a shape which will fit the place

[23] Breasted tr.

into which it is to be introduced. But if the fracture be farther within, it is not possible to introduce anything, for if it is irksome to tolerate anything of this kind in the lower part of the nose, it is even more irksome when the object is introduced farther in. At first, then, by reshaping the nostrils from the inside, they should be brought to their natural position. A fractured nose may be restored readily to shape, especially on the day of the accident, or even a little later. But physicians act irresolutely, and treat the fracture more delicately at first than they should. For the fingers should be introduced on each side along the natural line of the nose, which should be pushed forward and upward to combine elevation of the organ with reduction of the displaced fragments. But for these purposes no physician's finger is as satisfactory as are the index fingers of the patient himself: if he will take care and have resolution, his own fingers are the most natural instruments. Any of the fingers should be inserted and placed firmly along the whole nose to hold it immobilized, if possible until union occurs, or, failing that, for as long as the patient can. If he cannot do this himself a boy or a woman should do it, for the hands should be delicate. This is the most proper treatment of fracture of the nose attended with depression and without displacement to the side. I never have seen a case of fractured nose which could not be reduced when treated at once, before callus has formed, provided the treatment be applied properly. But although men would give much to escape defacement, they still do not know how to combine care and fortitude unless they suffer pain or fear death. But the formation of callus in the nose takes place speedily; usually it is complete in ten days, unless necrosis occurs.

"XXXVIII. When the fractured bone is displaced laterally, the treatment is the same. But it is obvious that the reduction is to be made not by applying equal force on both sides but by pushing the displaced portion into its natural position, and pressing upon it from without, and by introducing something into the nostrils; and boldly replacing the fragments which have been pushed inward, until the whole nose be

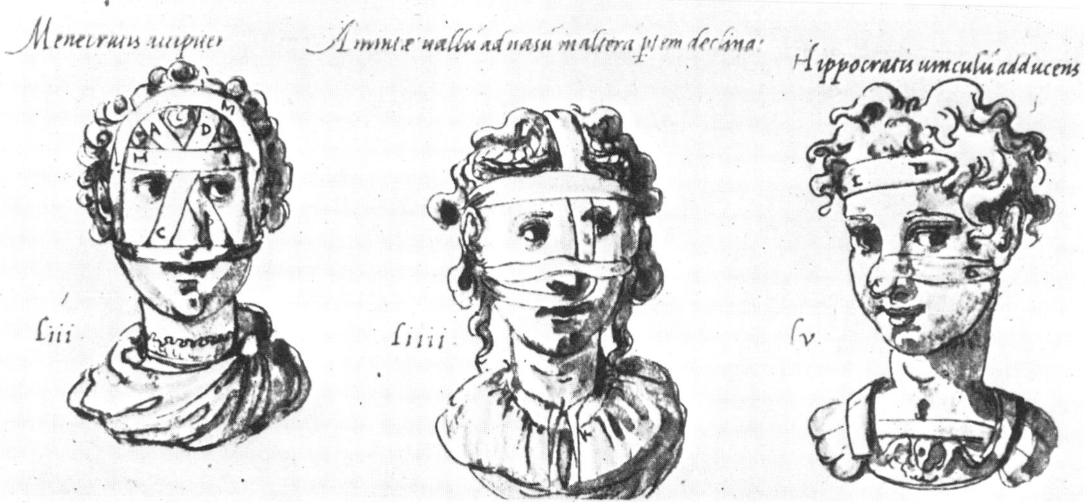

Figure 32. Illustrations from Latin manuscript 6866 of the Bibliothèque Nationale, showing bandages of the head described by Galen. (*liii*) The hawk bandage of Menecrates. (*liiii*) The bandage of Amyntas for correction of deviation of the nose. (One can see that this patient's injury caused a deviation of the nose to the left and that the bandage has been applied to the left side of the nose in order to correct the deviation.) (*lv*) The bandage used by Hippocrates to correct deviation of the nose to the right.

properly reconstituted. One should realize that if one does not restore the parts at once, it is certain that the nose will be distorted. But when you restore the parts to their natural position, either the patient himself, or some other person, is to apply one finger or more to the part which protrudes, and keep it in position until the fracture be consolidated. From time to time the little finger should be pushed into the nostril, to support the parts which are displaced inward. If inflammation occurs, a dressing of dough should be applied, but the little finger must be used still even after the application of the dough.

"If the fracture be in the cartilage, with lateral displacement, the end of the nose necessarily must be displaced. In such cases the methods of reduction mentioned before should be used and whatever is suitable should be introduced into the nostril.

"But there are many convenient things to be found which have no odor, and which are comfortable in other respects. On one occasion I introduced a slice of sheep's lung, as it happened to be at hand instead of sponges which absorb moisture. Also, an outer covering of Carthaginian leather may be used: cut a strip about the breadth of the thumb or as wide as may be needed, and paste it to the outside of the nostril which is depressed. Then apply tension to this piece of thong, a little more than what will be sufficient to make the nose straight and regular. Then the thong (which should be long enough) should be brought beneath the ear and upward around the head. Then the end of the thong may be pasted to the forehead, or, if long enough, carried completely around the head and secured. This is a mode of setting the nose naturally, is of easy application, and enables the counter-extension on the nose to be made greater or less, as one may choose. In a case where the fractured nose is turned to the side, the treatment is to be conducted in the manner just described; but the thong may be pasted to the end of the nose so as to make counter-deviation in the opposite direction.

"XXXIX. When the fracture is complicated by open wounds one need not be apprehensive. An ointment containing pitch, or any of the ointments used for fresh wounds, should be applied to the wounds, for in general they admit of easy cure, even when there is reason to fear that fragments of necrotic bone may be extruded. The parts are to be adjusted at once, fearlessly and accurately. Later, if necessary, they should be readjusted with the fingers more delicately, indeed, but this is necessary. For of all parts of the body, the nose is the most easily reshaped. And there is nothing to prevent one from having recourse to the fixing of the thongs and drawing the nose to the opposite side, even if there be a wound or the parts be inflamed, for these thongs give no pain."[24]

In another section of the Corpus Hippocraticum, *ΜΟΧΛΙΚΟΝ,* we read:

"II. When the nose is fractured, the parts should be reshaped at once. If the fracture be in its cartilaginous part, introduce into the nostrils a support formed of lint wrapped in thin Carthaginian leather, or anything else which will not irritate; strips of the leather should be pasted to the displaced parts, which parts thus can be elevated. Bandaging is harmful. Another method of treatment consists in bringing the parts into apposition at once and holding them so by applying a cerate with frankincense or sulphur. Afterward the parts should be kept in place with fingers introduced into the nostrils thus replacing the fragments; then Carthaginian leather may be used for maintaining the reduction. Callus forms even when there is a wound; and the same treatment should be employed even if particles of bone are extruded, for this is not a serious complication."[25]

The eight books on medicine by Aulus

[24] Tallmadge tr.
[25] Tallmadge tr.

Cornelius Celsus surely represent the finished Roman medical practice of his time. We quote from his chapter concerning fractures of the nose.

"VIII, 5. In fractures of the nose it is usual for both the bone and the cartilage to be fractured, whether the fracturing force comes from before or from the side. In either case the nose is depressed and the patient has difficulty in breathing. If the bone is fractured from the side the site of the injury is depressed; if the cartilage is fractured the nose is displaced to one side or the other.

"If the cartilage is depressed it should be elevated carefully, either by introducing a surgeon's probe or by two fingers pressing against each other; then a bandage folded lengthwise and covered with a layer of thin leather sewed on should be placed into the nostrils. Or the same method may be employed using a pack made of dried feathers, or from the wing of a bird, smeared with cerate or a paste made out of fine flour, covered with a layer of thin leather, so that the cartilages may remain reduced. If the fracture is horizontal each nostril ought to be packed in the same way. And if the fracturing force has been from the side the pack which is inserted ought to be bulkier in the nostril on the side to which the nose is deviated and less bulky in the other nostril. Externally a soft bandage should be applied. Its central part, which will lie over the nose, should be impregnated with the substances mentioned above to which should be added some burned incense. Each end of the bandage should be carried behind each corresponding ear and brought together on the forehead. By this means the bandage will remain in place as well as if it were adhesive, and will support the cartilages well. And if the fracture has injured the interior of the nose, as usually it does, especially when the lower cartilage is broken, the nostrils should be elevated in the same way and maintained in position by the same kind of bandage. The bandage should be removed after fourteen days. The injured nose should be treated daily with compresses of hot water.

"But if the bone is broken the fracture should be reduced with the fingers. If the fracturing force was from the front and the nose is depressed both nostrils should be packed. If the fracturing force was from the side only the nostril on the side toward which the nose is deviated should be packed. The bandage described above should be impregnated with cerate and fastened somewhat more tightly, for a callus is not desirable because it may cause an obstruction in the nostril. On the third day the injury ought to be treated with hot water, not only on its own account, but also because it is important to keep the nostrils clean. If there are several fragments each should be replaced with the fingers; the same kind of bandage should be applied externally and covered with cerate. Further bandaging is unnecessary.

"If any fragment does not unite with the others a complication arises whose presence can be discovered by a copious discharge from the wound in the nostril. The ununited fragment should be extracted with forceps and, when the inflammation has subsided some healing medicament should be applied. The worst cases are those in which a fragment of bone or cartilage protrudes through the skin; fortunately such cases are rare. But if one is encountered the fragments nevertheless should be replaced in the manner described and the skin should be covered with any of the substances ordinarily used in the treatment of recent wounds; no bandage should be applied."[26]

We conclude by reminding our reader that during World War I, when there was a high incidence of facial injuries, basic principles of management were formulated and widely adapted as the profession rose to the challenge of these mass casualties. Many great names are associated with the devel-

[26] Tallmadge tr.

opment of a systematic program of managing fractures of the facial bones.

The war's end gave no respite. The facial injuries of trench warfare were replaced by those of expanding industry and those of a nation suddenly "on wheels." In terms of treatment, the principles of reduction and fixation were well understood. The methods of accomplishment, however, were relatively complicated and frequently ineffective.

Fractures of the long bones in animals were treated first with external pin fixation by Lambotte (1913). The use of this method for the fixation of fractures of facial bones was made popular by Anderson (1936). The method gained in popularity from 1936 until about 1942, by which time its shortcomings had been recognized. And so the method gave way to that of open reduction and direct wire fixation.

The greatest progress in the management of facial fractures waited upon the introduction of antibiotic therapy, the development of improved anesthetic techniques, and the widespread use of blood transfusions. These advances paved the way to effective application of the open surgical techniques which are the keys to contemporary methods of management.

Milton Adams treated his first cases of extensive multiple facial fractures by open reduction and internal wire fixation in 1940 and published a monograph on the subject in 1942. His methods have been supplemented by the development of intramedullary pin fixation of the mandible, as practiced by Brown and McDowell (1942), and the use of transverse facial pin fixation for middle third facial fractures by Brown, Fryer, and McDowell (1952).

The development of Adams' technique initiated a new era in the management of facial bone fractures. His precise and effective methods led to superior results and to the elimination of clumsy, ineffective, uncomfortable extraskeletal appliances.

CHAPTER

3

GENERAL PRINCIPLES

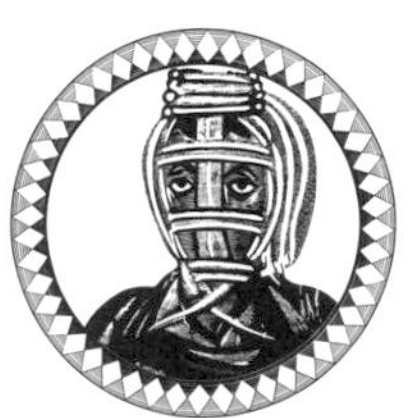

The essential principles of treating fractured bones have not changed since they were first defined by Hippocrates, or the Hippocratic writers, more than twenty-five centuries ago. These principles are reduction of the fractured segments and immobilization during the time of healing of the bone.

There are many ways to implement the principles of reduction and fixation. Methods vary considerably with the patient and with the training and skill of the operator. The method of choice should be the one that offers the simplest, most direct approach to successful reduction and positive fixation. Many fractures can be treated adequately by closed methods, but in our experience superior results have been achieved in the more serious injuries—with a minimum of effort and with the greatest degree of comfort to the patient—by open reduction with direct fixation.

In the management of facial injuries and fractures, it is the obligation of the physician to return the patient to his normal function and appearance, or as near to the normal as possible. In most cases, function as well as appearance and esthetics has to be considered. In some cases, however, the problems are entirely those of restoration of function or in others, entirely the restoration of appearance.

In a competitive society, economic, sociologic, and psychologic factors make it imperative that an intelligent, aggressive, expedient program be outlined and executed in order to return the patient to an active, productive life as soon as possible with minimal cosmetic and functional disability.

ETIOLOGY AND INCIDENCE OF FACIAL FRACTURES

Socioeconomic Factors

Today a wide range of statistical data indicates that socioeconomic factors have a strong bearing upon the incidence of facial fractures and associated injuries. On the one hand, reports from large metropolitan emergency hospitals serving highly transient, relatively low-income social groups show that a great percentage of facial fractures are caused by the impact of fists or weapons. On the other hand, hospitals in areas of higher socioeconomic level report more facial fractures resulting from transportational and recreational accidents.

Automobile Accidents and Other Factors

The costs associated with automobile accidents are staggering (National Safety Council, 1961). Reliable figures indicate that, including insurance, property damage, wage losses, and medical expenses, the cost in the United States is 6.5 billion dollars per year.

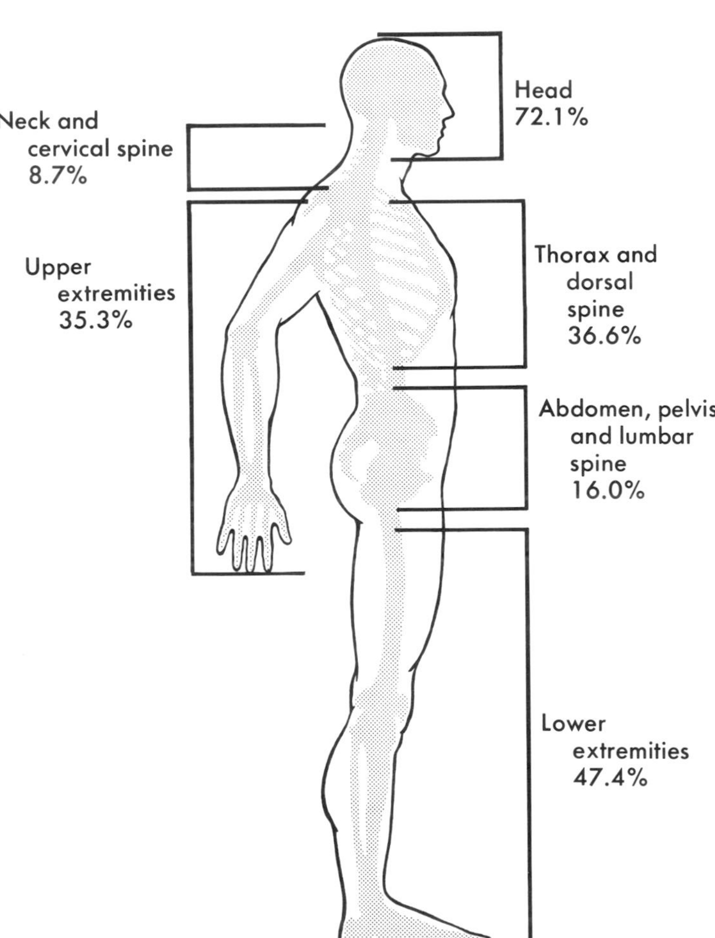

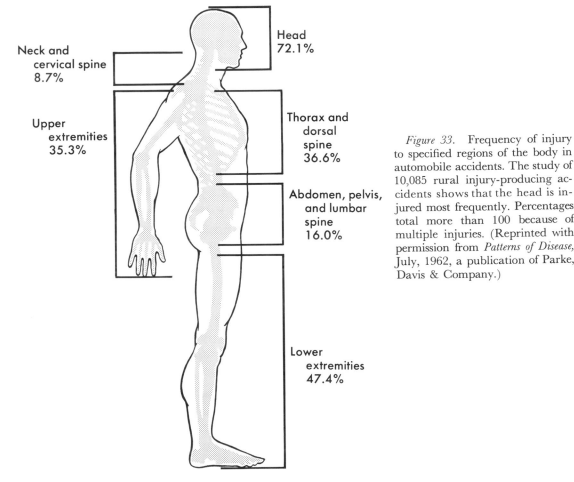

Figure 33. Frequency of injury to specified regions of the body in automobile accidents. The study of 10,085 rural injury-producing accidents shows that the head is injured most frequently. Percentages total more than 100 because of multiple injuries. (Reprinted with permission from *Patterns of Disease,* July, 1962, a publication of Parke, Davis & Company.)

Alcohol is a factor in over 50 per cent of automobile casualties. Poor judgment, emotional disturbances, physical disability, and other human factors account for most traffic accidents.

The report on Automotive Crash Injury Research of Cornell University (1961) indicated that 72.1 per cent of victims of automobile accidents suffer injuries to the facial structures. Although most of these injuries involve only soft tissue, many include fractures of the facial skeleton (Fig. 33).

Braunstein (1957), in a study of 1000 injury-producing accidents involving 2253 occupants, found that 72.3 per cent of 1213 injured persons suffered a head injury. In 7.2 per cent of these patients, at least one facial bone was fractured.

An evaluation of several studies indicates that most facial fractures occur between the ages of 15 and 40 years. The incidence of facial fractures is relatively low among children and older people. Because of greater activity and greater exposure, three times as many males as females sustain fractures of the face.

In their analysis of 319 cases of mandibular fractures, Hagan and Huelke (1961) reported that 55.8 per cent of the fractures were caused by automobile accidents, 17 per cent by fist fights, and 14 per cent by miscellaneous misadventures. A study of 500 cases in England by Rowe and Killey (1955) showed that 11.6 per cent of the fractures were caused by automobile accidents, 18.6 per cent by fist fights, 15.8 per cent by motorcycle smash-ups, 14.8 per cent by bicycle accidents, and 12 per cent by falls; epileptic seizures, sports, and pedestrian mishaps were among the causes of fracture in the rest of the cases.

According to reports from Switzerland as well as England, fewer than 7 per cent of all mandibular fractures have occurred as a result of automobile accidents. These reports from abroad point out the close relationship of the incidence of facial fractures to the country's mode of transportation.

Anatomic Considerations

The type and extent of a fracture of the facial skeleton is determined to a considerable degree by anatomic factors: the size, shape, location, and density of the bone structures; and the relationship of the bones to other structures and to cavities (cranial cavity, nasal cavities, paranasal sinuses, and oral cavity).

Overlying soft tissue also helps to determine the kind of fracture and the manner and degree of displacement of fractured segments. Such soft tissue includes the strong muscles that move the mandible, the muscles of the tongue and of the floor of the mouth, the overlying periosteal tissues, and also the adipose and subcutaneous tissues beneath the skin.

Specific anatomic details of the structure of the head and neck are not discussed here; it is assumed that the reader is well versed in surgical anatomy.

The Effect of the Impact

Fractures of the facial bones vary with the nature of the injuring force. The impact of a fist over the zygomatic area may cause separation at the suture lines, a typical fracture of the zygoma. By contrast, the violently explosive force of an automobile smash-up or a gunshot injury may result in extensive comminution with a multiplicity of fractures, even with loss or extensive displacement of bony structures. The injuring force of a fall, with impact upon the region of the symphysis of the mandible, may result in the subcondylar fracture of one or both necks of the mandible—without extensive displacement of bone segments. A more violent force in the same area, however, could cause multiple fractures of the symphysis and body of the mandible as well as of the condylar areas.

(Text continued on page 52.)

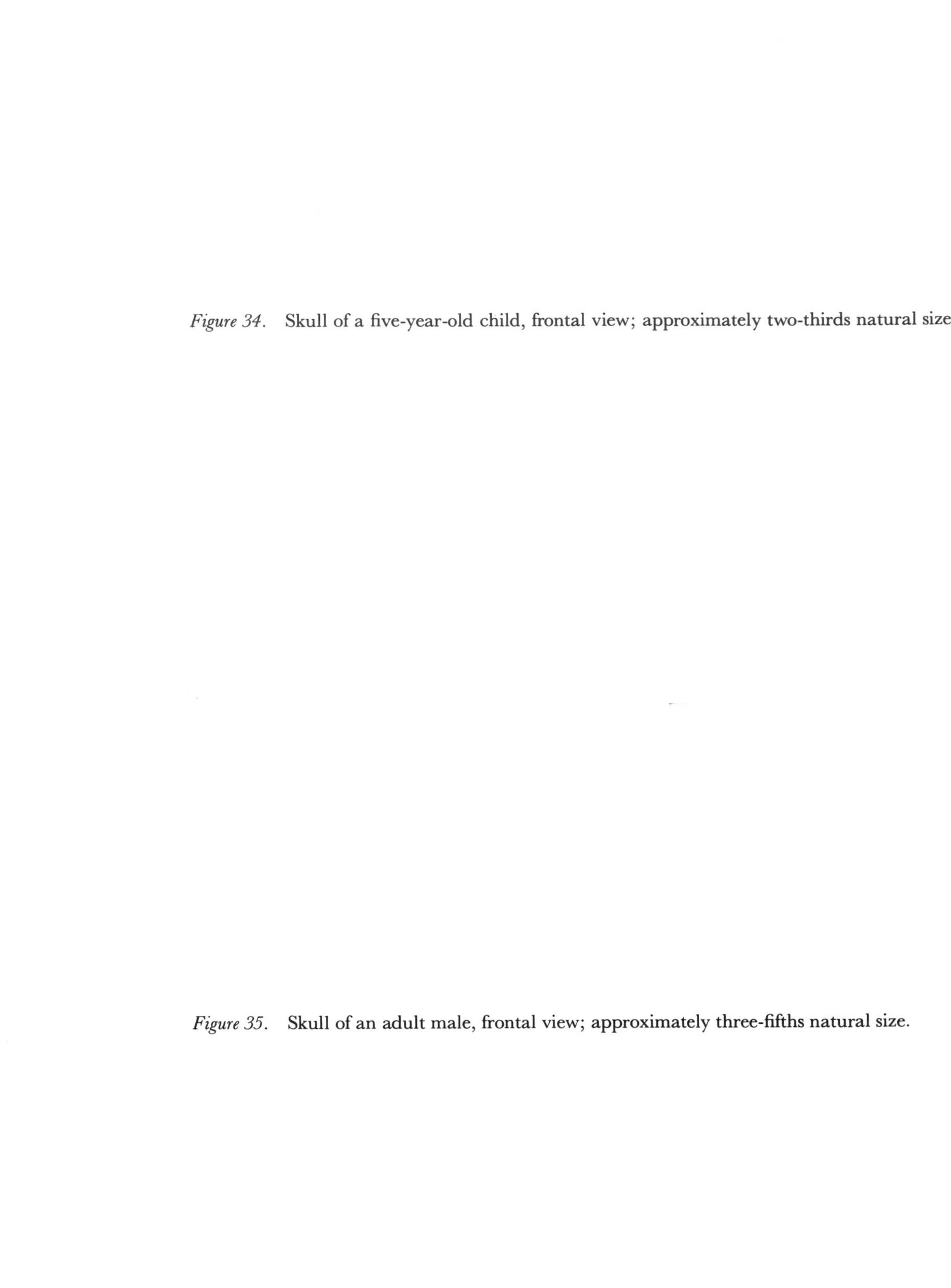

Figure 34. Skull of a five-year-old child, frontal view; approximately two-thirds natural size.

Figure 35. Skull of an adult male, frontal view; approximately three-fifths natural size.

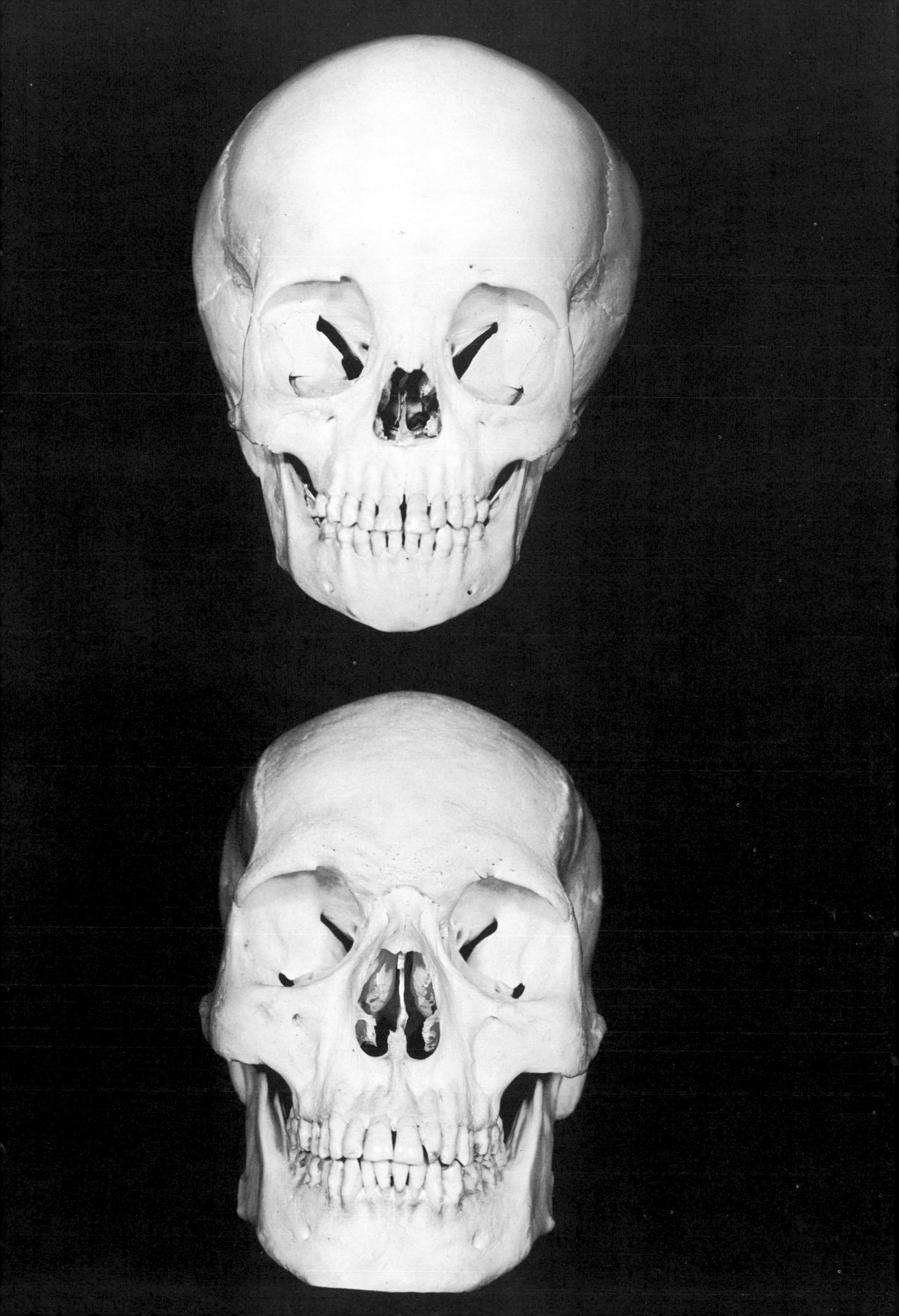

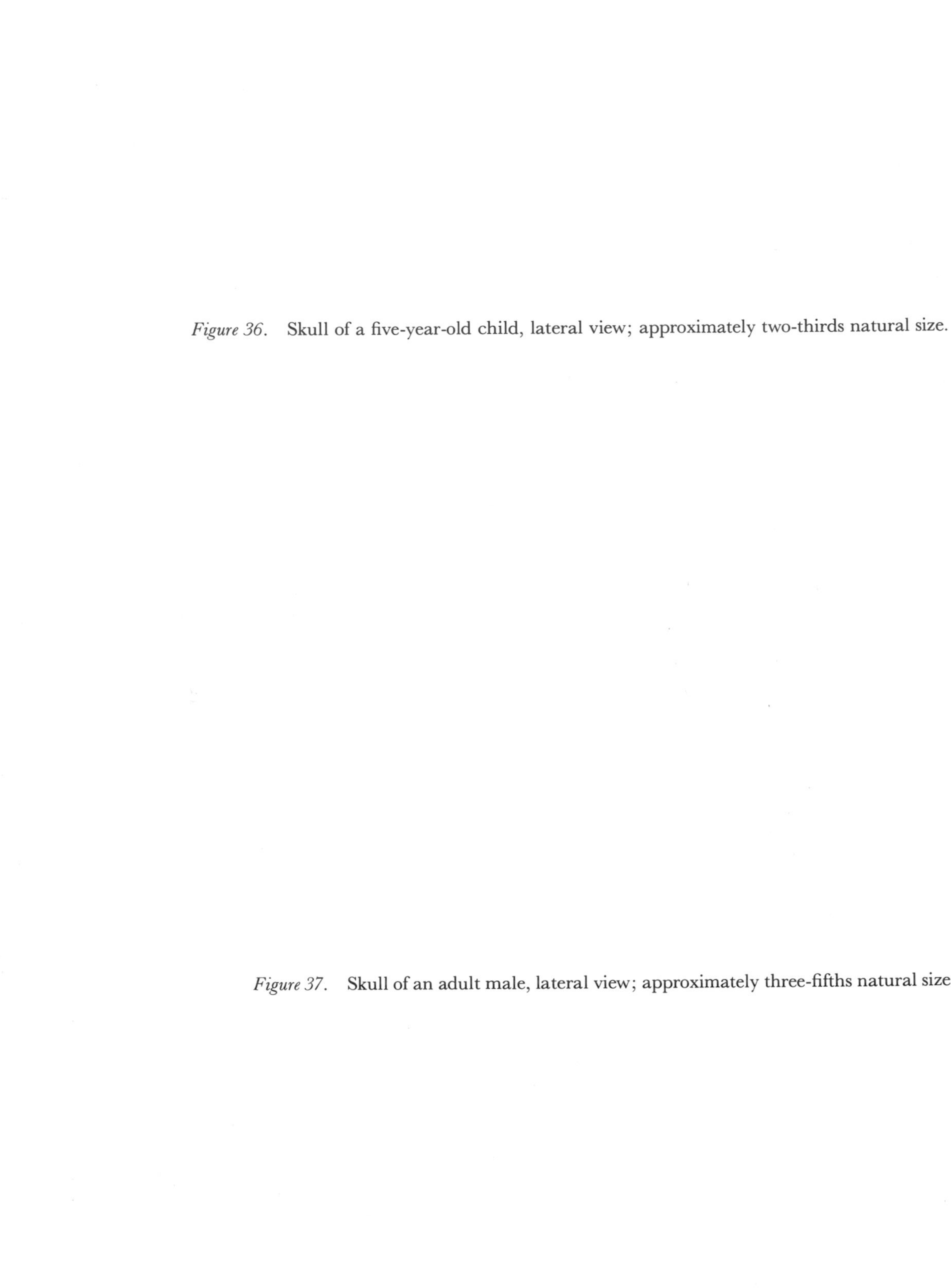

Figure 36. Skull of a five-year-old child, lateral view; approximately two-thirds natural size.

Figure 37. Skull of an adult male, lateral view; approximately three-fifths natural size.

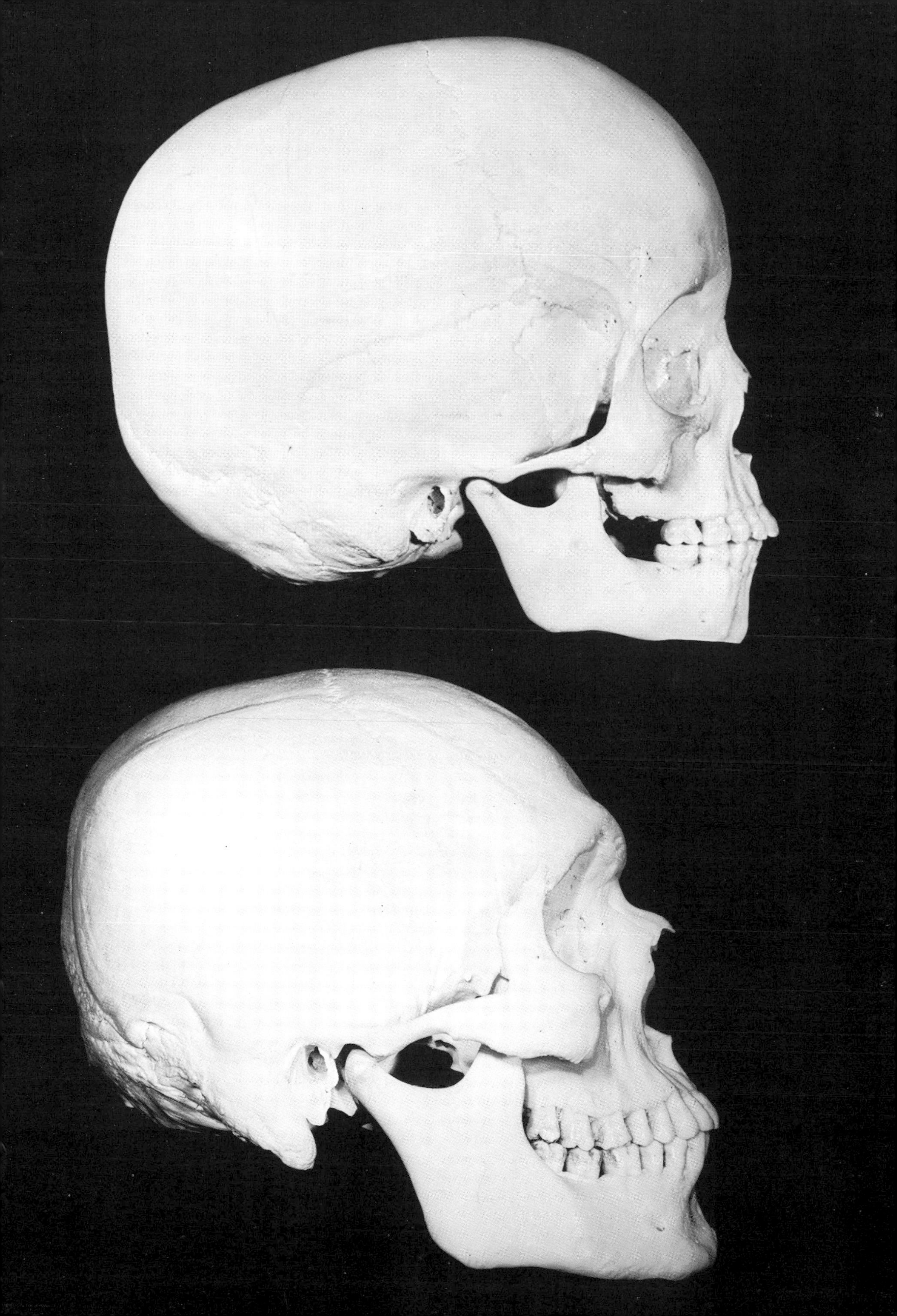

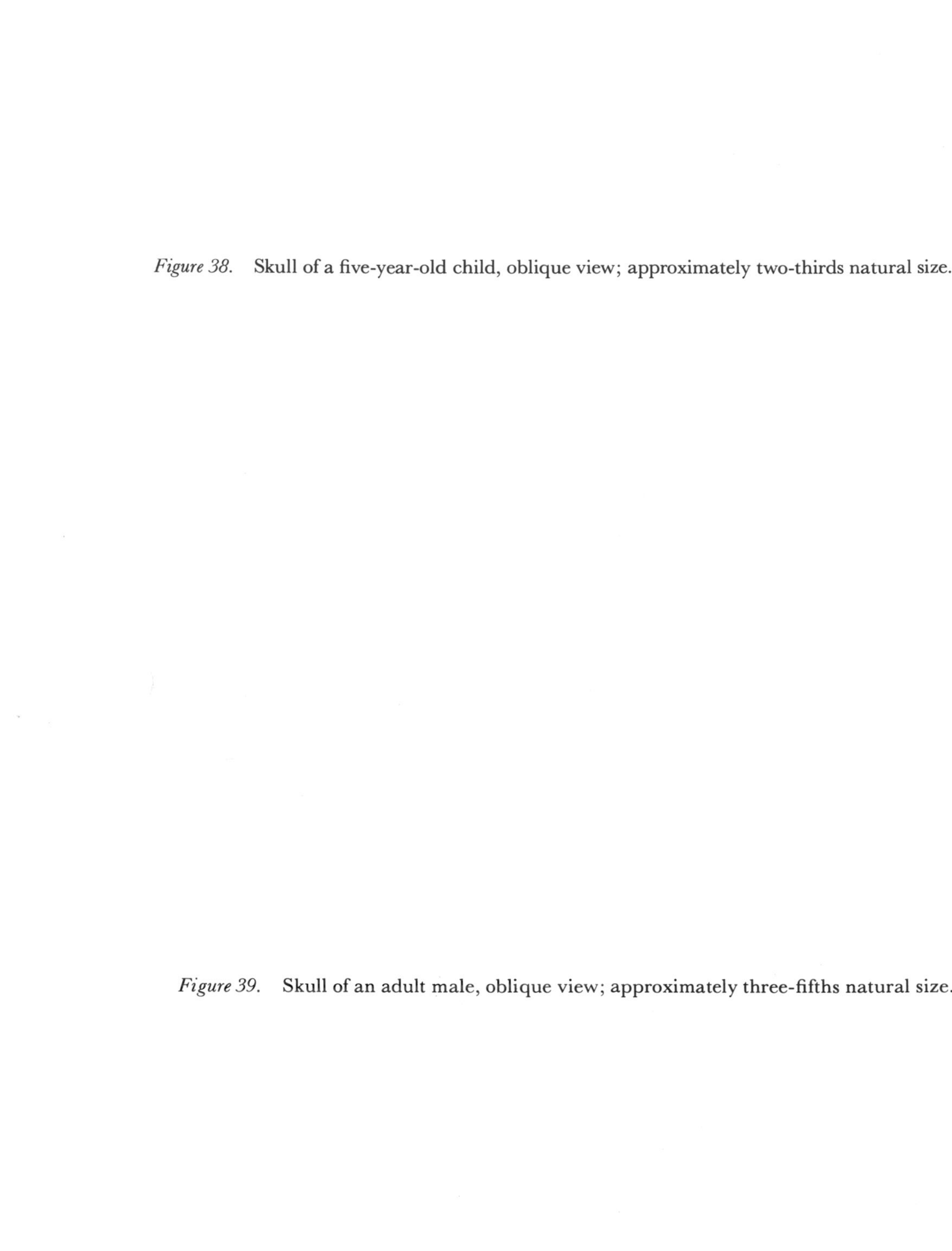

Figure 38. Skull of a five-year-old child, oblique view; approximately two-thirds natural size.

Figure 39. Skull of an adult male, oblique view; approximately three-fifths natural size.

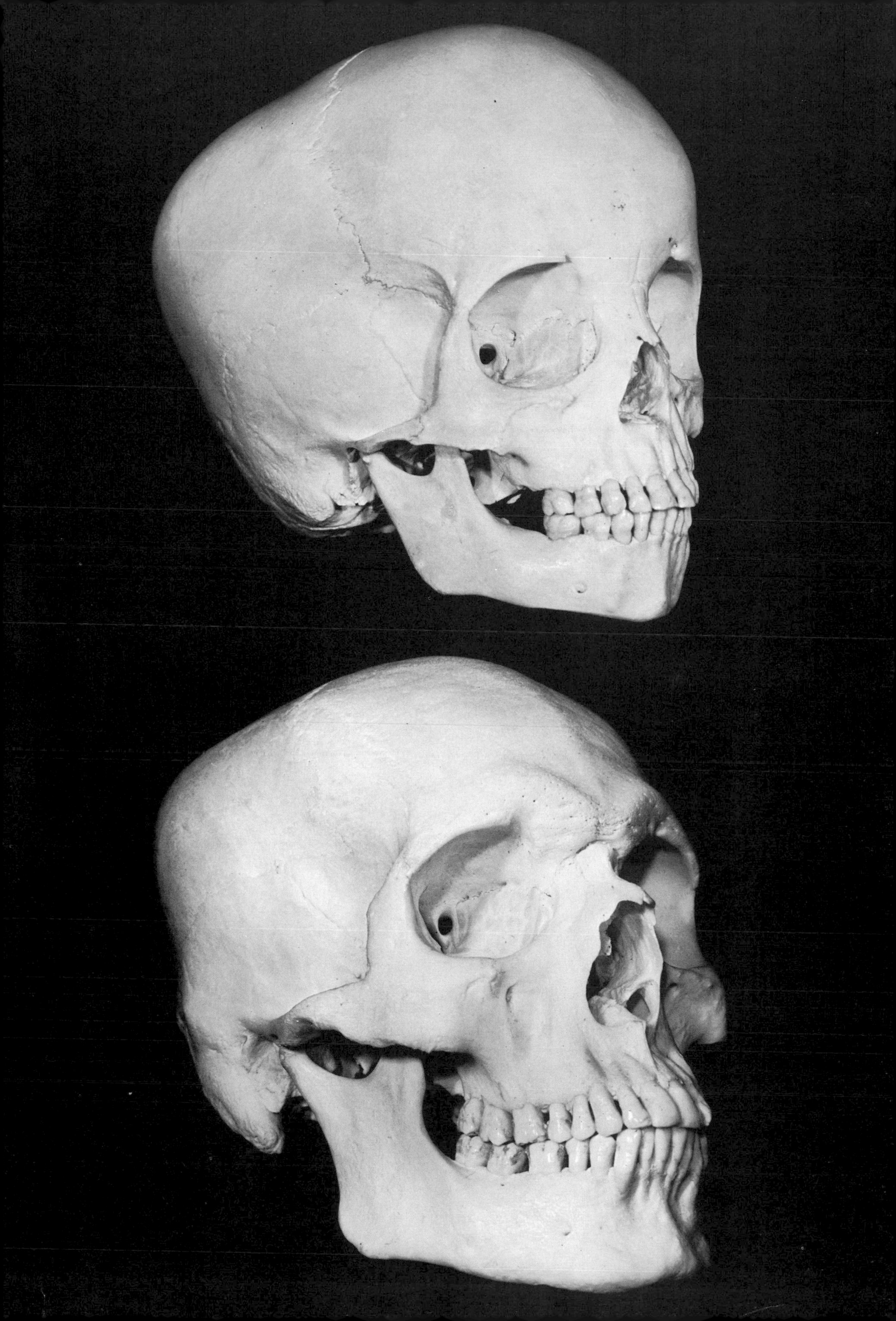

Fractures of the Lower and Middle Thirds of the Face

Rowe and Killey (1955) showed that fractures of the mandible alone occurred in 67.2 per cent of their 500 patients. Fractures of the maxilla and associated bones occurred in 23.6 per cent, and fractures of the mandible, maxilla, and associated bones in combination were found in 9.2 per cent of the cases. Of the 500 patients, 76.4 per cent sustained fractures of the mandible and 32.8 per cent had fractures of the middle face.

McCoy et al. (1962), in a study of 855 patients with fractures of the facial skeleton, showed that the middle third of the face was involved in 40 per cent of the cases. In 4.8 per cent of these cases there were associated mandibular fractures, and 28 per cent had associated nasal fractures. The mandible alone was fractured in 38 per cent of the cases and the nasal bones alone in 22 per cent.

Multiple Injuries

Facial fractures are associated frequently with injuries to other areas. The patient who has been involved in a high-speed automobile accident is most likely to have multiple body injuries. By contrast, the patient with a facial fracture caused by the blow of a fist may have scarcely any associated injuries.

When facial injuries are caused by violence, injuries to the airway or central nervous system should be suspected. Cranial, thoracic, and abdominal injuries are not uncommon, and fractures of the extremities occur quite frequently in association with facial injuries.

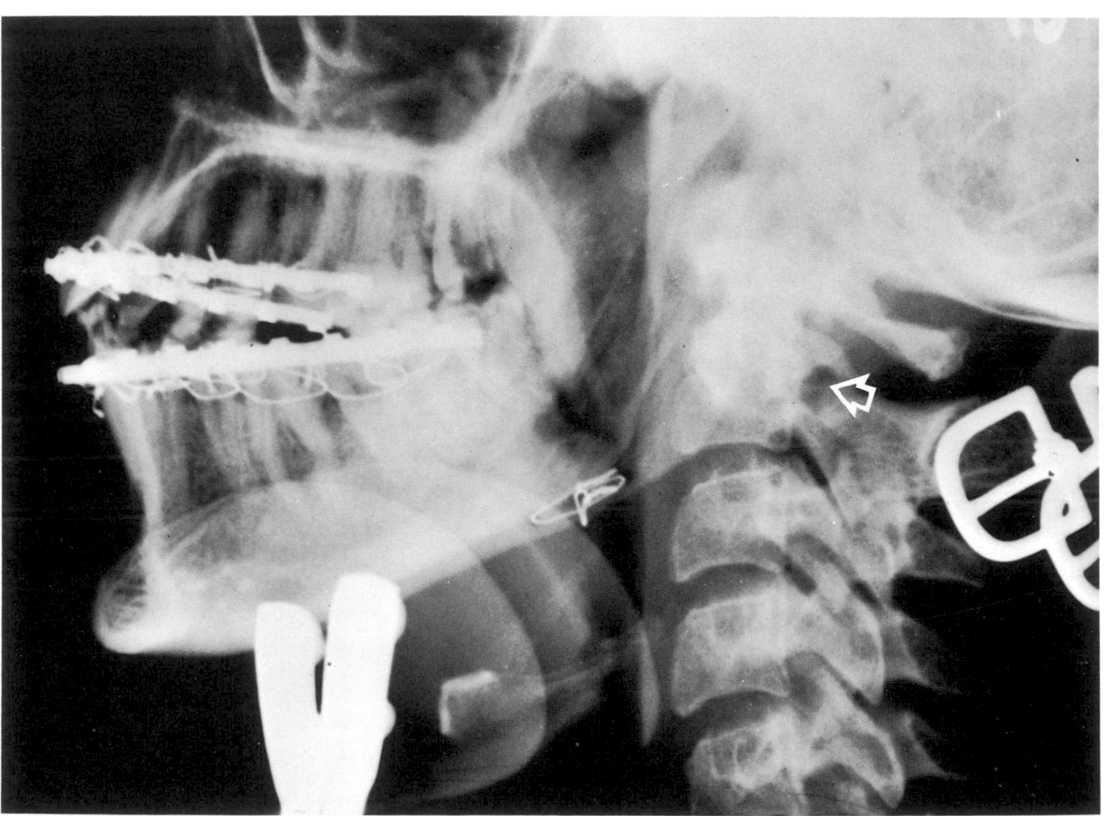

Figure 40. Roentgenogram of a patient with a fracture of the mandible complicated by a fracture of the second cervical vertebra. Head halter immobilization.

In automobile accidents, multiple injuries appear to occur with increasing frequency (Johnston, 1961). Although injuries to the neck and cervical spine account for the highest percentage of fatalities, they represent only 8.7 per cent of all injuries due to automobile accidents; 15.3 per cent of injuries to the neck and cervical spine are fatal and 8.1 per cent are dangerous (Cornell University, 1961).

In Kansas, multiple injuries occurred in 10 per cent of the cases in which drivers were killed and in 12 per cent of the cases in which passengers were killed in motor vehicle accidents over a period of two years (Franzen, 1962).

A combination of craniocerebral injury and injury to the long bones has been reported to be the most frequent type of multiple injury, followed in frequency by injury to the thorax and injury to the extremities (Johnston, 1961).

Prevention of Facial Injuries

The responsibility for finding methods of preventing trauma rests with various public bodies, with industry, and with the medical profession.

In the field of transportation, extensive research is being directed to the means by which the frequency of accidents can be reduced and injuries prevented. As a result, vehicular safety devices are being introduced continuously. Improved design, safety belts, shoulder harnesses, roll bars, collapsible steering wheels, shorter steering posts, and crash pads are some of the factors involved in increased safety of the automobile.

Graduates of high school courses in driver education are better drivers, as is shown by their lower accident and violation rates (National Education Association, 1961).

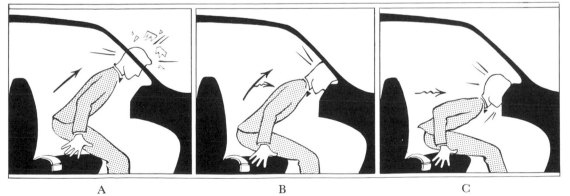

Figure 41. Mechanism of guest-passenger injury. The subject is unprotected by seat belts. There are three mechanisms by which injury is produced by sudden deceleration of an automobile: *A*. The guest-passenger is thrown upward and forward, striking his head against the windshield, and sustains injuries and cuts of the head and neck. *B*. The passenger strikes his head against the windshield and is then deflected downward, the face striking the instrument panel. This combination produces cuts and crushing facial injuries. *C*. The passenger is thrown straight forward, striking his face with full force against the instrument panel of the car. Crushing and tearing injuries result from this type of injury.

In the field of sports, facial fractures can be reduced in number through improved supervision and through use of properly designed headgear, bite appliances, and masks. Attention to safety education and protective devices designed into machinery and equipment have helped minimize industrial mishaps.

CLASSIFICATION OF FACIAL FRACTURES

The fractures that occur in the maxillofacial area may be classified as simple, compound, comminuted, and greenstick fractures. Also to be included are fractures involving loss of bone fragments or large amounts of soft tissue.

Age is an important factor in determining the type of facial injury and its management. In the younger age group, the fracture as well as its treatment and final results is greatly influenced by the presence of teeth, the absence of local and general disease, and the greater healing capacity of the tissues. A child's facial fracture, because of the greater percentage of organic structure of the bones, may be a greenstick type of fracture.* An adult, when subjected to a comparable force, would be more likely to suffer a complete break of bone with the probability of greater displacement.

TRANSPORTATION OF THE INJURED PATIENT

Problems involved in moving and transporting a patient with multiple injuries have been described adequately by others. We shall deal only with the specific problem of handling those who have suffered a facial injury.

At the scene of an accident, it is imperative that an attempt be made to arrest serious hemorrhage from facial wounds and to assure an adequate airway during transportation to a hospital. Most hemorrhage responds to pressure or the application of a simple dressing.

In most instances, the airway may be kept patent by removing blood clots, debris, broken dentures, and foreign bodies and by protracting the tongue and placing the head in a dependent position.

Stabilization of fractured segments by the Barton or other type of head bandage reduces pain, minimizes shock, and otherwise gives the patient a feeling of security during transportation.

Bandaging and packing of open wounds and, if possible, wire stabilization of large fracture segments, even if only temporary, adds comfort and may minimize complications during movement.

The conscious patient who is able to sit up with his head forward will be better able to control mucus and blood, and by the cough reflex keep his airway open. The force of gravity in the "head forward" position will assist in preventing tissues from falling back into the pharynx.

Inasmuch as definitive management of a facial injury is not a surgical emergency, patients should be in satisfactory general condition before transfer from one hospital to another for special care.

PHOTOGRAPHY

The adage that one picture is worth a thousand words is applicable in the field of facial injury management. Good black-and-

* Apologies to Robert Louis Stevenson: *Good and Bad Children* (verse 1):

"Children, you are very little,
And your bones are very brittle;
If you would grow great and stately,
You must try to walk sedately."

GENERAL PRINCIPLES

Figure 42. Outline of facial fractures.

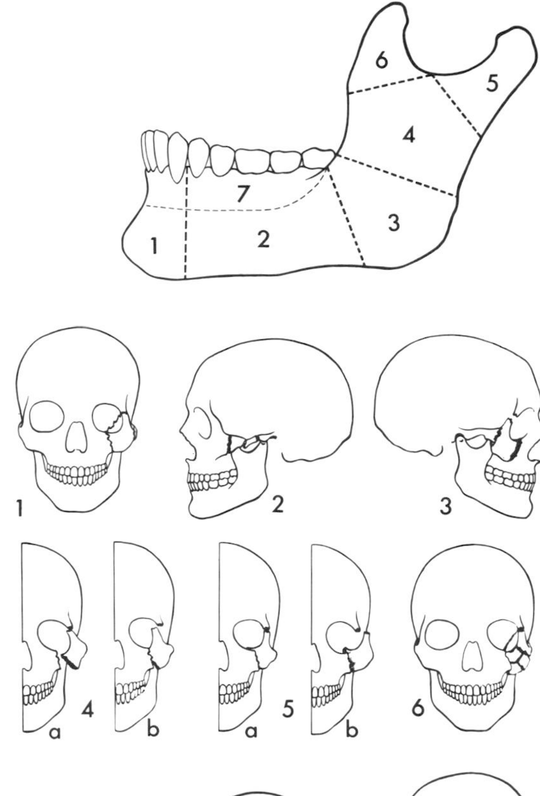

The Mandible (Chapter 6)

1. Region of the symphysis
2. Region of the body
3. Region of the angle
4. Region of the ramus
5. Region of the condylar process
6. Region of the coronoid process
7. Region of the alveolar process

The Zygoma (Chapter 7)

1. Group I: No significant displacement
2. Group II: Zygomatic arch fractures
3. Group III: Unrotated body fractures
4. Group IV: Medially rotated body fractures
   a. Outward at zygomatic prominence
   b. Inward at zygomaticofrontal suture
5. Group V: Laterally rotated body fractures
   a. Upward at infraorbital margin
   b. Outward at zygomaticofrontal suture
6. Complex fractures

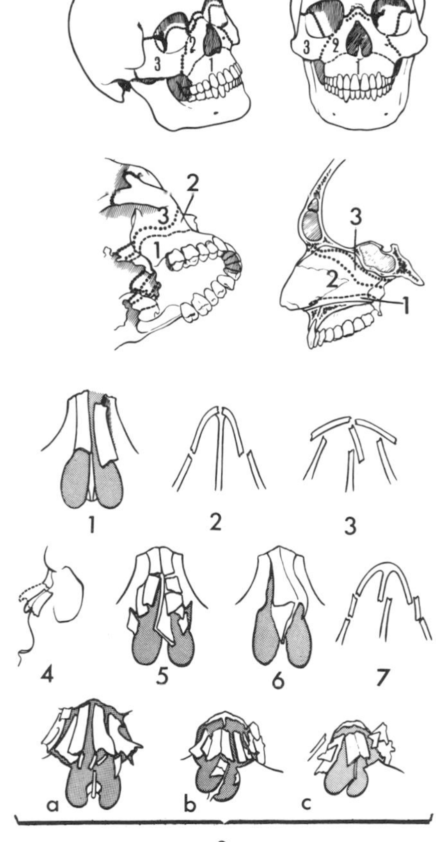

The Maxilla (Chapter 8)

1. Le Fort I (transverse fracture; Guérin fracture)
2. Le Fort II (pyramidal fracture)
3. Le Fort III (craniofacial disjunction)

The Nose (Chapter 9)

1. Inferolateral displacement
2. Separation of nasal bones in midline and frontal process of maxilla
3. Open book fracture
4. Posteroinferior displacement
5. Comminuting fracture of the nasal bones
6. Fracture of nasal septum with separation of nasal bones from frontal process of maxilla.
7. Cross-sectional diagram of a fracture similar to that in 6
8. Three examples of smash fracture of the nose (a, b, c)

white and colored photographs with satisfactory composition are most useful in supplementing the written word. They may be of extreme importance in medicolegal and insurance cases as well as being valuable for teaching. Good portable photographic equipment should be part of every surgeon's equipment.

Clothing should be removed from the area of injury and the patient draped with a towel or hospital gown. Dressings should be removed and the wound thoroughly cleaned before photographs are taken. The photographs should be taken with the patient in front of a plain backdrop so that other objects in the room are not included in the photograph. Standard positions will give the most uniform and most satisfactory pictures. The area photographed should be large enough to include other anatomic structures as landmarks.

The following views have been found most useful for recording injuries to the facial area: the front view, which includes the face from the scalp to just below the chin; profile views taken at direct right angles to the sagittal plane; and views of the teeth from the front and both sides, using mouth retractors to insure maximum exposure of the teeth and the occlusion in the photograph. A view taken from below the chin up to the base of the nose to include the prominence of the cheeks and forehead is useful in demonstrating fractures of the nose and zygomatic region.

These same views should be taken postoperatively, for comparison, in order best to evaluate the effectiveness of the surgical treatment.

HISTORY

In all cases an adequate history is important to both diagnosis and treatment. Knowledge of the details of the cause and type of injury is an aid to determining the extent and location of the fracture. A history of systemic disorders, such as cardiac, vascular, or respiratory disease, may influence the choice of treatment as well as its result.

EXAMINATION AND DIAGNOSIS

Evaluation of Clinical Findings

The examining physician must be concerned primarily with the overall welfare of the patient. Examination and diagnosis of injuries in the maxillofacial area would be of small value to a patient in danger of expiring from intra-abdominal hemorrhage.

The first objective should be to ascertain patency of the airway. Next the patient should be checked for external or internal hemorrhage. Every patient with a severe facial injury should be suspected of having suffered neurological damage. The neurological evaluation should include exact determination of the patient's state of consciousness.

Clinical evaluation is most important in detecting facial bone fractures. For accurate inspection of the mouth, nose, and throat, all secretions, blood clots, detached tissue, loose teeth, and foreign materials should be removed. Suction equipment is an important adjunct to diagnosis.

Signs and Symptoms

The presence of a fracture often is suggested by malocclusion of the teeth. External palpation of the mandible, orbital margins, nose, and maxilla may disclose irregularities of contour that indicate fractures. Intraoral palpation of the mandible and maxilla may also reveal significant irregularities. (See Figure 43 on pages 58 and 59.)

Fractures of the maxilla or zygomatic region may be suggested by loss of visual acuity, malfunction of the extraocular muscles, or diplopia. Bleeding from the nose, mouth, or ears may indicate damage to the adjacent bony structures. Use of the nasal speculum, the otoscope, and the tongue depressor may disclose the source of the hemorrhage.

In accidents involving injury to associated structures, the damage often includes fractures of the cribriform plate and other areas, accompanied by loss of cerebrospinal fluid. Concussion, cerebral laceration, intracranial hemorrhage, and damage to the orbital contents are not uncommon associated findings. Other areas that may require definitive care are fractures of the hyoid bone, of the styloid process, and of the thyroid cartilage.

In the patient who has a fair complement of teeth, malocclusion is one of the most frequent findings leading to the diagnosis of fractures of the jaws. The patient most often is conscious of abnormalities of occlusion and frequently volunteers the information that the teeth do not come together properly.

If examination reveals that the teeth do come together in good anatomic relation, fractures of the maxilla and mandible usually are not present. Abnormal mobility of osseous structures may be highly suggestive of fractures of the upper and lower jaws. If the mandible can be moved beyond its normal distance of excursion in any direction, fracture should be suspected. Mobility of the maxilla when pressure is applied indicates fracture of the maxilla.

The presence of edema, hematoma, and ecchymosis in the lower face is suggestive of fractures of the mandible. Dysfunction and open-bite deformity may indicate fractures of the mandibular neck. Lateral deviation of the jaw may indicate subcondylar fracture of the mandible or a telescoping fracture of the body of the bone. Pain and tenderness in the region of the temporomandibular joints suggest fractures in this region. An open bite may indicate fracture of the maxilla with posterior displacement. Bleeding from the nose or cerebrospinal rhinorrhea may suggest fractures of the nose or a pyramidal fracture of the maxilla or craniofacial disjunction resulting from involvement of the cribriform area. Ecchymosis, edema, and subconjunctival hemorrhage may indicate nasal or zygomatic fractures. Diplopia is almost always indicative of a displaced fracture of the zygoma or the orbital floor. Blood or cerebrospinal fluid draining from the auditory canal suggests a mandibular condyle fracture with fracture of the roof of the articular fossa and tympanic bone. Retrusion of the anterior portion of the mandible suggests fractures in the region of the symphysis or bilateral subcondylar fractures.

Fractures of the body of the mandible can be detected easily by supporting the angle of the mandible and applying up and down pressure on the anterior mandibular region. Crepitation may be a diagnostic sign but should not be forced because it is exquisitely painful.

Paralysis of any of the cranial nerves, unconsciousness, unequal and nonreactive pupils, paralysis of the extremities, abnormal reflexes, convulsions, delirium, or irrationality may be indicative of intracranial lesions with fractures of the skull.

Evaluation of Laboratory Findings

Diagnosis of fractures of the bony structures of the face is made principally on the basis of the clinical and roentgenographic findings. Laboratory evaluation may be helpful in differentiating between cerebrospinal fluid and nasal mucus secretion, a differentiation that is difficult clinically. If a sufficient amount of fluid can be collected, a

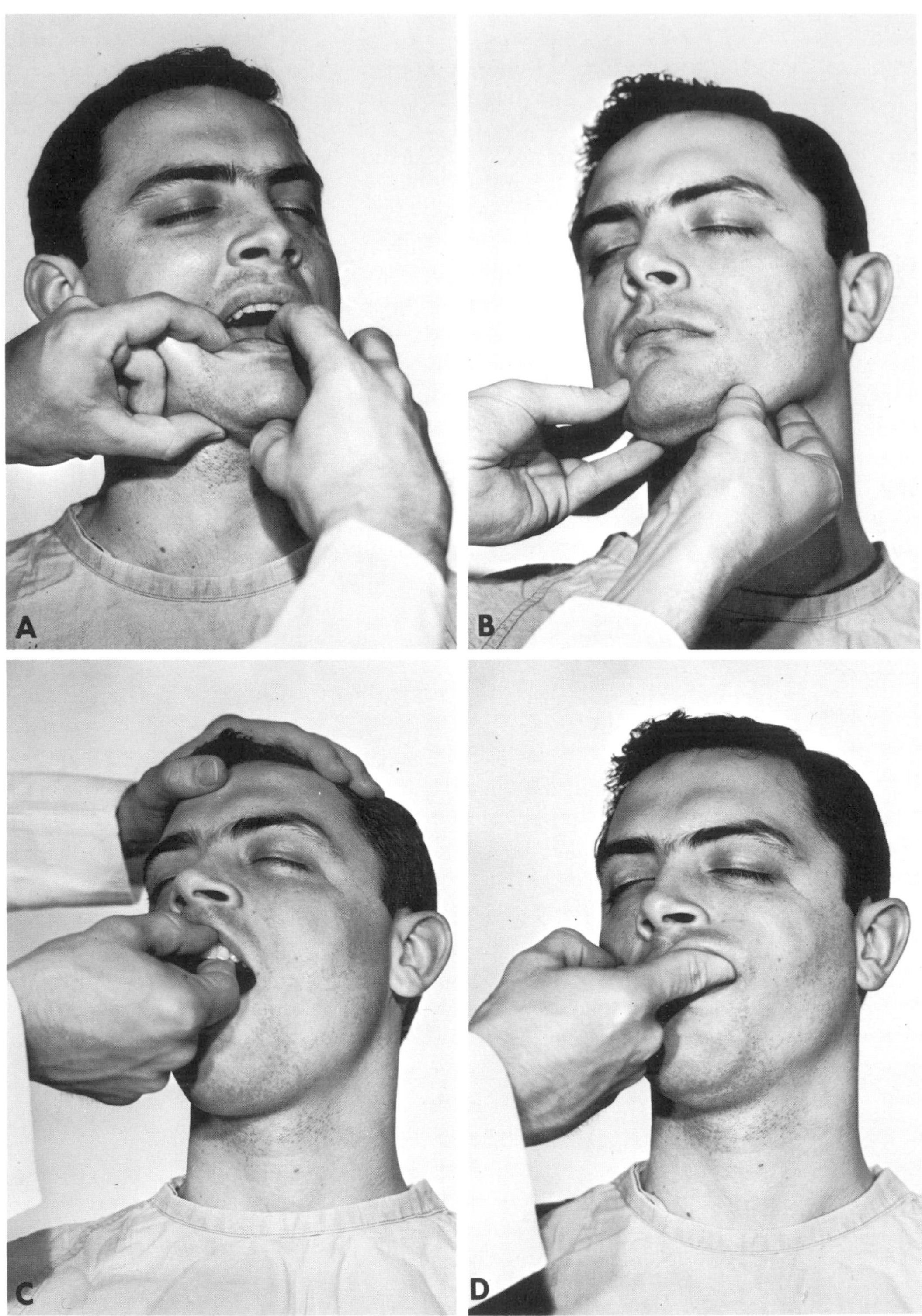

Figure 43. Methods of palpation of the bony skeleton of the face in detecting fractures. *A.* Intra- and extraoral palpation of mandible. *B.* Palpation of inferior border of mandible. *C.* Testing stability of maxilla.

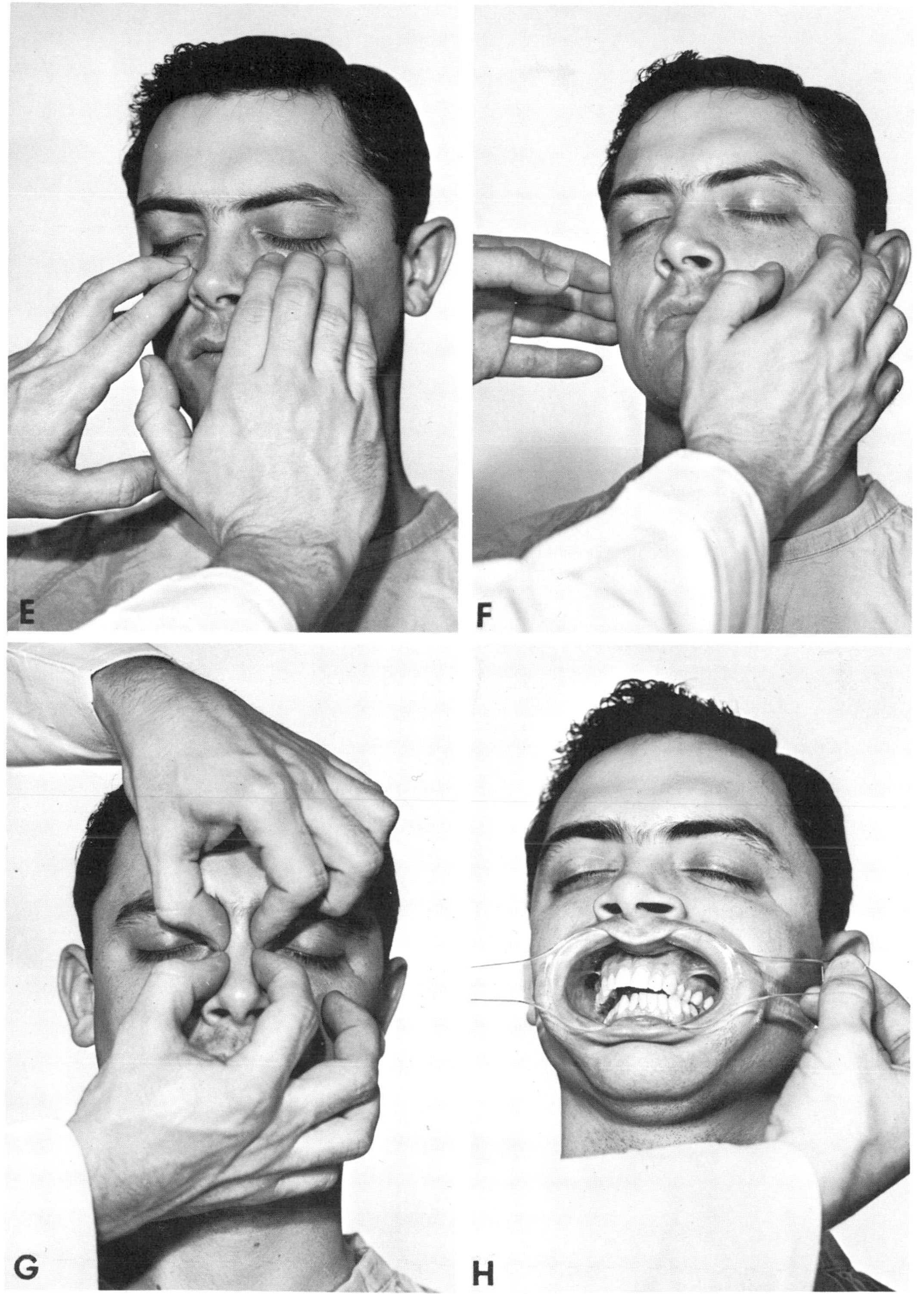

D. Intraoral palpation for zygomaticomaxillary irregularities. *E*. Palpation of infraorbital margins. *F*. Palpation over zygomatic arches. *G*. External palpation of nasal bones. *H*. Inspection of dental occlusion.

chemical test can be carried out. Cerebrospinal fluid will be found to be free from mucin and to contain sugar. Nasal secretions contain mucin but are free from sugar. If the test demonstrates the presence of sugar in the fluid, it may be considered as cerebrospinal fluid. The presence of blood in the cerebrospinal fluid obtained by spinal tap may indicate skull fracture, intracranial hemorrhage, or injury to the central nervous system.

Routine laboratory procedures should include a blood examination (hemoglobin, hematocrit, white blood cell count, and differential) and urinalysis. Specimens can be taken while the patient is being prepared for x-ray examination so that the results will be known upon completion of the radiographs. The time saved will permit additional laboratory tests if such are required. It is desirable to have the reports of basic laboratory examinations recorded on the chart before taking the patient to the operating room.

Consultations

In the case of the severely injured patient, consultation with various medical and surgical specialists should be held freely. When fractures involve the orbital area, a careful ophthalmological examination should be made. Neurological findings such as loss of consciousness, disorientation, abnormal reflexes, unequal or dilated or nonreactive pupils, and the presence of basilar skull fracture indicated by cerebrospinal rhinorrhea or hemorrhage into the external auditory canals demand neurosurgical consultation.

Bleeding into the external auditory canal, indicating the possibility of fracture of the tympanic plate and middle ear structure, may require the attention of the otolaryngologist.

It is axiomatic that the surgeon be conversant with the x-ray techniques that produce the best radiographs for recognition of facial fractures. Consultation with the radiologist will result in better interpretation and more accurate diagnosis.

Radiographic Evaluation

The roentgenogram is an invaluable adjunct to the diagnosis of facial and cranial fractures, but the prevention and treatment of shock must take precedence over radiographic evaluation. Routine x-ray examination is of little value to the patient expiring from intracranial hemorrhage or pneumothorax or from a ruptured viscus. When the patient's condition permits, facial x-ray studies should be made.

No matter how obvious the fracture, no matter how "clear cut" the diagnosis may appear to be, under no circumstances should definitive treatment of facial fractures be instituted without an adequate x-ray examination of all facial bone structures. X-ray examination is invaluable in detecting fractures which could not have been suspected clinically.

One should recognize that fractures of the facial bones are difficult to demonstrate by radiography. In the middle third of the face, superimposed bony structures may obscure the site of fracture. It is important that the radiographs be of highest quality and that a sufficient number of views be made to cover all areas involved. Because of frequently associated fractures of the extrafacial parts of the skull and of the cervical spine, these areas should be included in the x-ray examination. From the medicolegal standpoint, the importance of radiography cannot possibly be overstressed.

A posteroanterior view of the chest should be taken before subjecting the patient to

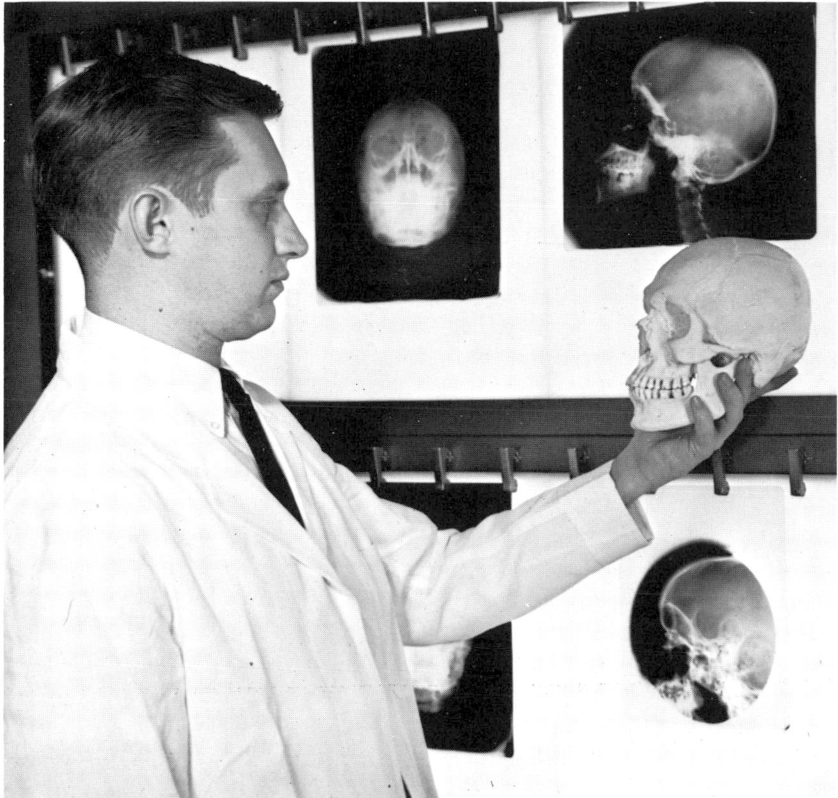

Figure 44. A human skull is useful in the study of roentgenograms for evaluation of facial fractures.

general anesthesia. This may rule out the possibility of overlooking pneumothorax or aspirated foreign objects, such as teeth or portions of dentures or other foreign bodies. Suppression of normal reflex activity due to a state of semishock may make it impossible for the clinician to observe the usual signs of foreign body in the respiratory tract.

Fractures of the mandibular neck are among the most difficult to detect by routine radiographic methods. In most instances, however, these fractures can be revealed by using the laminographic technique. Stereoscopic radiography is helpful in the detection of fractures of the facial skeleton. Special views may be required for the diagnosis of fractures in certain areas. Intraoral dental x-ray examination is required for detecting fractures of the teeth and the alveolar process.

(Text continued on page 86.)

Figure 45. **LATERAL PROJECTION OF SKULL**

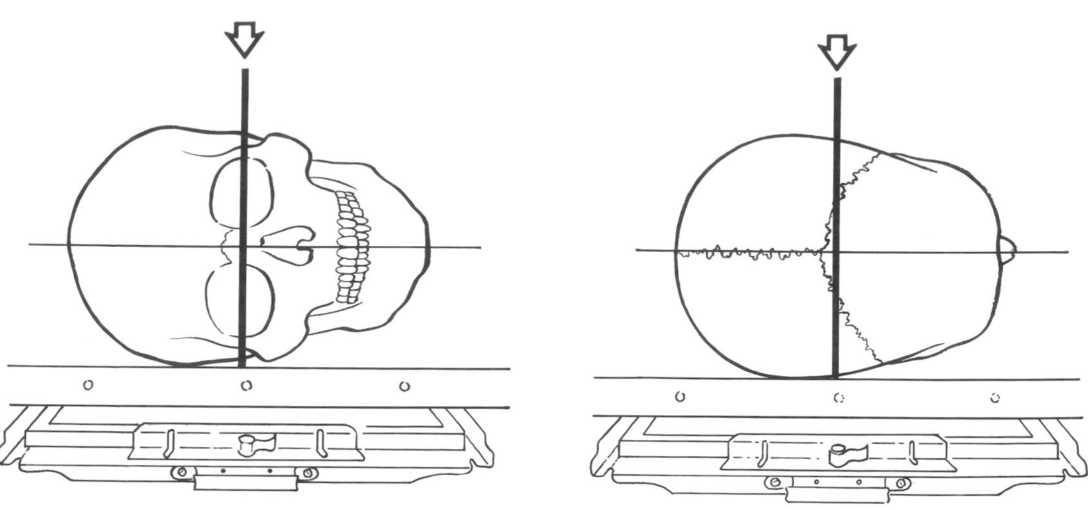

This view is taken with the side of the head in contact with the table. The midsagittal plane should be parallel to the table. The central ray is perpendicular to the center of the film and passes through the sella turcica.

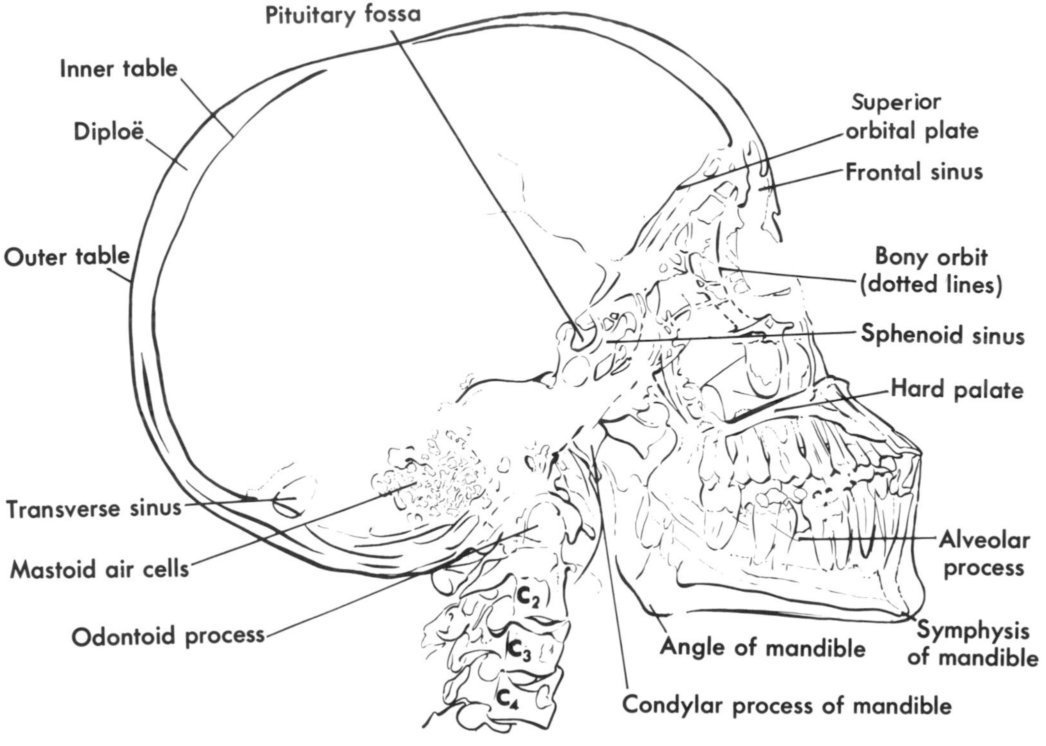

Diagrammatic Representation

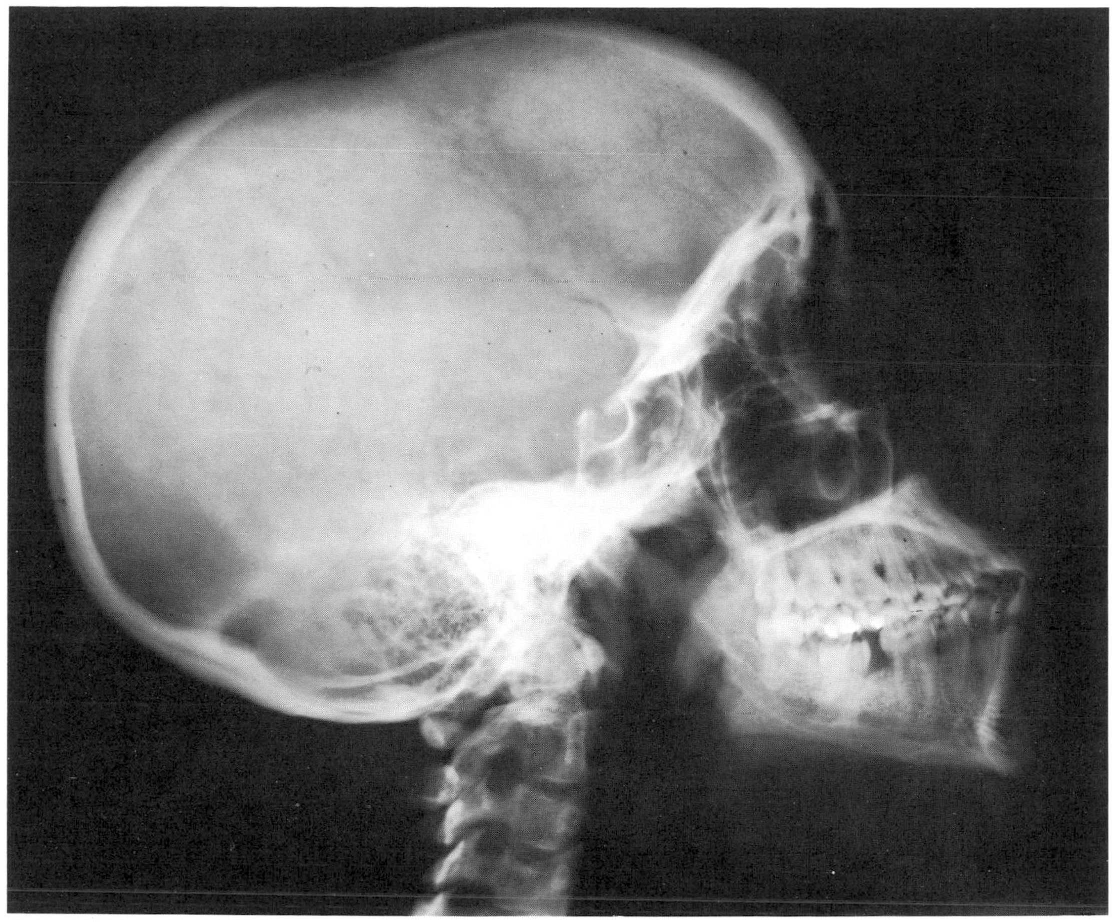

This projection shows a direct lateral profile of the facial bones and may show soft tissues of the face. It provides a profile view of the entire skull and is useful in studying fractures of the outer and inner plates of the frontal sinuses, as well as underdevelopment or overdevelopment of the mandible. This view may reveal foreign bodies in the oropharynx. It also demonstrates the relations of the maxilla to the mandible and is useful in evaluating posterior displacement in maxillary fractures. The upper cervical spine is shown on this projection.

The exposure factors have not been included because of their variability in different x-ray departments and because they are, for the most part, standard exposures and in common usage. Reference may be made to any standard manual of technique.

Figure 46. **POSTERIOR-ANTERIOR PROJECTION OF MANDIBLE**

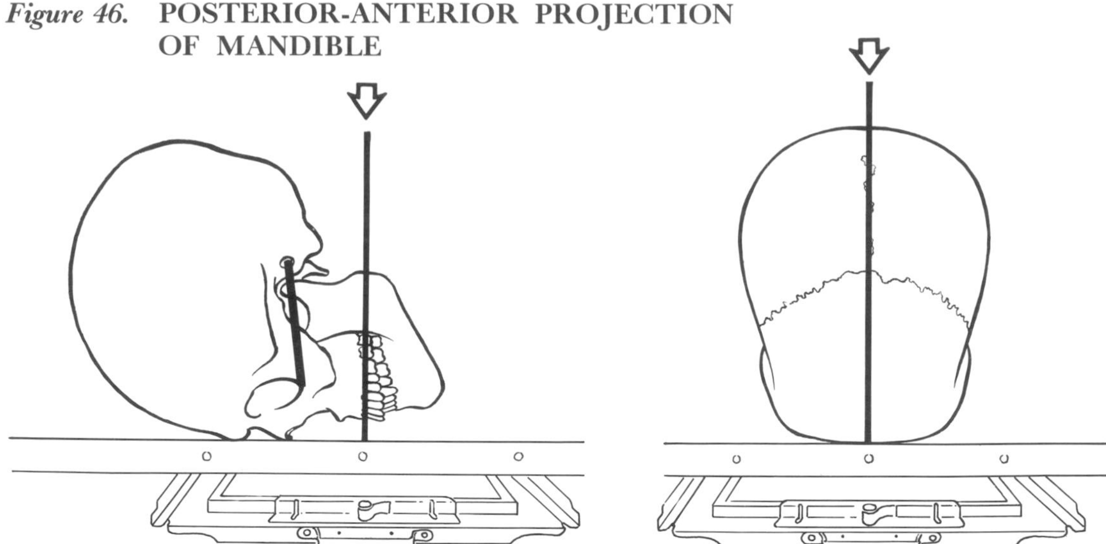

The patient is placed in the prone position with the forehead and tip of the nose resting on the table and the mouth aligned to the midpoint of the cassette. The midsagittal plane of the head is aligned vertically to the midline of the film. The central ray is at right angles to the cassette and is centered through the mouth. Respiration is suspended during exposure.

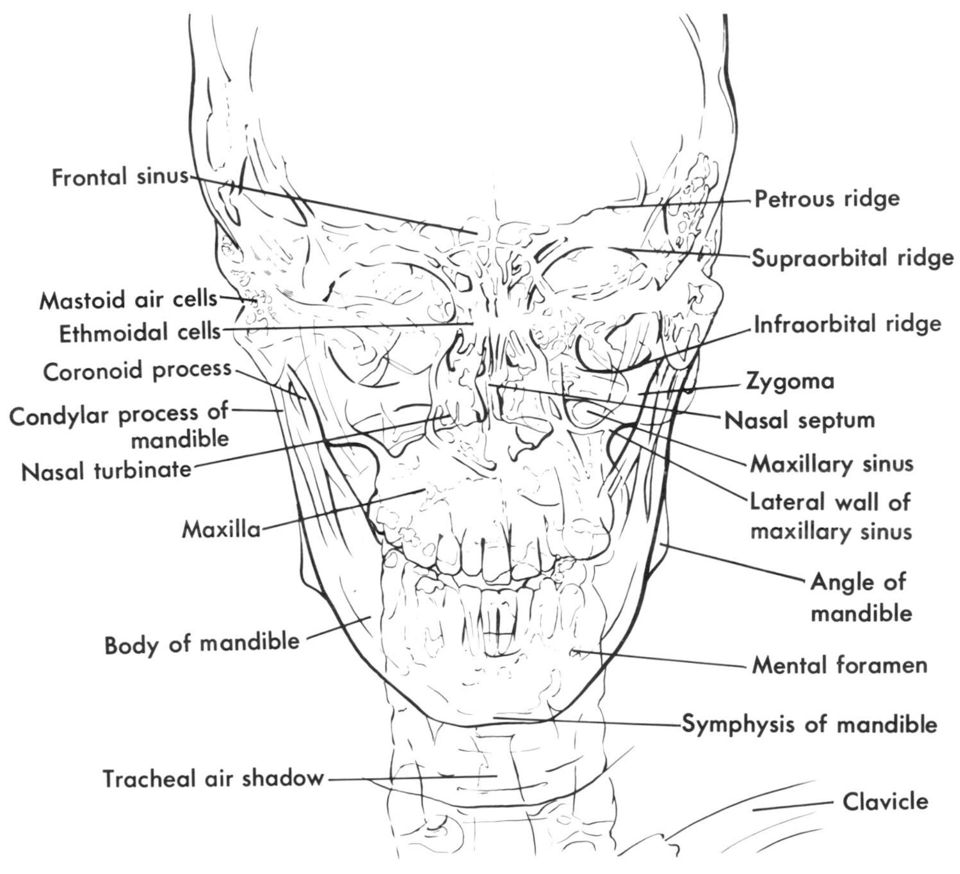

Diagrammatic Representation

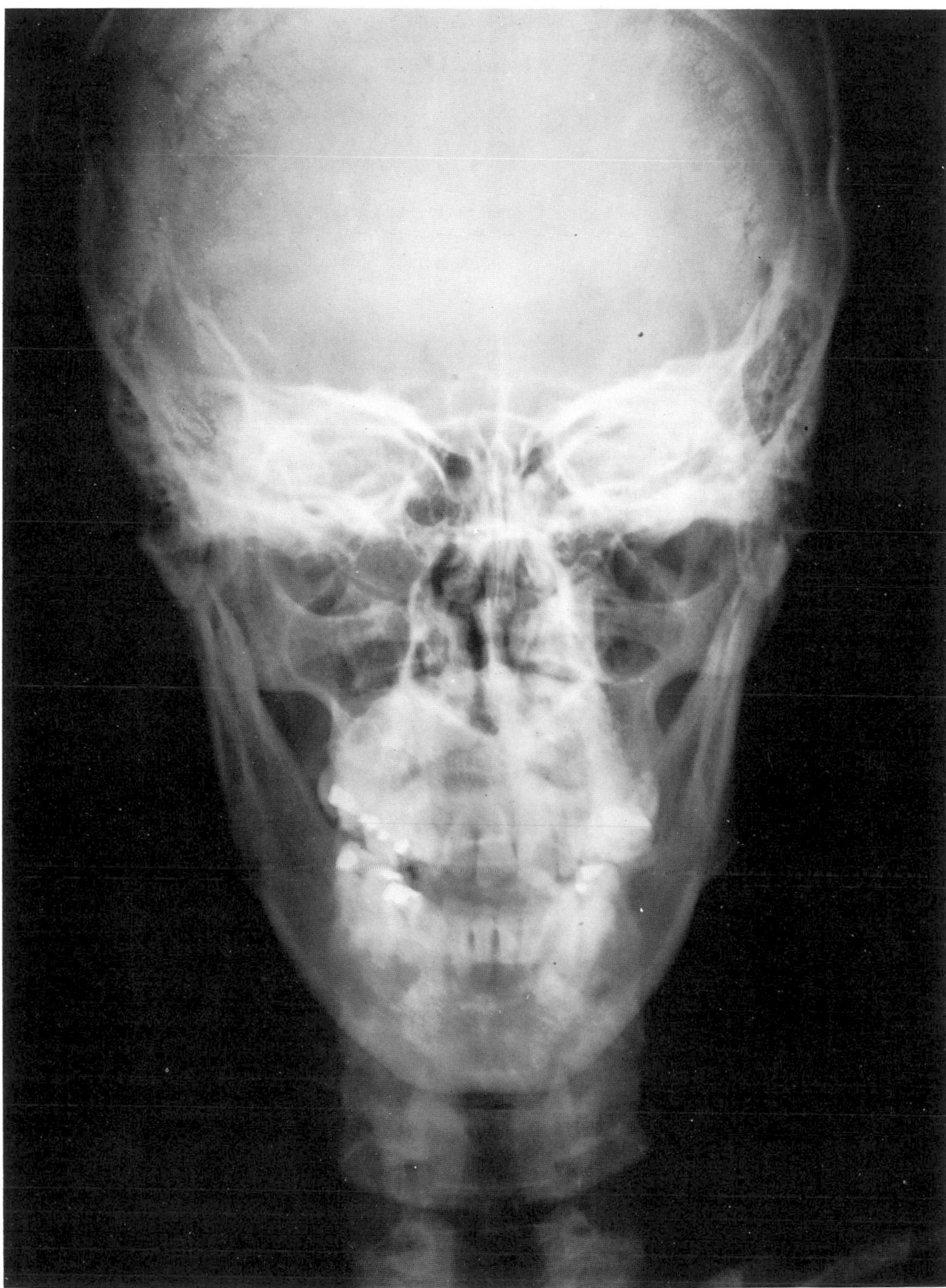

This view provides a general survey of the mandible, demonstrating the symphysis, the body, and the rami. Medial or lateral displacement of fractured segments and asymmetry of development of the mandible may be shown by this projection. This radiograph shows the lateral wall of the maxillary sinus and may demonstrate fracture-displacement of the nasal septum. This radiograph may be taken in the anterior-posterior projection if the patient is severely injured and is unable to assume the prone position.

Figure 47. LATERAL OBLIQUE PROJECTION OF MANDIBLE

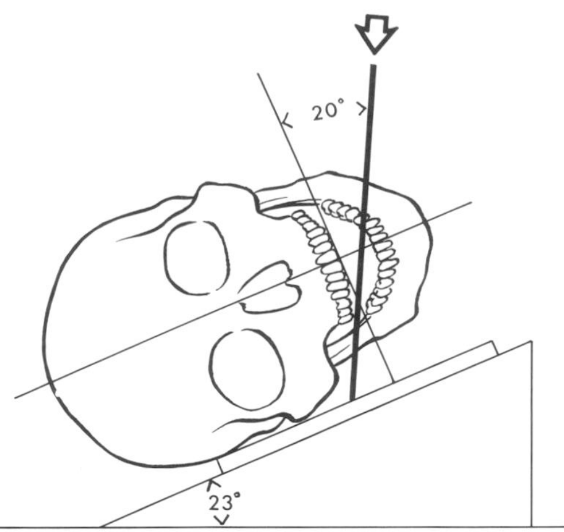

The patient's head is placed upon a block inclined 23 degrees, with the middle portion of the zygoma above the center of the film. The sagittal plane is parallel to the cassette, and the occlusal plane is at right angles to the cassette. The central ray is directed 20 degrees cephalad to the occlusal plane and toward the center of the cassette. The exposure is made with the mouth closed while respiration is suspended. The mouth is shown open in the illustration to demonstrate the occlusal plane.

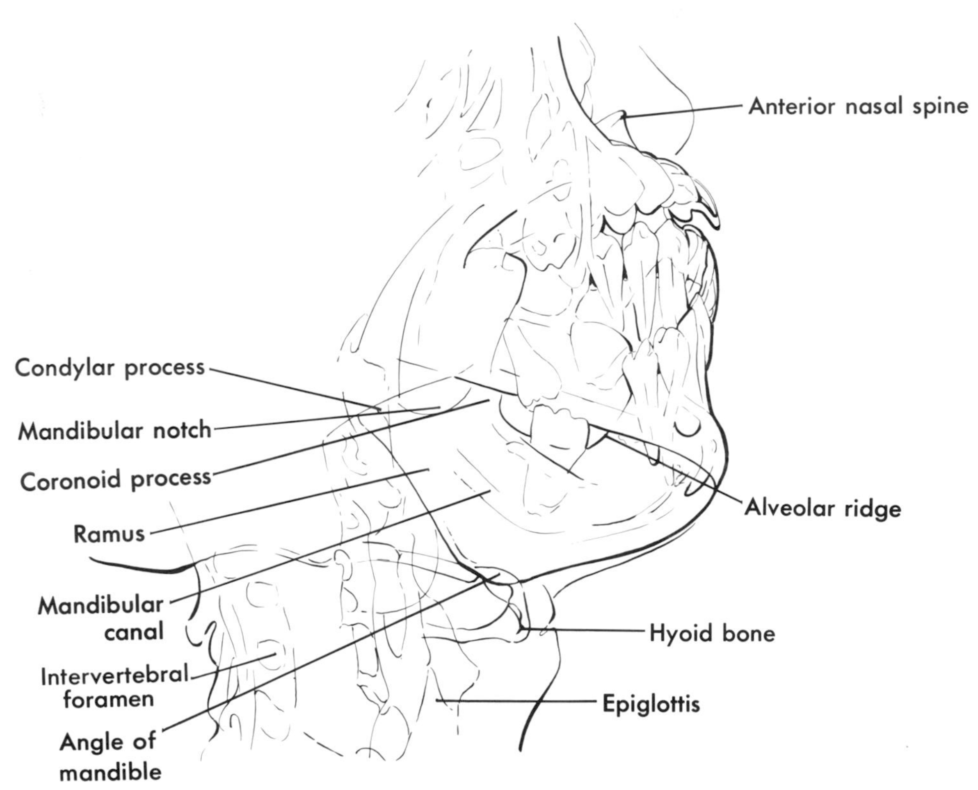

Diagrammatic Representation

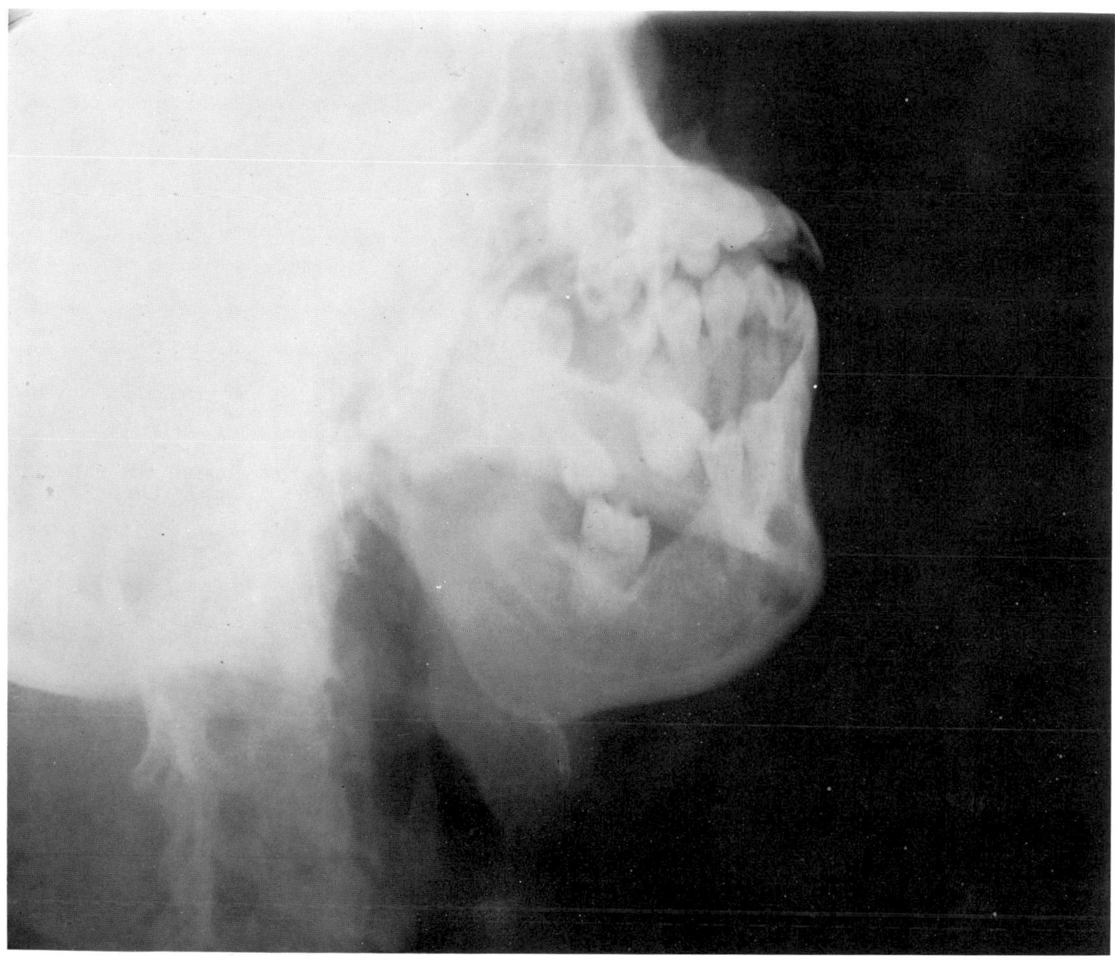

This projection shows the condylar and coronoid processes, ramus, and body of the mandible. It may show fractures of the alveolar process. The view is very useful in demonstrating fractures of the hyoid bone.

Figure 48. LATERAL PROJECTION OF TEMPOROMANDIBULAR JOINT

The patient is placed on the table, the head resting in the true lateral position with the temporomandibular joint slightly above the center of the midportion of the cassette. The midsagittal plane is parallel to the plane of the table, and the frontal plane of the head is perpendicular to the table. The central ray is directed at an angle of 25 degrees caudad, through the temporal region to the center of the film. One exposure is made with the mouth closed. The cassette is changed, and the second exposure is made with the mouth wide open. Respiration is suspended during exposure.

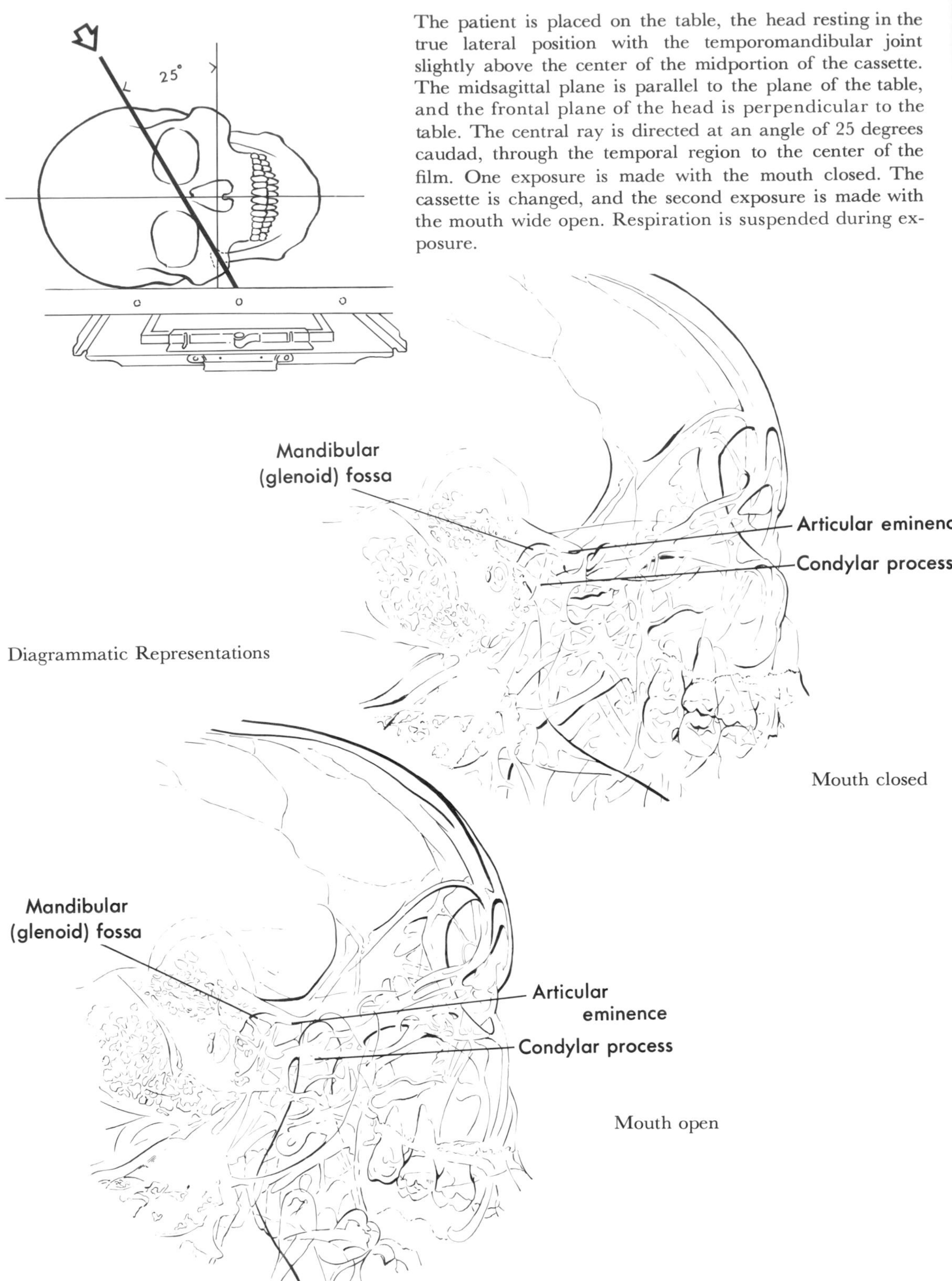

Diagrammatic Representations

Mouth closed

Mouth open

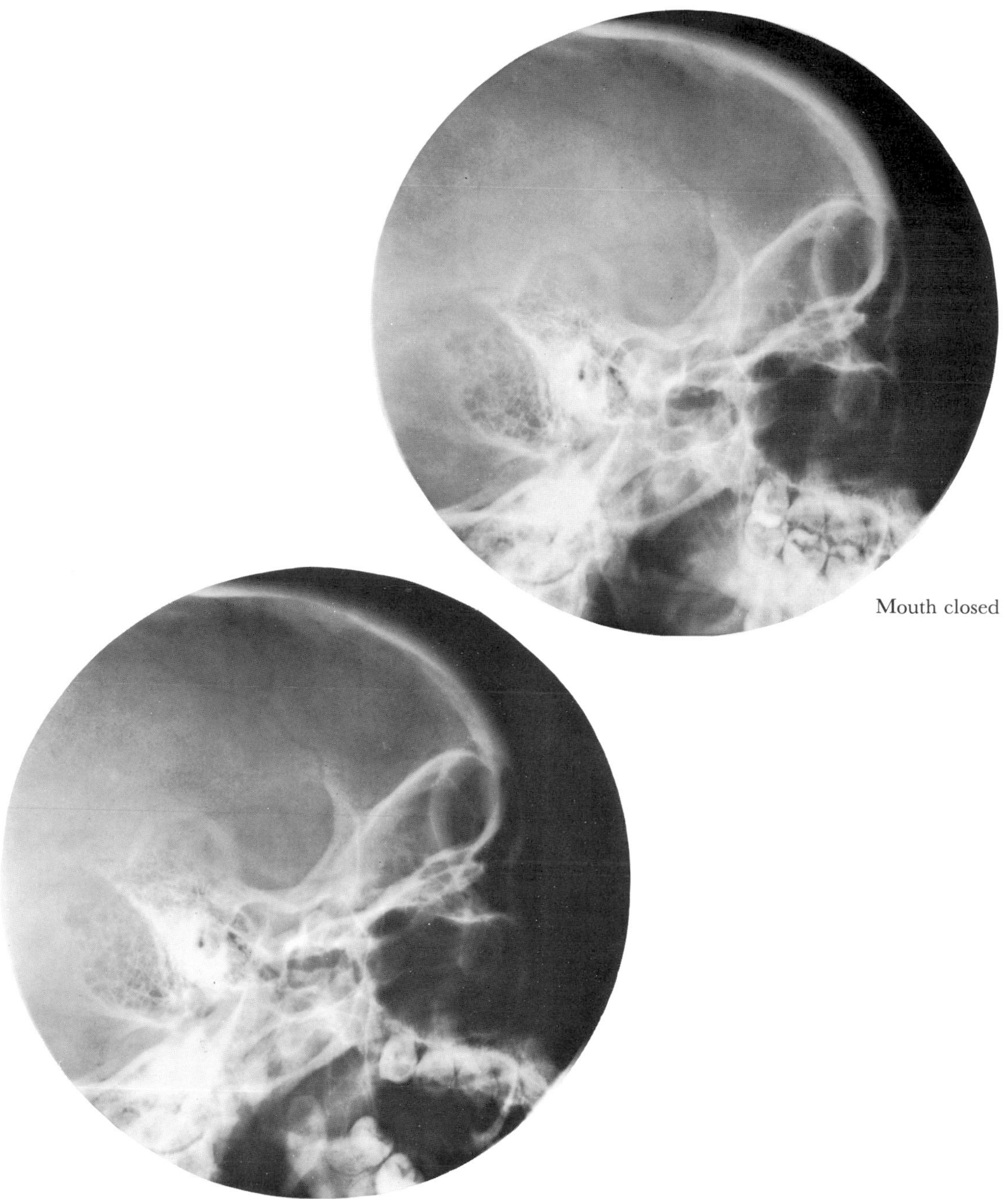

Mouth closed

Mouth open

These projections provide lateral views of the temporomandibular joint. They show developmental abnormalities and malformations in the temporomandibular joint and about the external acoustic porus, the arrangement of the temporomandibular joint, the relation of the mandibular condyle to the fossa, and the width of the joint space. The open view shows the extent of forward and downward movement of the mandibular condyle with relation to the mandibular fossa and the articular eminence. These views are useful in demonstrating dislocations and fractures, arthritic changes, bony malformations, and, by implication, impairment of motion in the temporomandibular joint.

Figure 49. ANTERIOR-POSTERIOR PROJECTION OF MANDIBULAR CONDYLAR PROCESSES INCLUDING ZYGOMATIC ARCHES (MODIFIED TOWNE'S PROJECTION)

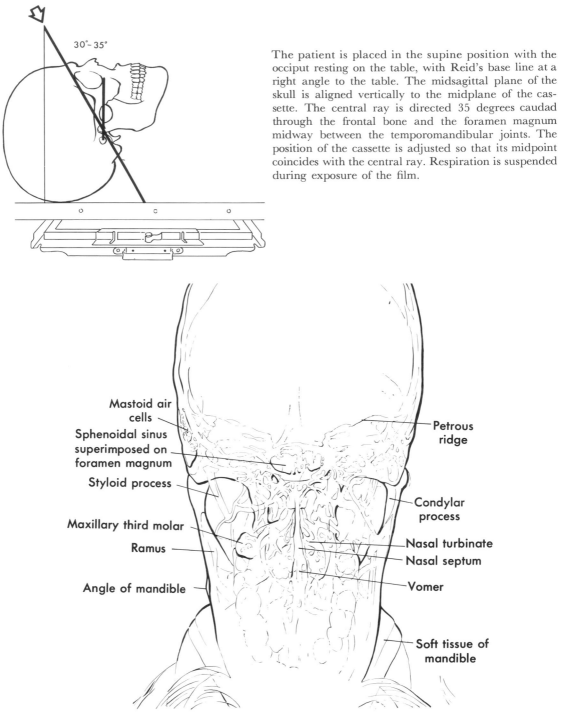

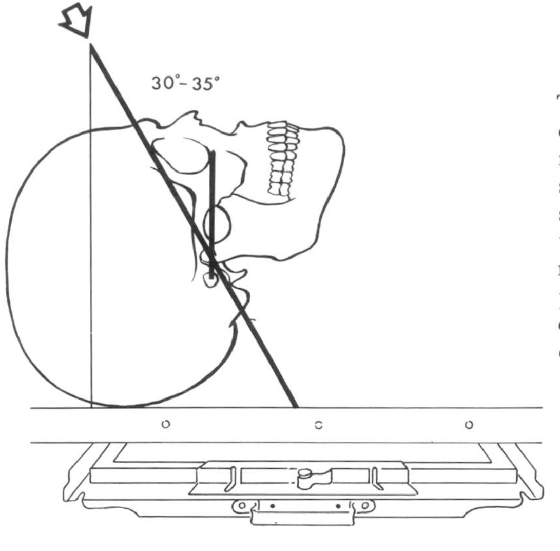

The patient is placed in the supine position with the occiput resting on the table, with Reid's base line at a right angle to the table. The midsagittal plane of the skull is aligned vertically to the midplane of the cassette. The central ray is directed 35 degrees caudad through the frontal bone and the foramen magnum midway between the temporomandibular joints. The position of the cassette is adjusted so that its midpoint coincides with the central ray. Respiration is suspended during exposure of the film.

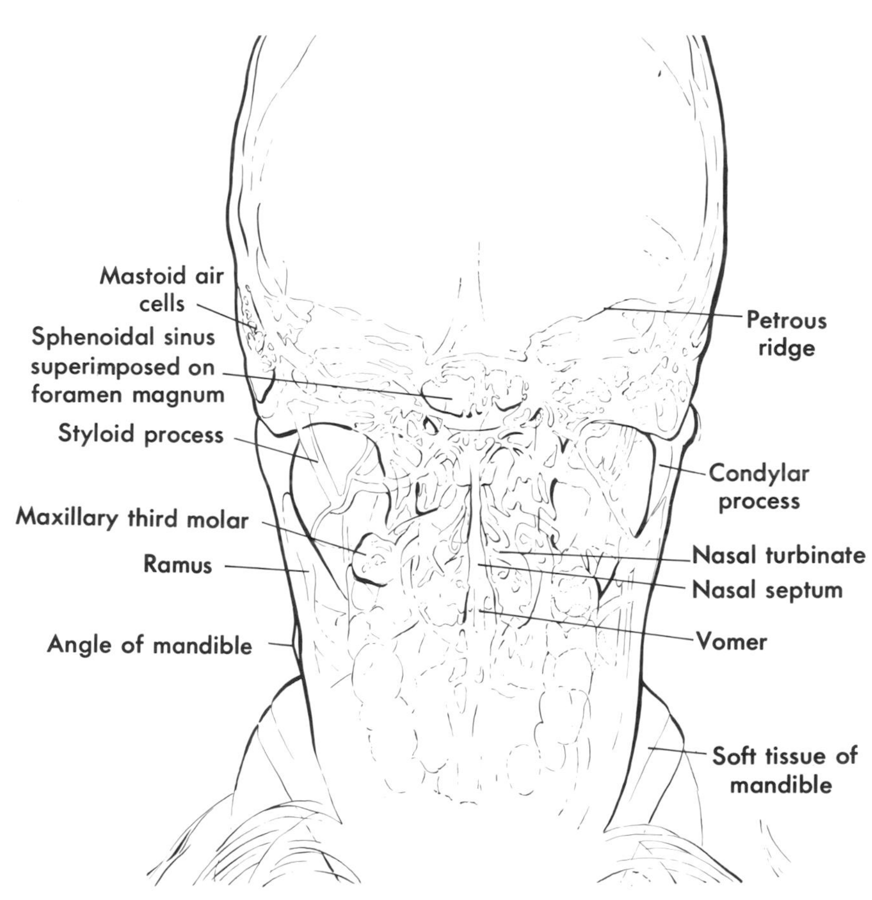

Diagrammatic Representation

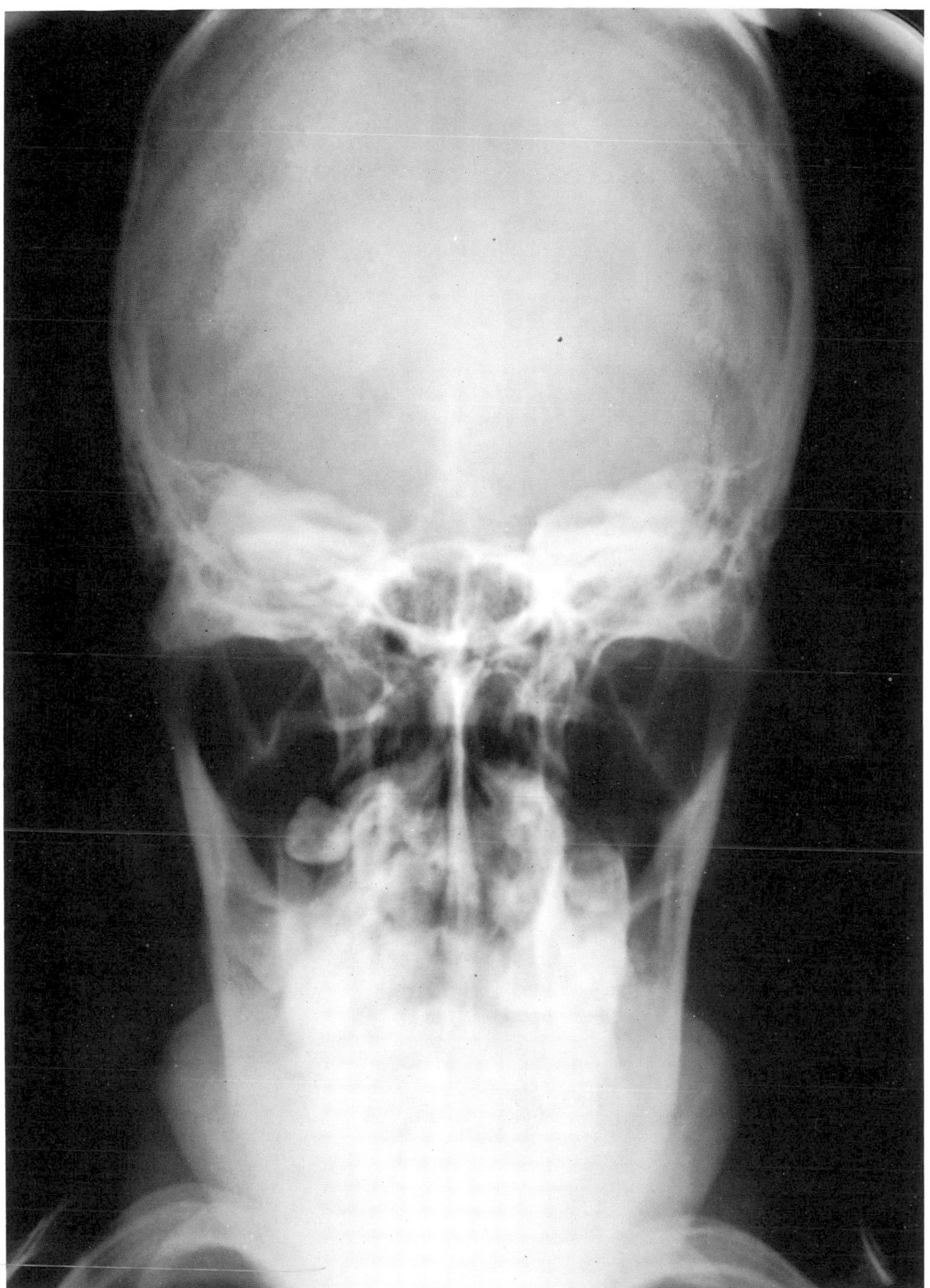

This view shows the condylar processes of the mandible, the occipital bones, and the posterior cranial fossa. This view is one of the best to demonstrate angulation of the condylar processes and may reveal basilar and occipital skull fractures. The nasal septum is well delineated. The zygomatic arches are often seen well by using hyperillumination.

Figure 50. INFERIOR-SUPERIOR PROJECTION, PARASYMPHYSIAL AREA, MANDIBLE

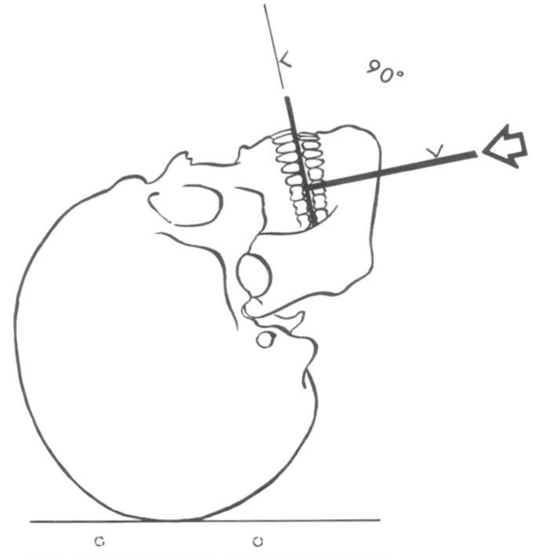

The patient is placed in the dorsal recumbent position on the table, and the film is held between the teeth. The central ray is directed through the midsagittal plane of the molar region 90 degrees from the occlusal plane.

Diagrammatic Representation

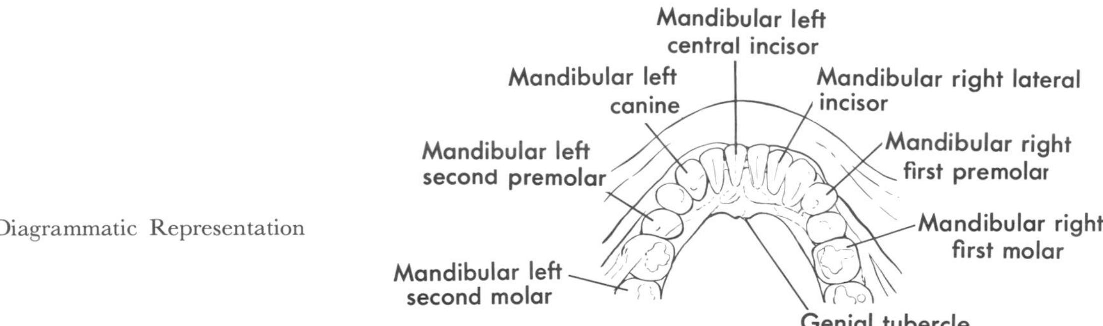

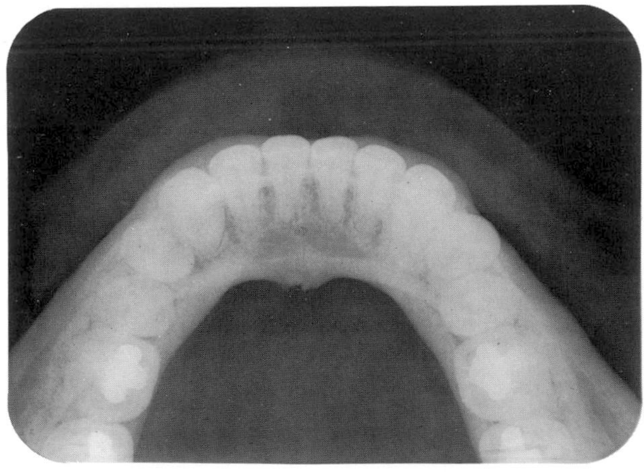

This projection of the parasymphysial area of the mandible shows the anterior portion of the mandibular body, the teeth, and the alveolar process of the mandible. This view reveals displacement of parasymphysial mandibular fractures. It affords an excellent view of bony detail and is helpful in evaluating neoplasms, developmental malformations, cysts, and osteomyelitis of the anterior part of the mandible. It will show symmetry or asymmetry of the mandibular arch and reveal telescoping of fractures of this portion of the mandible.

Figure 51. INFERIOR-SUPERIOR OBLIQUE PROJECTION, PARASYMPHYSIAL AREA, MANDIBLE

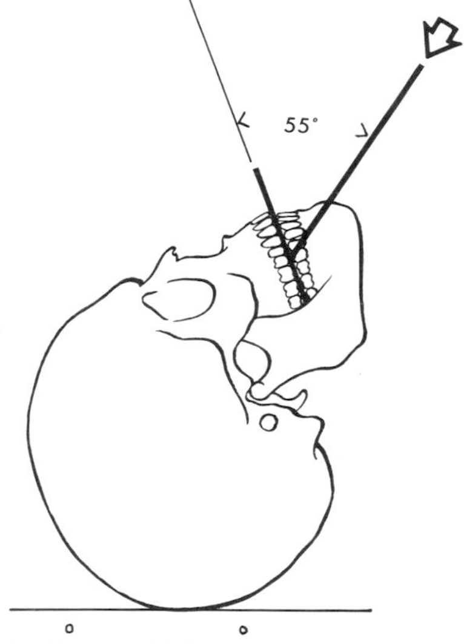

The patient is placed in the dorsal recumbent position on the table, holding the film between his teeth. His head is extended backward. The central ray is directed through the symphysis of the mandible at an angle of 55 degrees from the occlusal plane. Respiration is suspended during exposure.

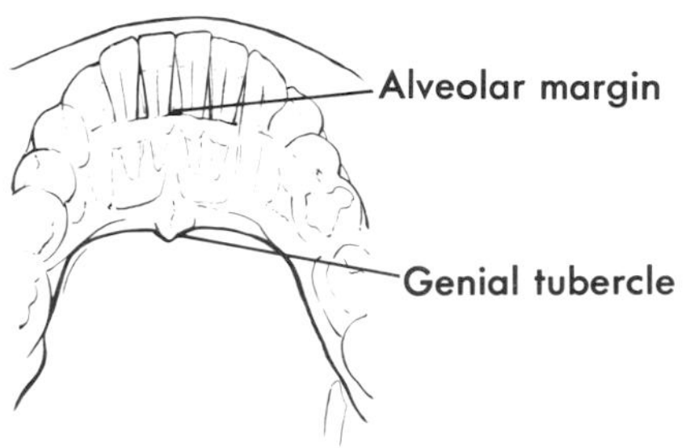

Diagrammatic Representation

This view shows the parasymphysial region, the incisor and canine teeth, and the alveolar process. This view may show alveolar fractures, telescoping of fractures, and irregularities at the inferior border of the mandible. It may also demonstrate cysts, tumors, or osteomyelitis.

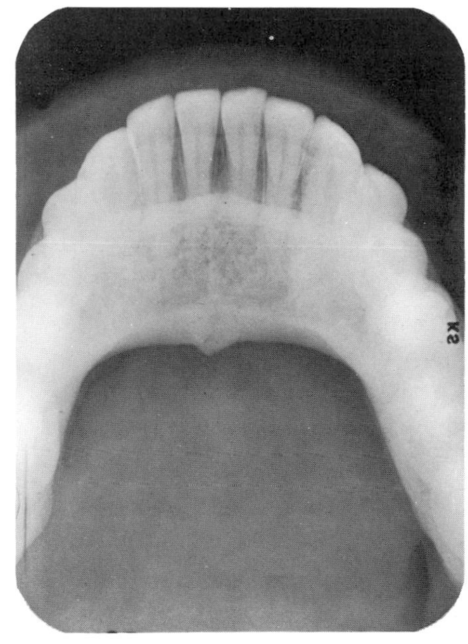

Figure 52. **POSTERIOR-ANTERIOR OBLIQUE PROJECTION OF FACE (WATERS' PROJECTION)**

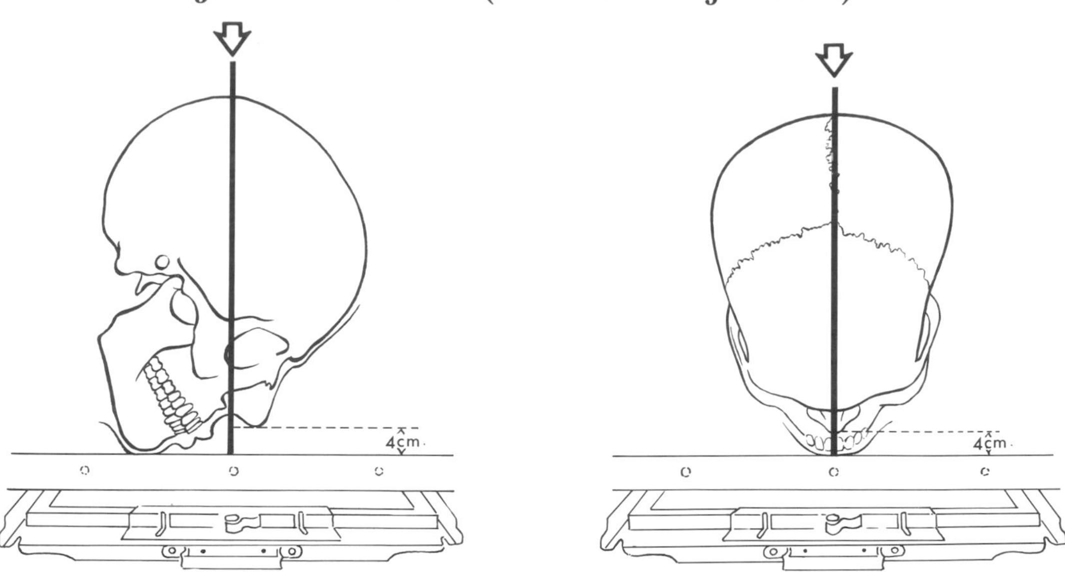

The patient is placed in the prone position with the face against the table. The midsagittal plane of the head is aligned vertically to the vertical midline of the film. The head is rested on the chin with the nasal tip elevated approximately 4 cm. from the table. The upper lip is placed directly over the center of the film, and the central ray is directed perpendicular to the midpoint of the film.

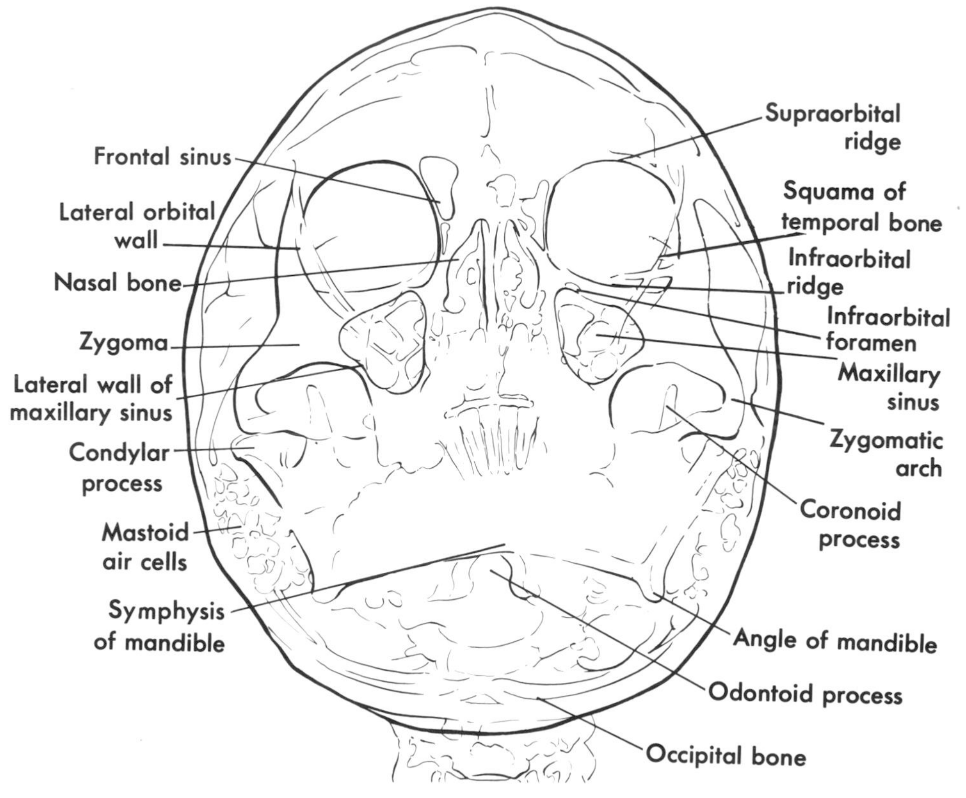

Diagrammatic Representation

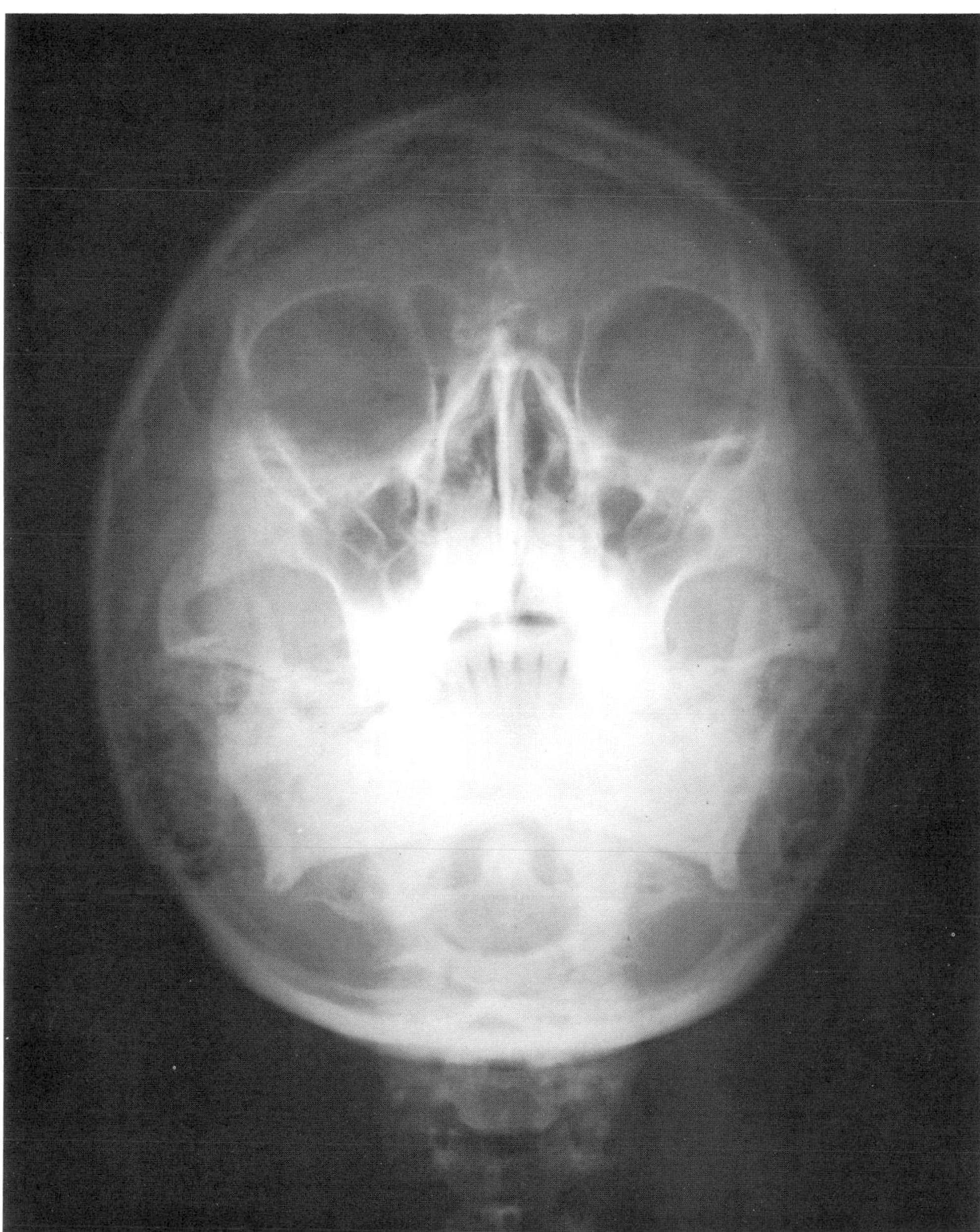

This is the best single view for demonstrating fractures of the maxilla, maxillary sinuses, the floors and inferior rims of the orbits, the zygomatic bones, and the zygomatic arches. It is also helpful in showing fractures of the nasal bones and the frontal processes of the maxillae. In this view there is minimal superimposition of structures. This projection is especially helpful when taken stereoscopically. When the patient is severely injured and is unable to assume the prone position, the reverse Waters' projection gives almost the same detail, but the structures appear somewhat larger because of the greater distance from the film.

Figure 53. ANTERIOR-POSTERIOR OBLIQUE PROJECTION OF FACE (REVERSE WATERS' PROJECTION)

The patient is placed upon the table in the supine position with the head resting on the occiput. The midsagittal plane is aligned to the midplane of the cassette with the lambda centered to the film. The central ray is directed in the midline at an angle of 30 degrees cephalad through the external auditory canal to the cassette. Respiration is suspended during exposure.

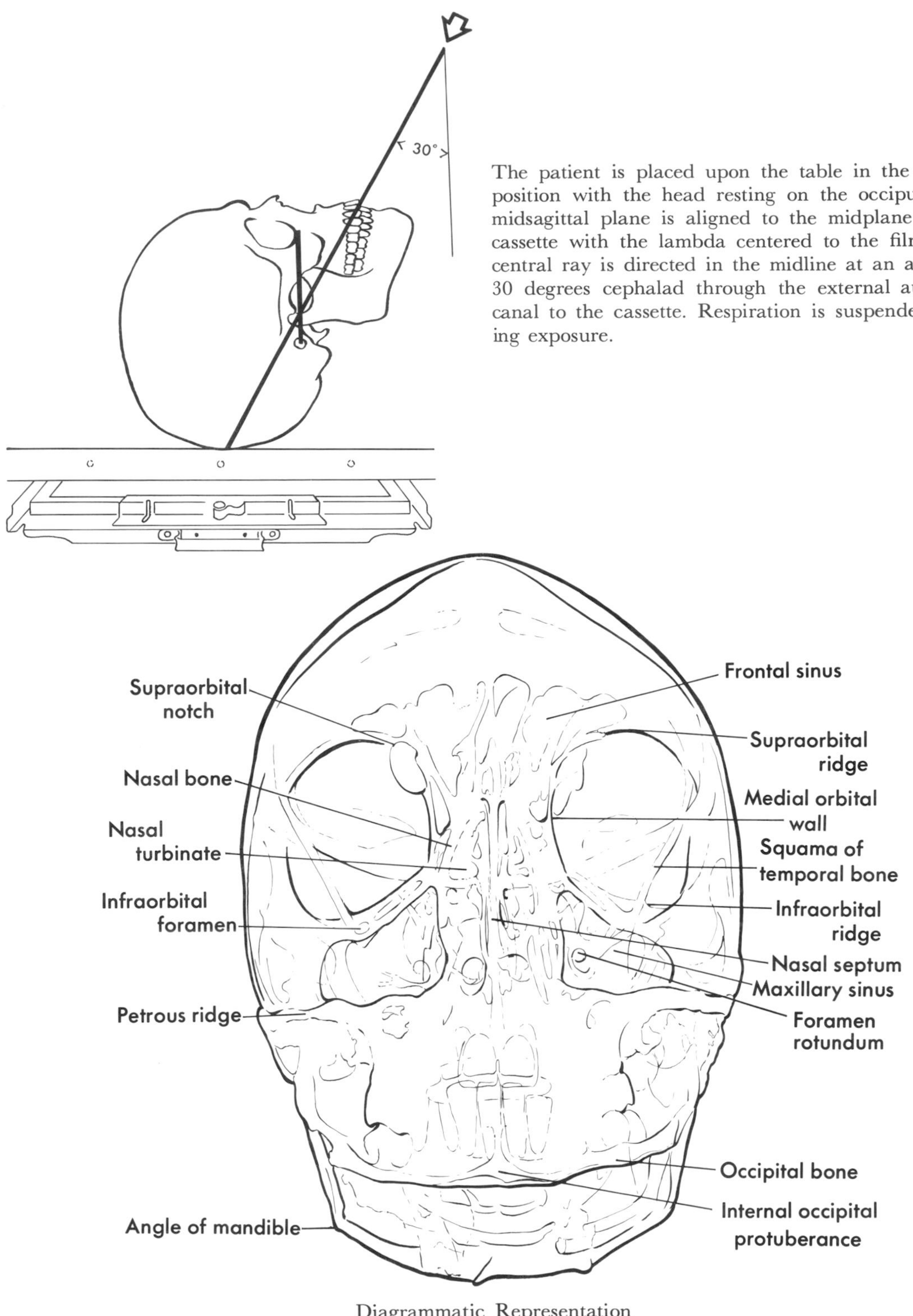

Diagrammatic Representation

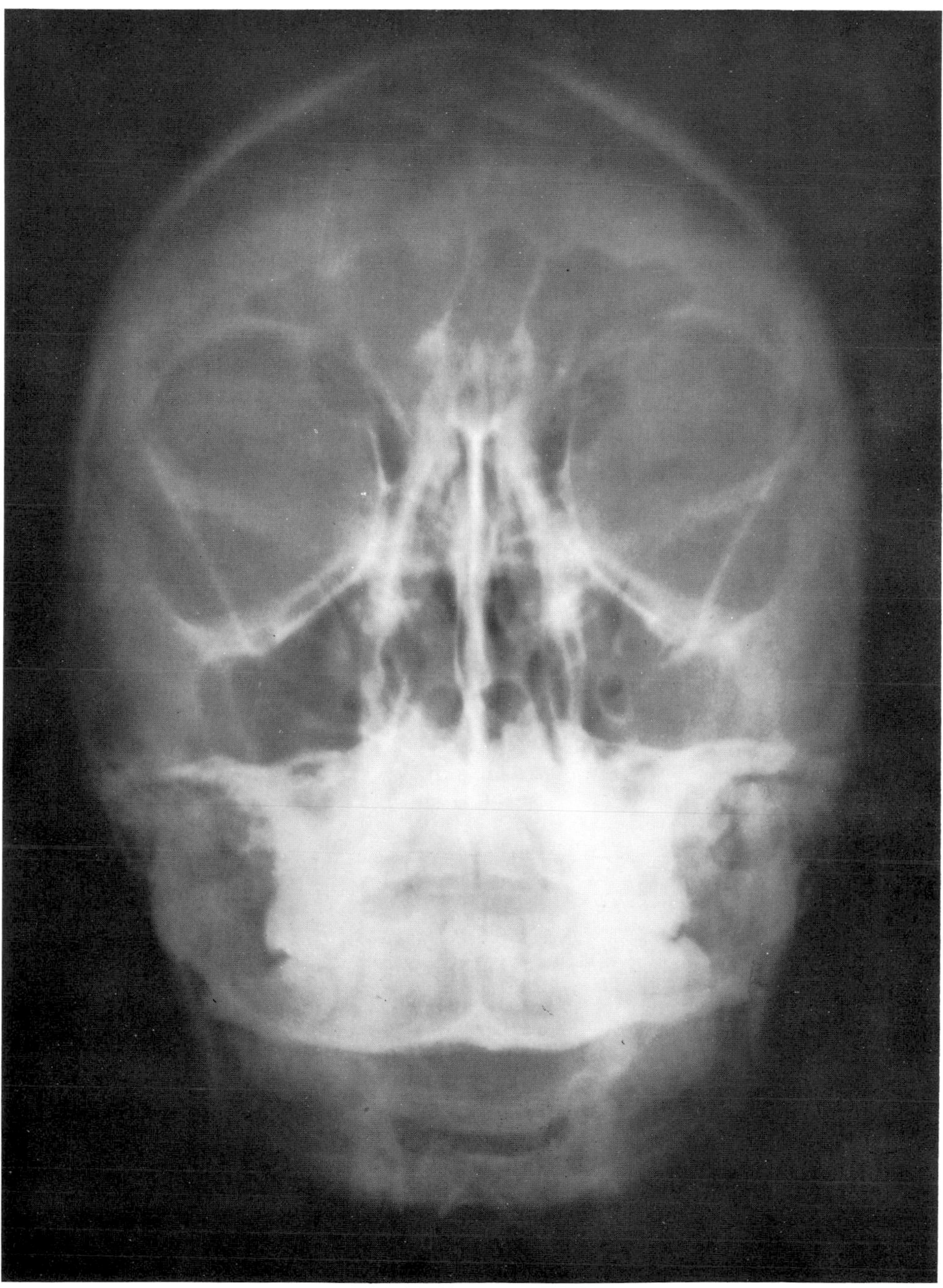

The reverse Waters' projection is used when the patient is severely injured or is unable to assume the prone position. The projection gives a good view of the facial bones, similar to that of the Waters' view except that the structures appear somewhat larger because of their greater distance from the film. This view may be taken stereoscopically.

Figure 54. SUPERIOR-INFERIOR PROJECTION OF HARD PALATE

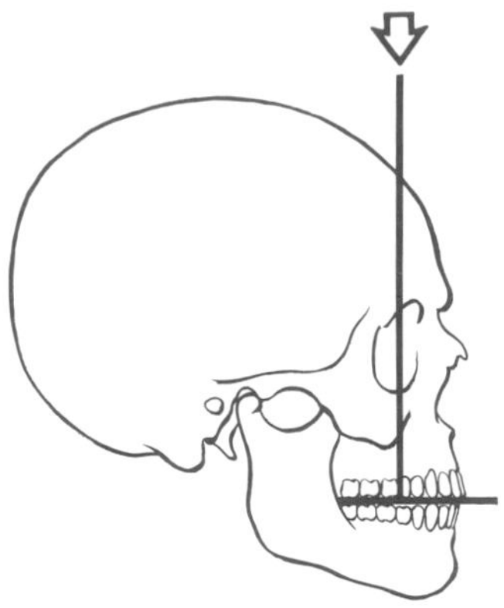

The patient may be supine or seated and holds the occlusal film between his teeth as far back in the mouth as possible. The central ray is directed at right angles to the plane of the film and centered to the midline in the anterior portion of the skull.

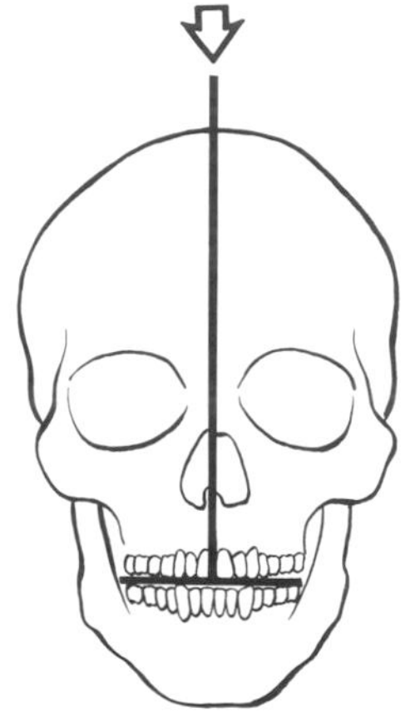

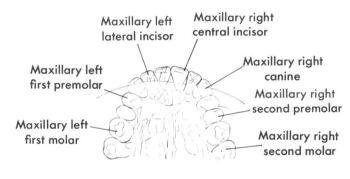

Maxillary left lateral incisor
Maxillary right central incisor
Maxillary left first premolar
Maxillary right canine
Maxillary right second premolar
Maxillary left first molar
Maxillary right second molar

Diagrammatic Representation

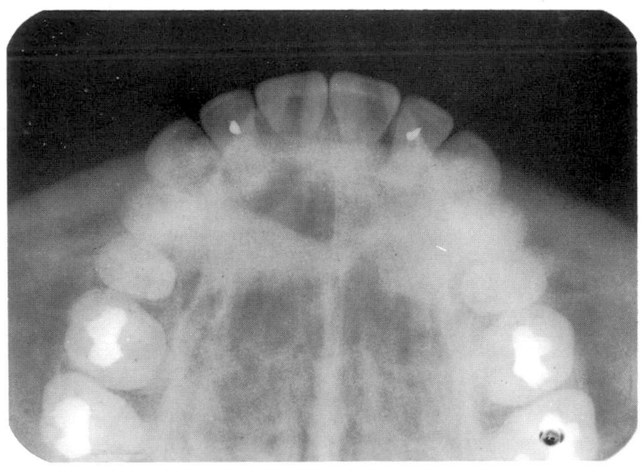

This projection shows the upper dental arch, nasal septum, fractures of the hard palate, malformations, cysts, or neoplasms. The palatine processes of the maxillae and the alveolar process may be seen well in this projection.

Figure 55. SUPERIOR-INFERIOR OBLIQUE PROJECTION OF HARD PALATE

The patient may be either supine or seated. The film is held between the teeth as far back in the mouth as possible. The central ray is directed in the midsagittal plane through the tip of the nose at an angle of 50 degrees caudad to the occlusal plane. Respiration is suspended during exposure.

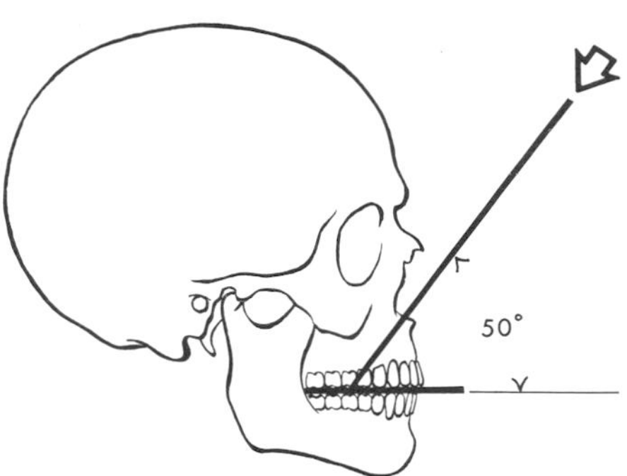

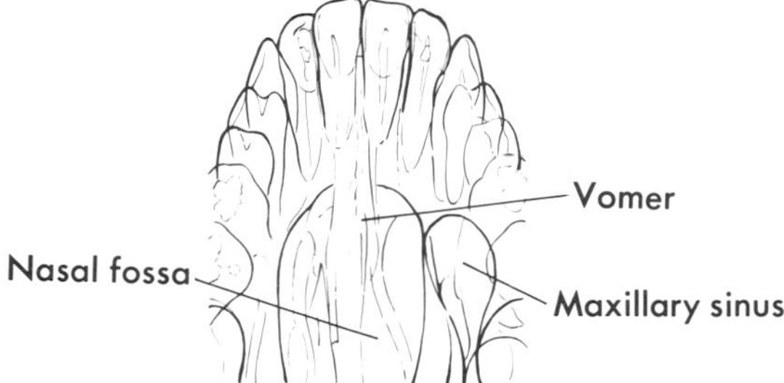

Diagrammatic Representation

This projection gives an excellent study of the anterior portion of the hard palate, teeth, and alveolar process. This view will show a Le Fort I fracture of the maxilla.

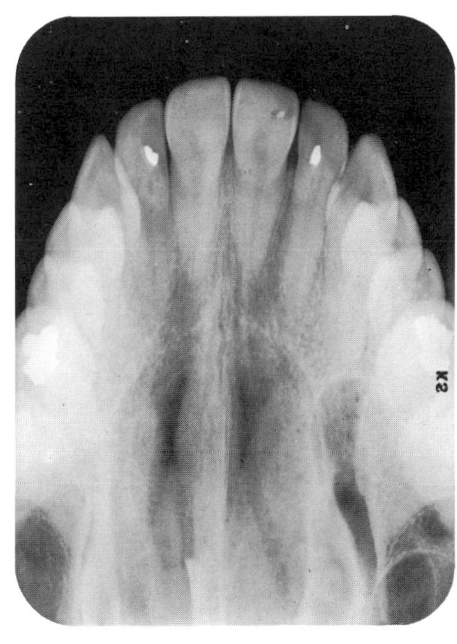

Figure 56. SUBMENTAL-VERTICAL PROJECTION OF ZYGOMATIC ARCHES

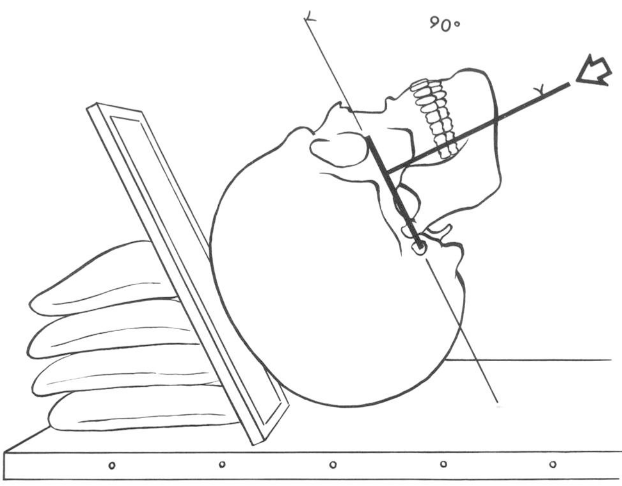

The patient is placed in the dorsal recumbent position with the shoulders elevated on pillows or sand bags to obtain maximum extension of the neck. The occiput is rested against the table with the midsagittal plane of the skull aligned vertically to the central vertical line of the film. The vertex is rested against the upright cassette. Reid's base line is parallel to the plane of the cassette. The central ray is directed midway between the angles of the jaw, perpendicular to the base line of the skull.

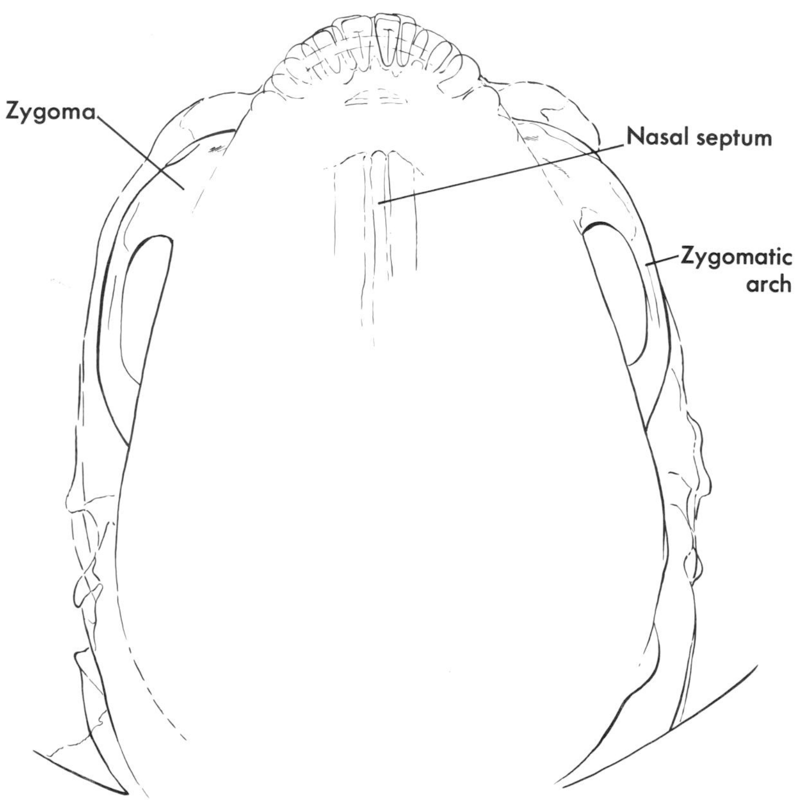

Diagrammatic Representation

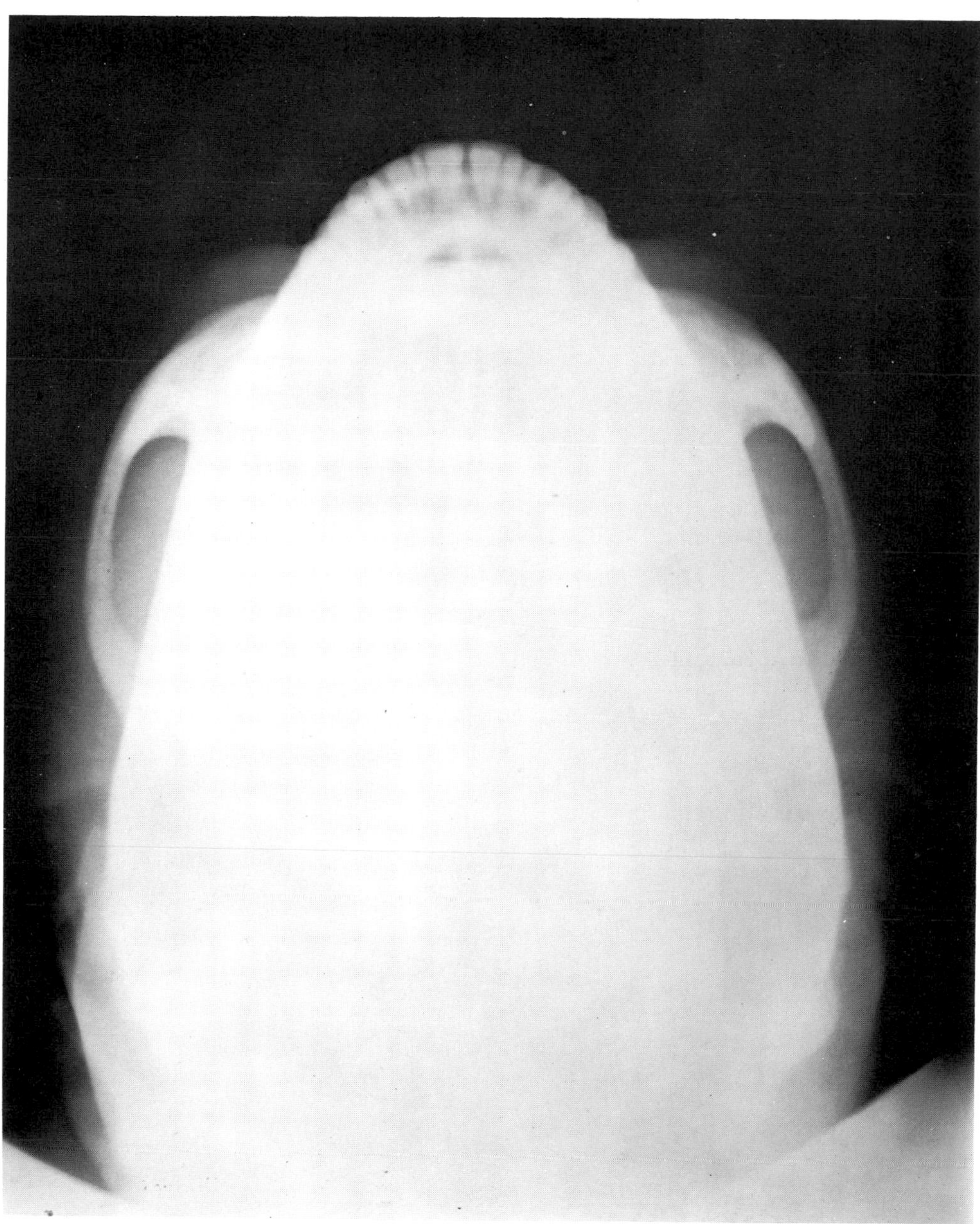

This is an excellent view to demonstrate the zygomatic arches and medial or lateral displacement of fractured segments. If the view is underexposed, it is useful only for outlining the zygomatic arches, but if taken to expose the base of the skull, it may reveal basilar skull fractures.

Figure 57. LATERAL PROJECTION OF NASAL BONES

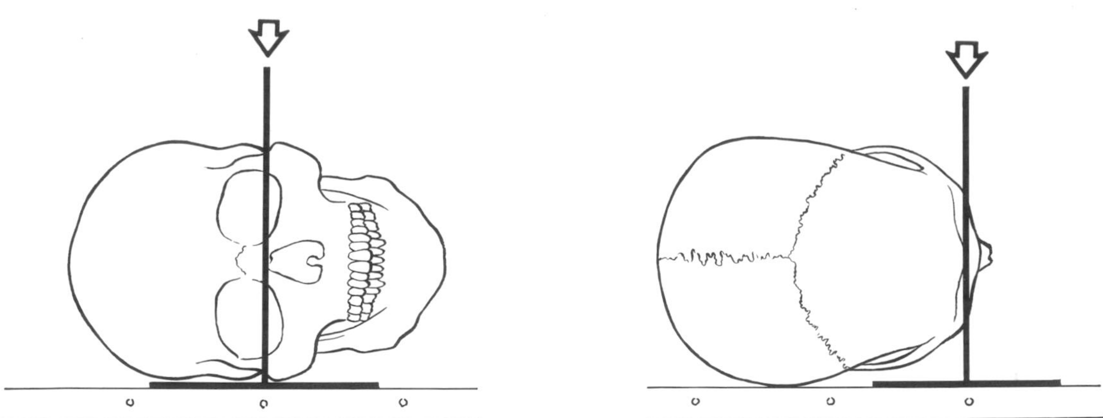

The head is placed in the precise lateral position over a film packet placed below the nose. The central ray is directed through the base of the nose at right angles to the plane of the film. Right and left lateral views should be taken. Respiration is suspended during exposure.

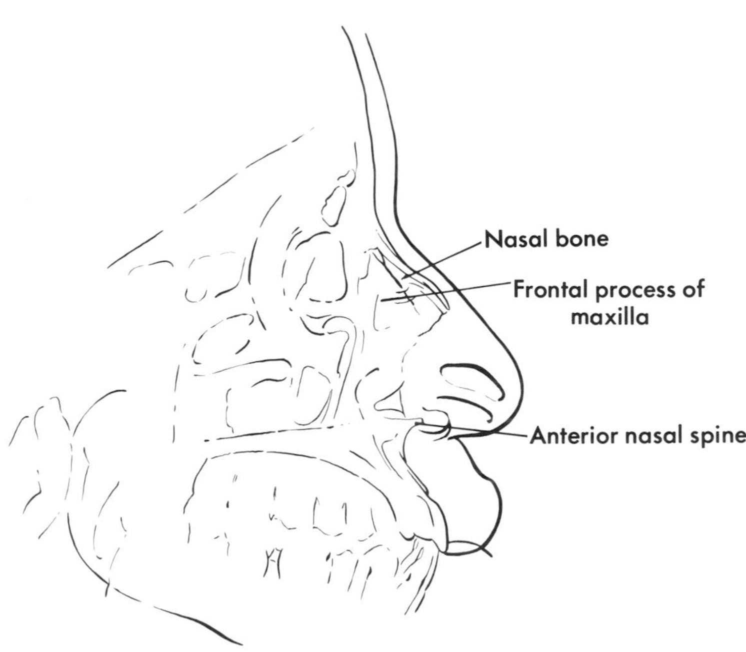

Diagrammatic Representation

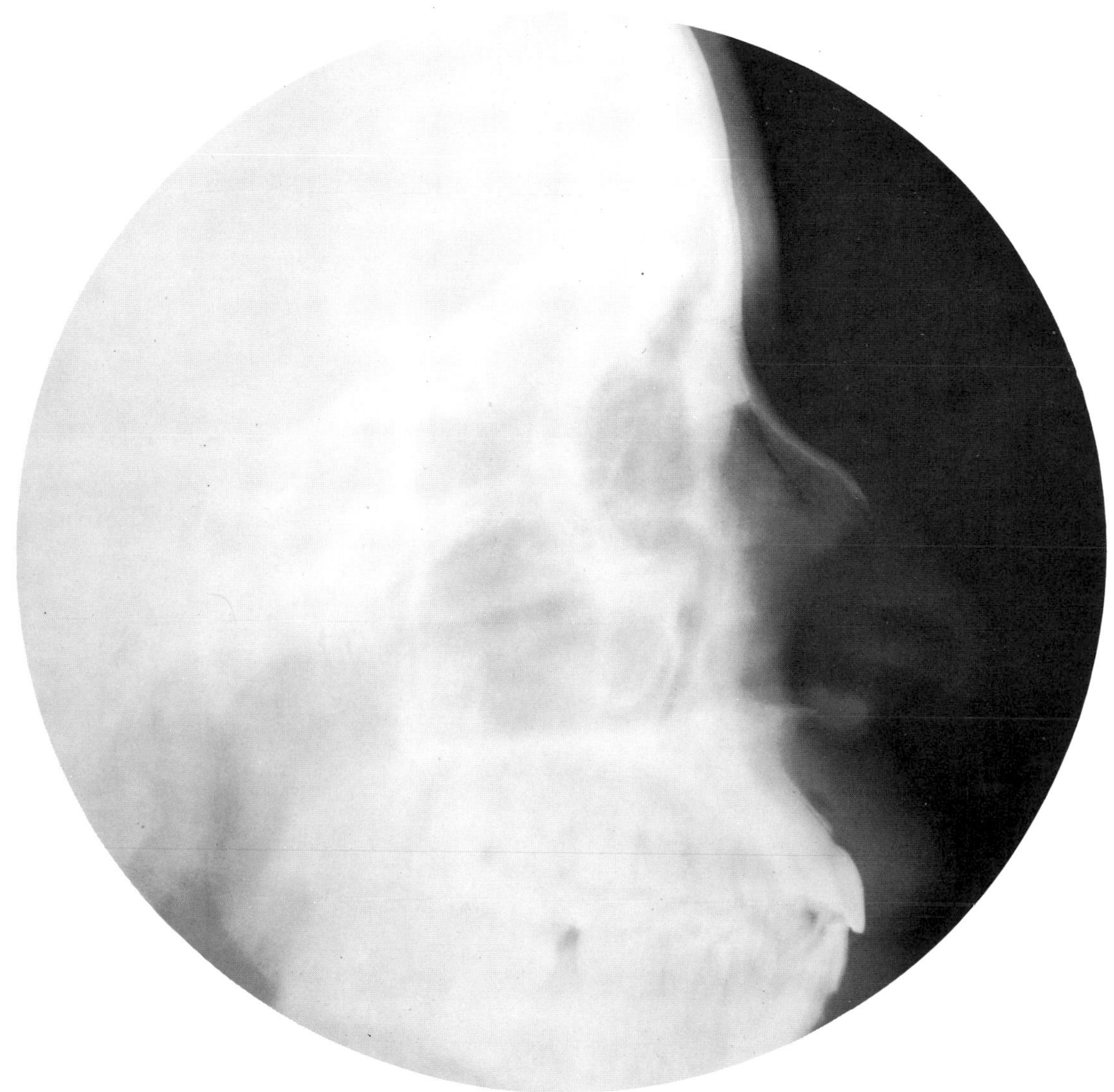

The nasal bone closest to the film is well demonstrated in the lateral view. Soft tissues and the anterior nasal spine of the maxilla are shown in profile. These views demonstrate fractures of the nasal bones, the anterior nasal spine, and the frontal process of the maxilla.

Figure 58. SUPERIOR-INFERIOR PROJECTION OF NASAL BONES

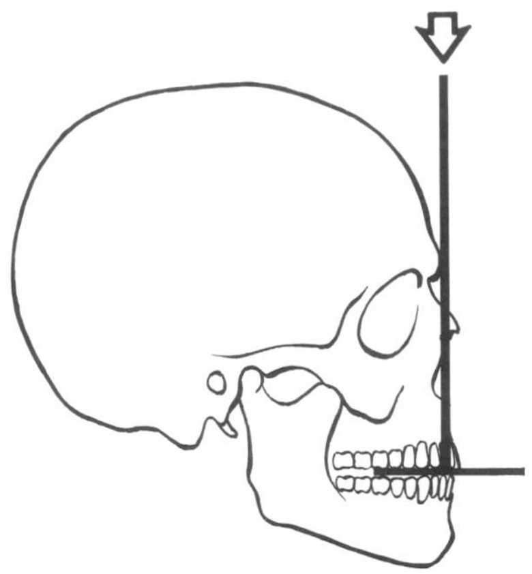

The patient is supine or seated, and the occlusal film is inserted into the mouth just far enough for the patient to hold it between the anterior teeth. The central ray is directed downward in the midline through the base of the nose at an angle of 90 degrees to the film.

Nasal bone

Nasal septum

Diagrammatic Representation

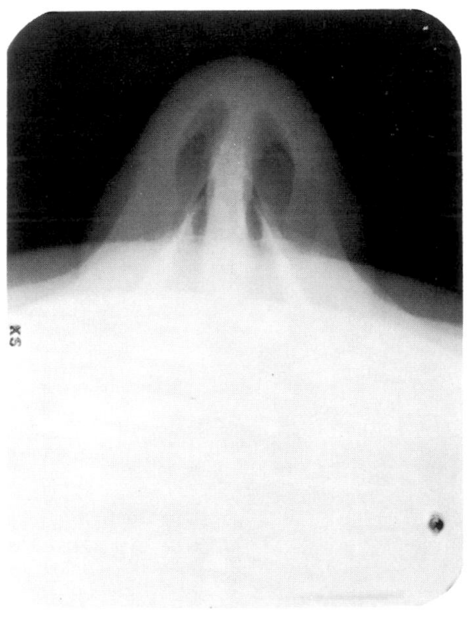

This view shows only the portion of the nose that extends beyond the forehead-chin line. This projection of the nasal bones may demonstrate fractures and medial or lateral displacement of fragments.

Figure 59. INTRAORAL DENTAL ROENTGENOGRAM

The film is inserted into the mouth with the long axis of the film directed longitudinally for exposure of the anterior teeth and transversely for exposure of the posterior teeth. The film packet is centered to the teeth. The packet is held by the patient with his thumb placed against the center of the packet with just enough pressure to hold the film firmly. However, the film should not be bent to conform to the arch. The extended fingers may be braced against the cheek for support to prevent movement of the film. The central ray is directed to approximately the midpoint of the film, at right angles to a plane that transects the plane of the tooth and the plane of the film.

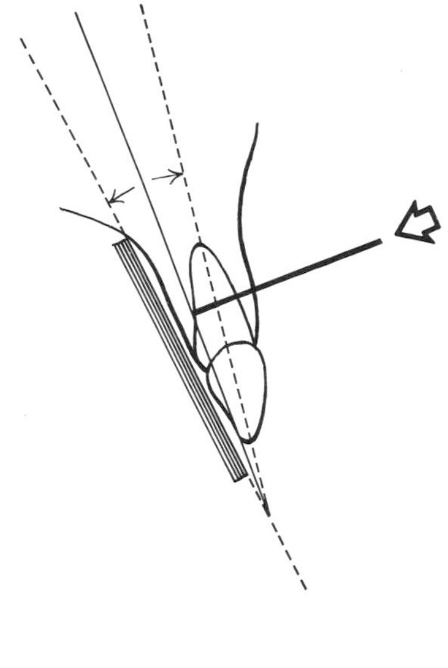

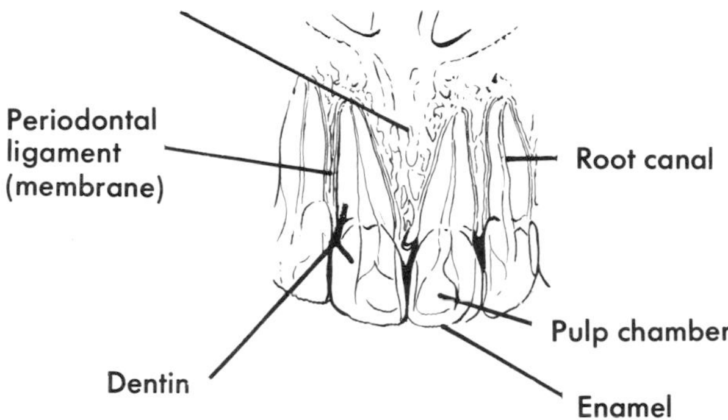

Diagrammatic Representation

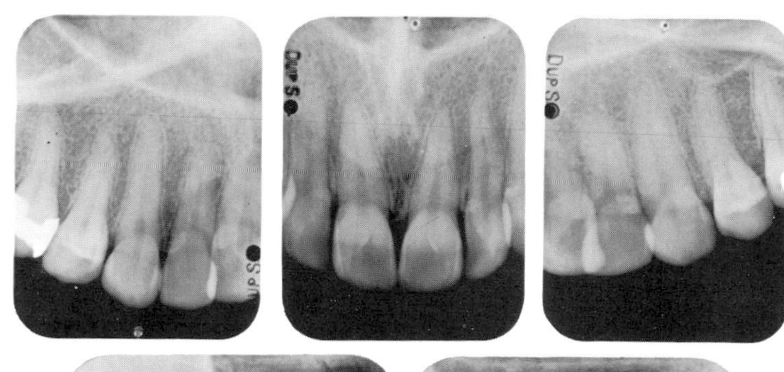

Dental radiographs show the teeth in detail and the surrounding alveolar bone and demonstrate fractures of the teeth, cysts, tumors, or infections of adjacent bone. Radiographs of the maxillary premolar and molar regions usually show a portion of the maxillary sinus.

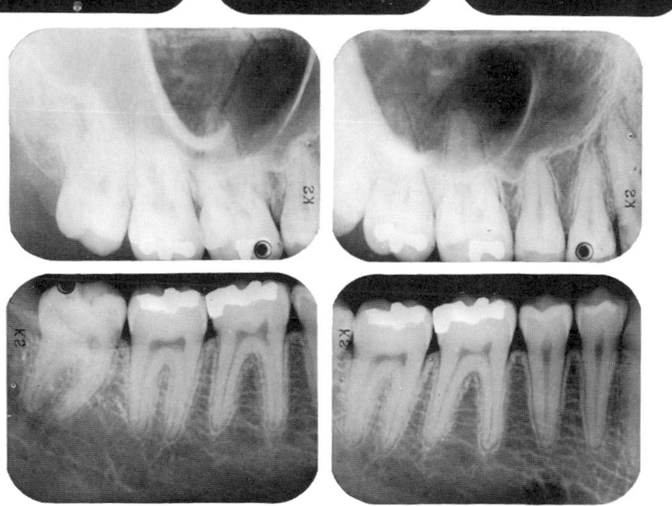

MANAGEMENT OF FACIAL FRACTURES

Timing of Treatment

When it is consistent with the patient's general condition, fractures of the facial bones should be treated as early as possible. When seen immediately after injury, fractures can be immobilized with a minimal amount of effort if the areas are not obscured by edema or hematoma.

Thus the method of management is indicated by the patient's general condition and his age, the extent of his injury, and the adequacy of the facilities. Management is also influenced by the presence or absence of teeth or by the availability of the patient's artificial dentures for use. Management of various types of fractures is considered in detail under the appropriate chapter headings.

The possibility of infection in fractures of the facial bones increases proportionately with the time interval elapsing between the time of the occurrence of the fracture and the time of reduction and fixation. If several hours have passed since the injury and an inflammatory reaction is suspected or edema or hematoma is severe, it may be advisable to administer anti-inflammatory drugs and wait until the edema is reduced in order to facilitate the surgery.

The management of facial bone fractures is seldom a surgical emergency. An injury which imperils life should receive first consideration. It is more difficult to reduce fractures of several days' duration, but it is possible to obtain good results, even after two to three weeks, if delayed treatment is indicated. Postponement may be necessary when the patient has been severely injured and is unable to withstand operative trauma. The most severely injured patient, however, may benefit if minor procedures are carried out at the bedside. These may consist of temporary fixation of fragments by intermaxillary wiring and removal of broken and loose teeth from the oral cavity or stabilization of the fractured segments by wiring the patient's teeth or artificial dentures. Support of fracture segments may be obtained with simple dressings or bandages.

If there are no signs of meningitis, the presence of cerebrospinal rhinorrhea should not deter the surgeon from manipulating and reducing fractures in the middle face. Should the cerebrospinal rhinorrhea persist for three to four weeks after reduction of the fractures, the neurosurgical consultant might recommend craniotomy and insertion of a graft of fascia lata in the floor of the frontal fossa.

Preoperative Care

Before anesthesia is administered or treatment attempted, the patient should have been evaluated thoroughly and all data recorded carefully. Except for emergency care, the patient should be in optimum condition for operative procedures. Shock, hypovolemia, dehydration, and electrolyte imbalance should receive consideration before an operation is undertaken.

If there is a history of rheumatic fever or valvular heart disease, administration of antibiotics should be a part of the preparation. When indicated, immunization for tetanus and gas organisms should be carried out. When infection is a complicating factor, antibiotic therapy should be instituted.

Diabetes mellitus should be treated and intravenous fluids used if there is evidence of dehydration. Steroid therapy should be instituted when indicated. An internist should be consulted to share in these problems of management.

The preparation of the patient is an important part of effective surgical procedure. In many instances the patient may be covered with dirt and grease. Every effort should be made to get the skin as clean as possible to reduce bacterial flora. If the patient has been hospitalized several days before the operation, special care should be given to preparing the skin. Harsh chemical irritants are to be avoided and mild detergents and irrigation with normal saline used. Frequent washing with a mild soap or detergent is adequate. Nursing personnel should be instructed to do this at three- or four-hour intervals.

The oral cavity should be cleansed frequently with a toothbrush and mild detergent supplemented with a mouth wash. Loose or infected teeth should be removed. The mouth should be swabbed and the teeth scrubbed with a small toothbrush. In instances in which oral sepsis exists, dental prophylaxis will be helpful.

Preoperative Medication

It is essential that preoperative medication be planned in a manner that gives the patient full physiologic action. When time is short, preoperative medication may be administered intravenously prior to general anesthesia. Choice of medication should be made in consultation with the anesthesiologist. The drying effect of atropine or scopolamine upon the respiratory mucosa makes these drugs the preoperative choice in the majority of cases.

Anesthesia

Special Problems in Surgical Emergencies

In the management of the post-traumatic surgical emergency the anesthesiologist meets three major problems: the management of the full stomach, the maintenance or establishment of a patent airway with adequate respiratory exchange and oxygenation, and the evaluation of the cardiovascular status and treatment of shock.

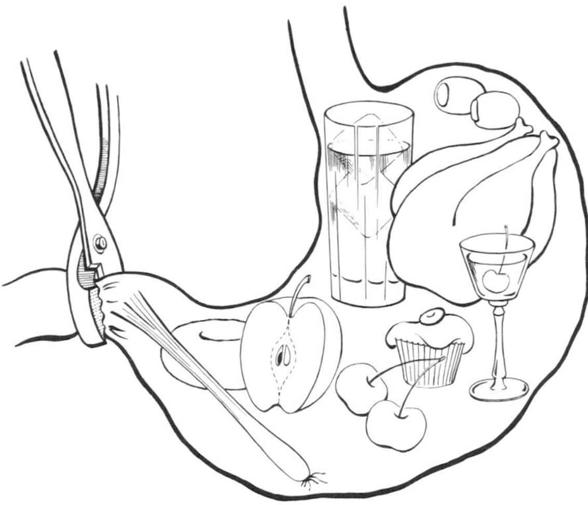

Figure 60. Cartoon illustrating pylorospasm incident to severe trauma and shock. Food may remain in the stomach for many hours following injury, and therefore the passage of several hours is not a guarantee that the stomach will be free of food. Vomiting with aspiration of stomach contents is a real danger at the time of administration of anesthesia.

Management of the Full Stomach

When the emergency patient enters the hospital for unscheduled anesthesia, it must be assumed that he has undigested food in his stomach. After an accident or an injury, digestive processes cease and pylorospasm ensues (Fig. 60). Experience has shown that food may remain in the stomach for 24 to 48 hours after an injury instead of the 4 to 6 hours that is the usual emptying time of the stomach under normal circumstances. Several methods are employed in dealing with the problem of the full stomach. Since the problem is encountered frequently and the consequences are of extreme danger, the methods will be presented and briefly discussed.

Preoperative removal of gastric contents. Levine tubes or even large-bore Ewald tubes may remove some liquid contents and decompress the stomach, but large undigested particles will be left and the risk will remain.

INDUCED VOMITING. Mechanical irritation of the pharynx or the administration of some emetic drug is upsetting to the patient emotionally as well as physiologically, and is not necessarily reliable—chunks of undigested food may be retained.

USE OF THE GASTRIC TUBE. A gastric tube with a balloon inflated in the stomach and pulled back against the cardia has been reported to be an efficient way of blocking the upward passage of stomach contents. Such a tube is not always easy to pass and may produce other undesirable hazards in the poor-risk emergency case.

RAPID INDUCTION AND ENDOTRACHEAL INTUBATION. The commonest technique used to prevent aspiration of the stomach contents utilizes rapid induction of anesthesia and insertion of an endotracheal tube with an inflatable cuff. Usually the tube goes in and the cuff is inflated before reflux occurs. If considerable intragastric pressure exists or if intubation is accomplished with difficulty, the danger from aspiration is great. Another hazard is that a strain is put upon the cardiovascular system by the rapid induction of the anesthesia. Rapid induction in the emergency or poor-risk patient may produce profound hypotension, relative hypoxia, myocardial infarction, and myocardial failure.

ENDOTRACHEAL INTUBATION OF THE CONSCIOUS PATIENT. The safest and most certain technique of preventing aspiration is to insert an endotracheal tube and inflate the cuff before the induction of anesthesia. In this fashion, an airtight and watertight system can be established in the trachea before the patient is put to sleep. This may be difficult to accomplish in some patients and may be a most frightening and upsetting procedure for others. The discomfort can be minimized by an intraluminal transtracheal injection of 1 cc. of 5 per cent cocaine through the cricothyroid ligament.

Each of the methods described has some disadvantage. In spite of all thought, deliberation, and careful preparation, some patients will vomit and aspirate either solid or liquid material. The symptoms of aspiration and its treatment depend largely upon the nature of the material aspirated.

ASPIRATION OF SOLID MATERIAL. Aspiration of solid material may produce laryngeal, tracheal, or bronchial obstruction with atelectasis, pulmonary collapse, mediastinal shift, cyanosis, dyspnea, tachycardia, or death. Treatment consists of using a bronchoscope for immediate visualization of the larynx, trachea, and bronchi and removal of solid material.

ASPIRATION OF LIQUID CONTENTS OF THE STOMACH. Stomach contents have a pH of 1.2. The lungs have a pH of about 8.0. The acid contents of the stomach are extremely irritating to the lungs and set up an immediate and intense chemical reaction initiating bronchospasm and asthma-like dyspnea followed by cyanosis, tachycardia, and radiographic findings of diffusely scattered, soft-mottled densities. The first 24 to 36 hours are critical. If patients survive this period, they recover without pulmonary sequelae and the radiographic findings will be negative in 7 to 10 days. Treatment consists of immediate and repeated irrigation of the tracheobronchial tree with 10 to 20 cc. of saline, which is quickly absorbed by the lymphatics, and the administration of cortisone for the first 48 to 72 hours.

Maintenance or Establishment of a Patent Airway with Adequate Respiratory Exchange and Oxygenation

The airway may be endangered or obstructed by head injury or local injury to the upper airway or chest. Passage of an endotracheal tube or a bronchoscope is often necessary. After initial oxygenation, a tracheotomy may be required. Ventilatory assistance also must be supplied if respiratory conditions demand it.

Evaluation of the Cardiovascular Status and Treatment of Shock

The patient's cardiovascular status must be carefully evaluated. Blood pressure may be maintained at normal or near normal levels by compensatory mechanisms, even in the face of considerable blood loss. Blood volume should be restored with whole blood if possible before the induction of anesthesia. Anesthetics must be administered carefully and in much smaller amounts than usual to the patient recovering from shock. Most anesthetic agents affect adversely the compensatory mechanisms and the cardiovascular system. They decrease vasomotor tone and motion, decrease the strength of myocardial contraction and cardiac output, and decrease the compensatory and homeostatic capacities of the autonomic nervous system. Anesthetic agents unwisely chosen or injudiciously administered may at any time, but especially in the post-traumatic surgical emergency, produce profound hypotension, tissue hypoxia, cerebral or myocardial infarction, hepatic necrosis, renal tubular necrosis, or death.

Choice of Anesthesia

In some cases it is possible to use a local anesthetic for the management of fractures of the face. However, general anesthesia, particularly in more extensive procedures, is less traumatic to the patient and more convenient for the surgeon.

The choice of anesthesia should be determined by consultation between the surgeon and the anesthesiologist. The choice between local or general anesthesia depends upon the available facilities, the condition and emotional stability of the patient, the competence of the person administering the anesthetic, and convenience for the surgeon.

For general anesthesia, the endotracheal methods have proved to be the safest and most effective. The nasal endotracheal route is useful, especially in the management of mandibular fractures. The management of nasal, zygomatic, and maxillary fractures usually requires the use of the oral endotracheal technique. In extensive fractures that involve several bones of the face and require nasal packing and intermaxillary fixation, administration of general anesthesia by means of a tracheotomy is the most effective method.

Use of a pharyngeal pack in conjunction with a cuffed endotracheal tube may prevent aspiration of foreign objects, blood, and mucus. All members of the operating team should be aware of the presence of the pack and be sure of its removal before the teeth are brought into fixation. Failure to remove the pack could cause lethal obstruction of the airway at the time of extubation.

To control oozing and hemorrhage in the operative site, local infiltration of weak solutions of epinephrine (1:100,000) is usually indicated. Muscle relaxants may be useful to permit reduction of fractures of the mandible. Selection of the relaxant and the timing of its administration should be left to the judgment of the anesthesiologist.

Surgical Equipment

To perform safe, effective surgical procedures, adequate equipment is essential. Instruments should be of the highest quality. They should be kept in excellent repair and kept sharp and readily available as a complete set (Fig. 61). It is disconcerting to discover that some instruments or supplies are missing when needed during the operation, for this results in loss of valuable time and

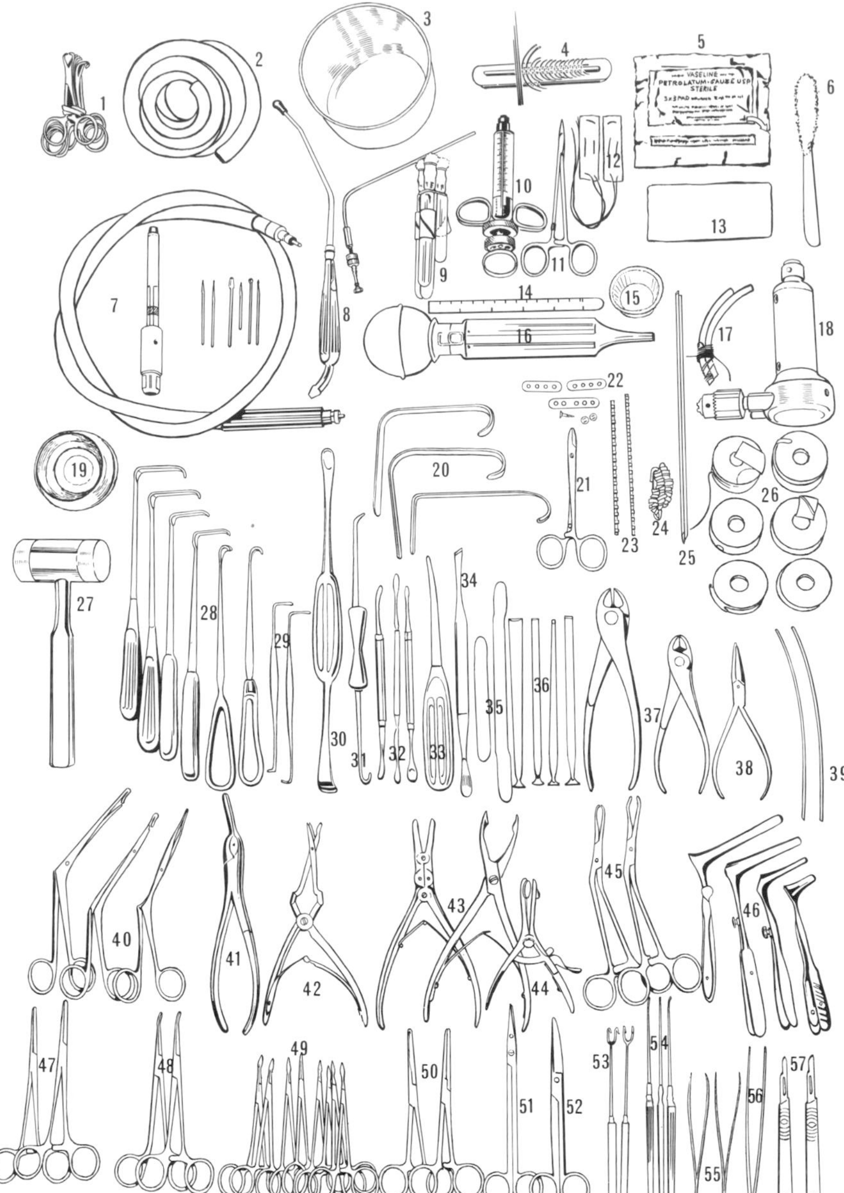

Figure 61. Equipment

1. Small towel clips
2. Rubber tubing
3. Metal basin for saline solution
4. Assorted skin needles
5. Petrolatum gauze
6. Cotton applicator
7. Handpiece, assorted burs and cable
8. Suction tips
9. Assorted hypodermic needles
10. Graduated 10 cc. syringe
11. Needle holder
12. Intranasal packs
13. Wide mesh gauze for collodion dressing
14. Metal ruler
15. Paper container for collodion
16. Asepto syringe
17. Intranasal rubber tubes
18. Motor-driven bone drill
19. Glass container for marking ink
20. Tongue depressor—lip retractors
21. Wire twisting forceps
22. Metal bone plates with screws
23. Erich arch bars
24. Latex rubber bands
25. Kirschner wires
26. Spools of stainless steel wire—gauges 20, 22, 25, 28, 30, and 32
27. Surgical mallet
28. Assorted retractors
29. Senn retractor-rakes
30. Haight elevator
31. Dingman elevator-hook
32. Periosteal elevators
33. Dingman zygoma elevator
34. Periosteal elevator
35. Ribbon retractors
36. Osteotomes
37. Wire cutting pliers
38. Wire bending pliers
39. Dingman passing needles

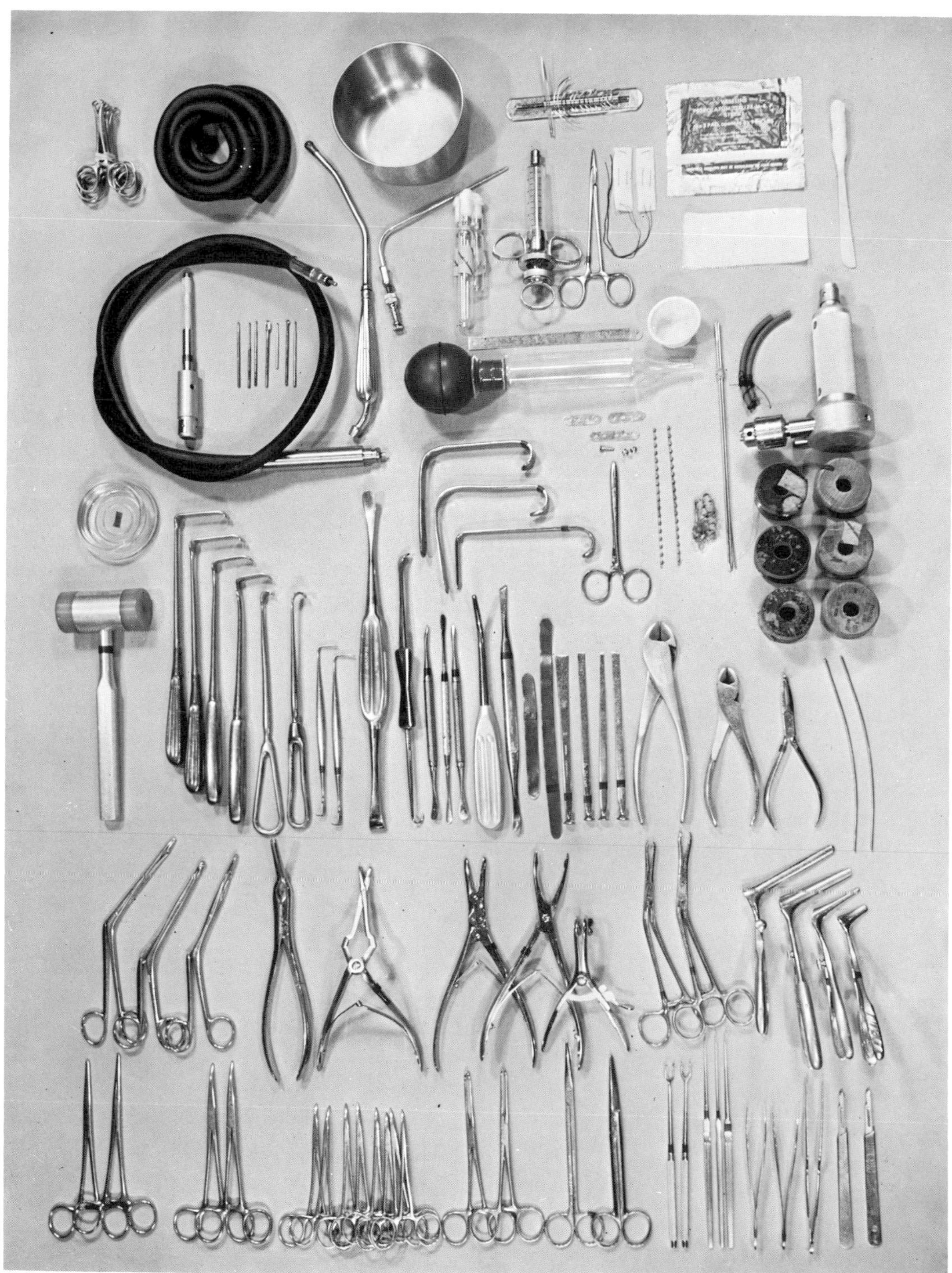

40. Septum biting forceps
41. Asch forceps
42. Jansenn-Middleton septal forceps
43. Rongeurs
44. Denhardt side-mouth gag
45. Dingman bone-holding forceps
46. Assorted nasal specula
47. Kocher forceps
48. Kelley forceps
49. Curved mosquito forceps
50. Allis forceps
51. Metzenbaum scissors
52. Straight Mayo scissors
53. Double tissue hooks
54. Single tissue hooks
55. Adson-Brown thumb forceps
56. Bayonet nasal dressing forceps
57. Scalpels

disruption of the continuity of the procedure. It is recommended that a kit containing all the necessary supplies, instruments, and equipment be utilized only for the management of facial fractures. In this way, the instruments are kept together and are readily and conveniently available. The instruments and supplies shown and coded in Figure 61 have been found the most useful in the treatment of facial fractures.

Preparation of the Patient in the Operating Room

In positioning the patient on the operating table, the convenience of the surgeon should be the first consideration. It is preferable that positioning take place prior to administration of anesthesia, especially if moving the anesthetized patient will require additional personnel.

The most useful type of operating table is one with a jointed headpiece that allows for flexibility of the patient's head and the neck. Additional maneuverability of the head and neck can be achieved by placing a sandbag under the shoulders. In all of this, it is obvious the arrangements must be such as to prevent any chance of sudden head movement while the patient is under anesthesia.

Hands and arms should be comfortably fixed at the side of the table, care being taken to avoid contact with sharp corners and edges. Now preparations can be made for whatever parenteral fluid therapy may be indicated.

Although all male patients should be shaved, it is unnecessary generally to cut the

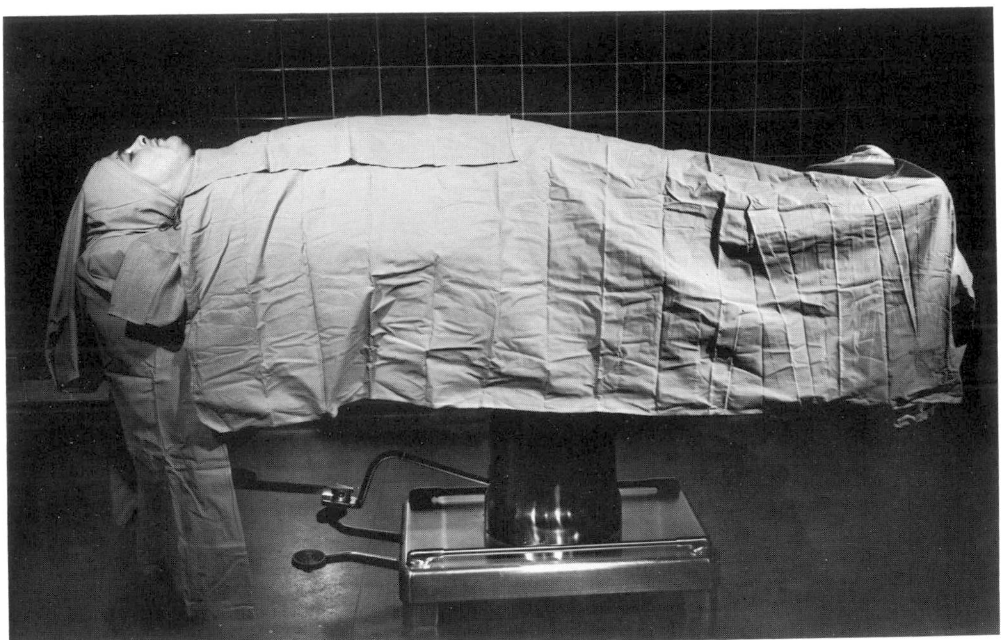

Figure 62. The position and draping of a patient on the operating table for the treatment of facial fractures. The face and neck should be exposed and the patient covered adequately with neat, nonbulky drapes.

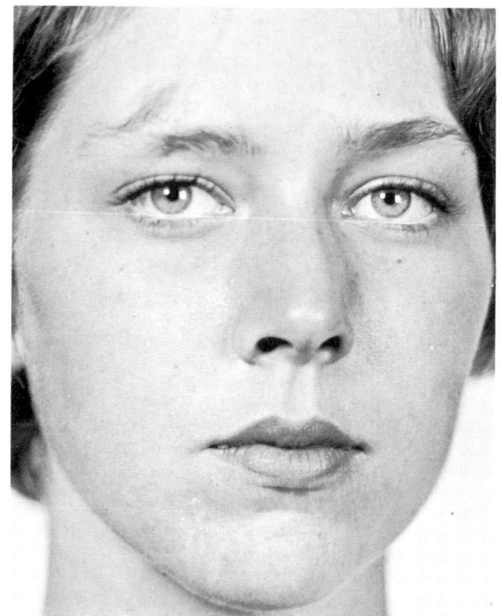

Figure 63. Misplaced eyebrow following suture of facial laceration. Eyebrows should not be shaved because they are important landmarks in locating incisions and in the repair of soft tissue lacerations.

patient's hair. In this respect, it is important to emphasize that eyebrows and lashes never should be cut (Fig. 63). First of all, they make excellent landmarks for suturing. Second, the slow growth of these hairs would tend to condemn the patient to a long period of poor appearance. The hair can be prepared adequately with the usual detergent solutions.

Skin Preparation

Draping of the patient should allow generous access to the operative field. In most cases, the eyes are left in the operative field for observation. To protect the eyes against chemical conjunctivitis from accidental exposure to detergents used on the face, methyl cellulose solution is helpful. If the operative procedure should involve danger of damage to the eyes, the lids can be pulled together easily with a small suture passed through the skin of the upper and lower lid margins.

Planning the Surgical Approach

The treatment of less extensive injuries may require only closed reduction and fixation by means of arch bars with intermaxillary rubber band traction. In severe cases, it may be necessary to use a combination of intermaxillary fixation and open reduction with direct bone wiring. When open reduction and intermaxillary fixation are done as a single procedure, the arch bars should be applied before beginning the open operation. The patient should be scrubbed and redraped for the open operative procedure.

Locations of incisions should be indicated on the skin with marking ink. To minimize scarring, it is desirable to plan incision lines in natural skin folds, or wrinkles, or in areas where the incisions will be obscured by bony prominences, e.g., below the inferior border of the mandible.

Incisions made within the brow heal with minimal scars. Incisions made in the neck or submandibular area should be made in or parallel to the flexion creases. Submandibular incisions result in inconspicuous scars if placed approximately 2 cm. below the border, in the shadow of the mandible. In the area of the lower eyelid, the wrinkle lines indicate the desirable location for incisions. To approach the infraorbital margin, the incision is best made low in order to avoid entering into the orbital fat. This is not dangerous, but the herniated fat in the operative field causes inconvenience during the surgical procedure.

Incisions in the region of the zygomatic arch should follow the natural lines of the skin. After passing through the subcutaneous tissues the dissection of the deeper structures should be done in the direction of the long axis of the branches of the seventh nerve. Glabellar incisions should be transverse, following the skin folds.

Extensive edema may distort the tissues and obscure the normal bony landmarks and flexion creases. Extra care should be taken to avoid misplacement of incisions. This is true especially for the mandible and upper cervical areas where misplaced incisions may result in unsightly scars on the face or over the mandible after edema subsides.

Operative Procedure

Before the incision is made the tissues should be infiltrated with an anesthetic solution containing epinephrine; a solution of 1 to 100,000 epinephrine will reduce bleeding, if a period of 10 to 15 minutes is permitted to elapse after the injection.

Lacerations over the site of the fracture may provide adequate exposure for open reduction. If inadequate, they should be lengthened in the line of the skin folds.

Observation of basic surgical principles will reduce postoperative complications. These principles include careful, aseptic handling of tissues, removal of foreign and devitalized matter, prevention of hematomas through adequate hemostasis, obliteration of dead space by careful closure of wounds in layers, precise closure of the skin with fine needles and sutures, and immobilization of the wound by splints or dressings when indicated.

If the acutely injured patient with many lacerations is in good general condition, it may be desirable to reduce the fractures and fix them by direct wiring through the wound. Reduction is followed by immediate closure of the wounds.

If the patient is in poor general condition, the wounds should be cleansed and loosely closed or covered with a dressing, and further management of the injuries should be deferred until the patient is a satisfactory surgical risk.

Postoperative Care

The habit of meticulous attention to all details of the postoperative care of the patient is a mark of character that distinguishes the accomplished surgeon.

Postoperative care is directed toward promotion of early and primary healing of tissues and prevention of infection. Frequent cleansing of the wound margins with 3 per cent hydrogen peroxide will prevent clots, crusts, wound maceration, and infection and will minimize scar formation. Fresh, light, sterile dressings should be applied after each cleansing of the wound.

The importance of adequate nutrition and vitamin administration has been demonstrated well by studies in wound healing and tissue repair. Early ambulation and return to normal physiologic activity is recommended practice.

The patient ought to be returned from the operating room to the recovery room or intensive care unit where he remains until he has complete control of his reflexes and has recovered sufficiently to be safely returned to his hospital room.

If the teeth are in fixation, the endotracheal tube may be left in place until the patient regains control of his reflexes. Immediately before extubation, a Levine tube may be passed into the stomach for aspiration of residual stomach contents. This precaution is designed to prevent aspiration if nausea and vomiting occur.

During hospitalization, suction equipment must be available to keep the respiratory tract free of blood and mucus. Even in those cases in which the patient vomits, adequate suctioning can remove most semisolid material. Suctioning of the pharynx by way of the nasal passage, using a soft rubber catheter, is quite effective. Even when the teeth are in tight occlusion there is sufficient space for the escape of fluids from the mouth.

The necessity for emergency removal of rubber bands by cutting with a pair of scissors is rarely required if adequate postoperative care has been administered.

Late Revision

When the results of primary surgery fail to meet the highest standards, secondary operations become necessary. Less-than-optimum results may be caused by infection, loss of tooth or bone structure, unsightly scarring, atrophy of underlying fat or subcutaneous tissues, loss of soft tissue, or nonunion or malunion of bone.

Corrective procedures include excision and revision of scars; restoration by means of bone, cartilage, or dermal fat grafts; and reconstruction of tissues lost due to injury or complications. Occlusal equilibration by selective grinding of the teeth or prosthetic dental replacements may be also part of the final rehabilitating process.

CHAPTER

4

TRACHEOTOMY

PART 1

GENERAL CONSIDERATIONS

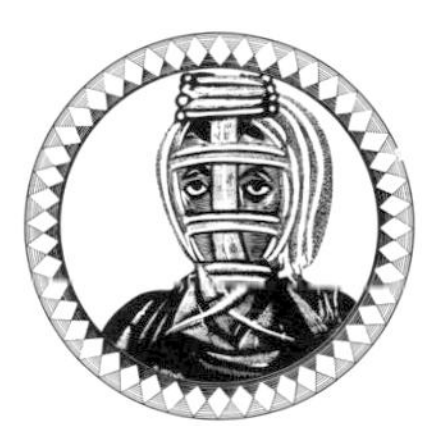

By definition tracheotomy* is the formation of an artificial opening into the trachea. In practice tracheotomy is indicated whenever the life of the patient is threatened by airway obstruction in or above the larynx. Obstruction may be due to the lodging of foreign bodies in the larynx, by laryngospasm, or by edema or tumors in the hypopharyngeal and supraglottic areas. Inadequate aeration also may result from malfunction of the muscles of respiration caused by tetanus, poisoning, poliomyelitis or other lesions of the central nervous system, or severe trauma to the head. Trauma, infection, or a tumor in the neck may damage or encroach upon the airway and result in obstruction.

Elective tracheotomy is important in the management of facial fractures. It provides an efficient and convenient route for the administration of an anesthetic, removes the anesthesiologist and the anesthetic equipment from the operative field, and in-

*Tracheostomy can be defined as the surgical formation of an opening into the trachea, the edges of the opening being sutured to an opening in the skin of the neck. If the term is defined in this way, it has a specific meaning and should not replace the old and well-founded term tracheotomy.

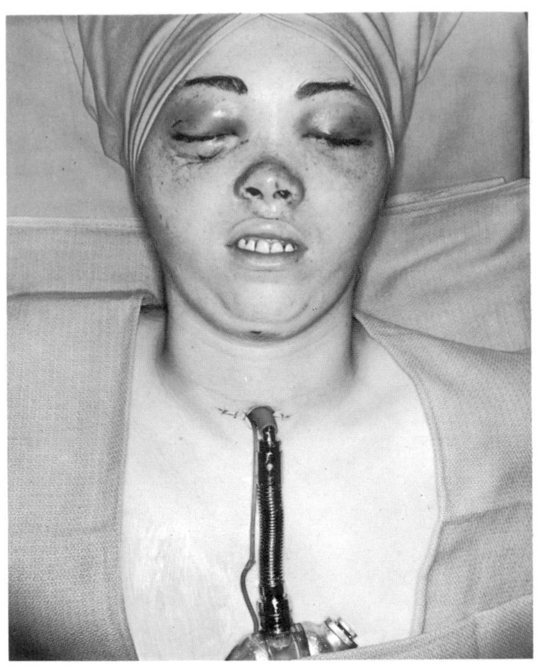

Figure 64. Patient with facial smash injury with multiple comminuted fractures of the middle third of the face. Anesthesia is administered by way of tracheotomy, leaving the entire facial area unencumbered for the surgical procedure.

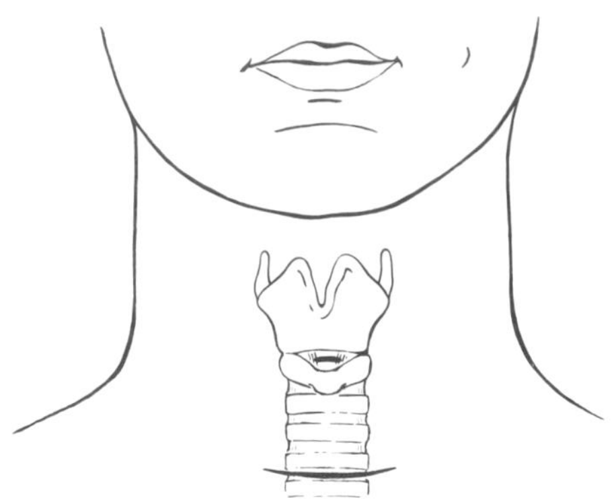

Figure 65. Diagram showing lines of incision for coniotomy (above) and inferior tracheotomy (below). Transverse incisions give adequate exposure and result in minimal postoperative scarring.

sures an adequate postoperative airway (Fig. 64). This surgical procedure is especially helpful during the postoperative course when intermaxillary fixation and nasal packing have been necessary.

Whenever it becomes evident that a patient may need a tracheotomy, or even when there is reasonable suspicion of such need, it is best to start the operative procedure immediately. There is small wisdom in waiting and turning an elective into an emergency procedure.

TYPES OF TRACHEOTOMY

There are two basic types of tracheotomy. Coniotomy, or superior tracheotomy, is performed above the thyroid isthmus through the cricothyroid ligament. Inferior tracheotomy is performed below or through the isthmus of the thyroid gland (Fig. 65).

Both types of tracheotomy offer significant advantages. Coniotomy is an emergency measure only; it is apt to produce undesirable complications, such as fibrosis, and renders more difficult the insertion and maintenance of the tracheal tube. As soon as possible, an inferior tracheotomy should be performed and the coniotomy repaired. If, however, the coniotomy has served its purpose (e.g., the removal of a foreign body above the level of the conic ligament), then the inferior tracheotomy would be superfluous. The inferior approach is the method of choice in most instances of elective tracheotomy.

POSITIONING THE PATIENT FOR TRACHEOTOMY

Whether the tracheotomy is an elective or an emergency procedure, positioning of the patient is important. The patient should be placed in the dorsal recumbent position with the shoulders elevated on sandbags or pillows and the neck in extreme extension. In this way the tracheal structures are brought to a satisfactory level for the operative procedure.

CONIOTOMY (SUPERIOR TRACHEOTOMY)

Coniotomy is most effective in cases in which assistance is not available and the patient is in extreme need of an airway. The high tracheotomy is performed through the cricothyroid (conic) ligament. (It is through this area that a large needle with a large lumen is sometimes inserted to provide an airway.) Although complications are more likely to occur with this method than with inferior tracheotomy, it is extremely effective in emergencies. The procedure is easy to perform as the overlying subcutaneous tissues are thin and the isthmus of the thyroid and the major vessels are not encountered.

Coniotomy, also known as intercricothyroid laryngotomy, was performed and described first by the French surgeon and anatomist Vicq d'Azyr (1805). Later it was described in detail by Tandler (1916). The operation was popularized in the United States by Sicher in 1949 (Sicher, 1960).

Technique of Coniotomy

With the patient in the dorsal recumbent position and the neck extended, the cricothyroid notch is located with the index finger. This is readily done by passing the finger from the chin down over the anterior midline surface of the neck (Fig. 66*A*). The first prominence encountered will be the thyroid cartilage, and a short distance below, the finger will drop into a shallow notch. This is the space between the thyroid and cricoid cartilages (Fig. 66*B*). With the palpating finger firmly pressed against the larynx, the cut is made quickly, transversely through the skin and the cricothyroid membrane. To avoid passing the knife too deeply and injuring the posterior wall of the larynx, a short grip should be taken on the knife with the thumb and index finger so that only about one-half inch of the blade is free. The incision through the cricothyroid ligament should extend approximately one-fourth inch. When the elastic cricothyroid ligament is cut transversely, the vertical fibers retract and insure patency of the opening.

The patient should be watched carefully, until he is placed under continuous expert care, in order to prevent the skin margins from occluding the opening. To avoid blocking of the opening into the larynx by the skin, adhesive tape can be used. If convenient, the skin margins may be separated by fixation with sutures. Since there are no vessels of consequence overlying the cricothyroid ligament, postoperative bleeding usually offers no problem. If bleeding seems to be a disturbing factor, it can be controlled by digital compression.

The results of coniotomy are dramatic, and the procedure has been responsible for the saving of many lives that otherwise might have been lost.

INFERIOR TRACHEOTOMY

If time permits, inferior tracheotomy is the method of choice in emergency situations when the operating conditions are favorable.

Most writers upon the subject of tracheotomy state that there are no significant structures that are likely to complicate the performance of inferior tracheotomy. It must be mentioned, however, that there are occasional anomalies of the venous system in this area and that the anatomic structures are seldom constant. Communicating vessels between the external jugular veins may be encountered at any level. In children or barrel-chested adults, with horizontal first rib structures, these veins will be found at a higher level.

Generally, communicating veins are not troublesome if identified, ligated, and cut,

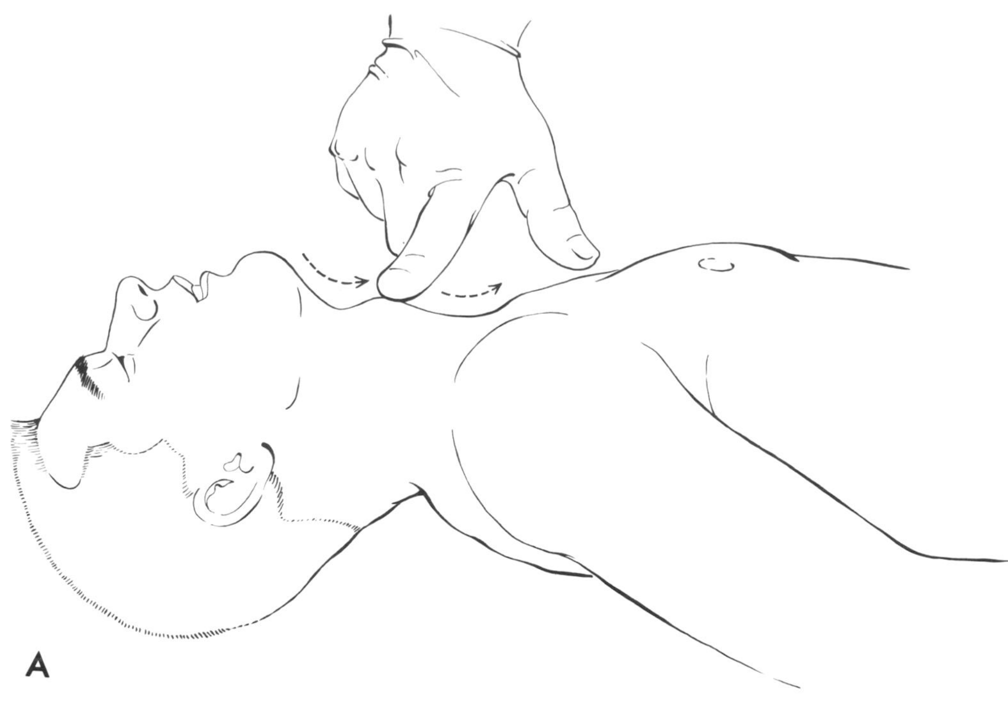
A

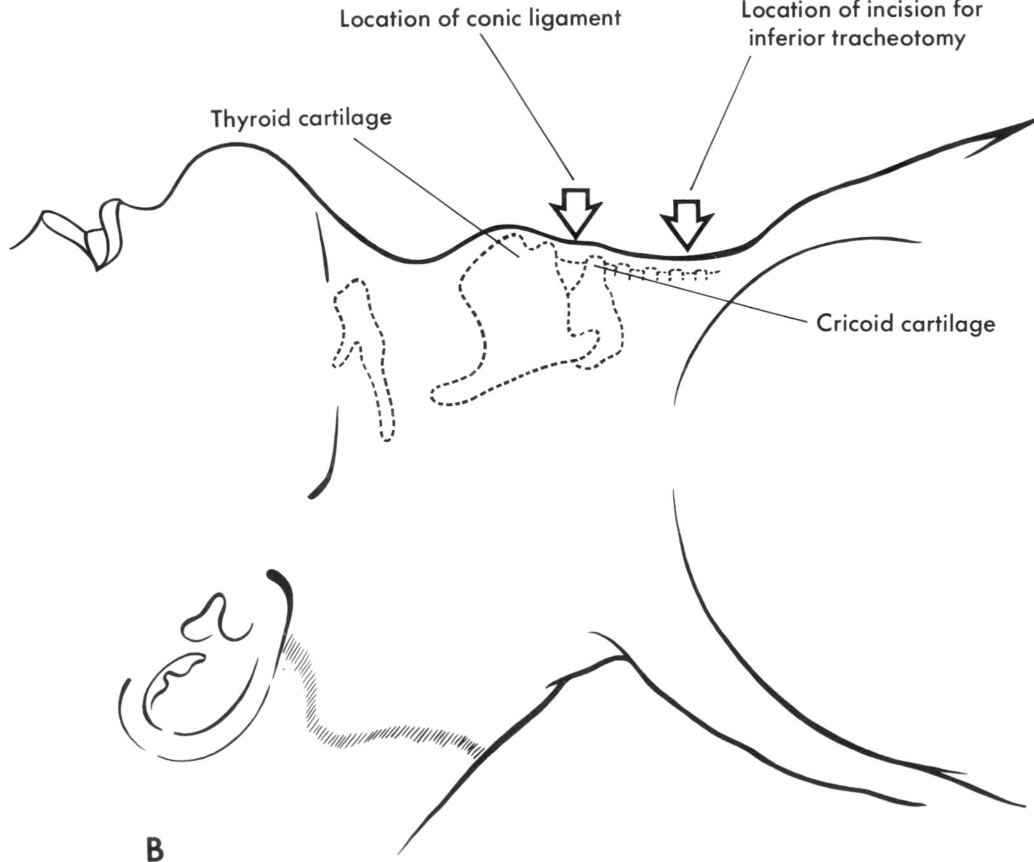
Location of conic ligament
Location of incision for inferior tracheotomy
Thyroid cartilage
Cricoid cartilage
B

but they can cause difficulty if inadvertently cut in the course of the dissection. When cut, the veins retract into the soft tissues and make bleeding difficult to control.

Sicher (1960) points out that the inferior thyroid veins are not always lateral to the midline. Sometimes large, distended veins may be found in the midline.

In some cases a low thyroid artery may pass in front of the trachea to the middle part of the thyroid gland. Although this anomalous artery usually arises from the arch of the aorta, sometimes it is a branch of the brachiocephalic artery or a branch of another of the other larger arteries in the base of the neck.

The inferior thyroid veins may be distended in patients suffering from severe dyspnea. This distention results from the lack of "milking action" of the surrounding musculature, which action is incident to normal respiration. The presence of such engorged veins makes inferior tracheotomy more difficult in emergency situations.

In adults, the brachiocephalic artery, contained in the same fascial layers as are the inferior thyroid veins, is rarely seen. But in children the heart and its great vessels are located at a higher level. Difficulty in this area can be avoided by blunt dissection, especially when passing through the pretracheal space, and by careful retraction of tissues with smooth retractors.

If the airway of the injured patient is partially obstructed because of hypopharyngeal edema, it is unwise to administer drugs that might decrease the reflex activity of the respiratory tract. If the tracheotomy is to be performed as an elective procedure in a patient with a patent airway, the usual preoperative medication can be administered.

Marking of the skin incision should be done with the patient's neck in normal position. When marked in the extended position, the incision is apt to be too low, and this results in skin tension on the tracheotomy tube and possible displacement of the tube.

A transverse incision in a skin fold of the neck gives good exposure for carrying out the tracheotomy and results in the least noticeable postoperative scar.

The operation may be performed under local or general anesthesia. Local anesthesia should be administered by infiltrating the area of the incision and by injecting an anesthetic into the midline and the anterior wall of the trachea. An anesthetic solution containing epinephrine prolongs anesthesia and also is effective in reducing hemorrhage. Tracheotomy may be performed with general anesthesia using oral endotracheal intubation. The endotracheal tube should be removed at the moment when the tracheotomy tube is inserted into the trachea.

Technique of Inferior Tracheotomy

The transverse incision should be made in one of the skin lines of the neck overlying the

Figure 66. Method of locating position for coniotomy and inferior tracheotomy. *A*. The palpating finger is passed from the chin downward along the anterior surface of the neck. The prominence of the thyroid cartilage is palpated easily. Immediately below the prominence the notch between the thyroid and cricoid cartilage can be felt. This is the location through which coniotomy is carried out. The tracheal rings can be palpated below the cricoid cartilage. *B*. Location for coniotomy and inferior tracheotomy.

third or fourth tracheal ring. The incision may be 3 to 6 cm. long, depending upon the size of the patient and the thickness of anterior neck structures.

The transverse incision is carried through the skin and subcutaneous fascia to the level of the superficial cervical fascia. The dissection is continued by blunt dissection with scissors through the linea alba to separate the "strap" muscles of the neck. Any transverse veins encountered should be identified and retracted. If they interfere with exposure, they should be clamped, severed, and ligated. Dissection should be sufficient to identify the cricoid cartilage and the first four tracheal rings.

To expose the trachea, blunt retractors of moderate depth are required in order to provide retraction of tissues and protection to the vessels immediately below the level of the dissection.

The trachea is stabilized on each side by means of a small tissue hook. With the tracheal rings accurately identified by palpation and direct vision, a blade with the cutting edge directed cephalically is used to make an incision through the fourth tracheal ring. The blade is then carried upward through the third tracheal ring. To avoid cutting the posterior wall, the blade should not be inserted into the trachea more than one-quarter inch; a tracheoesophageal fistula may be produced accidentally, especially in children. The intercartilaginous fibers between the third and fourth rings should be cut, in a transverse direction, a length equal to that of the vertical cut.

If it is anticipated that the tracheotomy will be in use more than one week, a section of tracheal tissue should be excised to create a circular opening large enough to accommodate the tracheotomy tube. If the need is not expected to exceed a few days, the structures at the angles of the cruciate incision should be pulled forward and the tube inserted. A soft rubber catheter attached to suction equipment should always be available immediately to remove any blood or other fluid that might have escaped into the trachea.

The bore of the tracheotomy tube should be about three-quarters the diameter of the trachea. Its length should be sufficient to pass through the soft tissues and into the trachea far enough to prevent spontaneous ejection. Excessive length and curvature of the tube may cause contact with and erosion of the tracheal wall. A tube that is too long could pass into one of the main stem bronchi and cause obstruction and atelectasis.

An obturator is used during insertion. The instant the obturator is removed, the cannula should be inserted and the system inspected immediately to make certain that the flow of air is adequate.

The wound should be closed in layers, in a funnel-like manner, with the larger aspect of the opening toward the skin surface. This will assure adequate leakage of air around the tube, prevent subcutaneous emphysema, and permit easier removal of the tube for cleaning.

When elective tracheotomy is done under general anesthesia, one of three techniques may be used for intubation. Some anesthesiologists choose to intubate through the open tracheotomy wound using a special short-cuffed endotracheal tube. Others prefer to use the tracheotomy tube with a special attachment for connecting the anesthesia equipment. Still others pass the endotracheal tube through the outer tracheotomy tube.

Fabric tape is used to fix the tracheotomy tube to the neck. If the tube is to be connected with the anesthetic equipment, it should be fixed to the neck with sutures. At the termination of the anesthesia, the sutures are removed and the tube held with fabric tape.

POSTOPERATIVE CARE

The patient with a tracheotomy tube requires constant attentive care to keep him comfortable and assure continuation of an adequate airway. During the first few days, special nursing care should be available. Aspiration of the trachea should be done as frequently as necessary with a soft rubber catheter rotated gently upon insertion with the Y tube open, as advocated by Glas, King, and Lui (1962) (Fig. 67). While the removal of secretions is advised, it is important to avoid excessive suctioning, for this may produce trauma to the lining of the trachea.

Humidity is required to prevent the formation of inspissated plugs of mucus and encrusted blood clots. Humidified air or oxygen may be administered in the form of a mist and concentrated over the tracheotomy opening by a small plastic hood tied to the patient's neck with fabric tape. Alevaire with saline assists mucolytic action.

To foster lysis of the gluelike mucus, Meade (1961) recommends that an isotonic saline solution (0.45 per cent) be dripped into the trachea at a rate of four drops per minute.

Other points suggested in tracheotomy care are (Mörch, 1960):

1. Wash the hands thoroughly before and after manipulation.
2. Use sterile catheters and use them only once before resterilizing.
3. Have at least ten sterile catheters at the bedside.
4. Do not touch the distal part of the catheter with the hands. The catheter should touch only the interior of the tube.
5. Separate catheters should be available for oral-nasal suction.
6. The lumen of the catheter should be flushed with sterile water or saline to clear during use.
7. Only brief attempts, for 10 to 15 seconds, should be made at aspiration. The patient should be allowed to have a short rest between aspirations.

Since the patient is not able to speak, a pad of paper and pencil at the bedside will enable him to communicate his wants and

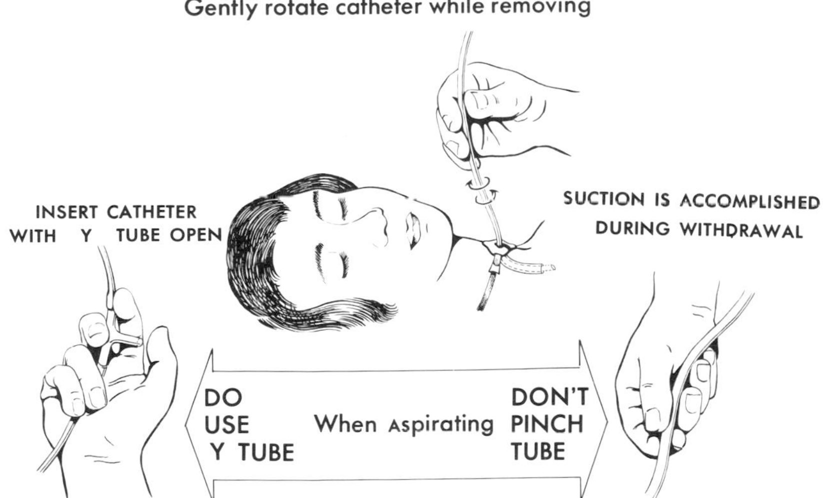

Figure 67. The correct and incorrect methods for tracheal aspiration. (After Glas, King, and Lui.)

needs. The patient may need help with feeding and may require sedation. After a few days, the patient will learn to manage without special aid. He may be taught to speak by placing a finger over the cannula opening.

The airway of the patient with a facial fracture is usually adequate upon removal of nasal packing and substitution of intermaxillary wires for rubber bands. The patient should then be able to speak and breathe through the spaces around and between the teeth. The tracheotomy tube may then be removed.

Prior to removal of the tube, it is a good precaution to test the patient's ability to breathe through his nose and mouth by placing a cork in the tracheotomy tube opening. If the patient can maintain an adequate airway for two or three hours with the tube plugged, it is safe to remove the tracheotomy tube.

The tracheotomy opening usually will close without operative intervention. When the tube has been in for less than one week, the opening will close in three to five days. Even in long-standing tracheotomy cases, the opening will close in one week to ten days. A small dressing will protect the opening until the wound heals.

COMPLICATIONS OF TRACHEOTOMY

Complications in as many as 30 per cent of the patients have been reported in some large series of cases with this seemingly simple, safe operative procedure. Complications may be classified under those occurring during the course of the operation, those occurring during the postoperative period, and those occurring several weeks or months after removal of the tracheotomy tube.

Operative Complications

1. Severe hemorrhage may occur from neck vessels cut during the course of the operation. Bleeding may be difficult to control if exposure is inadequate and assistance is not available.
2. The cricothyroid cartilage may be inadvertently damaged by cutting.
3. Through carelessness or inadequate exposure, a tracheoesophageal fistula may result if a cut is made through the posterior wall into the esophagus.
4. Damage to the pleura of one or both lung apices may result in pneumothorax.
5. The innominate artery may be cut, resulting in exsanguinating hemorrhage.

Postoperative Complications

1. Secondary hemorrhage may result from infection or erosion of a vessel.
2. Emphysema may spread through the subcutaneous tissues of the neck and the mediastinum.
3. The tracheotomy tube may become dislodged if it is not securely fixed to the neck or if the skin incision is too high or too low in relationship to the opening into the trachea.
4. During reinsertion of the tube after cleansing or following its avulsion, it may be placed outside the trachea in the structures of the neck.
5. Wound infections may occur.
6. If the tracheotomy tube is curved too much, it may result in erosion of the trachea, or if too long it may rest upon the carina and result in persistent coughing and erosion.
7. A tracheoesophageal fistula may result from erosion due to pressure of the tube against the common wall between the trachea and esophagus.

8. Aerophagia may result owing to pressure of the tube against the esophageal wall. The patient has a sensation that something is present in the upper esophagus and continually swallows air, which may cause distress, abdominal distention, gastrointestinal atony, paralytic ileus, or death. Glas, King, and Lui (1962) reported two such deaths in a study of 80 cases.

9. Recurrent obstruction may result from the collection of blood, purulent material, or mucus secretions in the tube.

10. Ulcerative tracheobronchitis may follow tracheotomy as a result of aspiration of mucus plugs, secretions, blood, or infected material.

Delayed Secondary Complications

1. Unsightly scars may occur in the line of incision, especially if a vertical skin incision has been made. An unsightly scar may occur following prolonged use of tracheotomy tubes. The scar becomes adherent to the trachea and moves with the trachea during swallowing.

2. Sloughing of the tracheal cartilages may result in tracheoatresia or stenosis several weeks or months following removal of the tracheotomy tube.

Most complications can be avoided by careful surgery and meticulous postoperative care.

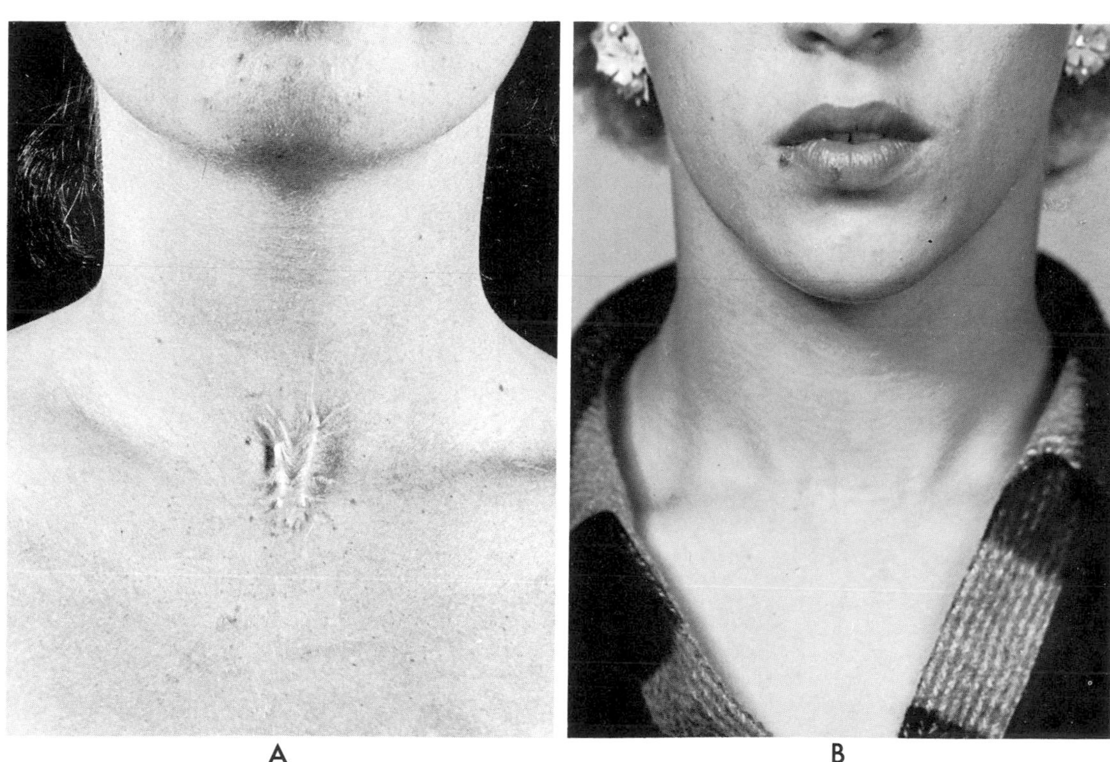

Figure 68. *A.* Unsightly scar from tracheotomy done through vertical incision. The opening was maintained for 12 days. The multiple radiating scars were the result of prolonged retention of the sutures. A transverse scar of this magnitude would be much easier to correct. *B.* Transverse tracheotomy scar on a patient in whom multiple facial fractures were reduced under endotracheal anesthesia administered through the tracheotomy. The transverse incision results in minimal deformity and is suitable if revision becomes necessary.

After removal of the tracheotomy tube, induration and fibrosis of adjacent tissues will be noted and a depressed scar may follow closure of the wound. In most cases, the scar will become less noticeable within a few months.

In some cases, scar contracture may bind the skin to the fascia overlying the trachea. This can be corrected by excision of the scar to the level of the trachea, identification and accurate approximation of the fascia and strap muscles, followed by accurate closure of the subcutaneous tissue and skin.

Correction of transverse neck scars usually gives satisfactory cosmetic results. However, a tracheotomy performed through a vertical incision may result in scar deformity in which it is difficult to attain a good result by revision (Fig. 68 *A*, *B*). Z-plasty procedures are used to rotate the vertical line of scar and to prevent recurrent contracture. This method leads to cosmetic improvement but increases the total length of the scar. For secondary correction it is more desirable to have a long transverse scar than a short, vertical scar.

Tracheotomy can be an exceedingly serious operation with complications in up to 30 per cent of the patients and a mortality of 3 per cent (Musselman, 1962). When performed carefully and methodically, tracheotomy is a safe procedure with benefits far outweighing any possible complications.

Tracheotomy

PART 2

OPERATIVE TECHNIQUE

Tracheotomy is classified generally among the simpler surgical procedures. The technical ease with which it may be accomplished is not an indication of its importance in emergency situations as a lifesaving procedure or electively as a significant adjunct to the management of extensive facial injuries.

The need for judicious and careful performance of tracheotomy has introduced factors of safety, convenience, and success to operative procedures that previously were impossible or, at best, extremely difficult to perform. These factors now benefit the patient with relatively small discomfort and with only occasional complications. Tracheotomy, nevertheless, is not performed without some danger or the possibility of serious complications. However, the benefits far outweigh these perils.

In the following pages, techniques are described for the performance of tracheotomy as an elective or an emergency procedure. Both low tracheotomy and coniotomy (high tracheotomy) are shown in step-by-step illustrations.

TECHNIQUE OF INFERIOR TRACHEOTOMY

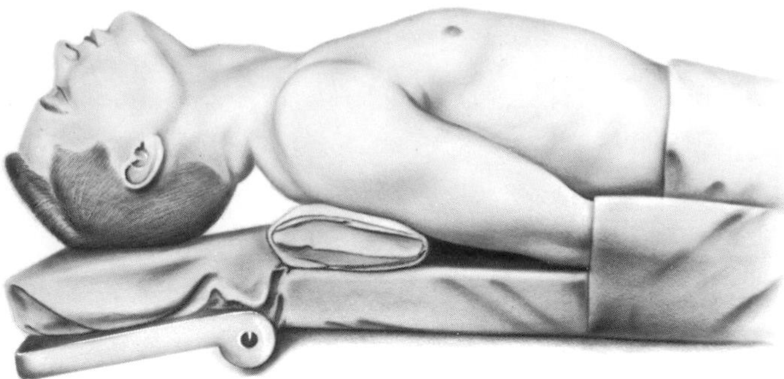

1.

Fig. 69. The patient is placed in the dorsal recumbent position with the neck extended as far as possible and the shoulders elevated and supported by a firm pillow or folded sheet. This placement on the table positions the trachea properly. If the index finger is passed down from the chin, in the midline, the first prominence encountered is the larynx; farther down is a small dip and a second but less prominent elevation which is the cricoid cartilage. It is between the thyroid and the cricoid cartilages that the coniotomy or high tracheotomy is performed. By passing the finger downward still farther, the trachea can be palpated in the midline between the cricoid cartilage and the sternal notch. The low tracheotomy is performed in this area.

2.

Fig. 70. The low tracheotomy incision is made below the isthmus of the thyroid gland through the third and fourth tracheal rings. If the thyroid gland is encountered in the approach to the trachea, it should be retracted upward or partially incised if necessary. The incision through the skin is made in the transverse direction or parallel to one of the lines of the skin of the neck.

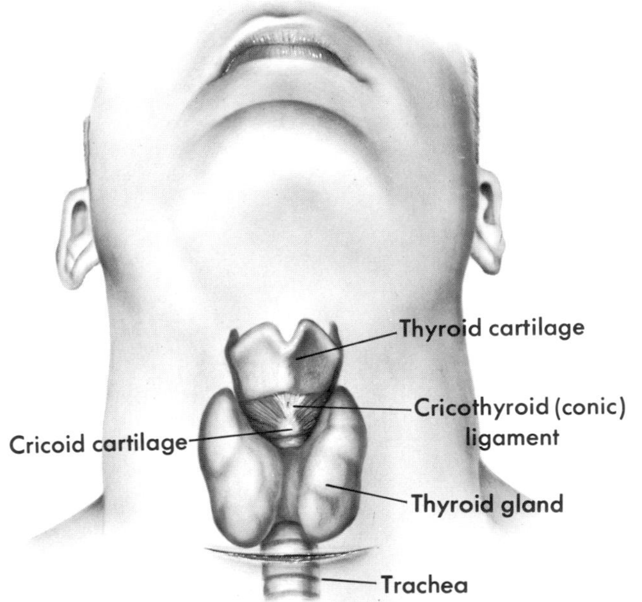

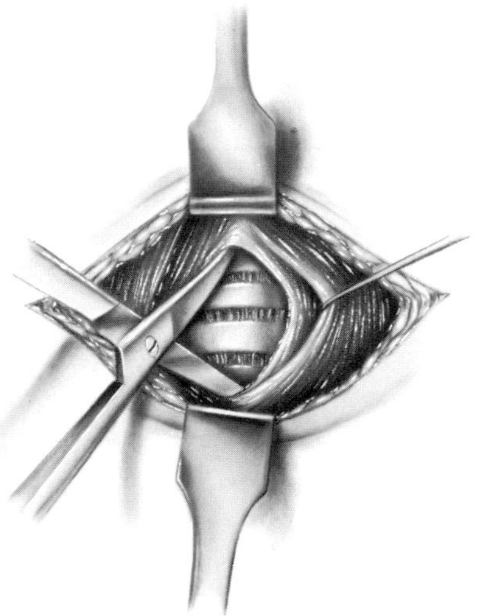

3.

Fig. 71. After incising transversely through the skin, the subcutaneous fascia, and the superficial cervical fascia, the dissection is performed in a vertical direction by blunt dissection with a scissors through the linea alba. The glistening fibers of the trachea come into view. Dissection through the linea alba is relatively bloodless. Exposure of the area should be adequate so that bleeding, if it occurs, can be managed without difficulty. The strap muscles have been separated to gain access to the anterior wall of the trachea.

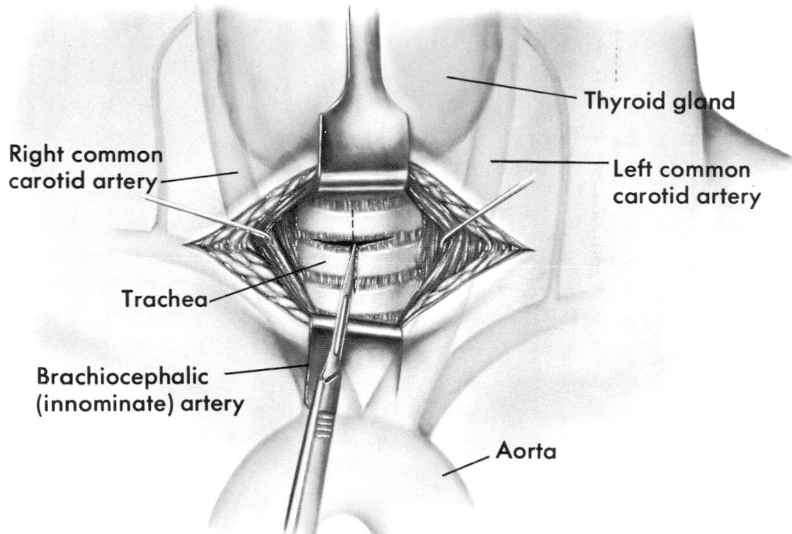

4.

Fig. 72. With the cutting edge of the knife directed upward, the fourth tracheal ring is incised and the knife is carried upward through the third tracheal ring. In children the trachea is narrow, and insertion of the knife too deeply may injure the posterior tracheal wall and the esophagus. A transverse incision, approximately the same length as the vertical incision, is made between the third and fourth tracheal rings. To prevent rotation of the trachea during incision, it is stabilized by hooks, which engage the tracheal fascia or tracheal rings.

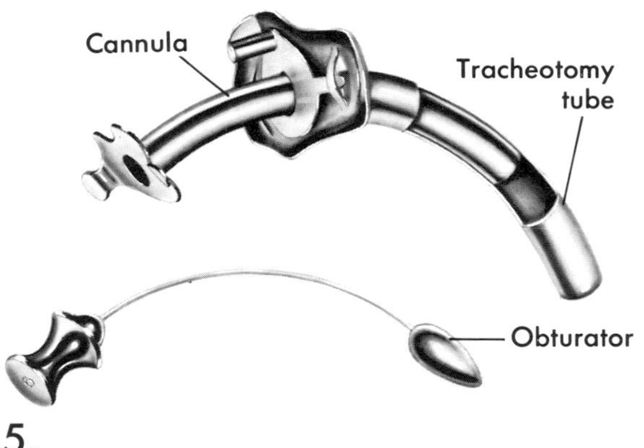

5.

Fig. 73. The tracheotomy tube must be selected carefully for size. Its circumference should be approximately three-fourths that of the lumen of the trachea. The length of the tube is determined by the thickness of the overlying soft tissue and the distance the tube is to be inserted into the trachea. A tube that is too curved or too long may cause complications. Tracheotomy tubes are available in both metal and plastic materials.

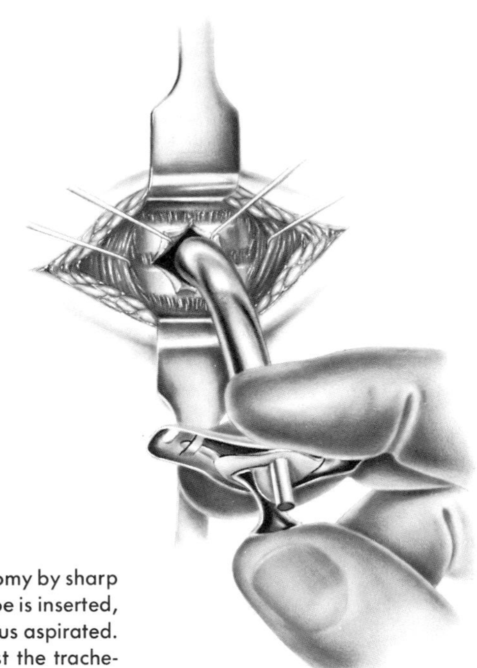

6.

Fig. 74. Retraction of tissues around the opening of the tracheotomy by sharp hooks is advisable and is helpful in inserting the tube. When the tube is inserted, the obturator should be removed immediately and blood and mucus aspirated. All retractors are released and the tissues allowed to fall against the tracheotomy tube.

7.

Fig. 75. A tracheotomy tube that is too long may irritate or erode the carina or extend into one of the main stem bronchi. Such complications are serious.

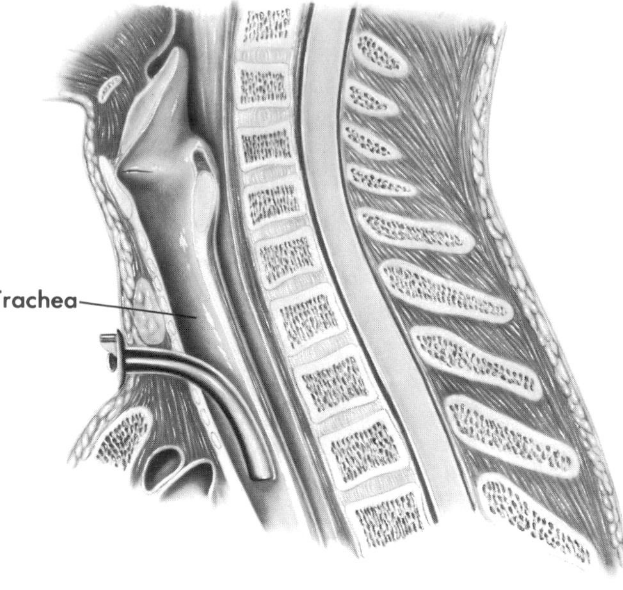

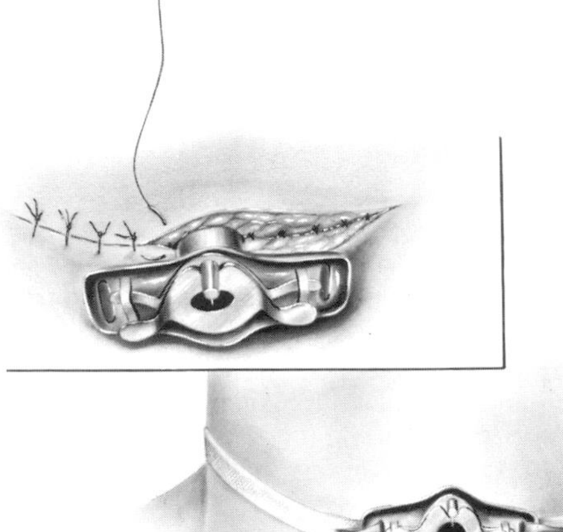

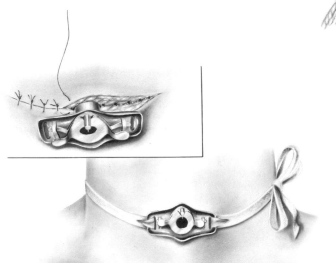

8.

Fig. 76. The wound is closed loosely in layers utilizing absorbable sutures for the deeper structures. The skin is closed with nylon on atraumatic needles. If anesthetic equipment is to be attached to or passed through the tracheotomy tube, the tube should be sutured to the skin temporarily. If the anesthetic is not administered through the tube, the tube can be held by fabric tape tied firmly but comfortably about the neck.

TECHNIQUE OF SUPERIOR TRACHEOTOMY (CONIOTOMY)

9.

Fig. 77. Technique of coniotomy. With a short grasp on the knife, to avoid cutting too deeply, a quick, transverse incision is made through the overlying skin and through the cricothyroid membrane. The technique is useful in cases of extreme emergency. The cricothyroid ligament is subcutaneous, and there are no important structures and few vessels in this region. The opening will remain patent because of the elastic vertical fibers of the cricothyroid ligament.

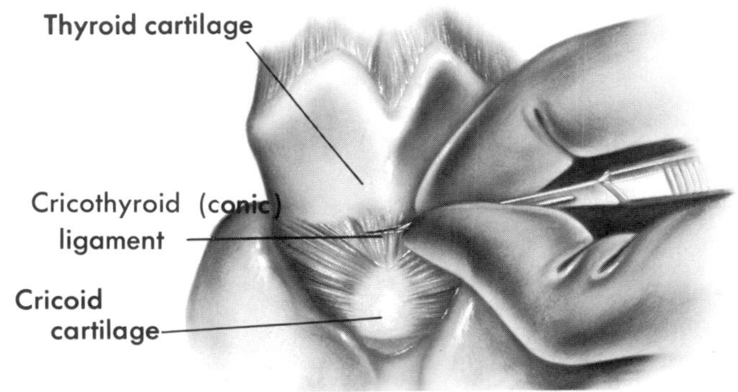

CHAPTER

5

OCCLUSION AND INTERMAXILLARY FIXATION

PART 1

GENERAL CONSIDERATIONS

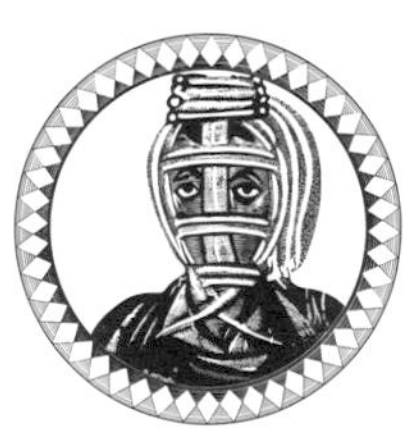

Occlusion is a dynamic concept, and, according to Sicher, occlusal positions are all those in which contact between some or all upper and lower teeth occurs. Median occlusion represents the interdigitation of mandibular teeth against maxillary teeth. To assure proper healing of fracture sites, median occlusion must be understood thoroughly, because reduction and fixation of many facial fractures depends upon restoration and maintenance of median occlusion for a given period of time.

Maxillary and mandibular first molars are guides for determining the correct establishment of median occlusion. A simple rule is in seeing that the mesiobuccal cusps of the maxillary first molars interdigitate with the mesiobuccal grooves of the mandibular first molars, with slight overbite and slight overjet of the anterior teeth. The teeth in the mandibular and maxillary arches should be arranged in such a manner that, when in median occlusion, the mandibular arch fits against the maxillary arch as a concave surface of a saucer fits into the convex surface of another. This line of occlusion is known as the "occlusal plane."

THE SIGNIFICANCE OF OCCLUSION

The primary objective in reduction of facial bone fractures is to return the structures to a normal position of function and contour. This means restoration of normal occlusal relations through proper positioning of the teeth and bony structures. Since the teeth bear an important relation to the alveolar processes and to the main structures of the maxilla and mandible, and since this relation is fixed and constant, the establishment of normal intermaxillary occlusion demands that the bone fragments to which the teeth are attached also be in relatively normal relation.

The normal intermaxillary relation is significant as a guide to repositioning the bones of the maxillary and zygomatic compounds in multiple facial fractures. Reestablishing fractured condyles of the mandible in their normal position (craniomandibular articulation) serves as a starting point for the reconstruction and repositioning of all facial bones.

THE TEETH

From infancy to adult life, two dentitions normally appear. The first, composed of 20 teeth, is called the deciduous dentition (milk teeth, primary teeth, baby teeth, temporary teeth). The permanent (or secondary) dentition is composed of 32 teeth.

The primary function of the dental apparatus is, of course, the mastication of food. Secondary functions include preservation of facial dimensions, aid in phonation, and esthetics of appearance.

The teeth are described according to general function. The anterior teeth are the incisors and canines. The incisors are cutting teeth and have sharp, chisel-like edges. The canines are spear-shaped and are used for apprehension and tearing. The posterior teeth are the premolars and molars; their function is grinding and comminuting.

It is important to note the functional gradation of the teeth from the anterior to the posterior parts of the mouth, starting with the sharp cutters and gradually blending to the wide, heavy, grinding teeth. This difference in function is reflected in the roots of the teeth. Incisors and canines have one root. Premolars have one or two. The molars in the mandibular arch have two roots and those in the maxillary arch have three. Thus, the heavier effects of mastication are readily distributed to the bones of the skull. The forces and stresses applied to the molar teeth are absorbed and transmitted to the base of the skull through a system of strong, massive buttresses—these are represented anatomically by the thick areas of the bony facial structures.

The teeth are seated in the alveolar processes of the mandible and maxilla with each root having its own socket (alveolus or phatne). Lining each alveolus is a layer of compact bone, the lamina dura.

In discussions of the crown of a tooth, two terms are commonly used. The anatomic crown includes all of the tooth covered by enamel. The clinical crown is that part of the anatomic crown that is seen by the examiner. In a young person the gingiva covers part of the anatomic crown. As the person grows older, recession of the gingiva may take place, exposing more of the anatomic crown and sometimes even part of the root. Then the anatomic crown and the exposed part of the root become the clinical crown.

Immediately beneath the enamel and cementum, the dentin (dentine) is found. Extending through both the root and the crown, the dentin surrounds a pulp-containing cavity. This cavity is divided into two portions: a wider coronal portion, which is the pulp chamber, and a narrower portion known as the root canal. If there is more than one root, each has its own canal.

Another important dental structure is the periodontal ligament (peridental membrane, pericementum, dental periosteum, alveolodental membrane). The integrity of this ligament is essential for the retention of the teeth in their alveoli. On occasions the tooth becomes solidly adherent to the alveolus (ankylosis). More commonly, however, disintegration of the ligament occurs, causing loosening of the teeth. This disintegration is the underlying process of what is known commonly as pyorrhea alveolaris (more properly termed periodontoclasia).

Even though the deciduous dentition is sometimes referred to as the "temporary teeth," one should not accept this term literally. The deciduous teeth normally are in use for five years (say, from age 2 to age 7), and some deciduous teeth are intact for about 12 years.

Deciduous teeth are necessary to a child's well-being. Their premature loss leads to improper mastication of food and jeopardizes normal development of the jaws and of the permanent dentition.

Though there are many minute differences between permanent and deciduous teeth, these are of little practical importance. The permanent and deciduous teeth have comparable morphologies. The principal differences between the deciduous and the permanent teeth are these:

1. Deciduous teeth are smaller.
2. Deciduous teeth usually are lighter in color.
3. The crowns of deciduous teeth are more bell-shaped and their necks are more constricted.
4. Deciduous teeth have a larger pulp chamber and wider root canals.
5. The roots of deciduous teeth are physiologically resorbed; the roots of the permanent teeth are not normally resorbed but may show resorption under stress (as in orthodontic movement).
6. There are 20 deciduous teeth and 32 permanent teeth.
7. Deciduous teeth include no premolars or third molars.
8. The deciduous dentition normally contains ten teeth in each arch. One arch has two central incisors, two lateral incisors, two canines, two first molars, and two second molars.
9. The permanent dentition has 16 teeth in each arch, two central incisors, two lateral incisors, two canines, two first premolars, two second premolars, two first molars, two second molars, and two third molars. The third molars, however, may never erupt, and may become impacted "wisdom teeth."

Mixed Dentition

From the age of 6 to 14 years a mixed dentition is present: deciduous and permanent teeth are present in both the maxillary and the mandibular arches. Individuals in this age group in whom facial fractures occur require special care in arch bar application to their teeth. During the phase of mixed dentition some deciduous teeth may be firmly fixed to the alveoli while others may be in various stages of resorption. Some may be very loose. Likewise, the permanent teeth are in various stages of eruption; some are completely erupted, others partially erupted. The practical application of this knowledge means avoiding ligation of loose deciduous teeth and partially erupted permanent teeth.

Teeth that have become loose as a result of trauma may have to be extracted if there is danger of avulsion and aspiration. Loose (or avulsed) teeth resulting from trauma may be transplanted and will reattach to the periodontal membrane if treatment is instituted soon after injury and major damage has not occurred to the alveolus or the tooth. Transplanted permanent teeth require firm fixation. Seldom is transplantation of deciduous teeth indicated. The complete deciduous and permanent dentitions serve well for arch bar fixation. However, in the mixed dentition, supplementary methods of arch bar fixation may be required (see Figs. 104, 105, and 106), as in the case of dental arches with scattered anodontia. Some stages of mixed dentition present the same picture as do arches with scattered anodontia. Loose deciduous teeth and teeth in stages of early eruption are useless for fixation and, for practical purposes, may be considered as areas of anodontia.

APPLICATION OF ARCH BARS AND INTERMAXILLARY TRACTION

Although reports of teeth being ligated one to another go back as far as 2500 years (Hippocrates), the practicable principle of intermaxillary fixation was not formulated until approximately 1887. Gilmer (1887) revived intermaxillary wiring as a method of fracture management (Fig. 78). This was a major step forward in accurate fracture management, which management requires return of the bone fragments to their proper relations and fixation of the teeth during healing.

No part of the human body is like the jaws in having appendages that project from bone, appendages that may be realigned for perfect or near-

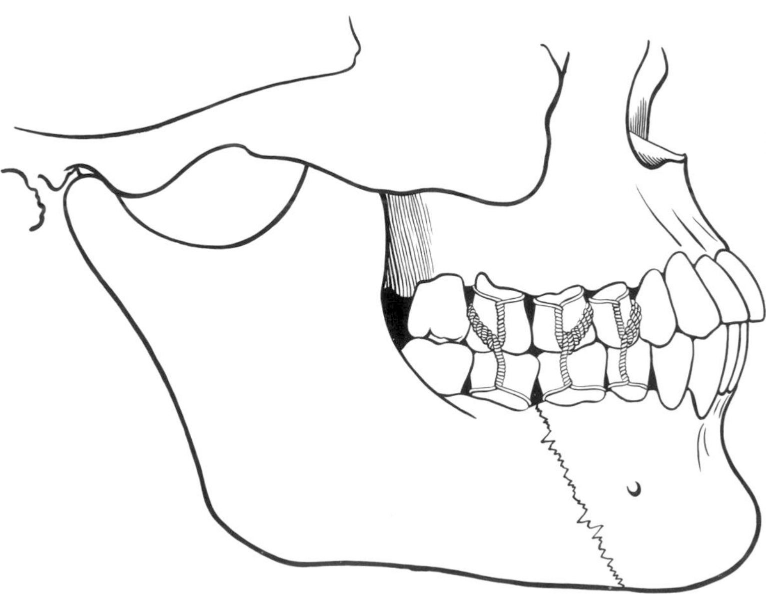

Figure 78. The Gilmer method of intermaxillary fixation with direct wiring between the maxillary and mandibular teeth. This method holds the teeth securely in position but has the disadvantage of requiring complete removal of the wires to open the mouth in emergency situations or to test the healing at the fracture site.

perfect reduction of fractures and locked into position. This surgically convenient feature is peculiar to the mandible and maxilla. Proper intermaxillary fixation is one of the most important factors in treating facial fractures, and the accurate fixation of the teeth is the keystone.

Although some clinicians choose to use intramedullary bone pin fixation or external pin fixation for mandibular fractures, we consider this to be unnecessary in cases in which reestablishment and fixation of occlusion would suffice to replace and fix the bone fragments. The use of intramedullary or external pin fixation is unwarranted if one merely has in mind achieving the questionable advantage of facilitating opening and closing of the mouth for eating. It is particularly unjustified in view of possible complications such as malunion, malocclusion, malfunction, and infection.

If the dentition is adequate for arch bar application and if the fractures of the mandible are multiple and oblique, with displacement, then intermaxillary fixation alone may not be adequate. In such a case, intermaxillary fixation should be used in conjunction with open reduction. This method is better than intramedullary pin fixation.

Intermaxillary traction is important in establishing and maintaining occlusal relations during the period of healing of the fracture. In some instances, especially when the fracture is of many days' duration, it is difficult to accomplish complete reduction manually. Application of traction between the arches with rubber band traction force will, in a few hours, stretch and move the fracture callus or fibrous tissue between the bone segments sufficiently to permit the fragments to assume their normal relations, thus bringing the teeth into occlusion (Dingman, 1939).

Methods of attaching rubber bands to the dental arches are numerous. If we fail to discuss here any reader's favorite method, this is not to be regarded as a criticism of its merit (Figs. 79–81).

A prefabricated arch bar with hooks can be shaped to the outer surface of the upper and lower dental arches. The Erich arch bar, made of a malleable metal, fulfills this requirement (Fig. 82). It provides an effective, quick, and inexpensive method of at-

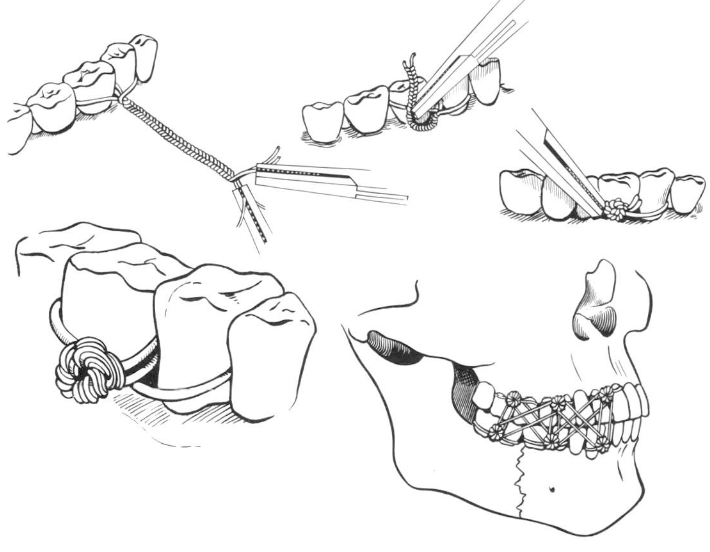

Figure 79. Steps in the construction of a Kazanjian button, an excellent method for attaching bony fragments holding only one or two teeth. A single button may be used in conjunction with arch bars, or the method may be used with intermaxillary rubber band fixation. (Modified from P. D. Wilson: *Management of Fracture and Dislocations*. J. B. Lippincott Company, 1938.)

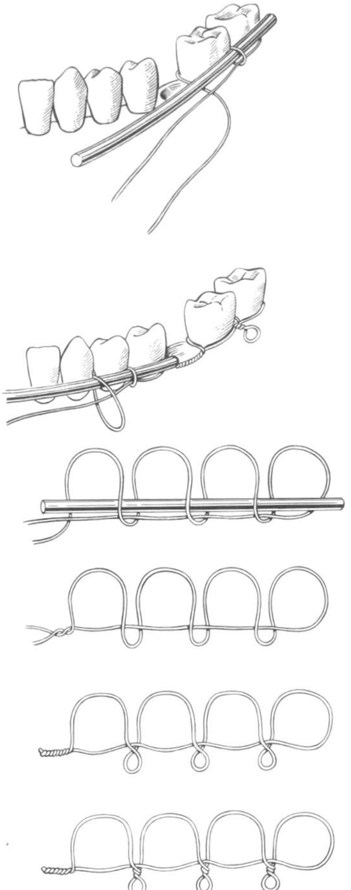

Figure 80. Details of methods of application of wire loops for intermaxillary fixation after the method of Stout.

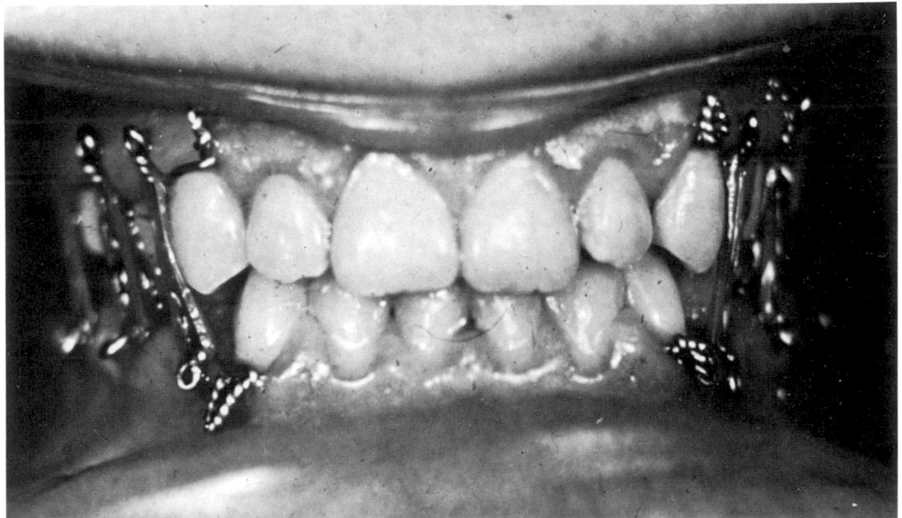

Figure 81. The Stout multiple loop wire appliance, with rubber bands for intermaxillary fixation.

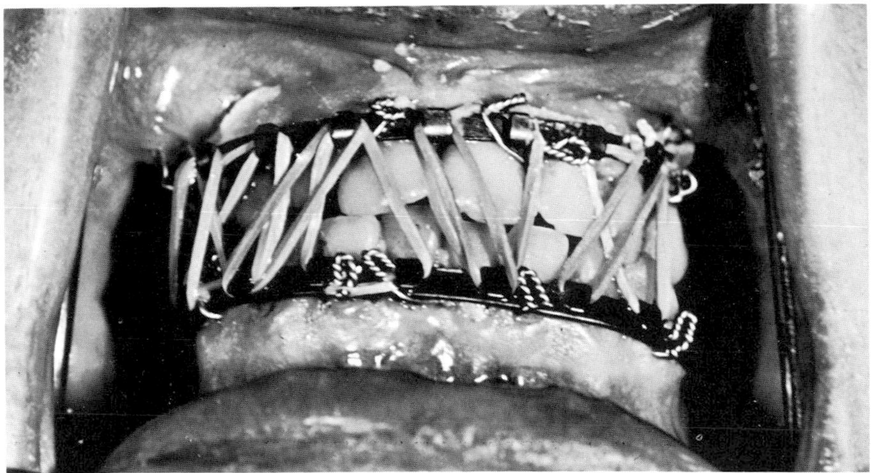

Figure 82. Intermaxillary fixation using Erich arch bars and rubber band traction.

taching rubber bands. The bar should be cut accurately to the length of the dental arch. Accuracy in this regard will prevent irritation of adjacent soft tissues by protruding ends. On the upper jaw, the hooks are arranged in an upward direction. The bar is attached to the lower jaw with the hooks in a downward direction (Fig. 83).

The arch bar is ligated to the teeth with No. 22 to No. 25 gauge stainless steel wire passing around the neck of a tooth to the lingual side and back through on the opposite side of the tooth. One end of the wire is above the bar and the other below. By twisting the two ends of wire together, the bar is attached securely and firmly to the

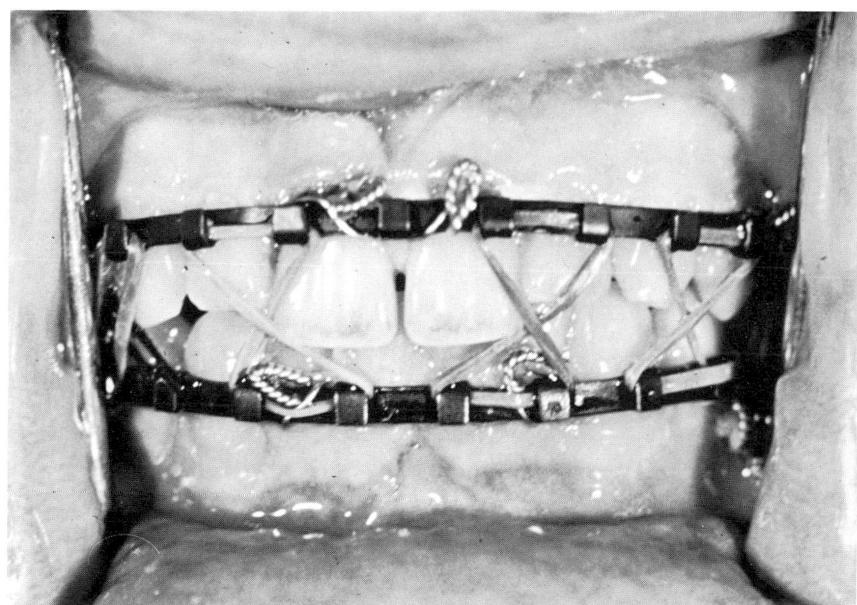

Figure 83. Maxillary and mandibular arch bars with intermaxillary rubber band fixation.

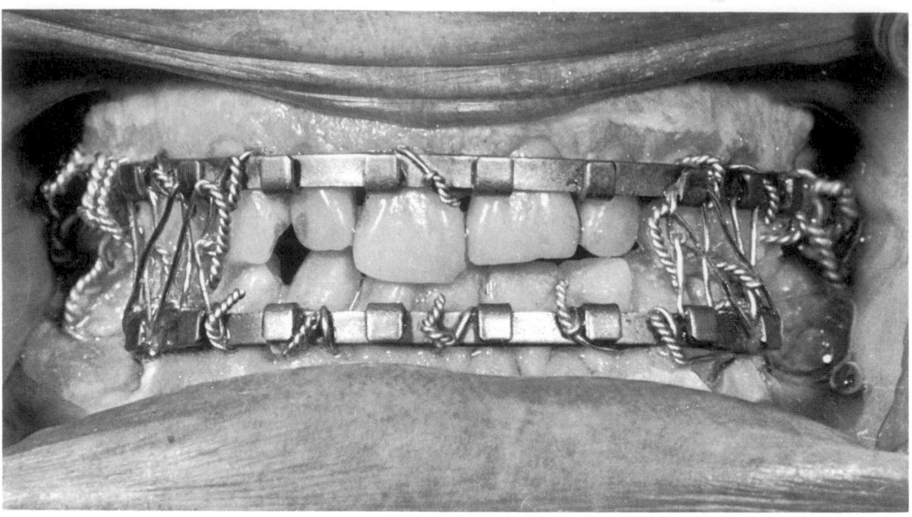

Figure 84. Erich arch bars used for intermaxillary fixation. Note the elongation and partial avulsion of the right maxillary central incisor due to wire ligature. Rubber bands are used in the early phase of the treatment. For reasons of hygiene, wire fixation may be substituted for the rubber bands after the teeth come into satisfactory occlusion. The elongated tooth should return to its normal position after removal of the arch bars.

necks of the teeth on the outer surface of the arch. To facilitate adjustment of loose wires and for ease of removal of wires after their usefulness has terminated, it is advisable to twist all the wires in the same direction (i.e., clockwise). The twisted ends of the wires should be cut long enough to prevent untwisting (usually 5 to 6 mm.). The cut end may be bent and tucked against the teeth or into the embrasures so that it will not irritate the gingiva or vestibular mucosa. *The wire should be twisted during the bending procedure to avoid its loosening.*

Because of the conical shape of the roots of the incisor teeth and their tendency to loosen under traction, they may be ligated, but traction should not be applied anteriorly (Fig. 84). In most instances the incisor teeth are not ligated. Satisfactory and adequate fixation is obtained by wiring the canine teeth and all posterior teeth. A special wiring technique is described for use on the upper and lower canine teeth, which do not retain the wire if it is applied in the usual manner (Fig. 85).

When ligation of the arch bars to the maxillary and mandibular arches is completed, small rubber bands of high quality are interlocked between the hooks of the maxillary and mandibular arch bars (see Figs. 101 and 102).

If it becomes necessary to apply heavy traction in the anterior region, a circumferential wire around the mandible and over the arch bar will provide the required stability (see Fig. 106). Similarly, in cases of the loss of teeth, or when, from trauma, loss of alveolar bone and teeth has occurred, there may be sufficient dentition remaining to serve as a guide to intermaxillary relations, yet still inadequate to provide good fixation for arch bars. In such cases the

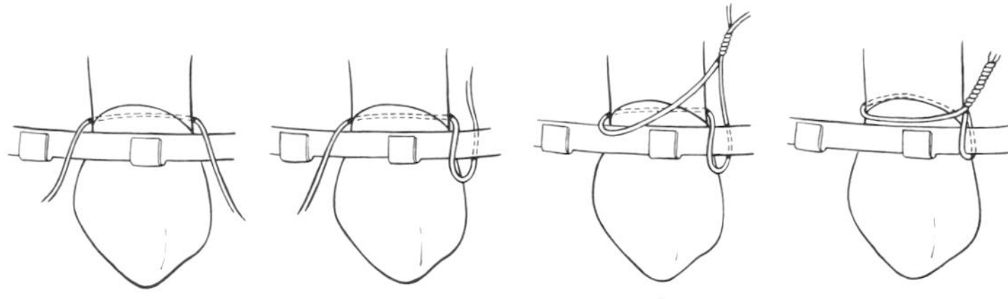

Figure 85. The conical shape of the canine teeth results in loosening of the wires if these are placed in the usual manner about the arch bar and neck of the tooth. The method illustrated here ensures stability of the bar. Wires placed in this manner usually are tight and will not slip.

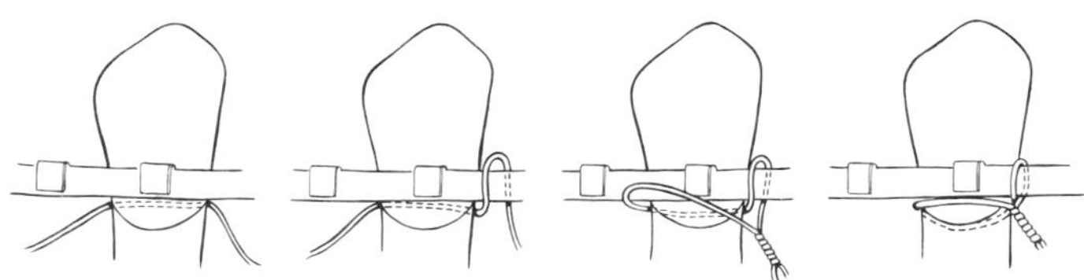

edentulous areas may be replaced by splints (or dentures, if the patient has them) and secured by circumferential wiring (Fig. 86).

The upper arch bar may be fixed more securely by passing a wire through a small hole drilled into the anterior nasal spine or into the bony margins of the pyriform aperture of the nasal cavity and then passing the wire around the upper arch bar (see Figs. 104 and 105). These bony fixations give

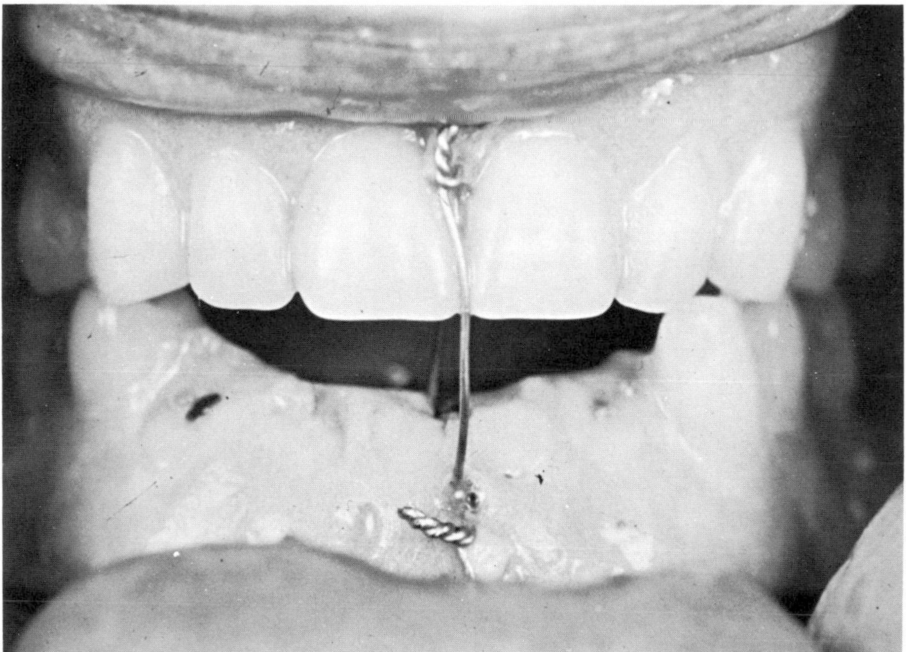

Figure 86. Fracture of the mandible treated by circumferential wiring. The lower denture is fixed to the mandible by circumferential wires, and the upper denture is fixed to the maxilla by direct wiring to the bone. The two dentures are fixed with a wire in the anterior region.

added stability and permit strong intermaxillary traction without dislodging or slipping of the bar on the few teeth available.

The removal of a tooth or teeth seldom is necessary to facilitate the feeding of the patient during the period of intermaxillary fixation. There is adequate space between teeth and the retromolar areas to permit ingestion of an adequate liquid diet.

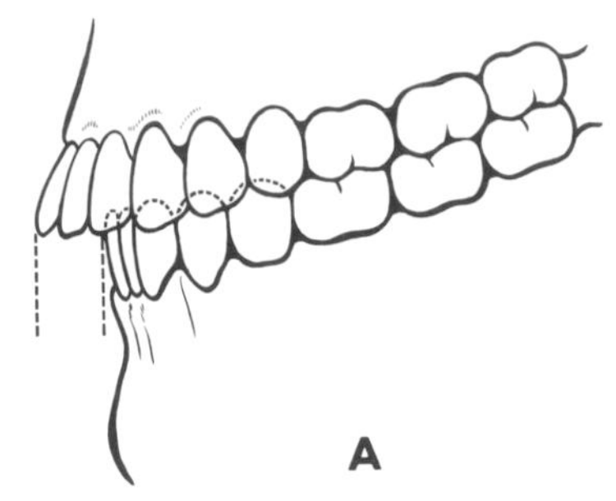

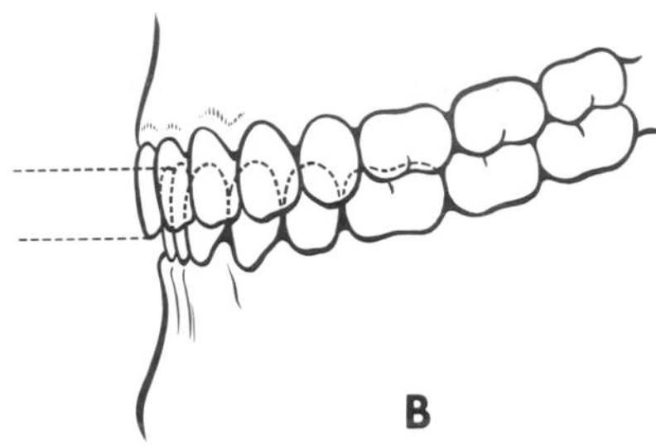

Figure 87. *A.* Overjet. The anterior-posterior interval between the lingual surface of the maxillary anterior teeth and the labial surfaces of the mandibular anterior teeth; this is exaggerated for diagrammatic purposes. *B.* Overbite. The superior-inferior overlapping of the maxillary anterior teeth and the mandibular anterior teeth; this is exaggerated for diagrammatic purposes.

MALOCCLUSION

In the treatment of facial fractures, it is important to have clear understanding of normal occlusion and a simple method of determining malocclusion. It is manifest that if facial fractures occur in a patient with malocclusion, reduction of the fracture should re-establish the preinjury state of malocclusion. There is no rationale to using a fracture to obtain normal median occlusion. The occlusion, though abnormal prior to injury, must be returned to its original state. Normal median occlusion exists when the mesiobuccal cusps of the maxillary first molars interdigitate in the buccal grooves of the mandibular first molars with slight overbite and slight overjet of the anterior teeth (Fig. 87 *A, B*). This is median occlusion or neutroclusion* (see Figs. 88 *A, B* and 108).

Distoclusion (Class II malocclusion) is that position in which the mesiobuccal cusps of the maxillary first molars interdigitate in the embrasure between the second mandibular premolar and the first mandibular molar. This may give the appearance of a slightly retrusive mandible and protrusive maxillary anterior teeth (see Figs. 89 *A, B, C* and 109).

Mesioclusion (Class III malocclusion) is that position in which the mesiobuccal cusps of the maxillary first molars interdigitate in the embrasure between the mandibular first and second molars. This produces an "underbite" and a protrusive appearance of the mandible (see Figs. 90 *A, B, C* and 110).

Figure 108 shows the generally accepted standard of median occlusion or neutroclusion for the majority of individuals. Figure 109, illustrating distoclusion, shows the retrusive mandible and the relations of the mesiobuccal cusps to the mandibular teeth. Figure 110, mesioclusion, shows the protru-

* Class I malocclusion has the same relations between the mesiobuccal cusps of the maxillary first molars and the mesiobuccal grooves of the mandibular first molars as neutroclusion. Class I malocclusion shows malposition of individual teeth.

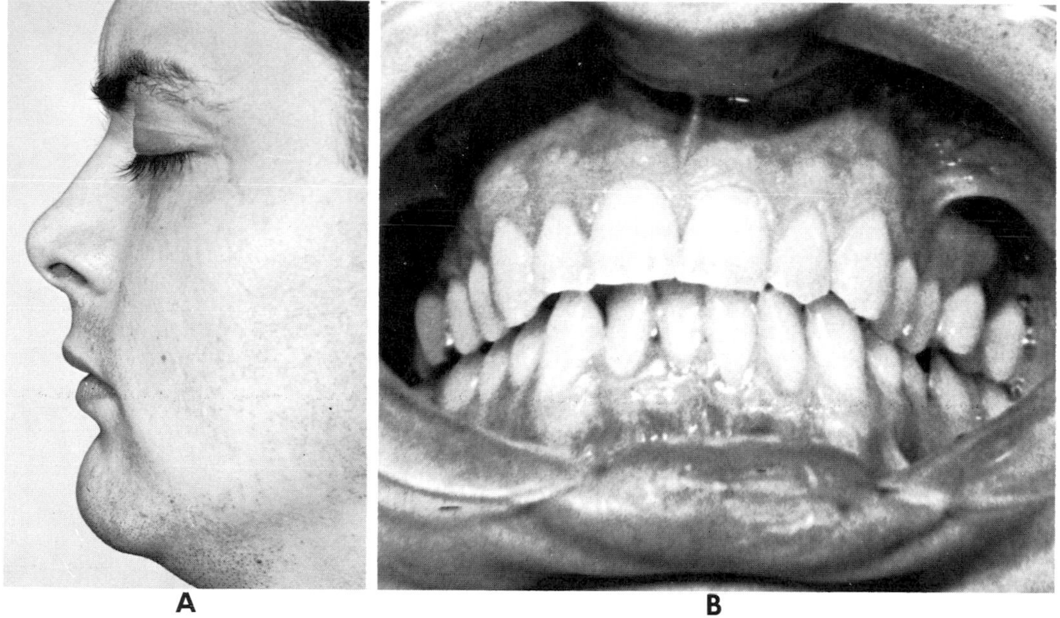

Figure 88. *A.* Profile view of patient with neutroclusion. *B.* Front view of teeth in neutroclusion. This is the normal physiologic occlusion for most patients. Note that there is slight overbite and overjet.

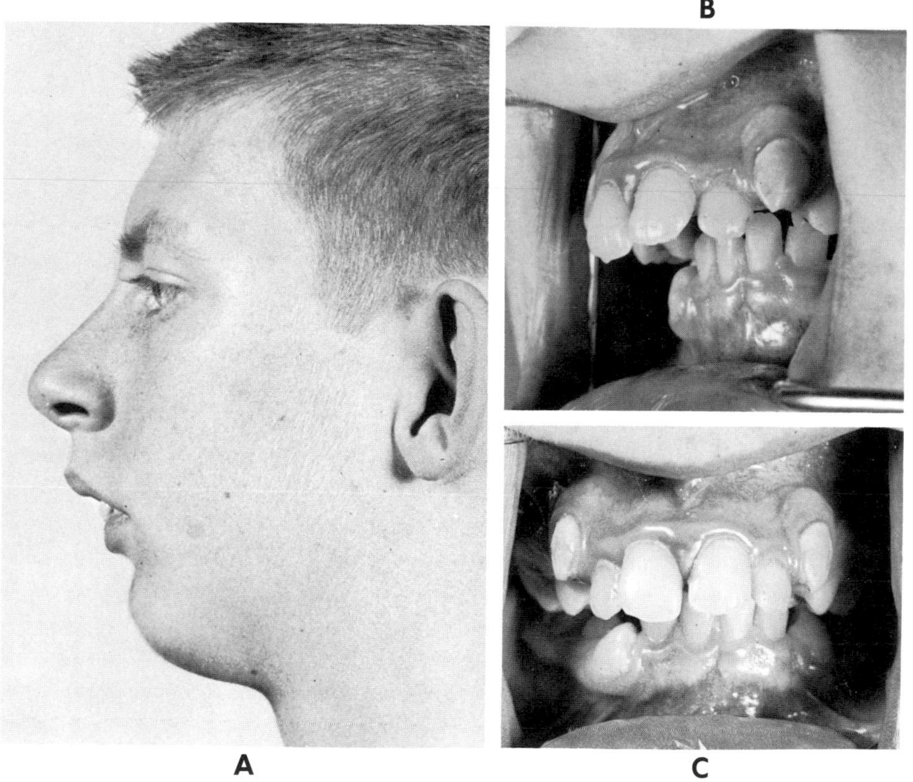

Figure 89. *A.* Patient with distoclusion; profile view showing underdevelopment of the mandible and retrognathic appearance. *B.* All the mandibular teeth are distal to the maxillary teeth. This is known as retrognathic or retrusive occlusion and is accompanied by lack of prominence of the symphysis of the mandible and a receded chin. *C.* Front view showing distoclusion.

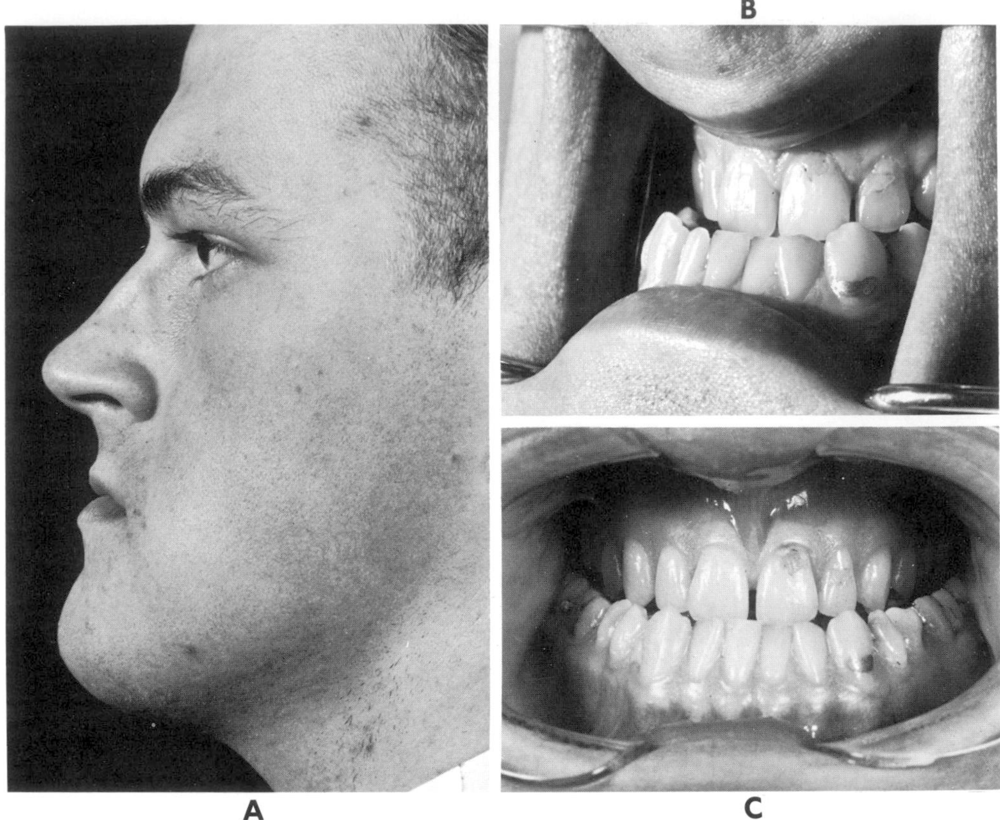

Figure 90. *A.* Profile view of a patient with mesioclusion, known as prognathic or protrusive occlusion. The chin is prominent on profile view. *B.* Oblique view of mesioclusion. The lower teeth occlude in front of the upper teeth. *C.* Front view of mesioclusion. All the mandibular teeth bite outside the maxillary teeth.

sive mandible and the relations of the mesiobuccal cusps to the mandibular teeth. Individual teeth within the classifications may show differences; however, if one uses the guide point of the mesiobuccal cusps in relation to mandibular teeth, one usually can identify the type of malocclusion.

Malocclusion, thus far described, has embraced only the abnormal anteroposterior relations of the dentitions. Another position of malocclusion must be understood to include differences in relations of width of the upper and lower arches. As shown in Figure 107, the buccal cusps of the *maxillary* posterior teeth and cusp of the canine tooth normally overlap the lower dentition and are in a more buccalward and labialward position. When the position is reversed and the buccal cusps of the posterior teeth and cusp of the canine tooth of the *mandible* are more buccalward, the condition is called "crossbite." Crossbite may occur unilaterally or bilaterally. Figure 107 shows the right side of the posterior dentition and canine (with molars in the inset) with normal median occlusion, while the left side (with molars inset) shows crossbite in the posterior teeth and canine. If crossbite existed preoperatively, the teeth must be returned to the preinjury malocclusion.

One may question how the status of the preinjury malocclusion may be determined when malocclusion also results from fracture and displacement of bone segments. This is not difficult when the open method of reduction and fixation of facial fractures is used together with intermaxillary fixation. When fragments have been fixed by open reduction, the teeth should be placed in occlusion. When the anatomic position of the bone fragments has been restored, the teeth usually will assume their preoperative occlusal relation. The occlusal surfaces of the teeth usually are well aligned so that all teeth interdigitate when intermaxillary traction is applied. In intermaxillary fixation (without open reduction and osseous wire fixation), rubber band traction should be applied; then the teeth will usually occlude without difficulty. During placement of the rubber band traction, closed reduction by manipulation may be useful; irregularities of bone may be palpated and repositioned. This is particularly true of simple fractures in regions of the mandible where teeth are present. It is not necessarily true when mandibular fractures are distal to the teeth. In multiple facial fractures, preinjury occlusion cannot be restored properly until the mandible is reduced accurately. Replacement usually requires open reduction and interosseous fixation, together with intermaxillary fixation.

Abraded surfaces on occlusal and incisal areas of the teeth often act as landmarks and thus are aids in replacing the teeth to the position of preinjury occlusion. Of course, facets of upper and lower teeth correspond to each other. In other words, preinjury occlusion can be established by relating mandibular and maxillary teeth using attrition marks rather than conventional patterns of maxillomandibular relations.

Examination of preinjury dental models, or photographs, or a reliable history from the patient or from his relatives to describe preinjury occlusion, are additional aids.

Occlusion and Intermaxillary Fixation

PART 2

OPERATIVE TECHNIQUE

No book dealing with the contemporary management of facial fractures is complete without a detailed discussion of physiologic dental occlusion and the methods of intermaxillary fixation.

Successful treatment of patients with fractures of the jaws calls for restoration of functional occlusion of the dentition. To obtain the best possible results, reduction must be accurate and fixation positive.

Of special importance is the exact and positive fixation of the teeth in functional occlusion. To this end, it is desirable that sturdy appliances be used and that these be fixed securely to the remaining teeth and bone segments.

There are numerous approaches to the problem of obtaining fixation of fractures of the jaws. Our experience indicates that the simple and direct procedures outlined on the following pages are highly effective and, in most instances, readily applicable without a detailed knowledge of the construction of dental appliances.

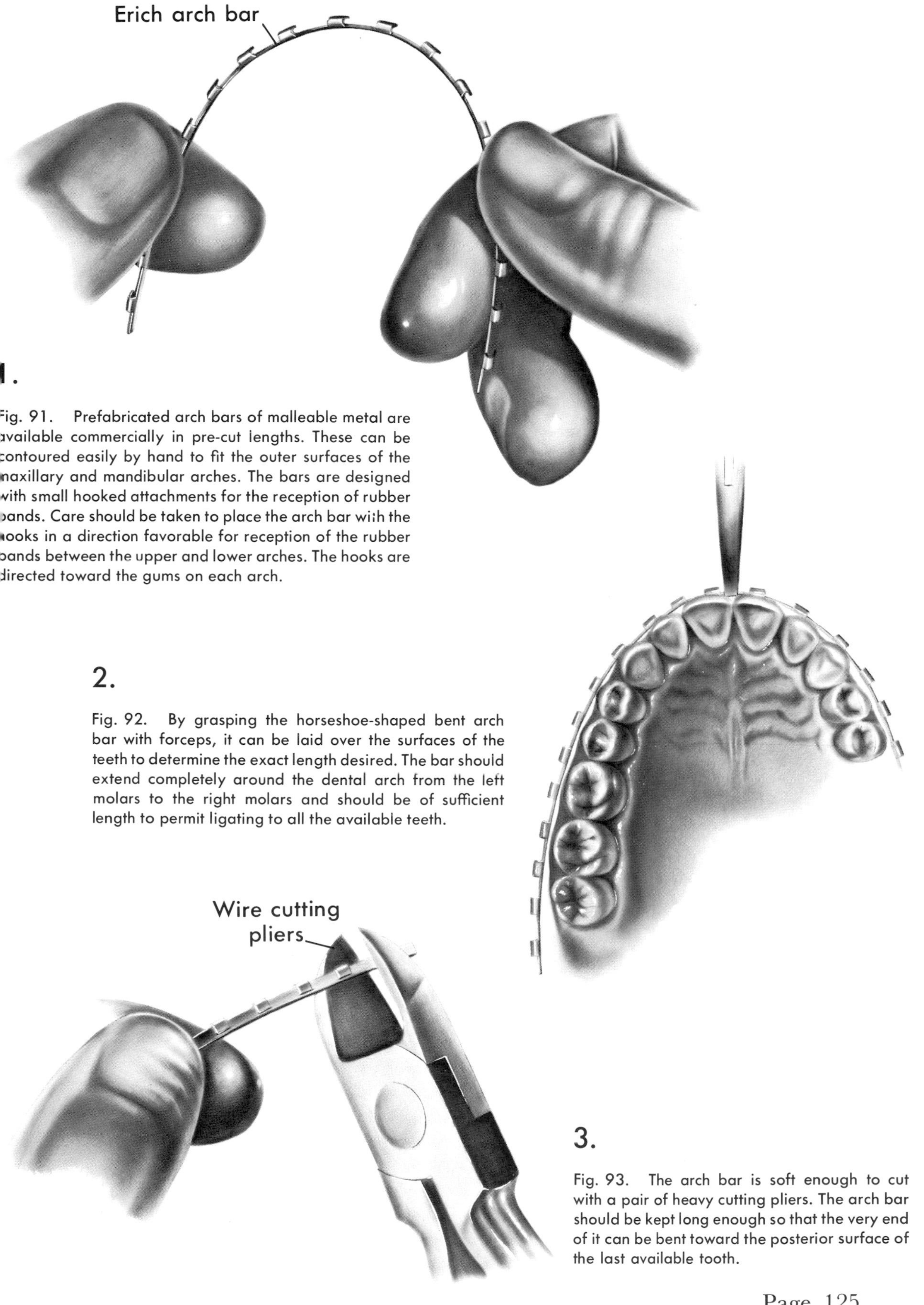

1.

Fig. 91. Prefabricated arch bars of malleable metal are available commercially in pre-cut lengths. These can be contoured easily by hand to fit the outer surfaces of the maxillary and mandibular arches. The bars are designed with small hooked attachments for the reception of rubber bands. Care should be taken to place the arch bar with the hooks in a direction favorable for reception of the rubber bands between the upper and lower arches. The hooks are directed toward the gums on each arch.

2.

Fig. 92. By grasping the horseshoe-shaped bent arch bar with forceps, it can be laid over the surfaces of the teeth to determine the exact length desired. The bar should extend completely around the dental arch from the left molars to the right molars and should be of sufficient length to permit ligating to all the available teeth.

3.

Fig. 93. The arch bar is soft enough to cut with a pair of heavy cutting pliers. The arch bar should be kept long enough so that the very end of it can be bent toward the posterior surface of the last available tooth.

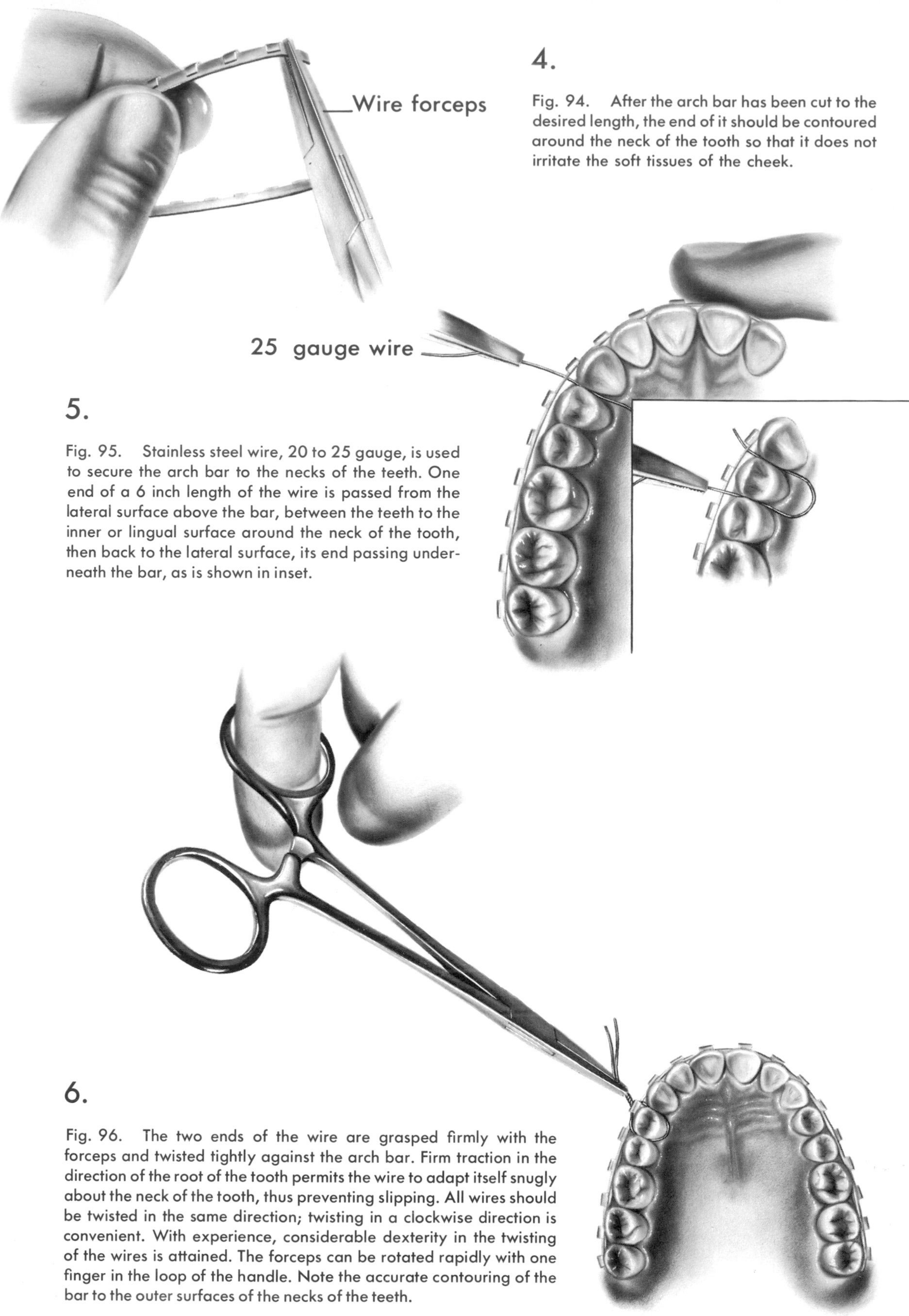

4.

Fig. 94. After the arch bar has been cut to the desired length, the end of it should be contoured around the neck of the tooth so that it does not irritate the soft tissues of the cheek.

5.

Fig. 95. Stainless steel wire, 20 to 25 gauge, is used to secure the arch bar to the necks of the teeth. One end of a 6 inch length of the wire is passed from the lateral surface above the bar, between the teeth to the inner or lingual surface around the neck of the tooth, then back to the lateral surface, its end passing underneath the bar, as is shown in inset.

6.

Fig. 96. The two ends of the wire are grasped firmly with the forceps and twisted tightly against the arch bar. Firm traction in the direction of the root of the tooth permits the wire to adapt itself snugly about the neck of the tooth, thus preventing slipping. All wires should be twisted in the same direction; twisting in a clockwise direction is convenient. With experience, considerable dexterity in the twisting of the wires is attained. The forceps can be rotated rapidly with one finger in the loop of the handle. Note the accurate contouring of the bar to the outer surfaces of the necks of the teeth.

7.

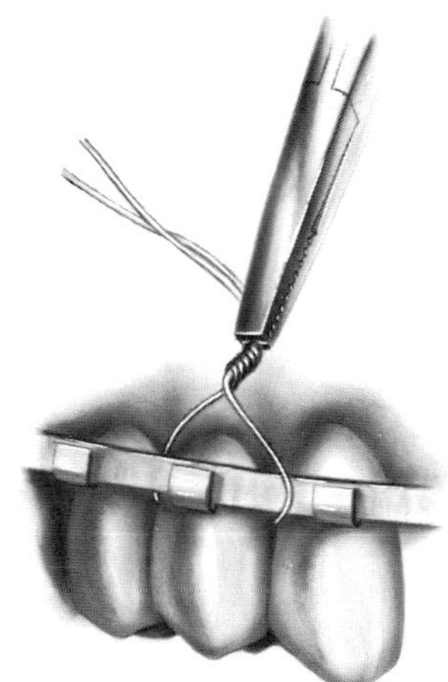

Fig. 97. The bell-shaped crowns of the posterior teeth permit use of the simple loop in wiring the arch bar to the teeth. The bell-shaped crown favors the seating of the wire loop under the gingiva and prevents downward slipping when traction is applied. This figure shows the wire passing over the top of the bar on one side, around the neck of the tooth, and upward under the bar on the opposite side. Pulling in an upward direction also favors seating of the wire at the smallest circumference of the crown of the tooth. This permits strong force to be applied with the rubber bands without dislodgment or slipping of the arch bar.

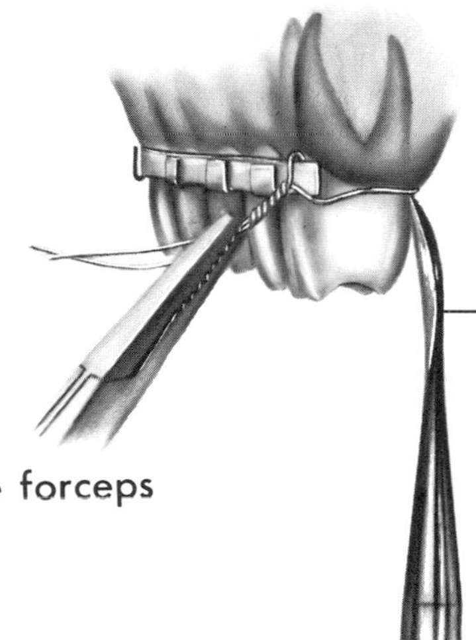

8.

Fig. 98. This cutaway section illustrates the placement of the wire around the neck of the tooth. If the wire has a tendency to slip downward while it is being twisted, it can be held firmly against the neck of the tooth, or pushed under the gingival margin, by the use of a sharp-pointed periosteal elevator. This places the wire in the position of least diameter about the neck of the tooth so that it will not slip. When applying the arch bar, it will usually be most convenient to start the wiring in the premolar region. The bar can be secured with one wire on each side to start the wiring procedure. This stabilizes the bar so that the wiring of subsequent teeth becomes less difficult. At this stage the bar can be rechecked for length and can be contoured to fit accurately against the necks of all the teeth in the dental arch.

9.

Fig. 99. The canine is a key tooth in retaining the arch bar, since its root is long and the surrounding bone is dense. Thus this tooth can withstand great stress. The shape of the tooth, however, is somewhat unfavorable for the retention of the ligature wire, because the crown is narrow at the gingival line and the wire has a tendency to slip, loosen, and permit movement of the arch bar. A special wire loop, as shown in Figure 85, is effective in maintaining stability of the bar. Both ends of the wire are passed above the bar, one on each side of the tooth, and one of the ends is twisted around the bar in the form of a loop. When this wire is tightened, it has a tendency to adapt itself, beneath the gingival margin, to the root of the tooth, where usually it remains secure without slipping. The simple wire loop as shown in Figure 97 is ineffective in ligating the arch bar to the canine teeth.

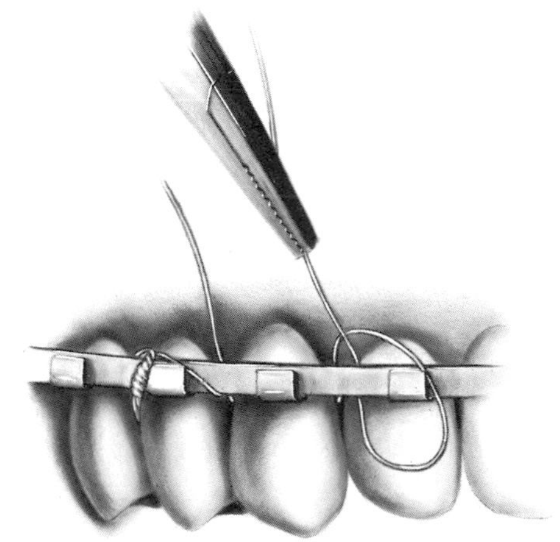

10.

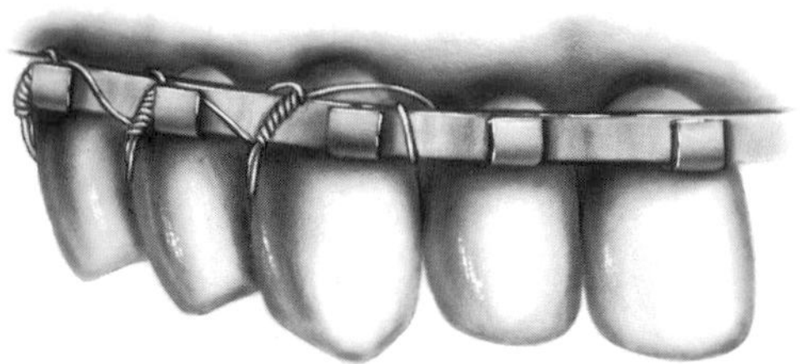

Fig. 100. As the individual wires are tightened securely about the necks of the teeth, they are cut at a convenient length with the wire cutter but are left long enough so that the ends can be tucked down between the teeth away from the soft tissues to prevent irritation. All the available teeth in the dental arch should be ligated to maintain accurate and adequate stability. However, the conical shape of the roots of the eight incisor teeth do not lend themselves well to the placement of ligatures. Strong intermaxillary forces with rubber bands may cause them to loosen from their sockets.

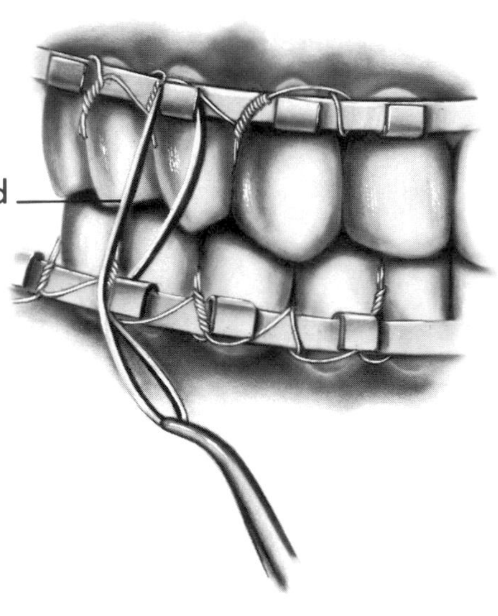

11.

Fig. 101. After fixing the arch bars securely to the circumferences of the upper and lower dental arches, they should be grasped with a forceps to test their stability. If either is loose, the wires should be tightened further and additional wires applied if necessary. Loosening of the arch bars, or movement of them during the postoperative period of fixation, is distressing and many times is difficult to correct by adjustment. Good quality, small rubber bands with high resiliency should be used. A few rubber bands on each side will exert strong traction. The direction of the rubber bands may vary with the individual case to produce the desired direction of movement of the segments.

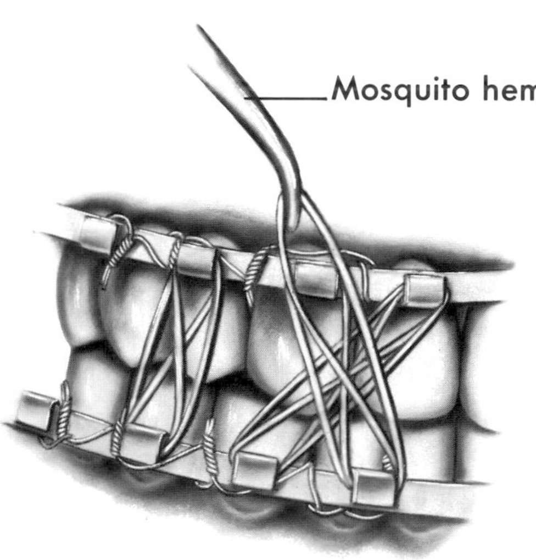

12.

Fig. 102. If the application of rubber bands in single loops does not seem to give adequate traction, the bands can be stretched and passed from the upper to the lower arch bar and again to the upper bar; in some instances bands can be stretched far enough so that they pass again to the lower arch bar. A small, curved hemostat is helpful in manipulating the rubber bands.

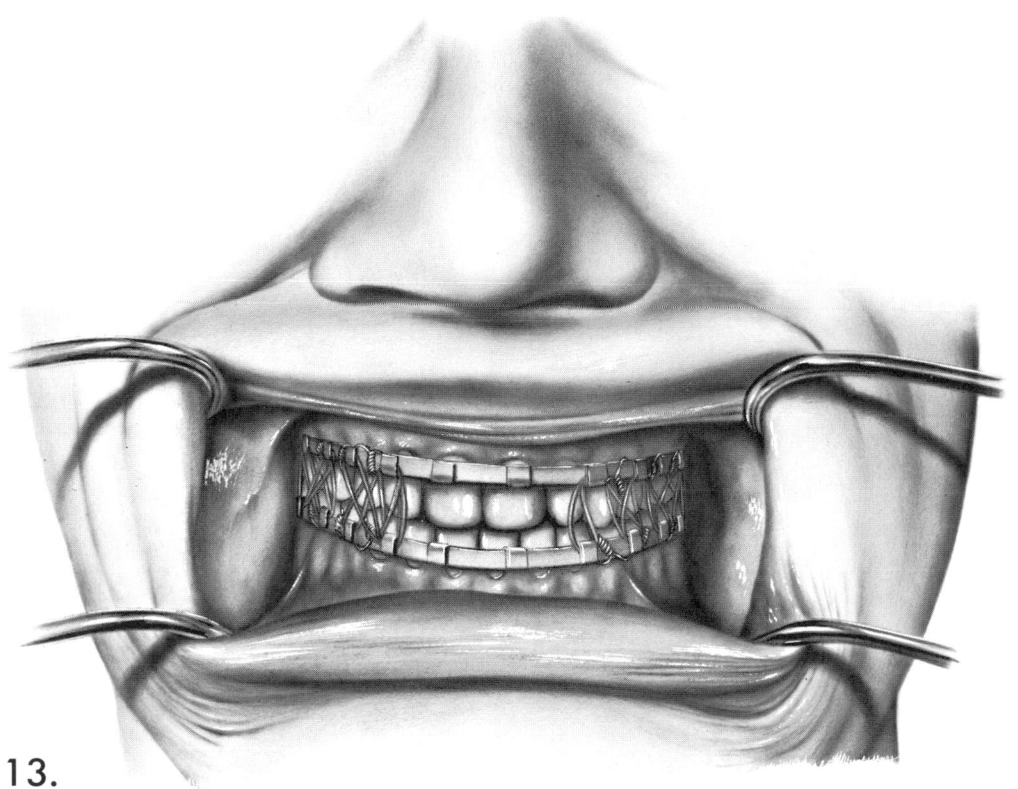

13.

Fig. 103. Arch bars placed carefully on the dental arches, and ligated securely with all sharp ends of wire turned in against the teeth, provide excellent anchorage for intermaxillary fixation and are quite comfortable. The neat, thin bars and fine wire take up little room in the mouth and the patient adjusts to them quickly.

SUPPLEMENTARY METHODS FOR STABILIZATION OF ARCH BARS

14.

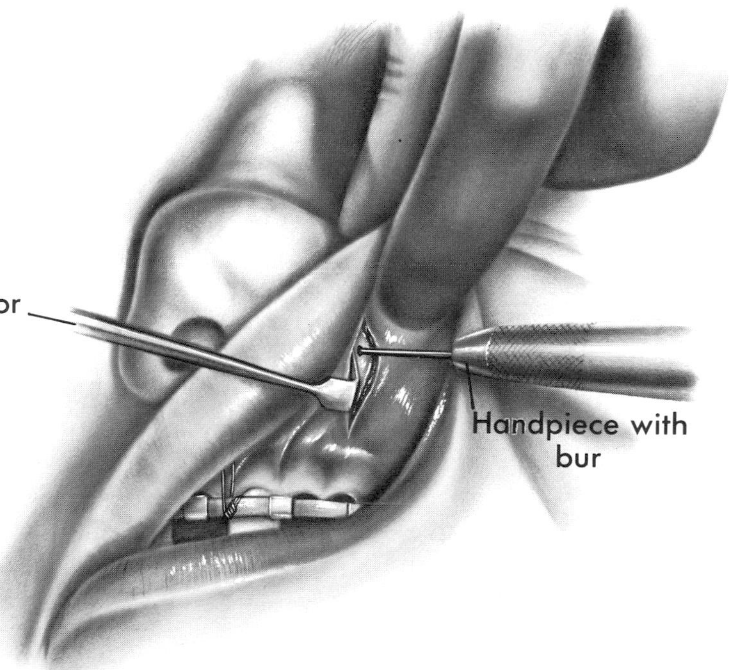

Fig. 104. If heavy traction is anticipated in the anterior maxillary region and there are insufficient teeth to support the arch bar, a wire may be passed through a small bur hole in the bony margin of the pyriform aperture of the maxilla for suspension of the maxillary arch bar. This illustration shows the vertical incision made over the canine area for exposure of the pyriform margin. A similar incision is made for an approach to the opposite pyriform margin. An incision at one side of the frenulum permits exposure of the anterior nasal spine. One or all of these suspension wires may be used if necessary.

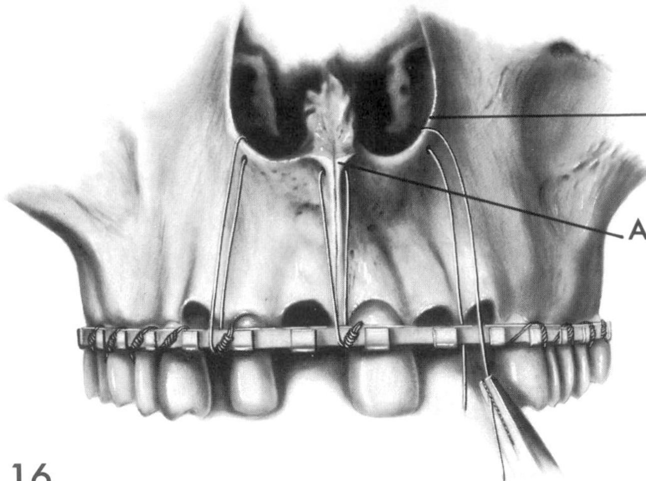

15.

Fig. 105. Shown here are suspension wires from the bon margins of the pyriform apertures and anterior nasal spine With three suspension wires, firm fixation of the arch bar ca be established. This allows great force to be applied betwee the upper and lower arch bars. Modifications of this metho are possible. If desirable, these wires may be attached to th lower arch bar for fixation of the mandible against the maxill

16.

Fig. 106. Instability of the mandibular arch bar may be overcome by passing a circumferential wire around the mandible and the arch bar in such a manner as to pull it snugly against the necks of the teeth. (The technique for circumferential wiring of the mandible is shown in Figure 131.) The wire passes completely about the circumference of the bone (see inset).

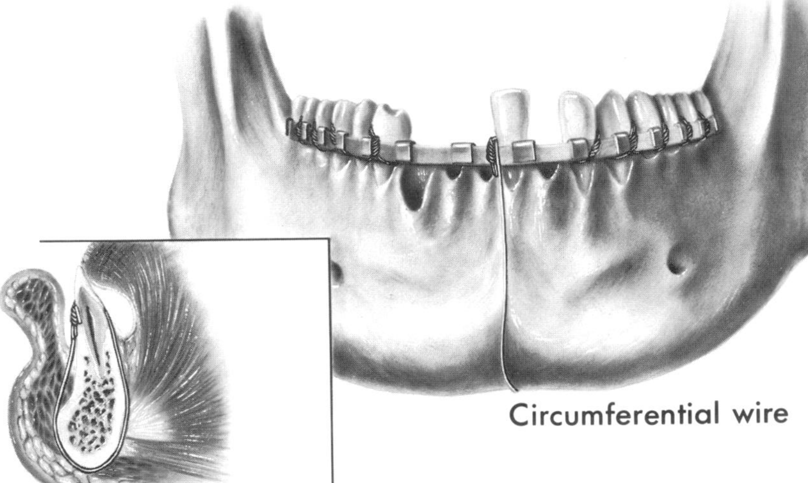

CRITERIA OF MALOCCLUSION

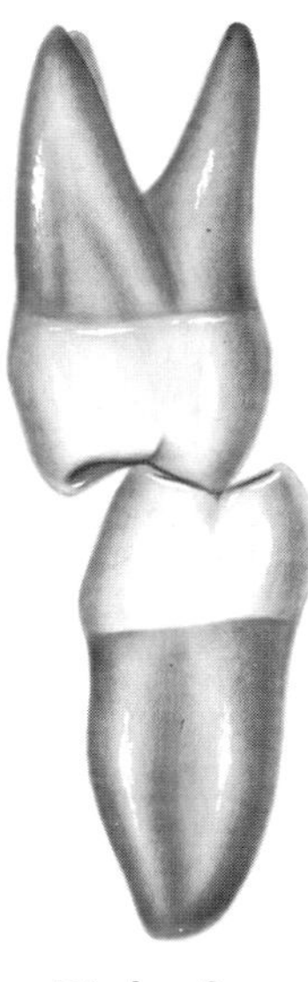

Left first molars

B

17.

Fig. 107. Variations of occlusion are present in many individuals. These variations are most often physiological and functional. Recognition of the pretraumatic occlusion is necessary so that the occlusion can be re-established. Recognition of the patient's pretraumatic occlusion is not easy. It might have been a normal bite, a retrusive or protrusive bite, or a crossbite, as shown. Inset A in cross section shows the normal occlusal relation in the molar region. Inset B shows medial positioning of the upper molar in relation to the lower. The occlusion of the right side of the dentitions demonstrates neutroclusion. The occlusion of the left side is in crossbite. Crossbite may be unilateral or bilateral.

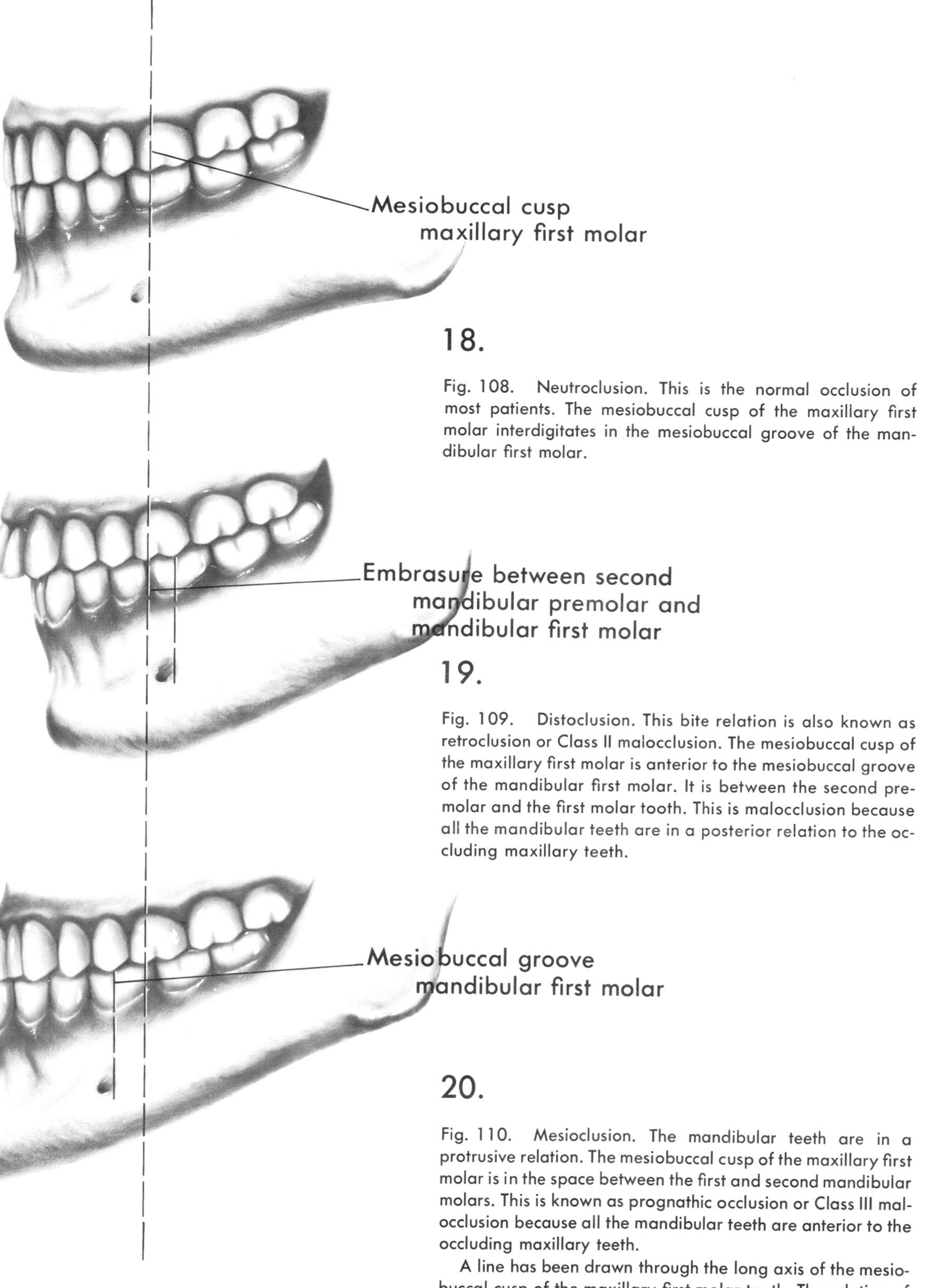

18.

Fig. 108. Neutroclusion. This is the normal occlusion of most patients. The mesiobuccal cusp of the maxillary first molar interdigitates in the mesiobuccal groove of the mandibular first molar.

19.

Fig. 109. Distoclusion. This bite relation is also known as retroclusion or Class II malocclusion. The mesiobuccal cusp of the maxillary first molar is anterior to the mesiobuccal groove of the mandibular first molar. It is between the second premolar and the first molar tooth. This is malocclusion because all the mandibular teeth are in a posterior relation to the occluding maxillary teeth.

20.

Fig. 110. Mesioclusion. The mandibular teeth are in a protrusive relation. The mesiobuccal cusp of the maxillary first molar is in the space between the first and second mandibular molars. This is known as prognathic occlusion or Class III malocclusion because all the mandibular teeth are anterior to the occluding maxillary teeth.

A line has been drawn through the long axis of the mesiobuccal cusp of the maxillary first molar tooth. The relation of the mesiobuccal cusp of the maxillary first molar tooth to the mandibular teeth is the principle upon which Angle's classification of occlusion is based.

CHAPTER

6

THE MANDIBLE

PART 1

GENERAL CONSIDERATIONS

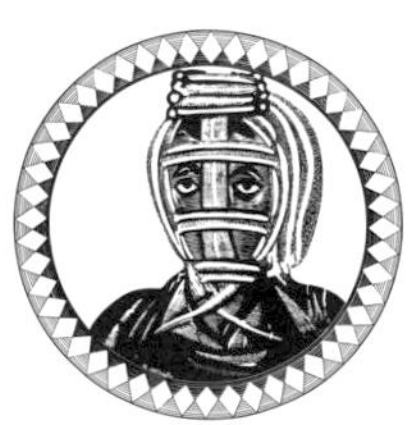

Fractures of the mandible make up approximately two-thirds of all facial fractures. Early reports in the literature of facial bone fractures were limited with few exceptions to fractures of the mandible. The incidence of middle-third facial fractures increased during the First and Second World Wars and with the development of high speed transportation facilities. With an increase in the number of facial fractures from transportation accidents, the ratio of middle-third facial fractures to fractures of the mandible is now considered about 1 to 2.

A detailed discussion of the anatomy of the mandible can be found in any of the standard books or atlases of anatomy, but certain points relative to the etiology and treatment of fractures of the lower jaw must be added. The prominence and position of the mandible in the facial skeleton predispose it to frequent trauma. Fractures of the facial bones, in some cases, may even be considered as a "shock-absorbing" lesser evil; impacts upon the mandible and other facial structures are dissipated by fracture which prevents more serious damage to intracranial structures.

SURGICAL ANATOMY OF THE MANDIBLE

The mandible is the heaviest and strongest of the facial bones. The lower jaw is a heavy, movable, U-shaped bone consisting of a horizontal portion, the body, which carries the alveolar process and the teeth, and two vertical portions, the rami, which articulate through the temporomandibular joints with the skull bilaterally. The mandible is attached to other facial bones by ligaments and muscles and articulates with the maxilla upon occlusion of the teeth. The jaw is moved by a posterior group of muscles attached to the rami and an anterior group of muscles attached to the body of the bone (see Fig. 115).

The Body of the Mandible

Embryologically the mandible develops

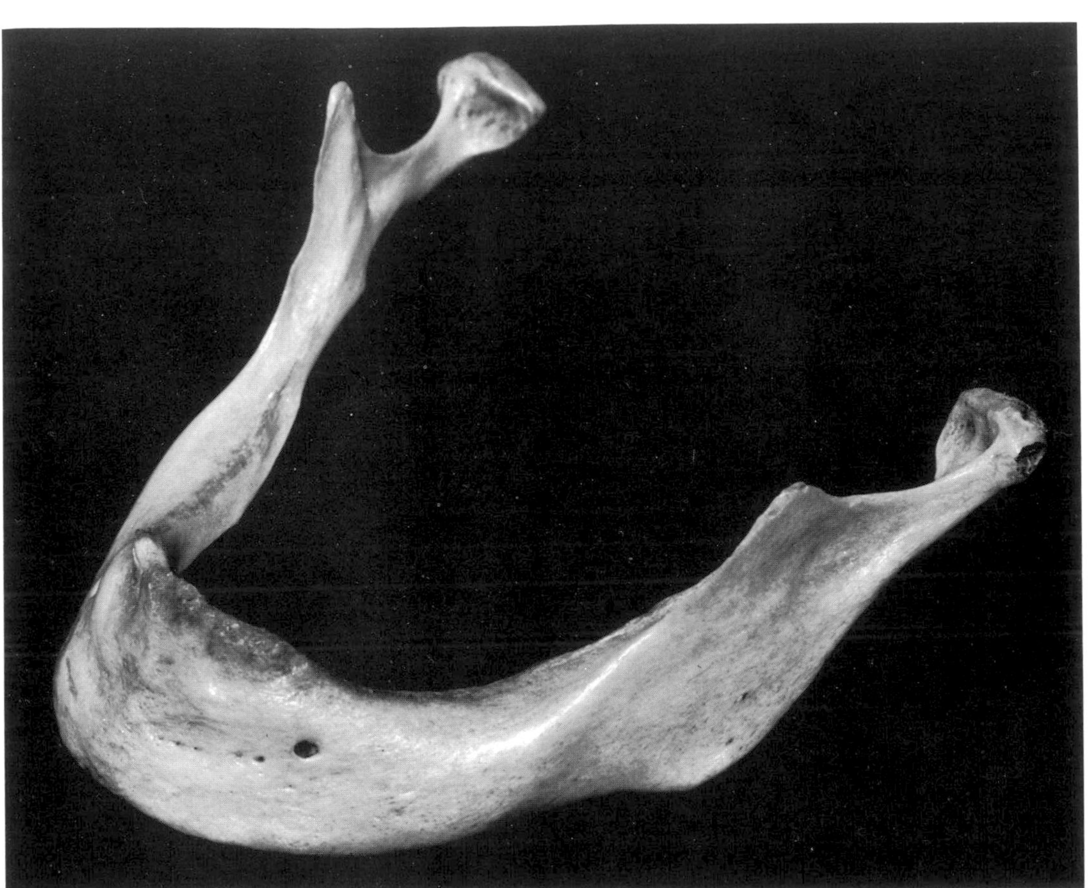

Figure 111. Photograph of an edentulous mandible. The posterior teeth were extracted before the anterior teeth were, as is evidenced by the greater resorption of the alveolar ridge posteriorly. Note the location of the mental foramen. If the individual had lived longer, the anterior portion of the alveolar ridge would have been resorbed equally to the posterior region, and the foramen would have been almost at the margin of the crest of the ridge.

from two bones which unite in the midline at the symphysis, usually represented by a ridge that extends from the alveolar process to the inferior border. Below and lateral to the symphysis is the heavy inferior border known as the mental protuberance, just lateral to which are bony prominences known as the mental tubercles. The muscles of the lower lip and chin attach in this area. The body of the bone is made up of a dense cortical structure on the lateral and medial surfaces with a small core of spongiosa through which pass the blood vessels, the nerves, and the lymphatics. The lower portion of the bone is heavy, thick, and dense and changes very little during adult life. The upper part of the mandibular body carries the alveolar process, which forms the dental sockets and supports the teeth. The alveolar process is composed of an oral (lingual) and a vestibular (labiobuccal) plate of compact bone but is mainly spongy bone. The alveolar bone changes throughout the life of the individual and becomes adapted to the movements of the teeth or to the loss of teeth. After extraction of teeth the alveolar process undergoes marked atrophy.

The deciduous or temporary dentition makes its first appearance at six months of age and is completed at 22 to 24 months of age. Until the age of six, the mandible contains 10 deciduous teeth, 5 on each side, and the tooth buds of the permanent dentition. The permanent dentition of the mandible is composed of 16 teeth, 8 on each side.

The mental foramen of the mandible is on the lateral surface midway between the inferior border and the alveolar crest and generally in the line of the long axis of the second premolar tooth. In the edentulous mandible with extreme atrophy of the alveolar bone, the mental foramen may be found on the upper border of the bone (Fig. 111). The mental nerve (a branch of the inferior alveolar nerve) and vessels pass through the mental foramen. The mandible is traversed by a canal, which begins on the inner surface of the ramus as the mandibular foramen and extends to the symphysis anteriorly. The canal opens upon the lateral surface of the mandible at the mental foramen. The inferior alveolar nerve passes through the mandibular canal to supply sensation to the teeth and bone of the mandible and to the soft tissues of the lip and labial vestibule by way of its mental branch. Fractures of the bone that involve the course of the inferior alveolar nerve usually result in damage to the nerve and anesthesia of the lower lip.

The body of the mandible is strengthened by a strong system of buttresses which extend into the region of the rami (Fig. 112). On the lateral surface the external oblique line passes from the body obliquely upward to the anterior border of the ramus.

The medial surface of the bone is thinner than the lateral table but is composed of the same dense, thick compacta. The medial surface is marked with ridges, spines, and fossae that accommodate the sublingual and submandibular glands and serve as attachments for the depressor group of muscles, which are attached to the inner and anterior surface of the mandible. The supporting structures of the floor of the oral cavity and the tongue attach to the inner surface of the lower jaw. The mylohyoid line is a low, irregular ridge that extends from the area of the socket of the third molar diagonally down and forward to end between the genial tubercles and the digastric fossa at the midline.

The reinforcement of the mandible is provided mainly by the strong compact bone at the lower border of the body. The most endangered part of the body is further strengthened by the mental protuberance or bony chin. The masticatory forces are led up toward the condyle of the crest of the

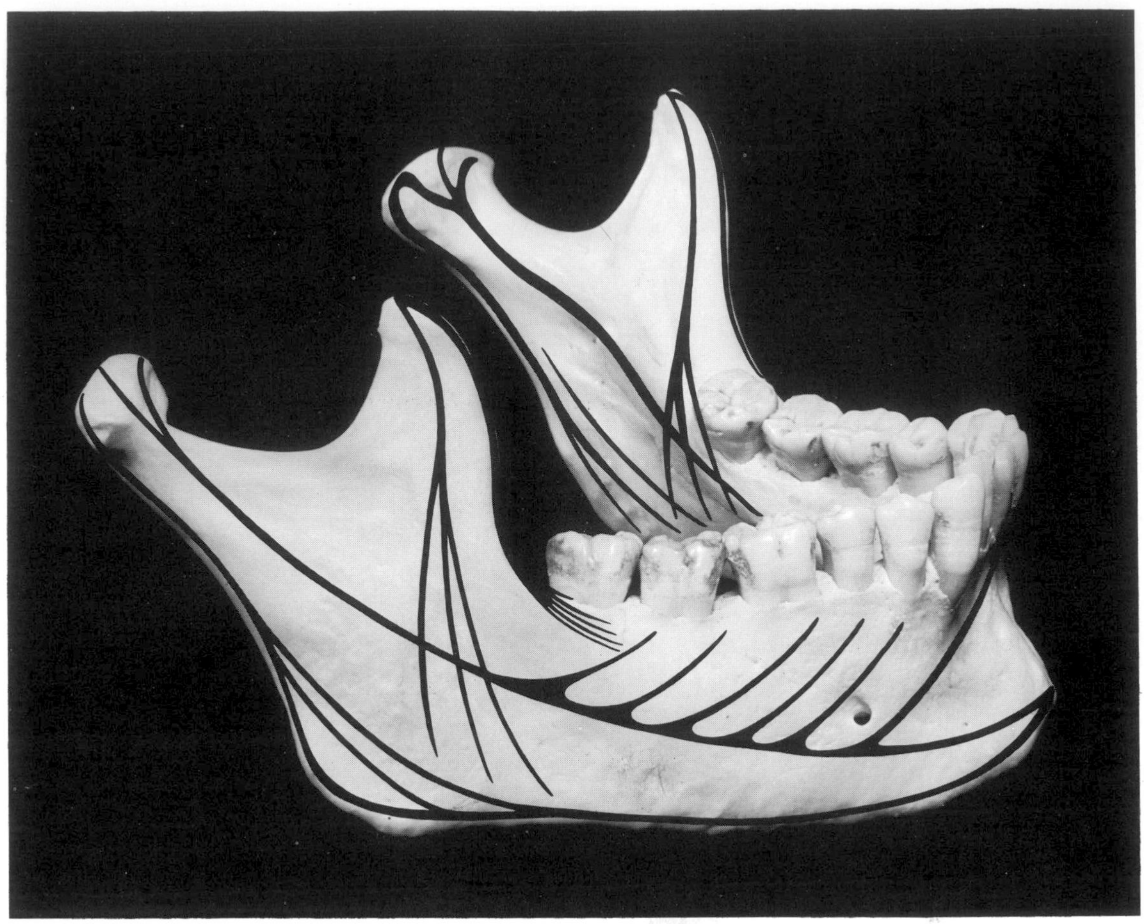

Figure 112. The trajectories of the mandible. The mandible is strengthened in response to the forces of the muscles of mastication by the development of massive compacta, as well as by trajectories of the spongiosa. (After Sicher: *Oral Anatomy*. 3d ed., St. Louis, The C. V. Mosby Company, 1960.)

mandibular neck, which is prominent on the inner side of the ramus and runs from the end of the alveolar process diagonally toward the head of the mandible (Sicher, 1963) (Fig. 112).

The Ramus of the Mandible

The vertical portion known as the ramus of the mandible joins the body at an angle of more than 90 degrees. The ramus is a broad, relatively thin, quadrilateral plate of dense bone which terminates in the coronoid process anteriorly and in the wider articulating or condylar process posteriorly. The flattened outer surface has oblique ridges at the inferior border; these provide strong attachments for the tendinous insertions of the masseter muscle (Fig. 113). The inner surface provides attachments at the angle for the medial pterygoid muscle and for the temporal and lateral pterygoid superiorly. The mandibular foramen is located at the midportion on the inner surface of the ramus. This foramen opens into the inferior alveolar canal and transmits the inferior alveolar nerve and vessels.

The posterior border of the ramus is

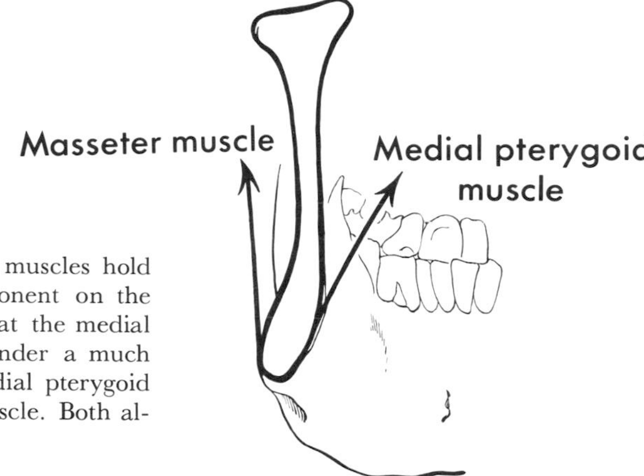

Figure 113. Masseter and medial pterygoid muscles hold each other in balance in their bending component on the mandibular ramus. Their angulation is such that the medial pterygoid muscle attacks the angular region under a much more favorable momentum. Therefore, the medial pterygoid muscle is always weaker than the masseter muscle. Both always act simultaneously.

rounded and strong and is united to the inferior border of the body of the bone to form the angle of the mandible. The anterior border of the ramus is continuous with the external oblique line of the mandible and terminates in the coronoid process, to which is attached the tendinous portion of the temporal muscle. The posterior border of the ramus terminates in the condylar process. The coronoid and condylar processes are joined by a sharp, concave ridge and separated by the rather deep mandibular notch. The condylar process of the mandible consists of a broad, transversely oval articular body, the mandibular head or condyle, that is supported by a narrow, thinner area known as the neck of the mandible. A shallow depression on the anterior aspect of the neck of the mandible is the site of attachment for most of the fibers of the lateral pterygoid muscle; some upper fibers attach into the capsule of the joint and thus to the disc. The articulating surface of the condyle is covered with fibrous tissue and articulates with the inferior surface of the articular disc of the temporomandibular joint. The fibrous capsule attached to the circumferential margin of the articular cartilage and to the neck suspends the mandible by its attachments to the articular tubercle and to the margins of the mandibular fossa of the squamous portion of the temporal bone.

The Temporomandibular Joint

In the management of fractures of the mandibular condyle, one must be completely aware of the structure and the function of the temporomandibular joints. They permit gliding and hingelike actions and are classified as ginglymoarthrodial articulations.

The temporomandibular joint is a compound joint made up of the articular surface of the mandibular head or condyle and the articulating portion of the temporal bone, the articular eminence or tubercle. An articular disc, enclosed within an articular capsule, is interposed between these bones. A heavy, smooth layer of fibrous tissue covers the surfaces of the articulating bones. The fibrous capsule that surrounds the joint is differentiated into inner and outer layers. The inner layer (synovial membrane) secretes a viscid fluid known as synovia, which serves to lubricate the joint and to furnish nutrition to avascular tissues of the joint. The outer layer is thicker and heavier and is supported by ligaments. The fibrous capsule, which encloses the joint, is attached to the entire circumference of the temporal articular area above and to the neck of the mandible and the posterior border of the ramus below. Anteriorly, the upper fibers of the lateral pterygoid muscle attach to the capsule and to the anterior border of the disc that here is fused to the capsule.

The articular disc is composed of fibrous tissue early in its development, but in adult life it is fibrocartilage. It is fastened to the inner circumference of the articular capsule by fusion anteriorly, but is attached loosely posteriorly where it attaches directly to the lateral and medial poles of the condyle. The upper surface of the disc is concave anteroposteriorly and slightly convex mediolaterally; the lower surface is concave in both directions. The disc is thick at its anterior and posterior borders and quite thin at its center. The joint is supported laterally by the strong temporomandibular ligament, which attaches the zygomatic process of the temporal bone to the lateral surface of the neck of the mandible. Wrongly, the stylomandibular and sphenomandibular ligaments generally are considered accessory ligaments of the joint. The weakest portions of the joint capsule are posterior and medial.

The blood supply of the temporomandibular joint is derived from superficial branches of the external carotid artery. The nerve supply is through the auriculotemporal and masseteric branches of the mandibular division of the fifth nerve. Nerve fibers are present in the connective tissue of the synovial membrane, but the articular surfaces of the cartilages have no blood or nerve supply.

APPLIED ANATOMY OF THE MANDIBLE

Although the mandible is dense and strong, it has areas of weakness which predispose to fracture in certain regions. The commoner areas of fracture are through the symphysial

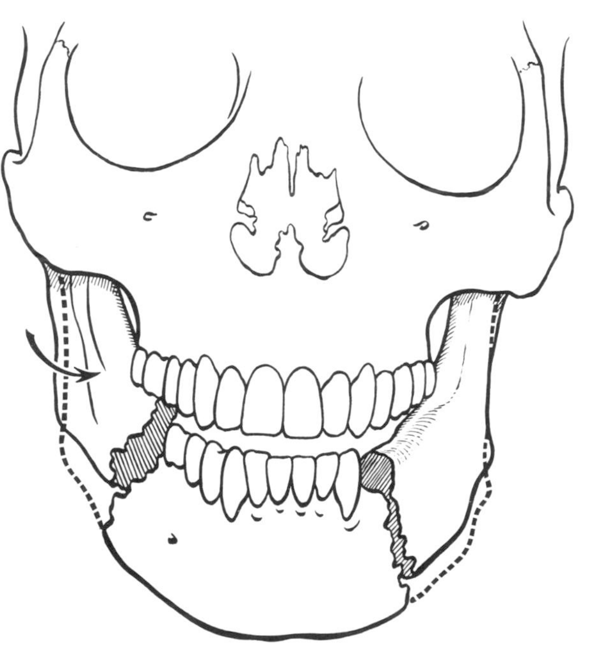

Figure 114. Diagram illustrating bilateral compound fracture of the mandible with edentulous proximal segments. Note displacement of the proximal fragment on the right against the maxillary teeth and partial displacement of the proximal fragment on the left. Impaction of fractures may prevent extreme displacement.

region lateral to the mental prominence, where the mandible is weaker because of the incisive fossae; through the region of the mental foramen; through the angle of the mandible; and through the neck of the mandible. The strength of the lower jaw also varies considerably with the presence or absence of teeth.

In childhood the body of the mandible is weakened by the presence of partially developed, unerupted permanent teeth, but this is compensated for by the youthful resiliency which protects the bone from fracture. With aging, the loss of teeth and resorption of alveolar bone result in a decrease in the vertical dimension of the mandible, making it more liable to fracture. The thinness of the angle of the mandible predisposes it to fractures in this region.

A direct blow upon the symphysis may result in fracture of one or both necks of the mandible. A blow to one side of the jaw may result in a fracture of the body on the side of the blow and a fracture of the neck on the opposite side. The thick, dense periosteum of the mandible is continuous with the alveolar soft tissues and continues to the necks of the teeth and the periodontal membrane. The periosteum is so intimately associated with the bone and the overlying thin periodontal tissues that fracture of the body of the mandible with the least bit of displacement, except in edentulous cases, is almost certain to be a compound fracture (Fig. 114). The periosteum and the heavy muscles of the ramus form a strong protective covering and give excellent support to fragments if fractures occur in this region.

Muscles Affecting Movement of the Mandible

Movement of the mandible depends upon two groups of muscles. An understanding of the function of these muscles is important in the diagnosis and treatment of fractures of the bone. The weak muscles of facial expression attached to the mandible have no appreciable influence on displacement of fractured segments (Fig. 115).

The Depressor-Retractor Group of Muscles

The anterior, or depressor-retractor, group of muscles attached to the mandible is the weaker of the two systems. The muscles of this group insert into the inner and inferior aspect of the mental region and exert a downward and posterior force which results in posterior and inferior displacement of fractured anterior mandibular segments.

Geniohyoid muscle. This paired muscle arises on the inner border of the mandible from the inferior mental spine and inserts into the body of the hyoid bone.

Digastric muscle. The digastric muscle consists of a posterior and an anterior belly connected by a long tendon. The posterior belly arises from the medial surface of the mastoid process and runs forward and downward to continue as the intermediate tendon. Where the tendon passes above the hyoid bone it runs through a pulley formed by the deep fascia. The pulley itself is attached to the hyoid bone and the tendon can slide in this pulley. At this point the tendon forms an obtuse angle and continues into the anterior belly that is inserted to the digastric fossa at the lower border of the mandible close to the midline.

The Elevator Group of Muscles

Masseter muscle. The masseter is an elevator of the lower jaw and extends from the medial and lateral surface and lower border of the zygomatic arch to the anterior and lateral surface and angle of the mandibular ramus. The superficial fibers run

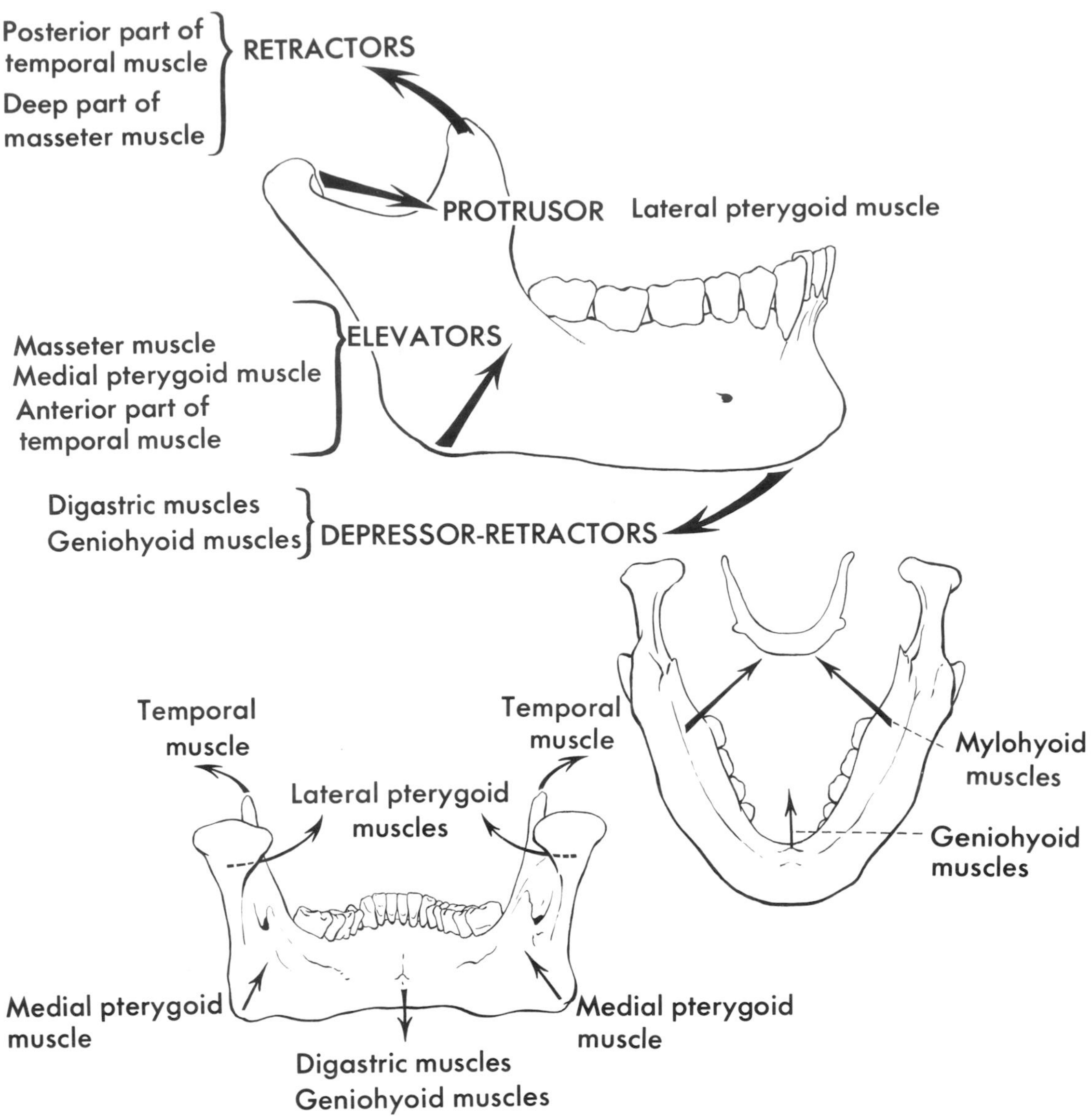

Figure 115. Diagrammatic representation of the main directions of the composite forces of the mandibular muscles.

downward and backward, whereas the deeper fibers run vertically downward.

Temporal muscle. This fan-shaped muscle arises in the temporal fossa and from the inferior temporal line. Its fibers descend medial to the zygomatic arch and insert on the coronoid process, the mandibular notch, and the inner surface of the ramus of the mandible. It elevates and retracts the mandible.

Medial pterygoid muscle. This powerful muscle originates from the pterygoid fossa of the sphenoid bone and the pyramidal process of the palatine bone and inserts on the inner surface of the ramus and angle of the mandible. It is an elevator of the jaw and is important in the movement of mastication. Its force is exerted upward, inward, and forward.

The Protrusor Muscle

Lateral pterygoid muscle. This muscle originates with two heads, the upper from the infratemporal surface of the great wing of the sphenoid bone and the lower from the outer surface of the lateral plate of the pterygoid process. It inserts with some bundles into the articular disc of the temporomandibular joint, but mainly into the anterior surface of the neck of the mandible. The uppermost fibers of the muscle pull the articular disc forward and medially. The lower fibers pull the head of the mandible medialward, forward, and downward.

The Mylohyoid Muscle

The mylohyoid muscle has hardly any influence on the movements of either the mandible or the hyoid bone because most of its bundles join in the midline at the mylohyoid raphe. The function of this muscle is to elevate the tongue, for instance, during swallowing. However, after a symphysial fracture of the mandible, this muscle running from the right to the left mandible will approximate the large fragments.

SURGICAL PATHOLOGY: FACTORS THAT INFLUENCE DISPLACEMENT OF FRACTURED SEGMENTS

An appreciation of the following factors is important in the diagnosis and treatment of mandibular fractures:

Direction and Intensity of Traumatic Force

A high velocity force may cause fracture with displacement only on the side of the mandible involved. A slower, less violent blow might result in a fracture at the point of contact without much displacement, with a subcondylar fracture on the opposite side. A direct blow on the chin may produce fractures of one or both mandibular necks or fractures through the region of the symphysis.

Site of Fracture

Fractures of the angle of the mandible may exhibit extensive displacement, while fractures of the ramus, in which fragments are protected by the heavy musculature, usually show little displacement.

Direction of Fracture Line

The direction of the fracture line greatly affects the degree of displacement of the fractured segments. When the line of fracture extends downward and forward from the molar region, it is said to be in a favorable direction for the alignment of the fragments. Progressive displacement of the posterior fragment is prevented by the position of the anterior fragment. If the line of fracture is in the opposite direction, displacement may occur from the action of the posterior group of muscles, for such action favors displacement. The presence of teeth in the posterior segment tends to minimize displacement because of their contact with the maxillary teeth.

The vertical direction of a fracture may or may not lead to displacement. Fractures passing from behind anteriorly and medially are favorable for displacement of the posterior fragment because of the medial pull on the proximal segment made by the posterior group of muscles. A fracture running in the other direction, from the lateral surface inward and backward, may present very little displacement because the forces exerted by the two muscle groups are such that the fragments are pulled together.

Muscle Pull in Fracture Displacement

The pull of the muscles attached to the mandible is a great factor in influencing the degree and direction of displacement of fractured segments. The anterior group of muscles tends to displace fragments downward, posteriorly, and medially, whereas the closing or posterior group of muscles pulls the mandible upward, forward, and medially (Fig. 116).

Presence or Absence of Teeth

Teeth on the proximal segment may prevent displacement by occlusal contact with the maxillary teeth. Proximal fragments in which there are no teeth may be widely displaced.

Extent of Soft Tissue Wounds

The extent of the soft tissue wounds may influence displacement of the fragments. Severe tears of the musculature and overlying soft tissues permit wider displacement of the fractured segments than occurs in cases in which soft tissues remain intact and give some support to the bony fragments. Fractures also can be displaced by the weight of soft tissues attached to bone if lacerations have been extensive and if large segments of soft tissue have been separated from their attachments. Suturing of soft tissues may give support to large segments of bone that have lost their complete support.

CLASSIFICATION OF FRACTURES OF THE MANDIBLE

Fractures may be classified in several categories. The following are the most common:

- A. According to the direction of the fracture and the favorability for treatment
  1. Horizontal
     a. Favorable
     b. Unfavorable
  2. Vertical
     a. Favorable
     b. Unfavorable
- B. According to the severity of the fracture

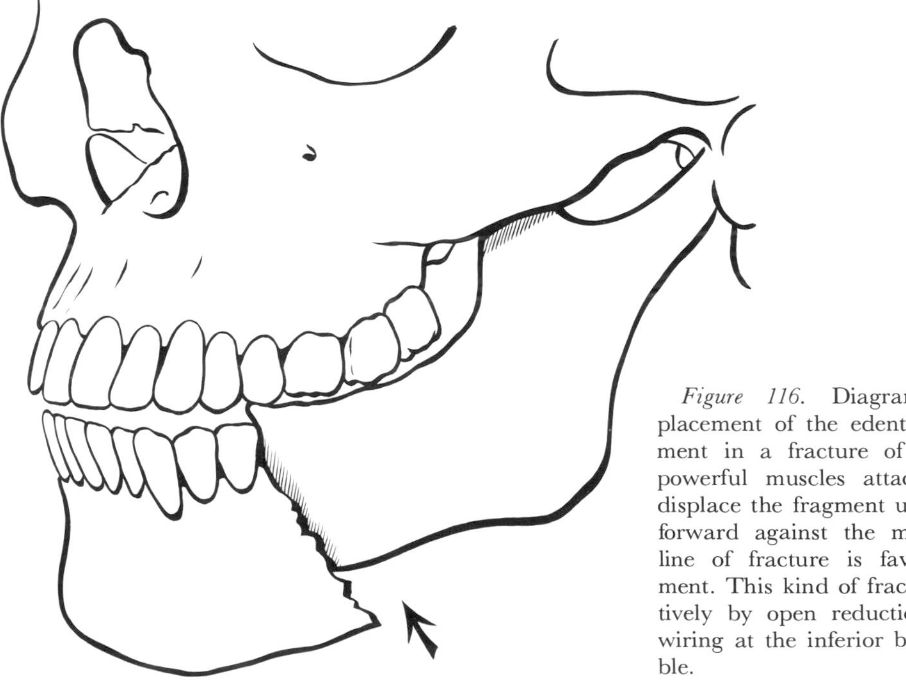

Figure 116. Diagram illustrating displacement of the edentulous proximal segment in a fracture of the mandible. The powerful muscles attached to the ramus displace the fragment upward, inward, and forward against the maxillary teeth. The line of fracture is favorable for displacement. This kind of fracture is treated effectively by open reduction and interosseous wiring at the inferior border of the mandible.

1. Simple fractures. In the simple fracture the soft tissues may be damaged but there is no open wound.
2. Compound fractures. Compound fractures are those in which there is a break through the overlying structures and skin or mucosa with direct communication of the fragments with the outside.

C. According to the type of fracture
   1. Greenstick fracture. In the greenstick fracture there is incomplete discontinuity of bone. The bone is bent to resemble a green stick which has been partially broken by force.
   2. Complex fracture. Complex fractures are those in which the fracture occurs in several directions—sometimes into a joint with severe injury resulting to surrounding tissues.
   3. Comminuted fractures. There are many fragments in a comminuted fracture. These fractures may be simple or compound.
   4. Impacted fractures. Fractures in which the fragments are driven firmly together are known as impacted fractures.
   5. Depressed fractures. These show depression and dislocation of the fractured segments, as in fractures of the zygoma.

D. Fractures classified according to the presence or absence of the teeth in the jaws*
   1. Dentulous
   2. Partially edentulous
   3. Edentulous

E. Mandibular fractures classified as to location
   1. Fractures of the symphysis region; those that occur in the region of the symphysis between the lower canine teeth.
   2. Fractures in the canine region.
   3. Fractures in the body of the mandible; fractures occurring between the canine teeth and the angle of the mandible.
   4. Fractures of the angle of the mandible; those occurring through the angle of the mandible behind the second or third molar tooth.
   5. Fractures of the ramus of the mandible; those fractures occurring between the angle of the mandible and sigmoid notch.
   6. Fractures of the coronoid process; fractures in which the coronoid process is fractured at a level above the mandibular notch.
   7. Fractures of the condylar process. These fractures include all fractures of the neck above the level of the sigmoid notch of the mandible.

Authors' Classification

A classification of fractures according to location is simple and correlates anatomic and clinical nomenclature.

Region of the Symphysis. This is the region bounded by vertical lines just distal to the lower canine teeth.

Region of the Body. The region of the body is the region which comprises the mandible from the canine line to a line coinciding to the anterior border of the masseter muscle.

Region of the Angle. The region of the angle is a triangular region bounded by the an-

* Rowe and Killey (1955) classified fractures according to the presence or absence of serviceable teeth in the segments of the mandible:
1. Teeth present on both sides of the fracture line (Class I).
2. Teeth present on only one side of the fracture line (Class II).
3. Fragments containing no teeth (Class III).

terior border of the màsseter muscle and an oblique line extending from the mandibular third molar region to the posterior superior attachment of the masseter muscle.

Region of the Ramus. This region is bounded inferiorly by the region of the angle of the mandible and superiorly by two equal lines which form a 90 degree apex at the midpoint of the sigmoid notch of the mandible.

Region of the Condylar Process. This region comprises the condylar process above the ramus region and includes the neck and the mandibular condyle.

Region of the Coronoid Process. This region includes the coronoid process above the ramus region of the mandible.

Region of the Alveolar Process. Fractures may not occur exclusively within a specific region but in most instances will be principally within one of the regions and ex-

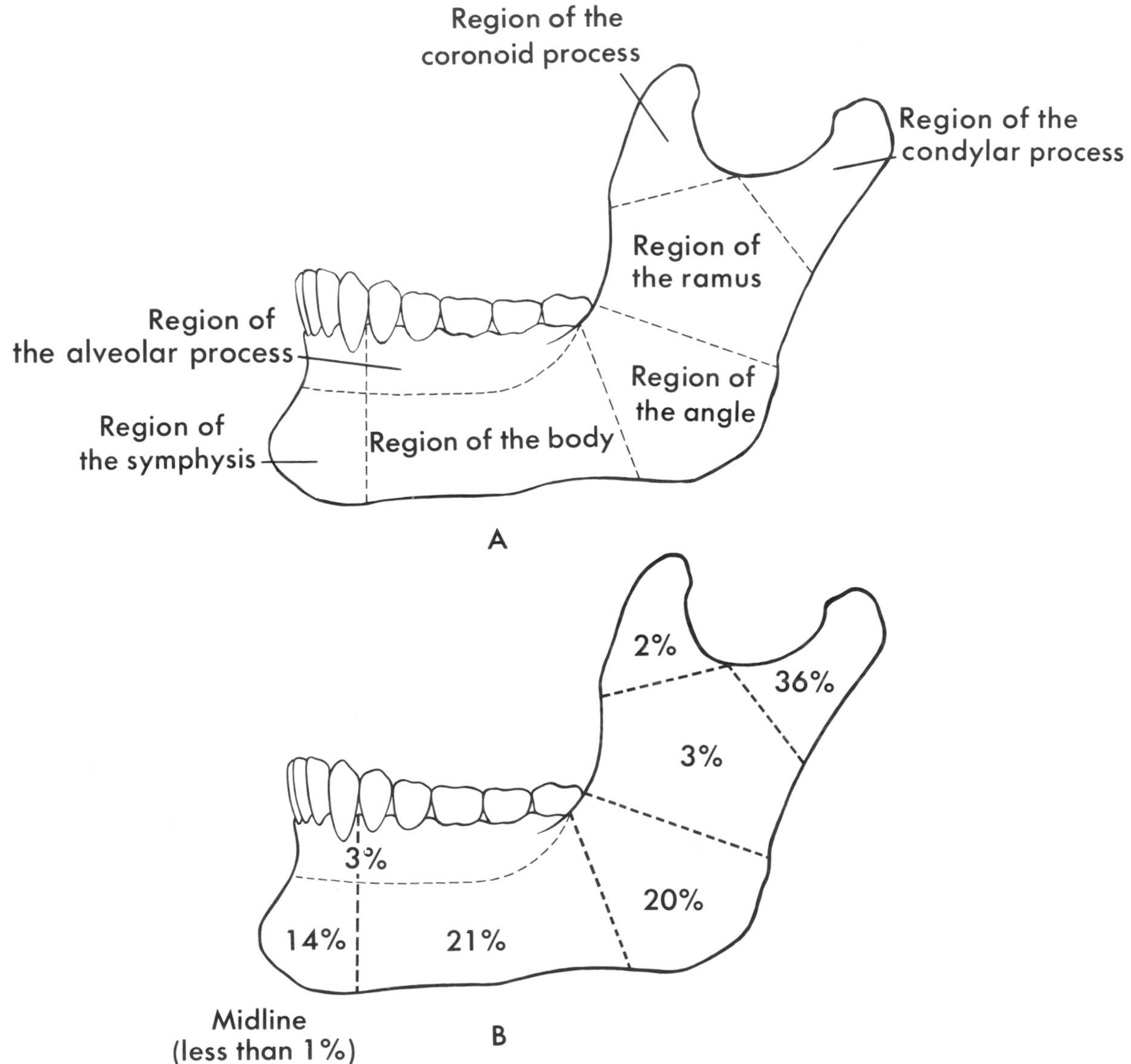

Figure 117 A, B. Frequency of fractures in various anatomic regions of the mandible.

tend partially into an adjacent region. If, for example, the main fracture is through the angle region but extends into the body, this may be described as an angle fracture with extension into the body region. If only the alveolar process is fractured, this should be described as a fracture of the alveolar process in the region of the symphysis, in the body, or as a combination of fractures in both regions. As a matter of illustration, fractures of the mandible may occur through the angle region on one side, through the body region of the opposite side, or through the neck of the mandible on the opposite side. Bilateral subcondylar fractures are usually associated with an oblique fracture in the region of the symphysis (see Fig. 158).

The highest percentage of fractures of the mandible occur through the weakest portion or the condylar process. These account for approximately 36 per cent of all mandibular fractures. The regions of the angle and the body each account for approximately 21 per cent, and the region of symphysis approximately 14 per cent. Less than 1 per cent occurs exactly through the midline of the mandible. Three per cent occur in the region of the ramus, 3 per cent are limited to alveolar fractures, and 2 per cent are in the region of the coronoid process (Fig. 117 *A* and *B*).

ETIOLOGY OF FRACTURES OF THE MANDIBLE

Most fractures of the lower jaw are caused by external violence, but a few follow severe muscular contractions as occurs in cases of electroshock therapy and in instances in which bone is weakened by pathologic conditions. Over one-half of fractures of the mandible are caused by automobile accidents, fist fights, falls, kicks, or sports trauma. Transportation accidents involving motorcycles, trains, and airplanes account for many fractures. Injuries from animals account for some and the remainder are due to miscellaneous accidents.

Predisposing Causes of Fracture of the Mandible

Generalized bone diseases such as hyperparathyroidism, osteomalacia, and fragilitas ossium which cause changes in the form and density of bone and so weaken its structure and predispose to fracture.

Localized bone diseases such as benign and malignant neoplasms, cysts, osteomyelitis, or hemangioma.

Anatomic considerations:

1. The thin regions at the angle or the neck of the mandible are frequent locations of fractures. Often not the weak areas but the junctions between the weak and strong parts are sites of fractures.
2. Edentulous regions with atrophy of the alveolar bone and loss of supporting structure predispose to fracture.
3. Weaker points. The mental foramina and the incisive fossae in the region of the symphysis are weaker points through which fractures may occur.

Exciting Traumatic Causes of Fractures

Direct force. A blow to the mandible may result in discontinuity of the bone at the site of impact.

Indirect force. Any force applied to the mandible may cause the mandible to bend, and if this bending surpasses the limits of the elasticity of the bone, it will cause a fracture. A fracture may be caused by a blow on the opposite side of the jaw or a blow at a point distant from the site of the fracture. Indirect force is the cause of most fractures of the neck. Fractures of the condylar process may result from a blow on the contralateral side of the chin, or a blow to the symphysis may result in fracture of both mandibular necks.

Muscular force. Fractures of the mandible may occur as the result of violent contraction initiated by accidental or intentionally induced electrical stimuli. Shock in psychiatric therapy and accidental electrocution has caused fractures of the spine and mandible. Bone weakened by disease, as in carcinoma or osteomyelitis, may fracture during mastication.

DIAGNOSIS OF MANDIBULAR FRACTURES

Importance of Detailed History

A full knowledge of the circumstances under which the injury was produced may be extremely helpful in arriving at a final diagnosis in fractures and injuries of the mandible. The direction of the force, the condition and state of consciousness of the patient at and after the time of injury, the presence or absence and use or non-use of a seat belt, and the position of the patient in the automobile, all may be helpful. A patient who gives a history of a severe blow to the symphysial region of the mandible might be expected to have fractures of the necks bilaterally. One who has sustained a blow on the side of the mandible could be expected to have a fracture at the site of injury associated with a subcondylar fracture on the opposite side. The patient who has been sitting in the passenger seat, unprotected by a seat belt, is quite likely to have fractures of the nose, or of the bones of the middle third of the face.

Clinical Examination

The clinical findings in fractures of the mandible vary considerably with the degree and extent of the injury. A fracture with minimal or no displacement of the fragments results in a small degree of edema and no other symptoms. Examination may reveal no evident abnormality of occlusion, but the patient may remark that the teeth do not come together as they did before the injury, and mastication may produce pain. Upon closer examination, tenderness on pressure over the skin or mucosa, ecchymosis, and abnormal mobility between the teeth on either side of the fracture line may be noted. Anesthesia of the lower lip may be present if the fracture is between the mental foramen and the inferior alveolar foramen of the mandible with injury to the inferior alveolar nerve.

In extensive fractures, the findings are more pronounced. Swelling, ecchymosis, and tenderness of the floor of the mouth and pain on slight motion of the mandible may be noted. Deformity of the lower facial area depends upon the extent of the edema and the degree of displacement of the fragments. Excessive salivation and drooling due to difficulty in swallowing usually are prominent features.

Abnormalities in occlusion usually are obvious and easily identified. Further evaluation is necessary to determine the extent of the fractures and the directions in which they run. Overriding of the fragments is most likely to occur in the regions of the symphysis and angle of the mandible. The displacement may be in a horizontal or vertical direction, depending upon the direction of fracture. The portion of the bone anterior to the fracture may be pulled downward, whereas the proximal fragment may be pulled upward out of position by the strong muscle pull on the ramus of the mandible.

In the body of the mandible, fractures usually are quite easily identified on inspection and manipulation, but fractures of the rami are more difficult to discover by clinical examination alone. A fracture of the body of the mandible on one side should suggest the possibility of a subcondylar fracture on thc opposite side. Puncture wounds and lacerations of the tongue or of the floor of the mouth or buccal mucosa should suggest the possibility that fragments of bone, teeth, or dentures have been imbedded in the soft tissues. All the oral soft tissues should be examined carefully as well as those of the pharynx.

Common Symptoms of Fractures of the Mandible

Pain. Pain usually is present on motion. It may be noticed immediately after the fracture occurs and then is due to injury of the inferior alveolar nerve, the periosteum, or the adjacent soft tissue.

Tenderness. On palpation, exquisite tenderness will be noted over the site of the fracture. Many fractures of the mandible can be localized by this symptom.

Disability. Because of pain and discomfort, the patient is unable to open his mouth and refuses to eat the usual food. The least movement may result in excruciating pain, and the fear of this keeps the patient from making an attempt to move the jaw in eating, speaking, or swallowing.

Swelling. The escape of blood into the soft parts at the site of the fracture results in swelling and facial asymmetry. Distortion and swelling occur almost immediately following injury.

Discoloration. The overlying tissues become red, bluish, or purplish as a result of hemorrhage into the adjacent soft tissues or the formation of a hematoma near the site of the fracture.

Deformity. Displacement of mandibular fragments may be suggested by the presence of asymmetry of the face and deformity of the mandible. Shifting of fragments to one side or the other may give a bizarre appearance to the lower face. Bilateral subcondylar fractures with upward and backward telescoping of the rami result in open bite in the anterior region with the appearance of elongation of the face.

Abnormal mobility. With fracture displacement of the neck on one side, the mandible will shift toward the fractured side when the patient attempts to open his mouth. On protrusive motion, the jaw shifts to the side of the injury because of lack of function of the lateral pterygoid muscle on the side of the injury.

Crepitation. The patient may notice a grating, cracking, or grinding sound as the fragments move in contact during opening or closing motions of the mandible.

Salivation. Pain and tenderness stimulate the salivary glands to overactivity. Drooling of saliva from the mouth is increased by the inability to swallow the excessive saliva.

Fetor ex ore. The patient may have offensive breath. Food, blood clots, and mucus undergo bacterial putrefaction; this gives a bad odor to the breath. This becomes obvious to friends, relatives, and the attending physician.

Clinical Findings in Fractures of the Mandible

The diagnosis of fracture of the mandible may be made if one or more of the following findings is evident:

Malocclusion. The most reliable finding in the dentulous patient with fracture of the mandible is malocclusion. Minimal dislocation of the fracture will be noticed immediately by the patient, who will complain that he is unable to get his teeth together properly. Upon inspection, malocclusion of the teeth will be discovered.

Mobility at site of fracture. Bimanual manipulation of the mandible will result in springiness or movement at the site of the fracture. This is especially noticeable in fractures of the body of the mandible. With one hand stabilizing the ramus of the mandible and the other manipulating the symphysial region, fractures usually can be identified easily if they are in the body of the bone. Fractures will be demonstrated by movement and discomfort at the site of the injury.

Dysfunction. The patient will request soft food, which requires a minimal amount of movement of the jaw for mastication. He is unable to move his jaw normally, and eating and speech are difficult because of pain on motion.

Crepitation. This sign is not reliable for the diagnosis of a fracture. The test may be extremely uncomfortable to the patient and no attempt should be made to elicit this finding.

Tumescence at the site of fracture. Almost all fractures are accompanied by some degree of swelling from hematoma or edema at the site of the fracture. This finding is associated generally with extensive ecchymosis.

Abnormal mobility of the mandible. This is a highly significant finding in patients with fracture of the mandible. Deviation to one or the other side may occur when the patient attempts to open his mouth or to protrude the mandible.

Injuries and Fractures of the Teeth of the Mandible

Damage to the teeth may occur in conjunction with fractures of the mandible or independently of any fracture. Management of the dental injury is important in the treatment of fractures of the jaws. Damage is most common to the exposed anterior teeth but is not necessarily limited to them. Frequently the cusps of premolar and molar teeth are sheared off as a result of lateral forces acting while the teeth are in occlusion. With the teeth set firmly in occlusion at the moment of the accident, a blow to the lateral surface of the mandible may result in fractures of the lingual maxillary cusps on the same side or of the buccal cusps of the maxillary teeth on the opposite side of the mouth, with exposure of the dental pulp. With the pulp of the tooth exposed, the patient may have extreme discomfort if the exposure is not recognized before the teeth are fixed in occlusion. Removal of the dental pulp or extraction of the tooth may be indicated before fixation.

The anterior teeth may be evulsed, or the crowns of the teeth may be broken off at the gum line. Fragments of teeth that will serve no useful purpose in stabilization of the fractures may be removed at the time of reduction, or, if they seem to be causing no difficulty, they can be removed after the fracture has healed.

Teeth in the line of fracture that will aid in stabilization of the fragments, or those which are unlikely to cause complications, should be retained. The presence of a single tooth or even the half of a tooth on the proximal fragment may aid in the stabilization and prevent dislocation of the segment. Although such a tooth may be worthless in itself, it should be retained at least until the fragments have shown evidence of bony union. Some teeth that are tender to the touch or loosened in their sockets may undergo spontaneous repair without pulpal necrosis. Teeth that are greatly loosened or are attached to a loose segment of alveolar bone, if retained, should be supported by ligation to the adjacent teeth or to arch bars.

Orthodontic bands may be helpful in stabilizing teeth of strategic significance. These teeth should be tested frequently to determine the vitality of their pulp. Their pulp may necrotize and the teeth may be discolored several months after injury. Loosening of the posterior teeth usually indicates fracture of the root or a portion of the crown. Teeth that cannot be salvaged should be extracted.

Reimplantation of evulsed teeth sometimes is successful, but usually it is inadvisable to attempt this in a patient with multiple fractures. Reimplantation is most likely to be successful in cases of developing teeth with open root canals. The blood supply in young teeth is abundant and regeneration may occur.

Roentgenographic Examination

Diagnosis of fractures of the mandible usually can be made on clinical evaluation, but additional information can be obtained by roentgenographic studies to determine the extent and direction of the fracture and the condition of the teeth of the mandible. The complexity and direction of the fractures, involvement of the root apices, pre-existing pathologic conditions of the mandible, the degree of displacement of bone fragments, the presence of foreign bodies and portions of tooth that may be displaced can be identified and determined by roentgenographic examination.

Radiographic Findings in Fracture of the Mandible

X-ray examination should be done carefully and thoroughly in all cases of suspected fracture of the mandible. Fractures in the body and angle of the mandible generally are detected on the usual standard roentgenographic position films (see p. 67). The condylar processes are especially difficult to demonstrate radiographically and particular attention should be taken to examine the condylar regions. Stereoscopic views or planograms may be necessary in some cases to demonstrate the site of fracture. Occlusal films and dental roentgenograms are helpful in detecting fractures of the symphysial region, the alveolar structures, and the roots of the teeth. Although the diagnosis of fractures of the mandible may be made on the basis of clinical findings alone, the precise characteristics and degree of displacement must await the evaluation of a carefully taken and complete set of roentgenograms.

Postoperative X-ray Examination

Postoperative x-ray examination is important in evaluating the effectiveness of reduction and position of the fragments after treatment. Follow-up radiographs during the course of treatment offers very little information, since radiologic evidence of bony union is not present in mandibular fractures for several months after reduction. Bony union is estimated on the basis of digital manipulation after a sufficient period of immobilization.

TREATMENT OF FRACTURES OF THE MANDIBLE

General Principles

Early reduction and immobilization of the fragments should be carried out as early as the patient's general condition permits. Early treatment permits manipulation and reduction of the fractured segments before granulation tissue forms and organization of clots occurs between the ends of the bones. After the process of repair has begun and is fairly well established, reduction is more difficult. Early reduction restores anatomic relations and reduces the size of the wound, decreases the pain resulting from motion at the site of fracture, and promotes early healing of the soft tissues and bone. The risks of infection and secondary hemorrhage are greatly reduced by early reduction and fixation.

Region of the Symphysis

Fractures occurring exactly through the midline of the mandible are rare and account for less than 1 per cent of all mandibular fractures. Midline fractures may show displacement from the force of the blow causing the fracture, but otherwise tend to show very little displacement. If displaced, these fragments usually respond easily to manipulation or reduction. They can be held by fixation with arch bars if teeth are present on both sides of the fracture. The broad approximating surfaces are held together by the force of the mylohyoid muscles.

The symphysial region is defined as the region between vertical lines passing just distal to the canine tooth of each side. Fractures in the symphysial region are most frequently oblique, beginning in the mental fossa and extending posteriorly and laterally. The direction of fracture obliquity provides gliding surfaces which permit telescopic displacement of the segments because of the clinically unfavorable pull of the muscles attached to the inner surface of the mandible (Fig. 118).

The diagnosis of fractures in the symphysial region usually can be made easily upon clinical inspection. Swelling and ecchymosis of the tissues of the floor of the mouth, with tenderness and pain at the site of the fracture and malocclusion, usually establish the diagnosis. Bimanual palpation of the mandible exhibits movement at the site of the fracture, and the arch may be narrowed as the result of telescoping of the fragments.

Radiographs of fractures in the symphysial region usually do not show much on posterior-anterior projection of the mandible; such fractures are shown best in occlusal views (see Figs. 50 and 51). The presence of a symphysial fracture should suggest the possibility of a subcondylar fracture on one or both sides, and roentgenographic examination of the condylar processes should be made in all cases of injury or fracture in the anterior mandibular region.

Fractures in the symphysial region, ex-

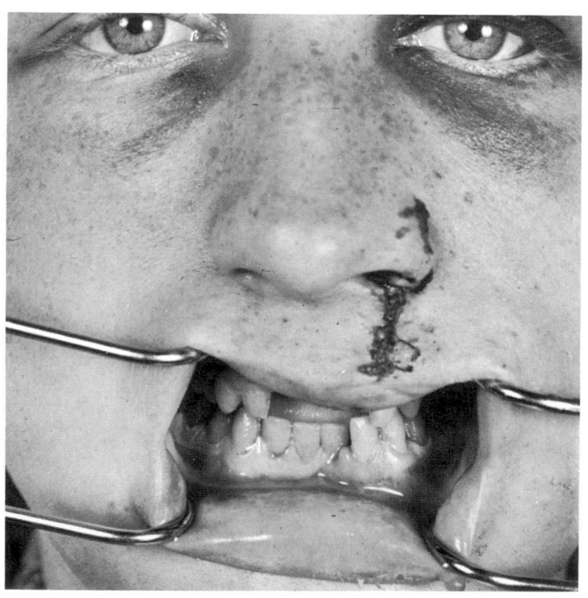

Figure 118. Fracture of the symphysial region of the mandible with overlapping of fragments and malocclusion.

cept for that small percentage that occurs exactly in the midline, do not respond well to simple reduction with intermaxillary fixation. In many cases, even though the teeth seem to be in some semblance of occlusion, there is moderately wide separation of the segments at the inferior border.

Extensive comminution of the symphysial region or bilateral fractures in this region may result in severe respiratory difficulty due to the posterior displacement of the mandibular segments. Lack of support of the muscles of the floor of the mouth, especially the genioglossus muscles, permits the

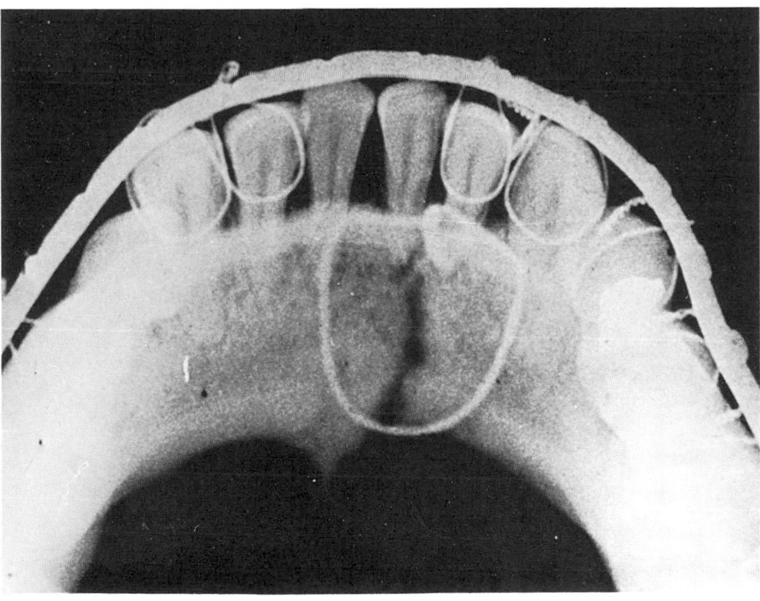

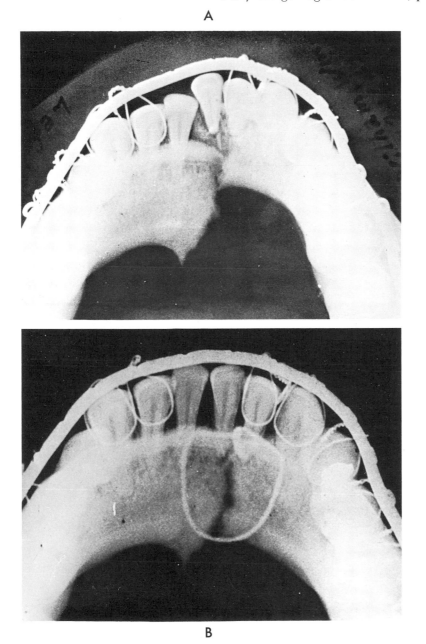

Figure 119. A. Fracture of the symphysial region of the mandible with displacement. The intraoral appliance failed to provide stabilization in the line of fracture. *B.* Stabilization of the fracture by open reduction and interosseous wire fixation.

tongue to fall into the posterior pharyngeal region, causing respiratory obstruction. In cases of severe comminution or loss of bone from the region of the symphysis, tracheotomy may be necessary as a lifesaving procedure. Obstruction may be relieved temporarily by protraction of the tongue and by placing the patient in the prone position and permanently by early reduction of the fracture.

Fractures of the symphysial region may be reduced by bimanual manipulation, by slow traction with rubber bands, or by open reduction (Fig. 119 *A, B*). When seen early, many fractures in this region may be reduced adequately by manipulation of the larger fragments. If the fracture occurred several days before treatment was possible, the formation of granulation tissue or callus between the fragments may make reduction by manipulation impossible. In some cases the application of an upper arch bar and of an arch bar on the lower fragments, with strong rubber-band traction, will pull the teeth and the bone fragments into their normal relations (Fig. 120). If the fragments overlap or telescope (bayonet apposition) and are greatly displaced by muscle pull, open reduction is the only satisfactory method of accurately repositioning the fragments. The kind of fixation necessary to immobilize fragments in fractures near the symphysis depends upon the direction of the fracture, the degree of displacement, and the muscular force operating to displace the fragments.

In some cases monomaxillary fixation with a single arch bar attached to teeth on both sides of the fragment will provide adequate stabilization (Fig. 121). Monomaxillary fixation usually is adequate for the relatively simple fracture in which displacement is minimal, and the obliquity of the fracture tends to prevent displacement.

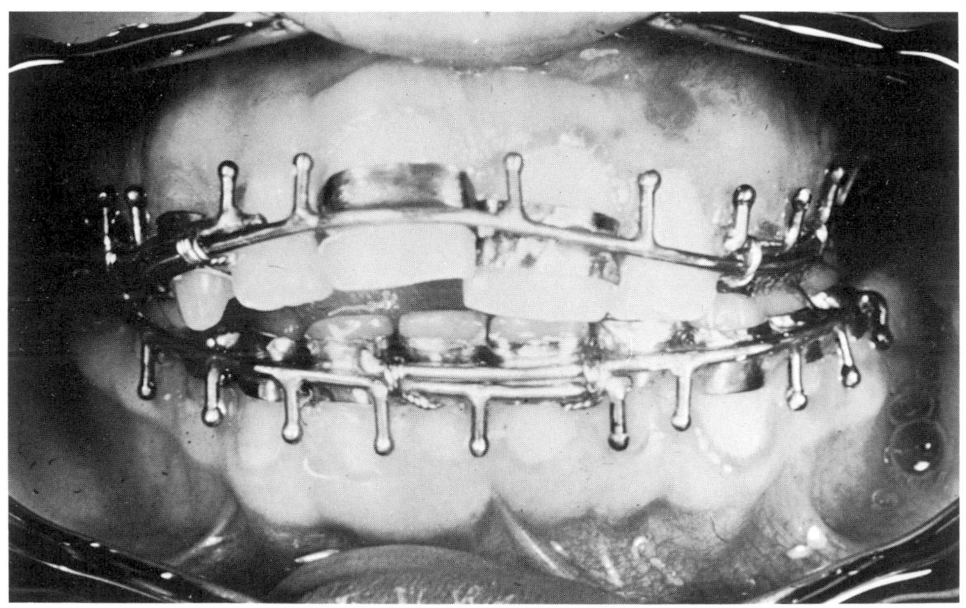

Figure 120. Orthodontic dental splint with bands about the crowns of the teeth. This is designed for the application of intermaxillary rubber band traction. Such splints are stable and effective, but are time consuming and expensive to construct. Commercially available arch bars are cheaper, can be applied more quickly and easily, and are equally effective.

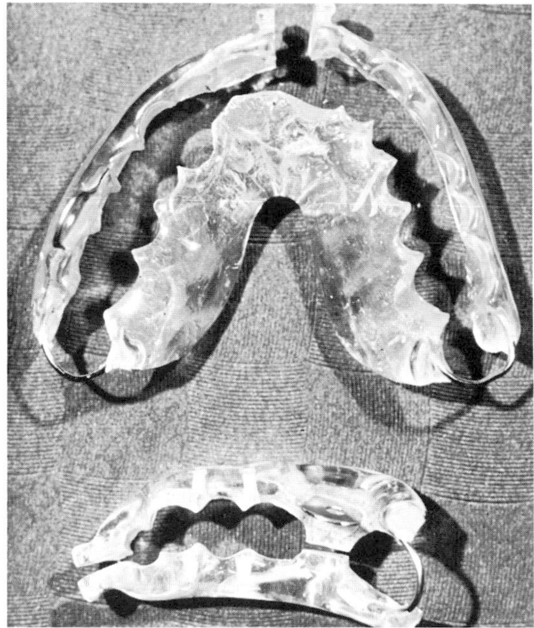

Figure 121. A Stout acrylic dental splint for monomaxillary fixation of mandibular fractures. The larger splint may be used for multiple mandibular fractures and the smaller splint for unilateral localized fracture.

Monomaxillary fixation may be satisfactory when there are no maxillary teeth.

Even though the single arch bar seems to be satisfactory for stabilizing fractures near the symphysis, it is best to use intermaxillary fixation if the patient has enough maxillary and mandibular teeth. Healing of the fragments stabilized by intermaxillary fixation results in a better final occlusion.

In some fractures of the symphysial region, in which there is displacement because of strong muscular forces, adequate fixation cannot be maintained by a single arch bar or by intermaxillary fixation. A combination of intermaxillary fixation and open reduction with direct interosseous wiring may be necessary (Fig. 122 *A*, *B*). Symphysial fractures in edentulous patients usually respond well to open reduction and interosseous wire fixation, or in some instances they may be stabilized adequately by using circumferential wiring about the patient's lower denture.

Open Operation

The direct surgical approach to fractures in the region of the symphysis is an effective means of treatment. The approach may be through the skin below the lower border of the mandible, or, in edentulous patients, through the mucoperiosteum overlying the alveolar ridge of the mandible. Both these approaches are made through areas in which there are no important anatomic structures that might be damaged.

The external operation is performed through an incision placed in the direction of the skin creases, at least 1 or 1.5 cm. behind the inferior border of the mandible. The line of the incision should be marked out with ink before the patient is anesthetized (Fig. 123). It is best, if possible, to mark the skin with the patient in the upright position. Edema may obscure the skin lines, and one must use care in making incisions in edematous tissues to avoid leaving a scar in a conspicuous area. The incision is made 4 to 5 cm. in length. It should be long enough to provide adequate exposure for visualization of the fracture. Too short an incision may result in damage to the soft tissues by overenthusiastic retraction of the wound margins.

The incision is made through the skin, the subcutaneous fascia, and the platysma muscle. The tissue is retracted forward, and the dissection is carried along the fascia of the digastric muscles to the bone at the inferior border of the mandible. The periosteum is incised along the inferior border of the mandible. On the anterior surface of the mandible the periosteum may be elevated without difficulty, but on the inner, or medial, surface of the mandible, sharp dissection is necessary to sever the attachments of the digastric muscles, which insert intimately into the bone of the digastric fossae.

On the inner surface of the mandible the

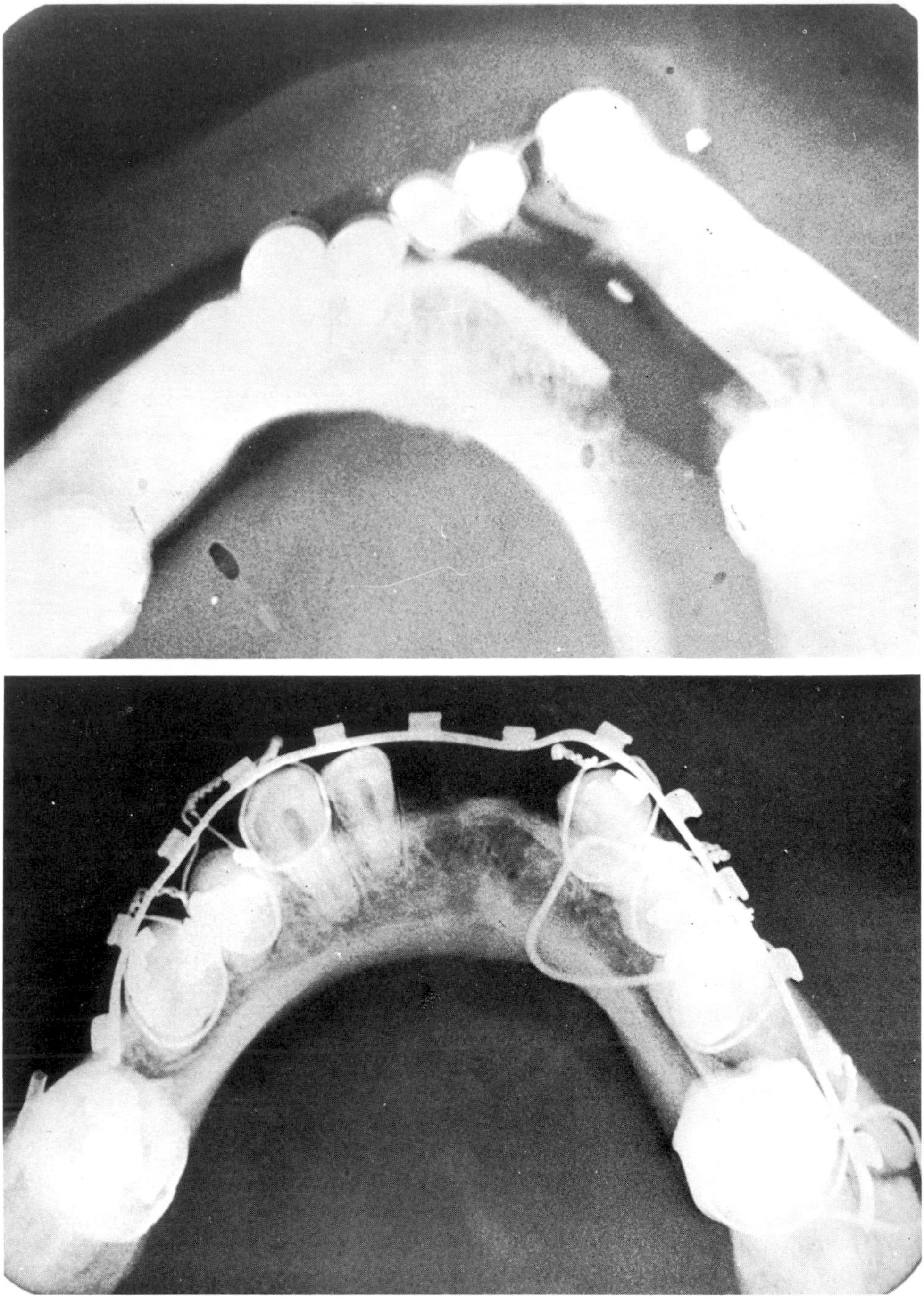

B

Figure 122. *A*. Compound fracture through the symphysial region of the mandible running backward to terminate in a splinter at the inferior border of the bone in the molar region. Mandibular anterior teeth have been dislocated, together with a section of alveolar bone. *B*. Mandibular reconstruction by means of open operation, interosseous wire fixation, and stabilization with an arch bar.

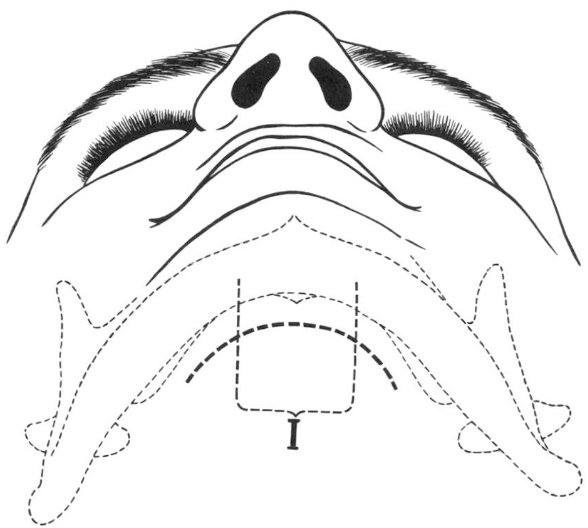

Figure 123. The surgical approach to the region of the symphysis of the mandible is through a curvilinear incision in the submandibular area, in or parallel to the skin folds. The skin line is purposely marked longer than the length of the intended incision (I) to facilitate lengthening of the incision during the operation if this becomes necessary.

dissection should be sufficient to permit placement of drill holes for the insertion of wires. On the outer surface the periosteum should be dissected sufficiently to permit visualization of the fragments. Intervening clots, bone spicules, muscle fibers, organized tissues, and foreign bodies should be removed carefully with a curette or scraped out with an elevator before attempting to reduce the fracture. The large fragments are grasped with a bone forceps and manipulated into position. If the line of fracture is at right angles to the outer surface of the bone, drill holes are placed on each side of the fracture site a short distance above the inferior border of the mandible. A 6 inch length of 25 gauge stainless steel wire is placed through the holes on each side of the fracture, and both ends are brought to the outer surface of the bone, where they are twisted tightly against the anterior mandibular surface.

If the fracture is oblique, the bone fragments should be placed in anatomic alignment and the drill hole passed through the overlapping parts of both segments. Twenty-two to 24 gauge wire is placed through the hole and twisted tightly around the lower border of the mandible. The twisted end of the wire is cut long enough to permit the end of it to be bent and inserted into one of the drill holes or pressed firmly against the surface of the bone in a position such that it will not irritate the overlying soft tissues.

To prevent the formation of a seroma or hematoma and to induce early healing, the periosteum should be sutured carefully over the border of the mandible with 000 or 0000 chromic catgut sutures. The digastric muscle should be replaced and held by sutures. A few 0000 plain catgut or fine white nylon sutures are used to approximate the platysma muscle and subcutaneous tissue. The skin is closed with 00000 single strand, synthetic sutures. The wounds usually are closed without drainage, but if there is any evidence of incipient infection, or if bleeding has not been completely controlled, it is advisable to insert a rubber drain into the depth of the wound.

Open reduction should not be attempted in the presence of frank infection. The infection should be brought under control before an operative procedure is done. Immobilization by means of intermaxillary fixation may help bring the infection under control by preventing damage to the soft tissues surrounding the fragments.

In the dentulous patient, open reduction and interosseous wire fixation of the mandible should be supplemented by the use of arch bars and intermaxillary rubber band fixation.

In cases of comminuted fractures in the symphysial region, in which there are not enough teeth for stabilization, these fractures may be treated by open reduction and direct interosseous wiring techniques; by the intramedullary pin fixation method of

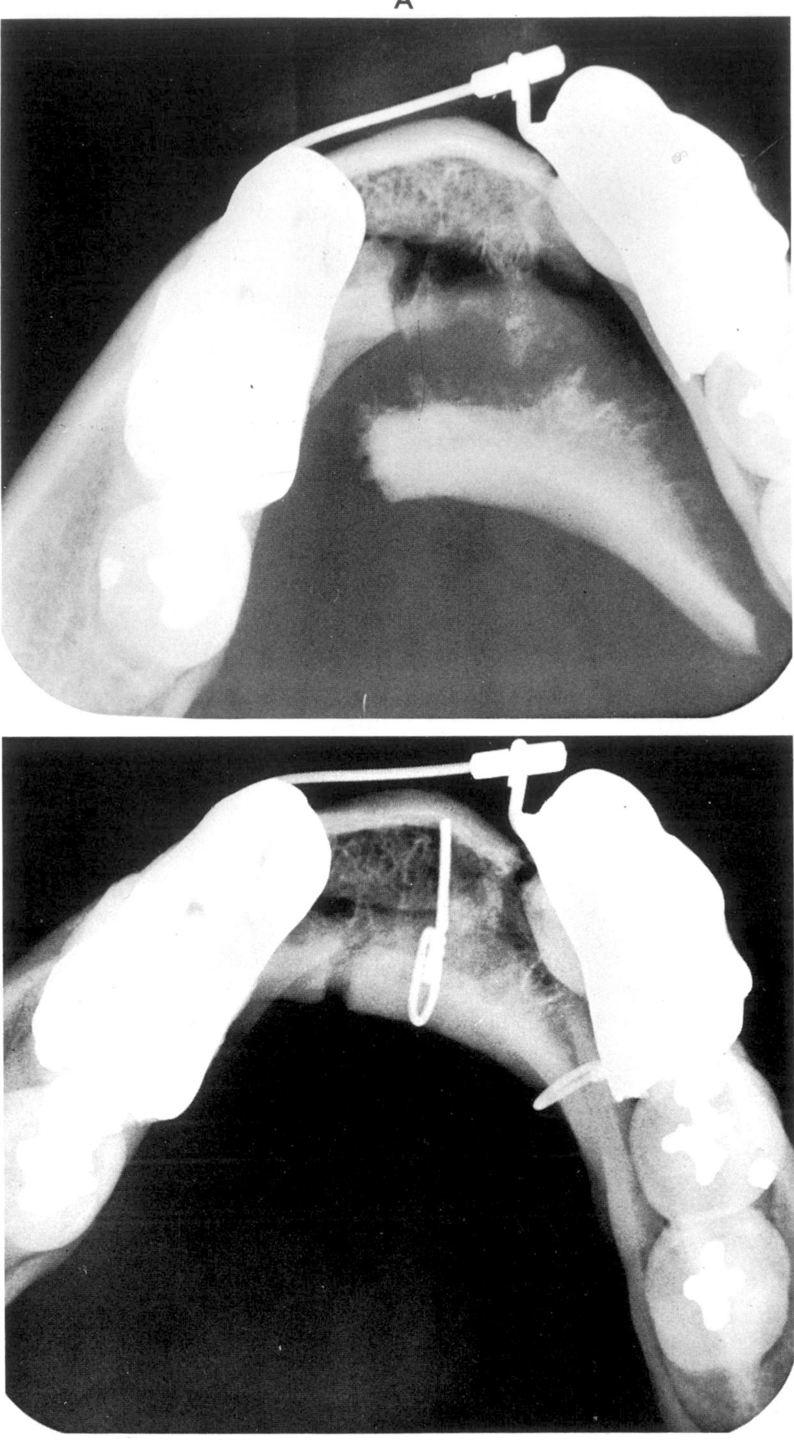

Figure 124. *A.* Fracture of the symphysial region of the mandible with displacement of a large segment of the lingual plate of the symphysis and the body. The fragment is pulled backward by the muscles of the floor of the mouth. An attempt was made to reduce the fracture by means of a cast-capped splint. The fragment in the floor of the mouth continued to give the patient difficulty and permitted the tongue to fall backward. The function of the tongue was greatly impaired. *B.* Open reduction was performed through a submandibular incision and the fragment was held with interosseous wire fixation.

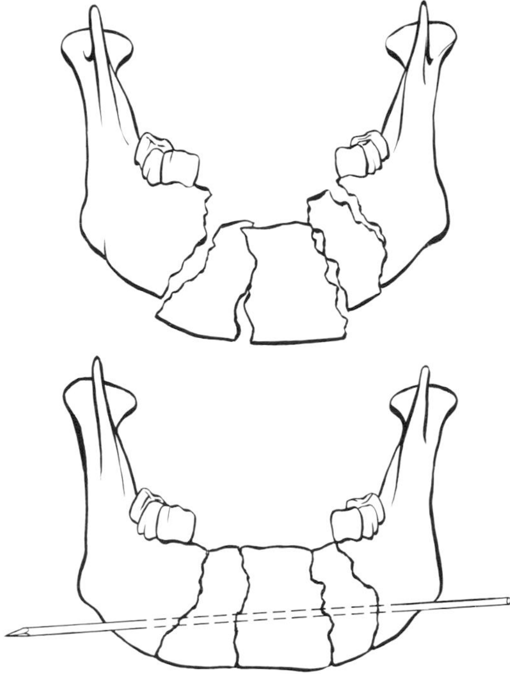

Figure 125. Multiple comminuted fractures of the mandible treated by the "shish kebab" method of Kiehn.

Brown and McDowell (1942) and Brown, McDowell, and Fryer (1949); by metal plate fixation; or by open reduction and the shish kebab wire fixation method (DesPrez and Kiehn, 1959) (Fig. 125).

Region of the Body

The body of the mandible is that segment which lies between a vertical line drawn distal to the mandibular canine and a line coinciding with the anterior border of the masseter muscle. The body supports the premolar and the molar teeth. It is the largest region of the mandible and sustains the second greatest number of mandibular fractures. Twenty-one per cent of all fractures of the mandible occur in the body, despite the fact that this is the heaviest, thickest, and strongest portion of the bone.

Fractures of the body of the mandible, because of the very intimate association of the periosteum with overlying soft tissues, invariably are compound fractures. Fractures with even minimal displacement, except in the edentulous patient, result in a tear of the mucosa with compounding of the fracture.

Fractures in the body usually exhibit all the classic signs and symptoms of fracture of the mandible. Except in cases of linear fractures without displacement (Fig. 126 *A, B*), anesthesia of the lower lip is a prominent and constant finding because of injury to the inferior alveolar nerve as it passes through the canal in the body of the mandible. Displacement of the fragments depends upon the presence or absence of teeth on each side of the fracture site, the direction of the fracture, the direction of the force of the blow, and the muscle pull on the fragments. In fractures through the body of the mandible with no teeth on the proximal segment, displacement is upward and medialward until the fragment impinges against the upper teeth or alveolar ridge. In bilateral fractures through the body of the mandible, especially in edentulous jaws, the anterior fragments are pulled downward and backward, and the posterior fragments are pulled upward and medialward resulting in separation of fragments. Most fractures of the body of the mandible are single, but they may be comminuted (Fig. 127 *A, B*) or associated with loss of bone as, for example, in gunshot wounds.

The choice of treatment of fractures of the body is determined largely by the presence or absence of teeth in the fragments. A large percentage of such fractures can be managed by simple intermaxillary fixation by any of the methods of dental wiring, or by the use of upper and lower arch bars and intermaxillary rubber band fixation (see Fig. 103). The problems of reduction and fixation are more difficult if the teeth are

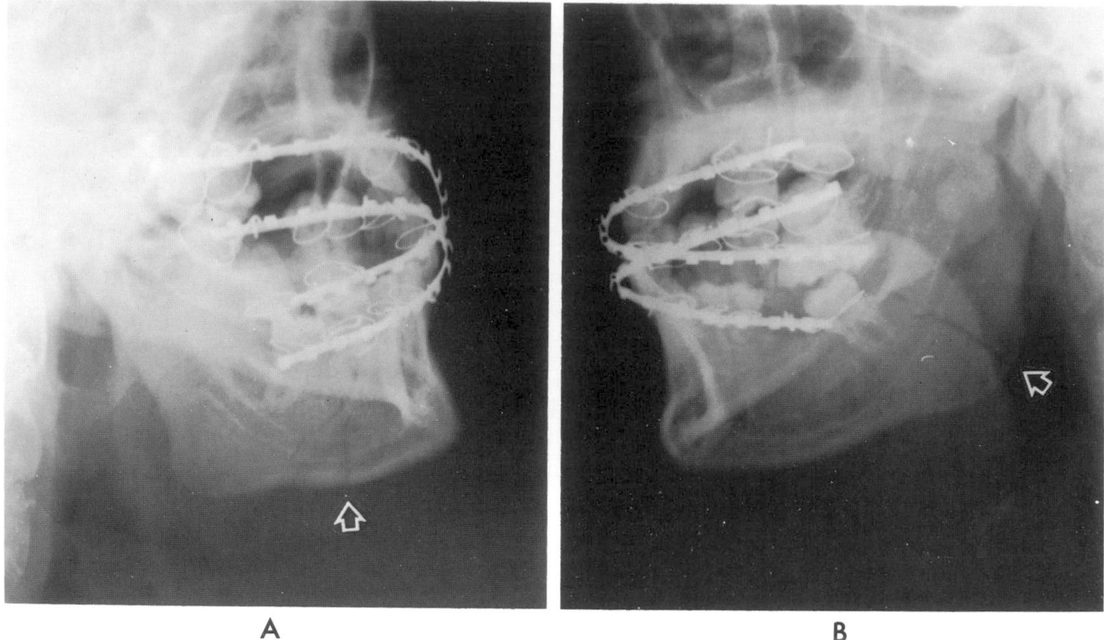

Figure 126. Bilateral simple fracture of the mandible. *A.* Fracture through the body of the mandible on the left side with fixation by intermaxillary traction. *B.* Fracture through the angle of the mandible on the right, stabilization obtained by fixing the teeth in occlusion.

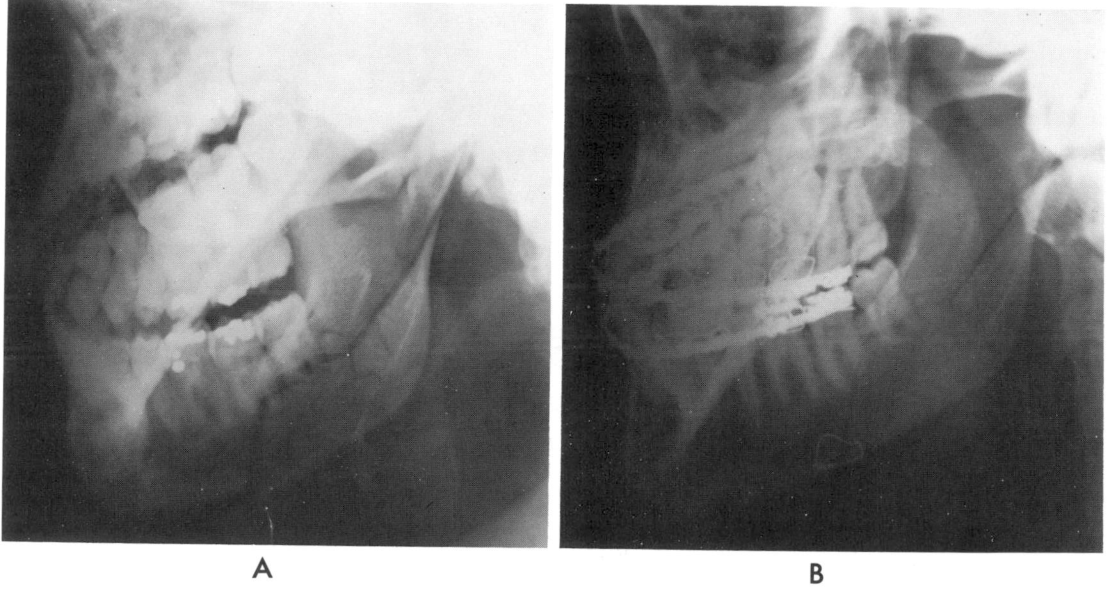

Figure 127. Compound comminuted fracture of the mandible, beginning at the alveolar border in the body and passing around the roots of the third molar across the region of the angle to end in the ramus below the neck of the condylar process. The mandible was very unstable and the fragments were loose. Stabilization was obtained by one interosseous wire at the inferior border of the mandible. *A.* Preoperative view showing direction and extent of the fracture. *B.* Postoperative view.

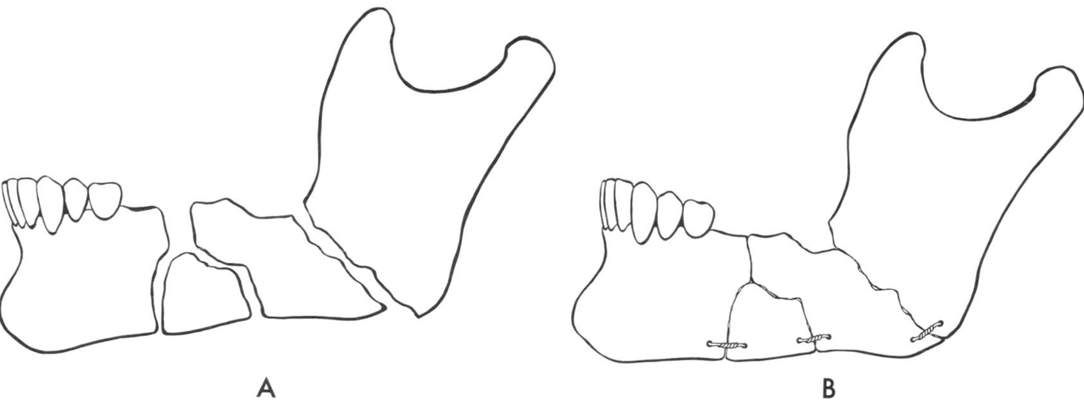

Figure 128. *A.* Multiple comminuted fractures of the body of the mandible. *B.* Immediate reconstruction by interosseous wiring of multiple fragments. The teeth should also be fixed in occlusion.

absent or lost by evulsion due to the injury. If the teeth are absent from the proximal or posterior segment, displacement due to muscle action is difficult to overcome and intermaxillary fixation alone will not provide proper stability. Open operation is the best method of management of such fractures. If no teeth are present on either side of the fracture, open reduction with interosseous wire fixation by the intraoral or extraoral approach is the method of choice. Intramedullary wire fixation after the method of Brown, McDowell, and Fryer is useful in managing edentulous fragments. Extensively comminuted fractures may require metal plate support for fixation of the major segments, and to bridge areas of bone loss or to stabilize extensive comminution when the fragments are too small to be wired in place (Figs. 128, 129 and 130).

The operation for open reduction and interosseous wire fixation for fractures of the body of the mandible should be planned carefully before the patient is anesthetized and draped. The skin incision should be planned so that the final scar will be below the border of the mandible. The skin should be marked in one of the creases of the submandibular region or parallel to the skin lines and one finger's breadth below the inferior border of the mandible. The central point of the incision should be directly opposite the site of fracture. An incision 4 to 5 cm. in length gives adequate exposure for reduction and fixation of fractures in this region. After marking the skin, local infiltration of an anesthetic containing 1 to 100,000 adrenalin solution into the soft tissue and into the region of the fracture will minimize the operative bleeding. Ten min-

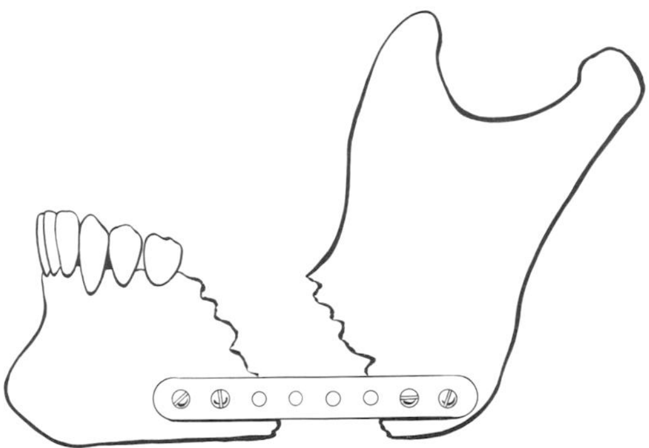

Figure 129. Metal plate method of fixation of fractured mandibular segments in a case of traumatic loss of bone. This method prevents displacement of the proximal bone segment and supports it until a bone graft can be inserted.

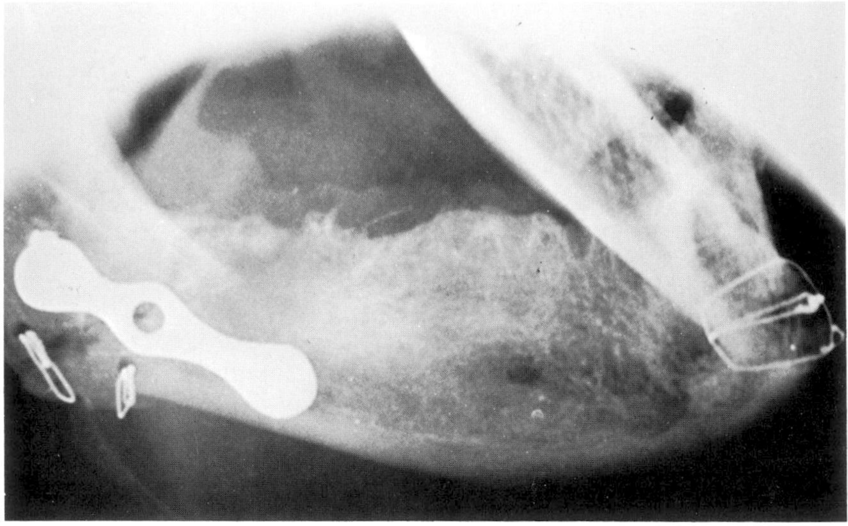

Figure 130. Bilateral fracture of an edentulous mandible. The fragments have been stabilized by means of interosseous wire fixation on the right, and interosseous fixation with the use of a metal plate with screws on the left.

utes should elapse following injection of the local anesthetic solution before surgery is started.

The incision is carried through the skin, the subcutaneous fascia, and the platysma muscle. The deep cervical fascia lies just below the platysma muscle, and it is on this plane that the branches of the seventh nerve may be seen. The fascia should be inspected carefully, and if branches of the seventh nerve are identified, they should be dissected free and retracted. The incision should not be continued through the cervical fascia at this level, since exposure of the submandibular gland complicates the procedure.

After incising the platysma muscle, the dissection is carried laterally and superiorly on the fascial plane to the inferior border of the mandible. In most cases the ramus mandibularis of the seventh nerve does not extend below the inferior border of the mandible, but in an occasional case it may extend below the border for a short distance. Care in dissection must be exercised, for damage to the ramus mandibularis causes paralysis of the depressor muscles of the angle of the mouth and the lower lip. In most cases, recovery from such paralysis takes place in 12 to 18 months, but in a few cases the paralysis may be permanent. With few exceptions the ramus mandibularis of the seventh nerve lies lateral to the facial artery and vein and crosses the blood vessels at the level of the inferior border of the mandible. In occasional cases the nerve passes deep to the facial artery. If the facial artery and vein interfere with exposure of the fracture and it is inconvenient or not possible to retract these structures, the vessels should be securely ligated, cut, and retracted out of the field.

Now the inferior border of the mandible can be palpated readily. The periosteum along the inferior border of the bone, if not already torn by the injury, is incised. The periosteum can be elevated easily, using a pointed instrument, to expose the site of the fracture. Stripping of the periosteum should be sufficient only to provide access to the fracture for reduction and wiring of the fragments; excessive periosteal elevation may deprive the fragments of their blood supply and increase the possibility of necrosis, though the inferior alveolar artery contributes to the blood supply of the bone.

Drill holes are made on each side of the fracture site through the cortical portion of the bone. If the drill is passed at too high a level, the mandibular branch of the fifth nerve coursing through the mandibular canal may be injured. The holes may be made safely 5 to 7 mm. above the inferior border of the mandible. If it seems necessary to make holes at a higher level, the course of the inferior alveolar nerve and the location of the roots of the teeth should be determined on the lateral jaw radiograph so that they will not be injured.

If the fracture is at right angles to the lateral surface of the mandible, a 22 to 25 gauge stainless steel wire passed through the drill holes and twisted tightly will usually provide adequate fixation. If the fracture is in an oblique direction, a wire passed through holes on each side of it may result in slipping and overlapping of the fragments if the wire is twisted tightly. Better fixation in oblique fractures can be obtained by passing one drill hole through both fragments of the bone. A single wire carried through this drill hole and twisted securely about the inferior border of the mandible gives more stable fixation. If a single hole and wire does not give good fixation, another drill hole made through both segments at a higher level, with a mattress-type wire passed through both of the holes, usually gives secure immobilization. If the single wire is used, a small notch made with a bone drill at the inferior border of the mandible will prevent slipping of the wire ligature in any direction.

When muscular action results in displacement, two drill holes may be placed on each side of the fracture and criss-crossed, or figure-of-eight wire application may be used to hold the fragments. When twisting wires, it is helpful to twist all the wires in the same direction. They may be twisted clockwise or counterclockwise but the pattern should be consistent in all cases. This simplifies removal of the wires if necessary later. Care is taken to avoid an excess wire loop on the inner surface of the bone. The wires are twisted tightly with a forceps and then cut about 1 cm. long so that the end can be bent and tucked into one of the drill holes. Twisting should continue while bending to prevent loosening of the wire loop. Placement of the wire end in one of the drill holes or pressing it firmly against the lateral surface of the mandible prevents irritation to the overlying soft tissues (see Fig. 168).

Usually it is unnecessary to remove interosseous wires, but an occasional one will cause a reaction which necessitates its removal many months after the fracture has healed.

The periosteum is important in bone healing and should be replaced over the bone. If the tissues have been dissected carefully, replacement can be done by suturing with chromic catgut sutures. Because of the possibility of contamination in wounds about the mouth and jaws, absorbable suture is used to close the soft tissue; 0000 or 00000 catgut sutures are used for soft tissue closure. A minimal amount of suture is buried in the wound. The knots are cut short and generally the reaction is minimal. The total reaction to fine catgut is less than that to nonabsorbable sutures such as silk, especially in contaminated wounds.

Even though there appears to be anatomic realignment of bone fragments, some degree of malocclusion, even though minor, usually exists. The supplemental use of arch bars with intermaxillary rubber bands is recommended to restore the exact occlusal relations of the teeth and to hold them in position during the course of healing of the bone.

A rubber drain may be used in the wound if there is evidence of gross contamination, difficulty in controlling bleeding at the site of fracture, or the presence of a compound fracture. With preoperative and postoperative antibiotic therapy, wound infection is rare, and the complication of osteomyelitis is seen only infrequently.

The Edentulous Patient

The edentulous patient may require special consideration in the management of fractures of the body of the mandible. An edentulous or partially edentulous patient is one who has lost all or most of his teeth as the result of injury or previous extractions, or who, if teeth are present, has an insufficient number and in improper relations to be effective for establishing good occlusion and providing adequate fixation. The artificial dentures of an edentulous patient may be invaluable in the management of fractures of the body of the mandible. Some patients wear an upper denture and a partial lower denture to supplement the few remaining natural lower anterior teeth. Patients with fractures with missing teeth should be questioned about dentures. Dentures often are broken at the time of injury and may be discarded by friends or relatives who feel that they are no longer useful. If the patient was known to have worn dentures at the time of injury and they are not present, search should be made to locate them at the scene of the accident. Pieces of the denture may be recovered and successfully repaired and utilized as fixation splints.

The incidence of fracture of the body of the bone in edentulous patients is lower than in patients with natural teeth. Older patients are less active in travel and sports, and pursue less hazardous occupations, which no doubt accounts for the decreased incidence of fractures in edentulous patients. Although relatively infrequent in occurrence, fractures of the mandible in the edentulous patient become serious problems in management.

The causes of fractures of the body of the bone in the edentulous patient are the same as are those for fractures in patients with teeth, except that a traumatic occurrence, with minimal force, may result in fracture of facial bones in the aged patient.

The edentulous mandible is weakened, the cortical plates thin, the trabeculae thinner, and the marrow spaces wider from disuse atrophy, but senile osteoporosis is also a factor in old patients. The mandible, therefore, is brittle and withstands less force than bones of the younger patients. Extractions of teeth must be done with the minimum force and in multirooted teeth is best done after dividing the tooth. Otherwise, the force of extraction may transcend the resistance of the bone in an old patient and may cause fractures, especially during extraction of premolar and molar teeth.

Neoplasm is a more frequent cause of fracture of the jaws in the older patient. Atrophy of the bone not only predisposes to fractures, but complicates the management because of the small bulk of bone for approximation. The decreased blood supply results in delayed healing and nonunion of fractures in the body of the mandible.

It is difficult to detect malposition between the maxilla and mandible in the edentulous patient. If the dentures are available, the occlusion can be checked as in the patient with a full complement of teeth.

Pain, deformity, malfunction, crepitation, edema, ecchymosis, and excessive salivation are the usual signs of fractures in the edentulous patient. Roentgenographic examination may demonstrate fractures less easily in the edentulous patient because of the decreased density of the bone which makes fractures less apparent in the films.

Fractures of the body of the mandible often can be managed by simple circumferential wiring of the lower denture to the mandible (Figs. 131–135). Fractures prox-

(Text continued on page 166.)

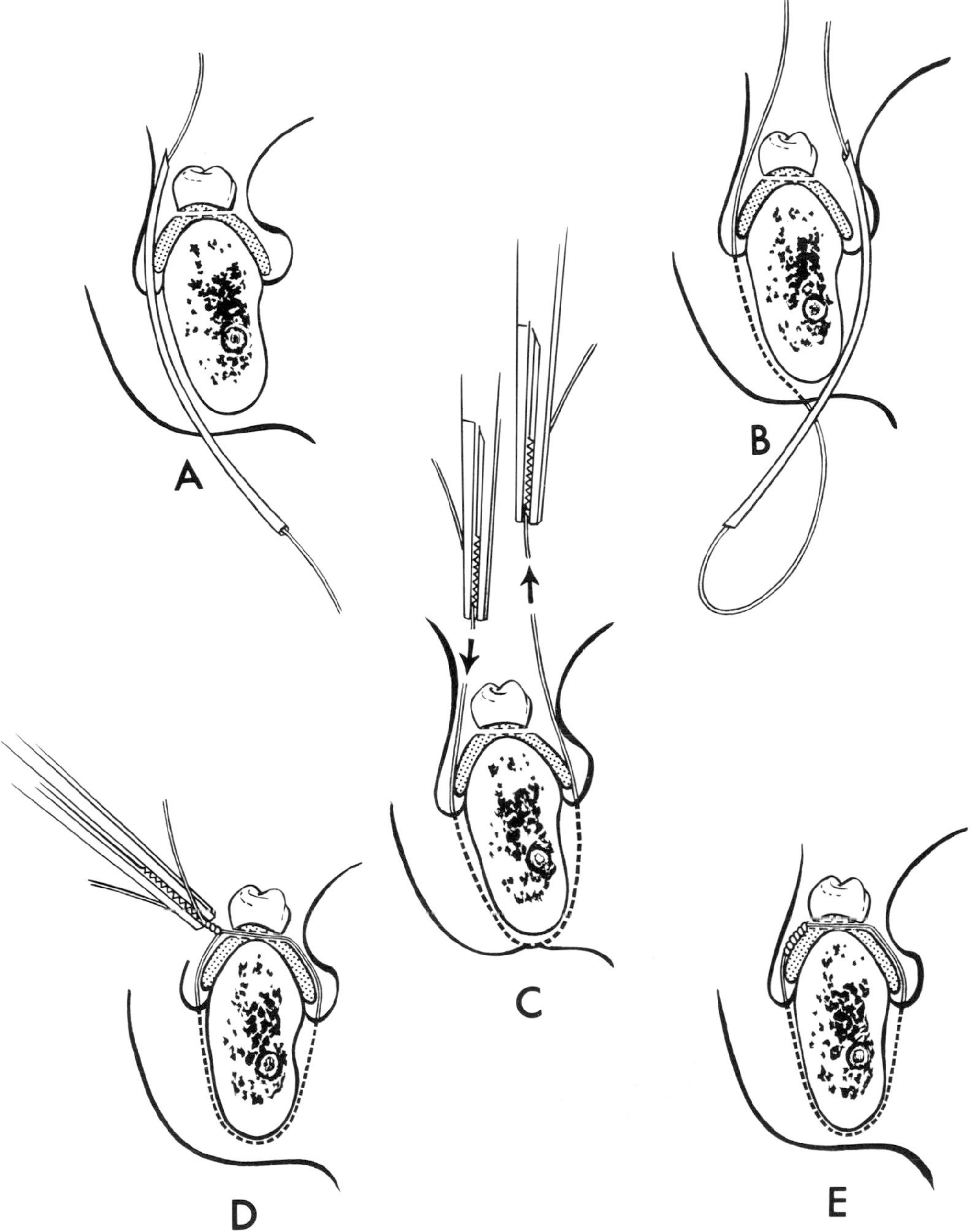

Figure 131. Circumferential wiring of the patient's artificial denture to the mandible. *A.* A curved passing needle, armed with a wire, punctures the skin at the inferior border of the mandible and passes upward on the lateral surface of the bone into the buccal vestibule. The passing needle is pulled through into the mouth and is slipped off the wire. *B.* Another passing needle, similarly armed with the wire, is inserted through the same puncture wound in the skin and is directed, on the medial surface of the mandible, into the lingual sulcus. The passing needle is slipped off the wire and is removed from the mouth. *C.* A seesaw motion is applied to the wire to cut through any small fibers of tissue that are trapped in the wire loop. This ensures contact of the wire with the inferior margin of the bone. *D.* The wire from the lingual side is passed through a bur hole in the artificial denture and twisted securely with the wire from the buccal side. *E.* The twisted double wire is cut, and its end is pressed firmly against the denture so that the end does not irritate the buccal mucosa.

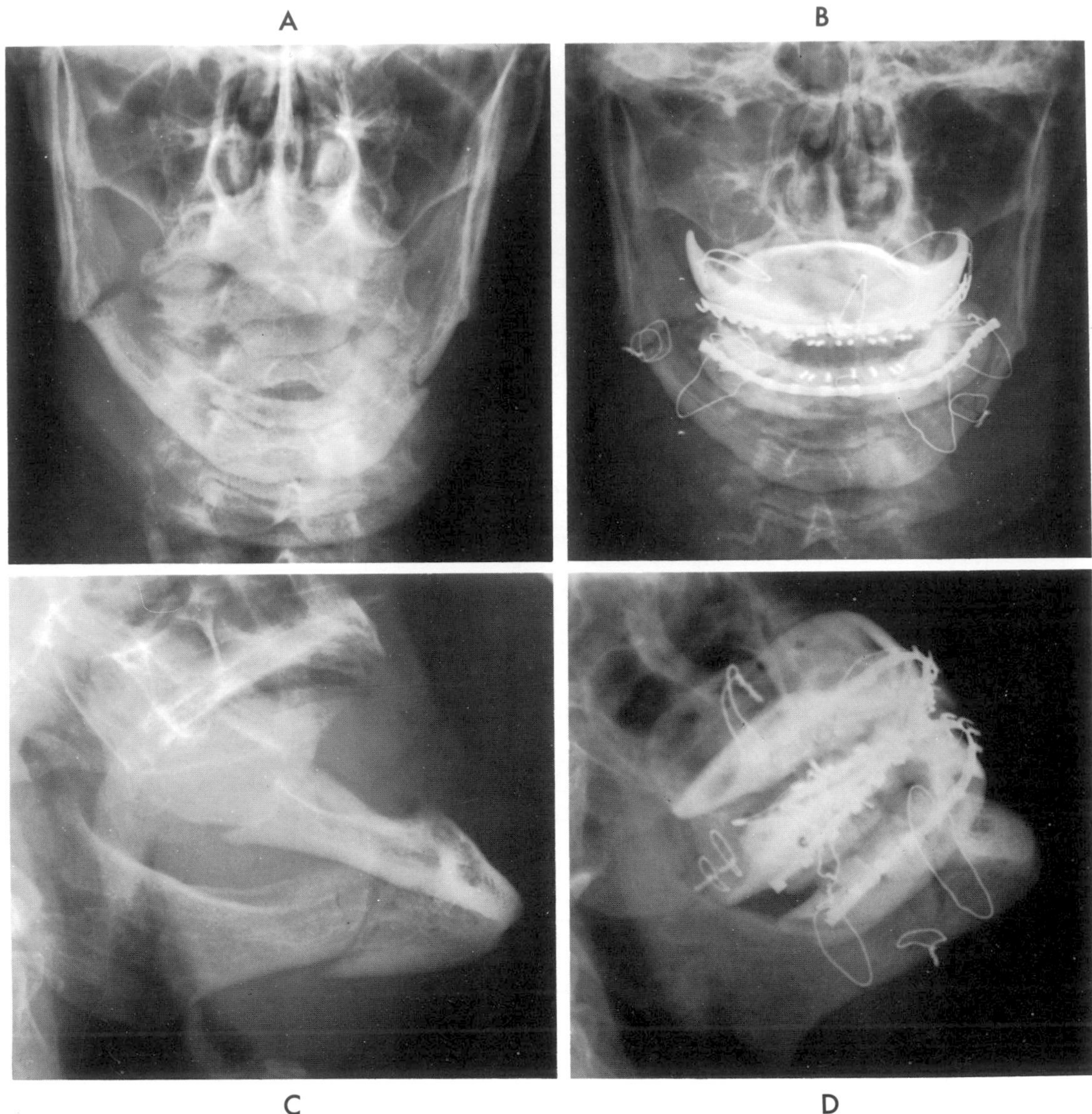

Figure 132. Bilateral fracture in an edentulous mandible treated by open interosseous wire fixation and stabilization, using the patient's artificial dentures, which were fixed to the mandible and maxilla by circumferential wires. *A.* Frontal projection showing bilateral mandibular fractures. *B.* Frontal projection showing bilateral interosseous wire fixation and stabilization with patient's artificial dentures. Arch bars were wired to the upper and lower dentures through drill holes between the teeth. The dentures were stabilized against the mandible by circumferential wiring and against the maxilla by wiring to the maxilla through drill holes in the bone. The teeth were brought into occlusion by rubber band traction. *C.* Lateral view showing bilateral fractures in edentulous mandible. *D.* Postoperative view showing bilateral interosseous wire fixation, circumferential wires holding dentures in place on the mandible and maxilla, and intermaxillary fixation with arch bars.

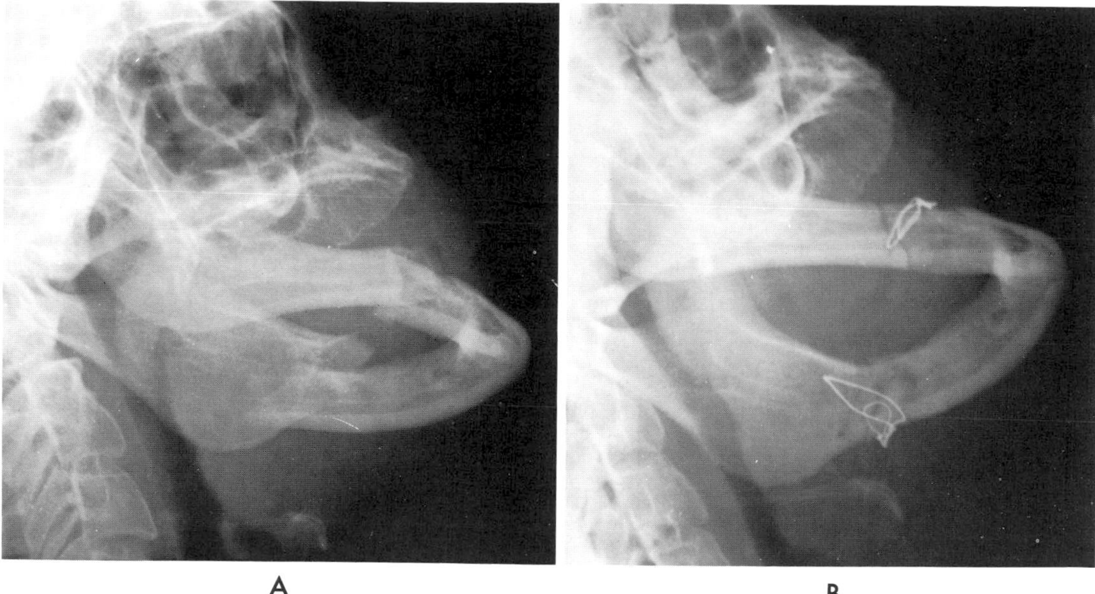

Figure 133. Bilateral comminuted fractures of an edentulous mandible, treated by extraoral open reduction and interosseous wire fixation. *A*. Preoperative roentgenogram showing bilateral fractures with downward and backward displacement of the anterior portion of the mandible. *B*. The fracture is stabilized with interosseous wires.

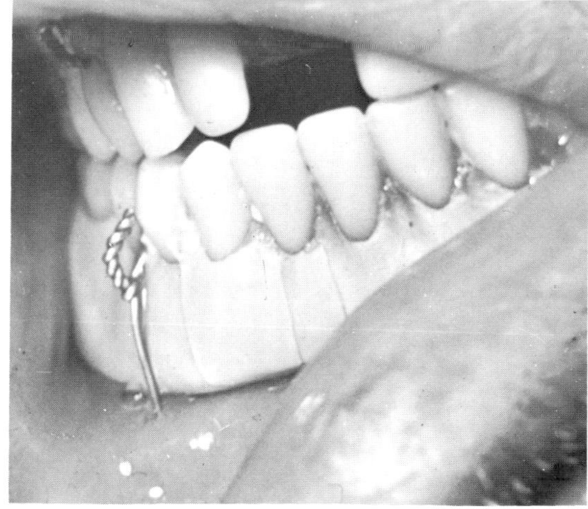

Figure 134. Broken artificial dentures may be repaired and used for circumferential wire fixation. Note in this oblique view the wire passing into the soft tissue of the labial vestibule; it passes around the mandible and comes up on the inner surface and through a hole in the denture. Twisting of the wire secures the denture firmly against the mandible.

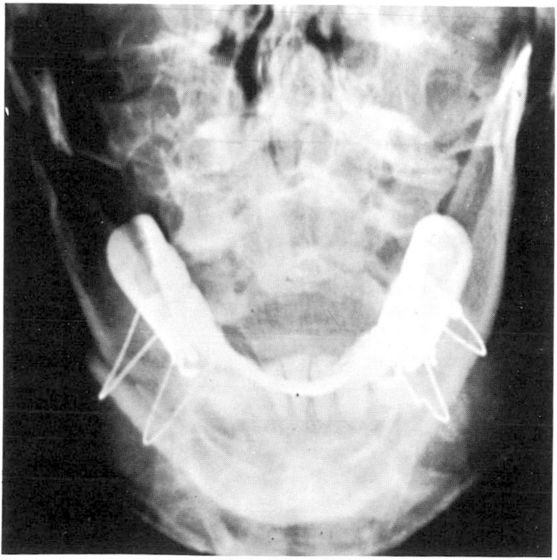

Figure 135. Fracture of the body of the right side of the mandible, stabilized by circumferential wiring using the patient's partial denture.

imal to the denture-bearing area and anterior to the angle of the mandible require open reduction and direct wiring technique. If the edentulous patient has no artificial dentures to use for circumferential wiring, a dental colleague can make a saddlelike splint to place upon the alveolar crest, around which circumferential wires are tightened to stabilize the segments. This type of appliance is known to the dentist as a base plate. To get an accurate base plate, the dentist makes an intraoral impression of the unreduced fragments and from the impression makes a plaster model. The plaster model is cut and reassembled in normal relations. The base plate is made to fit the reconstructed model.

If the use of a base plate does not seem to be practical in managing the fracture, direct wiring of the bone should be attempted. Because of the thinness of the bone of the anterior portion of the mandible, the muscle pull from the anterior group tends to pull the fragments out of position if the wire is placed at the inferior border (Fig. 136 *A, B*). It is possible to gain a mechanical advantage by placing the drill holes near the crest of the alveolar ridge. The muscles that close the mouth pull upward on the back fragment, and the muscles that open the mouth pull downward and backward on the front fragment. Their reciprocal forces hold the fragments in secure position. Open reduction can be done through an external approach or through the intraoral route.

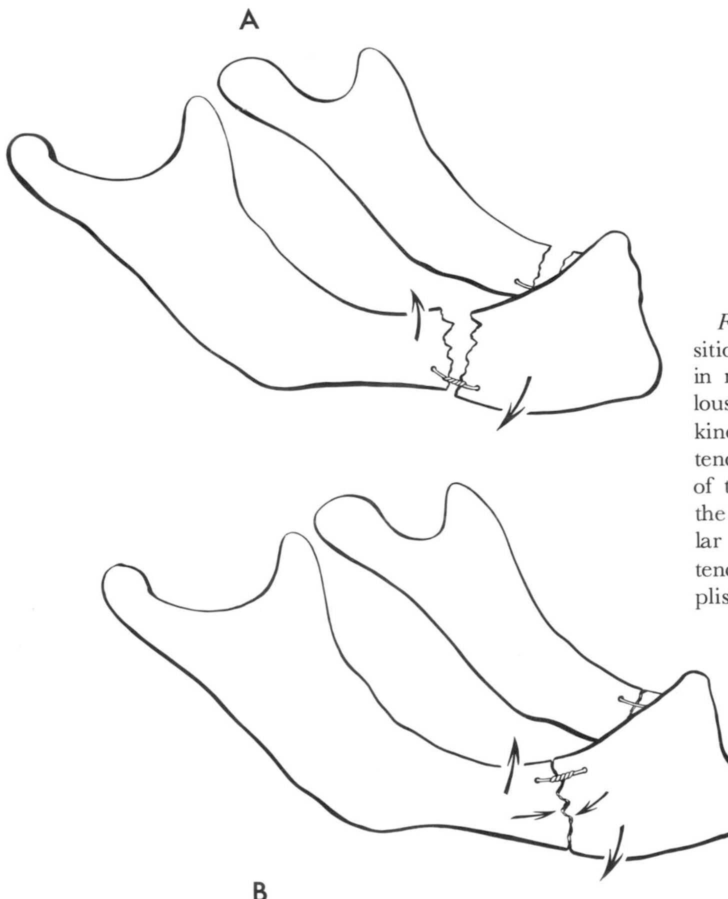

Figure 136. Correct and incorrect positions of placement of interosseous wire in reduction of fractures of the edentulous mandible. *A.* With this incorrect kind of wiring, the fragments have a tendency to separate because of the pull of the muscles attached to it. *B.* When the wiring is near the crest of the alveolar ridge, the pull of the muscles even tends to enhance the reduction accomplished by the correct wiring.

Intraoral Approach for Open Reduction and Interosseous Wiring in Edentulous Fractures

The incision is made on the crest of the alveolar ridge through the thin overlying mucous membrane to expose the alveolar crest (Fig. 137). The mucoperiosteum is stripped from the bone on the lateral and medial surfaces to expose the fracture. A

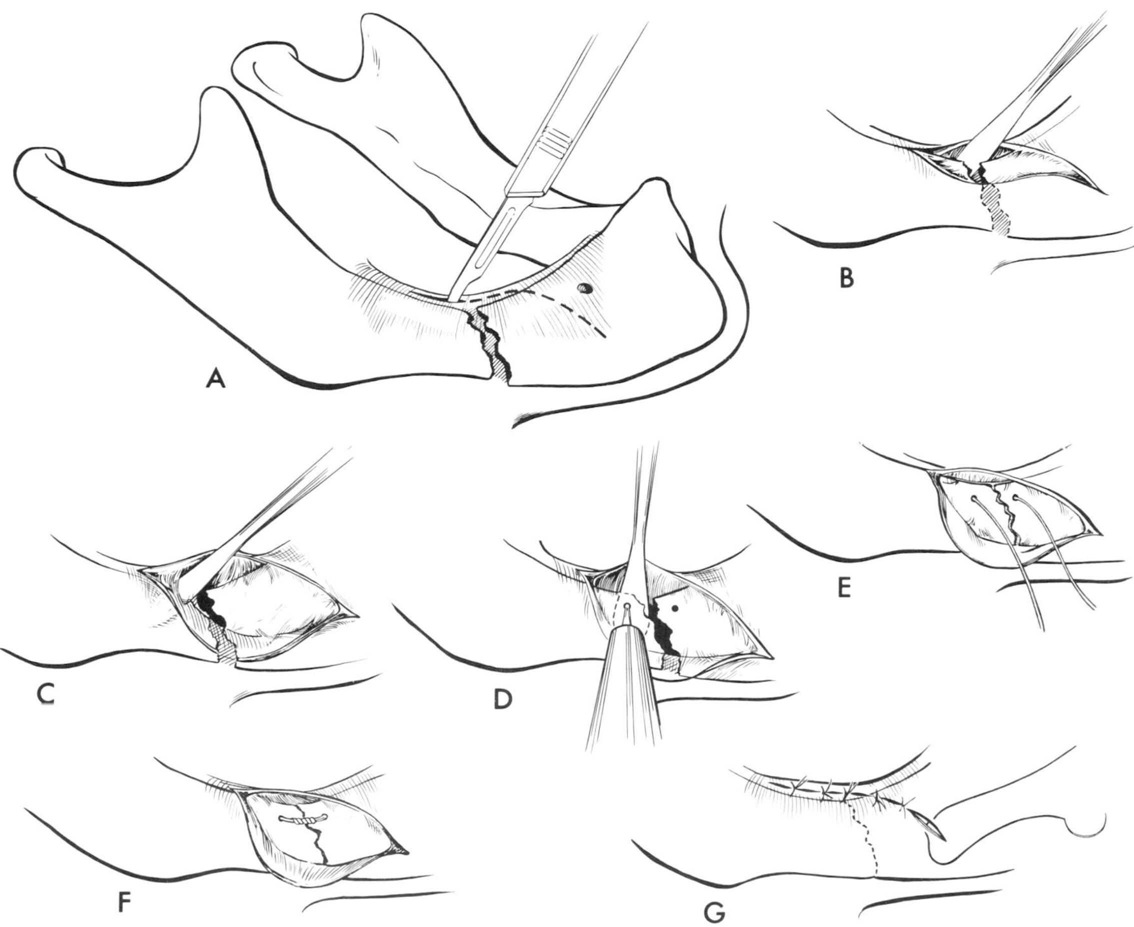

Figure 137. Steps in intraoral open reduction for fracture of the body of the mandible. *A.* An incision is made along the crest of the alveolar ridge and downward and forward, anterior to the site of the fracture. The flap should be large enough to give adequate covering to the fracture site after reduction, and designed so that the suture line does not lie directly over the line of fracture of the bone. *B.* The periosteum is elevated from the medial surface of the bone with a sharp elevator. *C.* The periosteum is stripped from the lateral surface sufficiently to expose the site of the fracture and to permit instrumentation without damage to the tissues. *D.* Bur holes are drilled on each side of the fracture site 5 mm. below the crest of the alveolar ridge and 5 mm. from the fractured margin. *E.* A wire of stainless steel is passed through the bur holes, both ends appearing upon the lateral surface of the bone. The loop of wire on the medial surface should be flattened against the bone. *F.* The wires are twisted clockwise to fix the fragments in position securely. The ends of the wires are cut off. The remaining twisted end is bent and inserted into one of the bur holes. The wire should be flattened against the bone surface to avoid irritation from an overriding denture. *G.* A single layer closure of the mucoperiosteum is made with silk or absorbable sutures. The wire may have to be removed if it interferes with the wearing of an artificial denture.

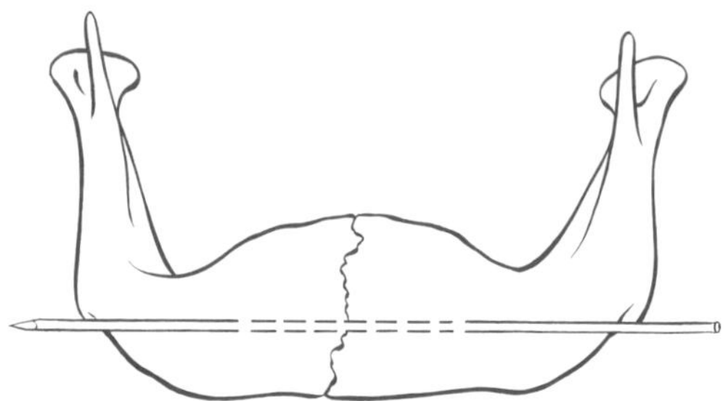

Figure 138. Intramedullary wire fixation is useful in the reduction of mandibular fragments. This method may be used alone or as an adjunct to other methods.

small hole is made through the upper portion of the bone on each side of the fracture site. Twenty-five gauge stainless steel wire is passed through the hole, and both ends are brought out to the lateral surface where they are twisted tightly against the bone and cut short. The ends of the wire are twisted so that the stump can be placed in one of the drill holes or pressed flat against the alveolar bone. The wire is best placed below the alveolar crest so that it does not interfere with the wearing of a denture. The mucosa is closed with silk or absorbable sutures. This fixation may suffice and may be all that is possible to obtain if the patient does not have dentures.

Intramedullary Kirschner wire fixation may be useful in the immobilization of fractures through the body of the edentulous mandible (Fig. 138).

Region of the Angle

The angle of the mandible is defined clinically as the region underlying the attachments of the masseter muscle, between the region of the body and the region of the ramus. The posterior limiting margin of the angle region is an oblique line extending from the distal aspect of the third molar to the superior posterior attachment of the masseter muscle. Fractures through the region of the angle make up approximately 20 per cent of all mandibular fractures. The bone in this region is thinner than it is in the body, but protection is offered by the splinting afforded by dense attachments of the masseter muscle on the lateral surface and of the medial pterygoid muscle on the medial surface. These muscles give protection to the angle region, and their dense attachments prevent displacement. Fractures of the angle may extend forward into the body of the mandible to the second or third molar tooth. Fractures occurring in the anterior portion of the angle are likely to be displaced by the pull of the posterior group of muscles. An angle fracture may be displaced medially or laterally, depending upon the plane and obliquity of the fracture and the direction of the force. Angle fractures are associated frequently with fractures of the body of the mandible on the opposite side (Fig. 141 *A, B*).

Subcondylar fractures should be suspected in all instances of angle fractures (Fig. 142 *A–D*).

Intermaxillary fixation may suffice to secure angle fractures if displacement is not great. In most patients with displacement, open reduction gives the best results. The operation may be done by way of the intraoral or the extraoral approach. The intraoral route is most effective for the management of fractures in the edentulous jaw. The external approach is the most practical and easiest if the patient has teeth in the region of the fracture.

The intraoral approach is essentially the same as that described under the section dealing with intraoral open reduction for fractures of the body of the mandible (p. 167), except that the incision is made farther back.

(Text continued on page 173.)

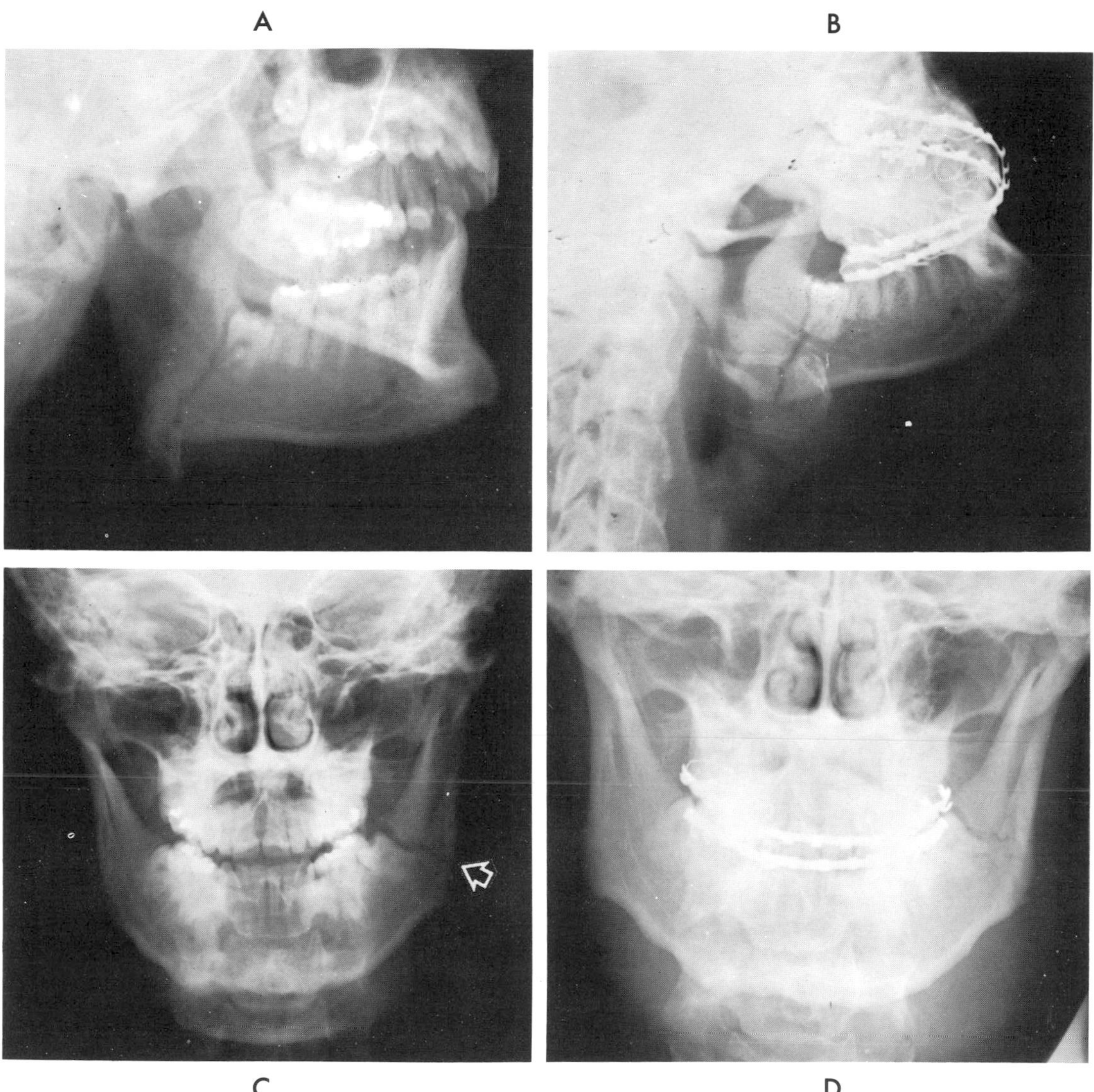

Figure 139. Fracture through the angle of the mandible and unerupted third molar tooth, with minimal displacement. The tooth in this instance helps to maintain the position of the proximal segment and should not be removed. *A*. Lateral view of the body and angle of the mandible showing direction of fracture. *B*. Treatment by intermaxillary fixation. *C*. Anterior view showing line of fracture. *D*. Anterior view showing fixation during the course of treatment.

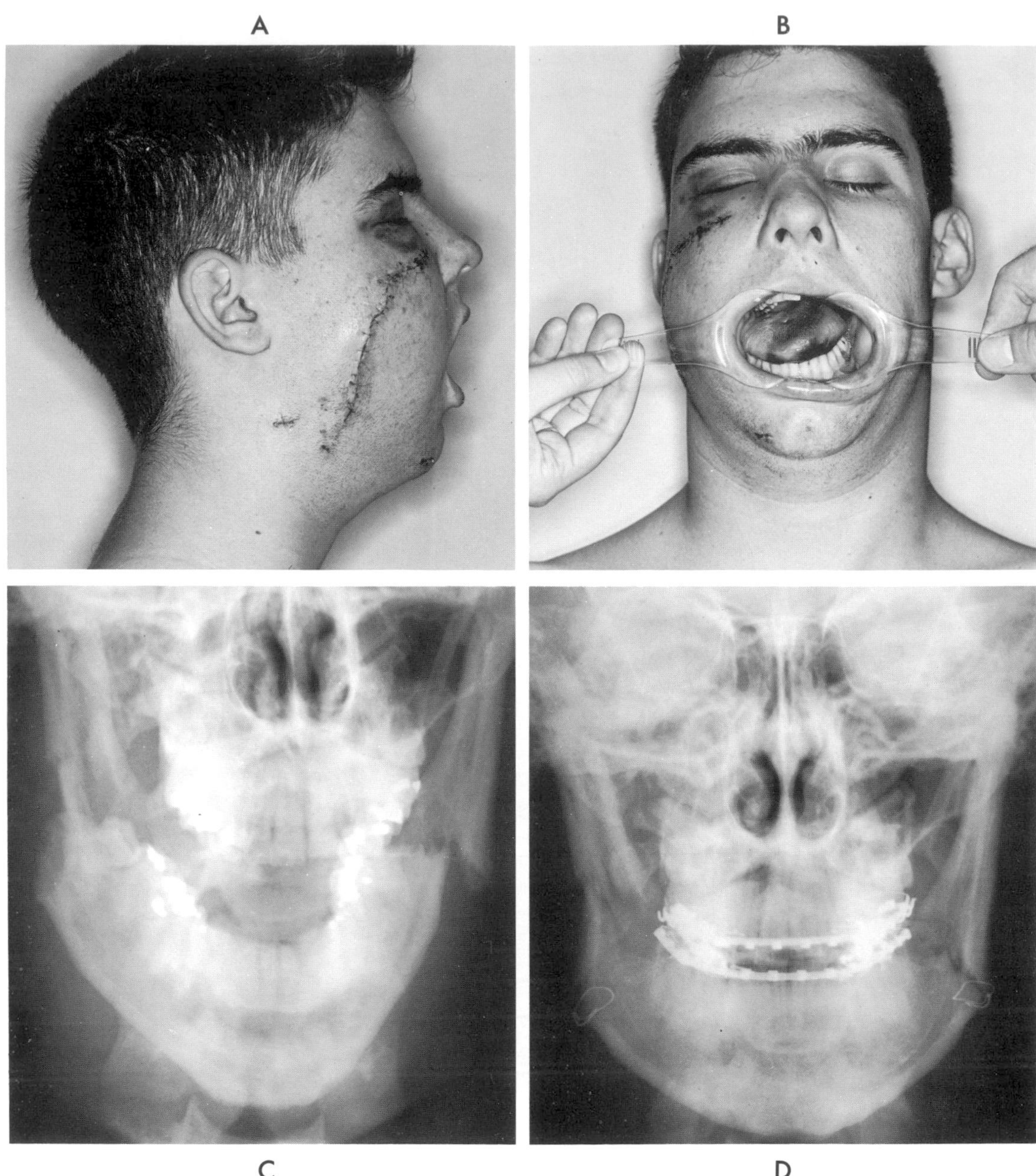

Figure 140. Compound fractures of both angles of the mandible. The patient's face was crushed between an automobile door and a truck. *A.* Profile view. The patient is unable to close his mouth because of dislocation of the fractured segments and the presence of a large hematoma and edema of the floor of the mouth and tongue. *B.* Open bite deformity caused by displacement of the anterior fragments. *C.* Roentgenogram showing fractures of the angles with displacement of the body of the mandible to the right side. *D.* The patient was treated by bilateral open reduction of mandibular fractures and intermaxillary fixation with arch bars and rubber bands.

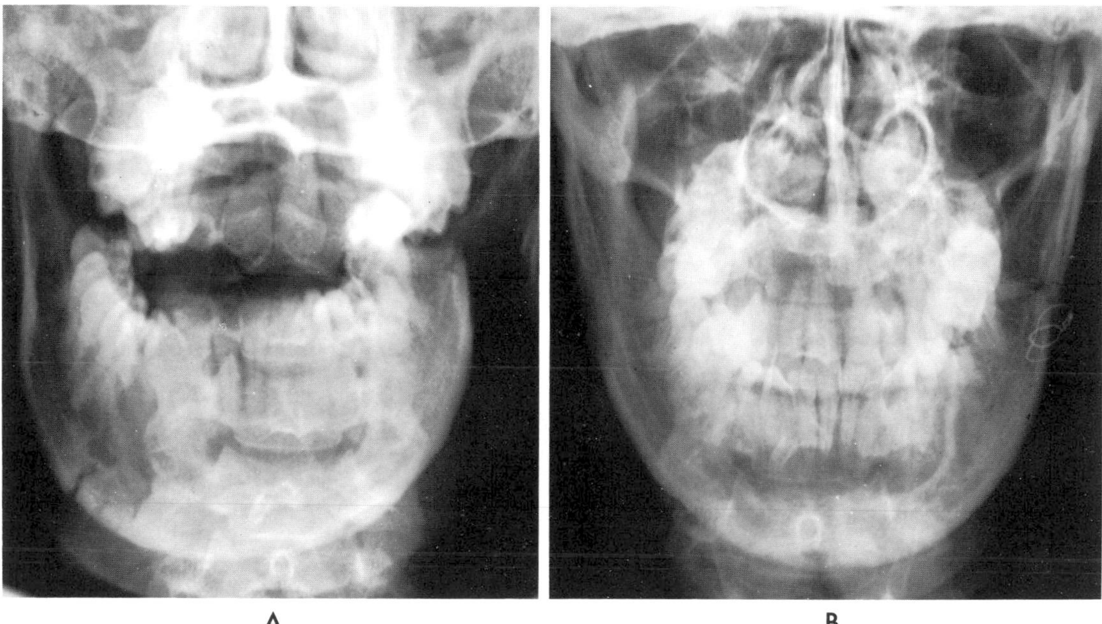

Figure 141. Bilateral mandibular fracture. The patient was struck from the left side. *A*. Fracture occurred above the angle of the mandible on the left and through its body on the right. The anterior segment of the mandible and the left body of the mandible were driven into the floor of the mouth. *B*. Treatment consisted of open reduction of the fracture of the angle on the left and closed reduction of right mandibular fracture. Fixation was maintained for six weeks following reduction.

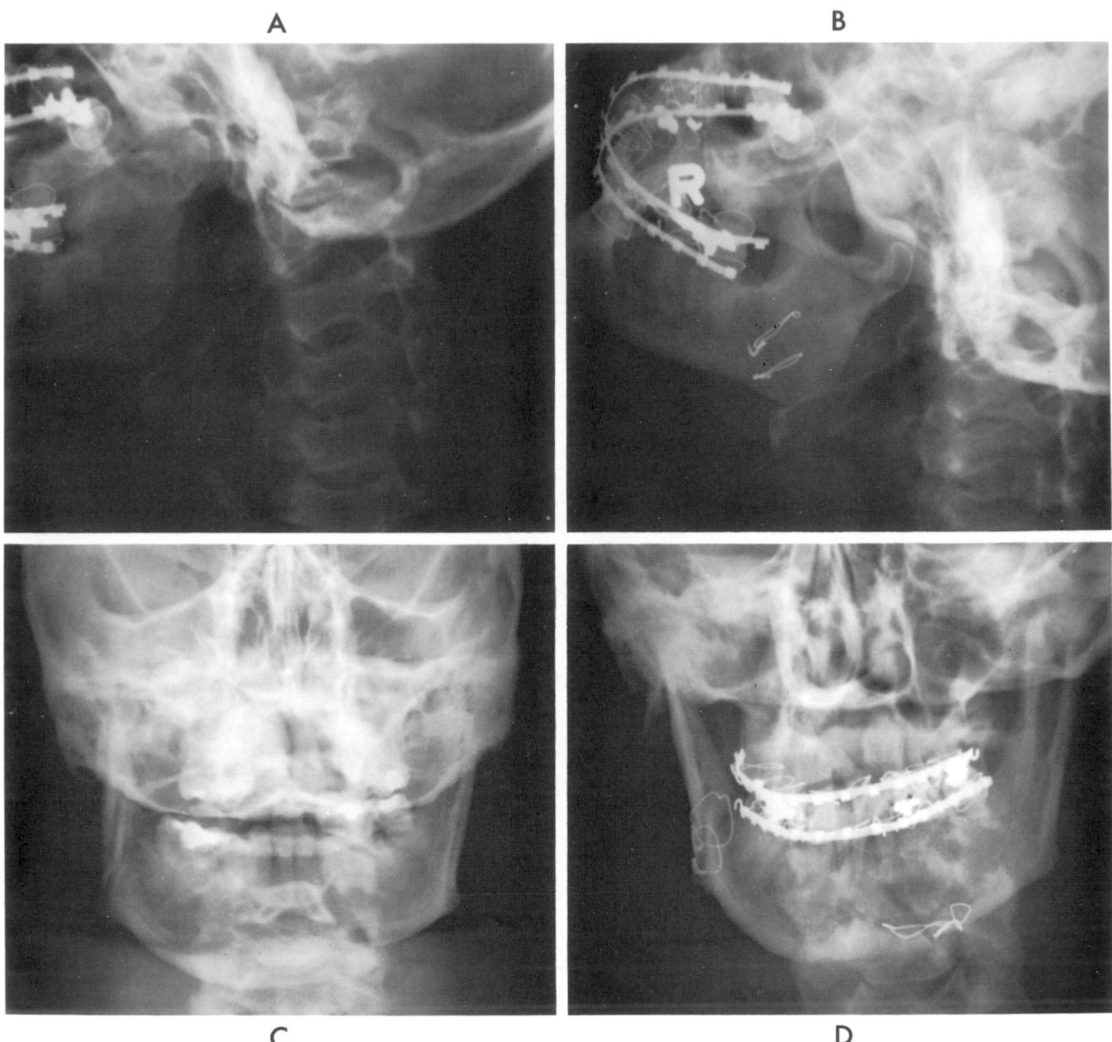

Figure 142. Fracture through the body and symphysial region on the left and through the angle of the mandible on the right. This kind of fracture results from a blow to the body of the mandible from the left front. The force causes a direct fracture at the point of impact and an indirect fracture through the angle of the mandible. In this case there is also a fracture with lateral displacement of the neck on the right. *A*. Lateral view showing fracture through the angle of the mandible and the neck on the right. *B*. Lateral view showing interosseous wire fixation for fracture of the angle on the right side. *C*. Preoperative front view showing fracture through the canine region on the left and through the angle of the mandible on the right. *D*. Front view postoperatively showing interosseous wires for fixation and intermaxillary fixation with arch bars. Note lateral displacement of the fractured condylar process on the right.

The Extraoral Approach

The skin is marked with ink on a line 1.0 to 1.5 cm. below and behind the angle of the mandible. The mark is continued in a curvilinear fashion in a skin line for approximately 4 cm. Local anesthetic solution containing epinephrine is injected subcutaneously and through the tissues to the bone. This aids hemostasis and simplifies the operative procedure.

Dissection is carried through the skin, subcutaneous fat, and platysma muscle to the deep fascia and then to the inferior border of the mandible. The insertion of the masseter muscle is identified and its fibers are incised at the inferior limits of their insertion. The intimate attachments of the tendinous portion of the muscle make dissection difficult. The fibers must be incised away from the angle for a short distance. Then a periosteal elevator will slip easily between the periosteum and the bone to elevate the masseter muscle. The periosteum on the medial surface of the mandible is elevated in a similar manner. Soft tissues, blood clots, and debris in the line of fracture are removed. A bone forceps is used to grasp the fragments on each side of the fracture site. Manipulation of the bone with the forceps reduces the fracture.

The forceps is used to maintain the position of the bones while a drill hole is placed 5 mm. above the inferior border of each fragment. The soft tissue on the medial surface should be protected with a ribbon retractor while the holes are drilled. A length of 25 gauge stainless steel wire is passed through the holes and both ends are brought to the lateral surface of the bone. The ends are twisted tightly together while the position of the fragments is maintained with a bone-holding forceps. The wire is twisted to secure the fragments in positive position. The twisted end is placed close to the bone on the outer surface of the mandi-

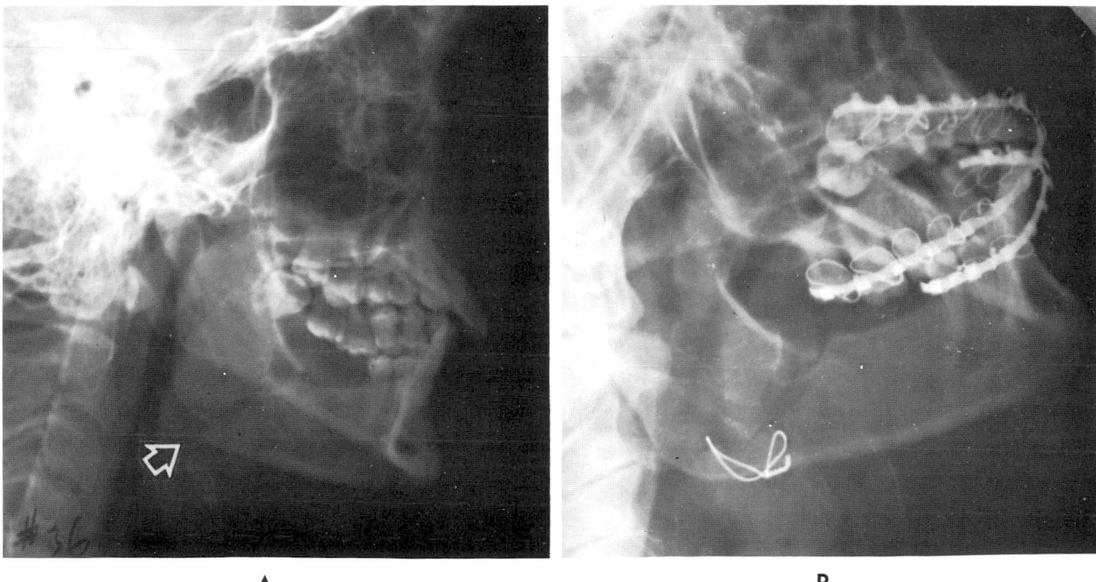

Figure 143. Fracture through the angle with the posterior edentulous fragment pulled upward by the muscles attached to the ramus of the mandible. *A.* Preoperative view. *B.* Fixation by means of figure-of-eight wire about the angle and inferior border of the mandible. Note that the fracture line passes through a tooth socket and that the tooth has been removed.

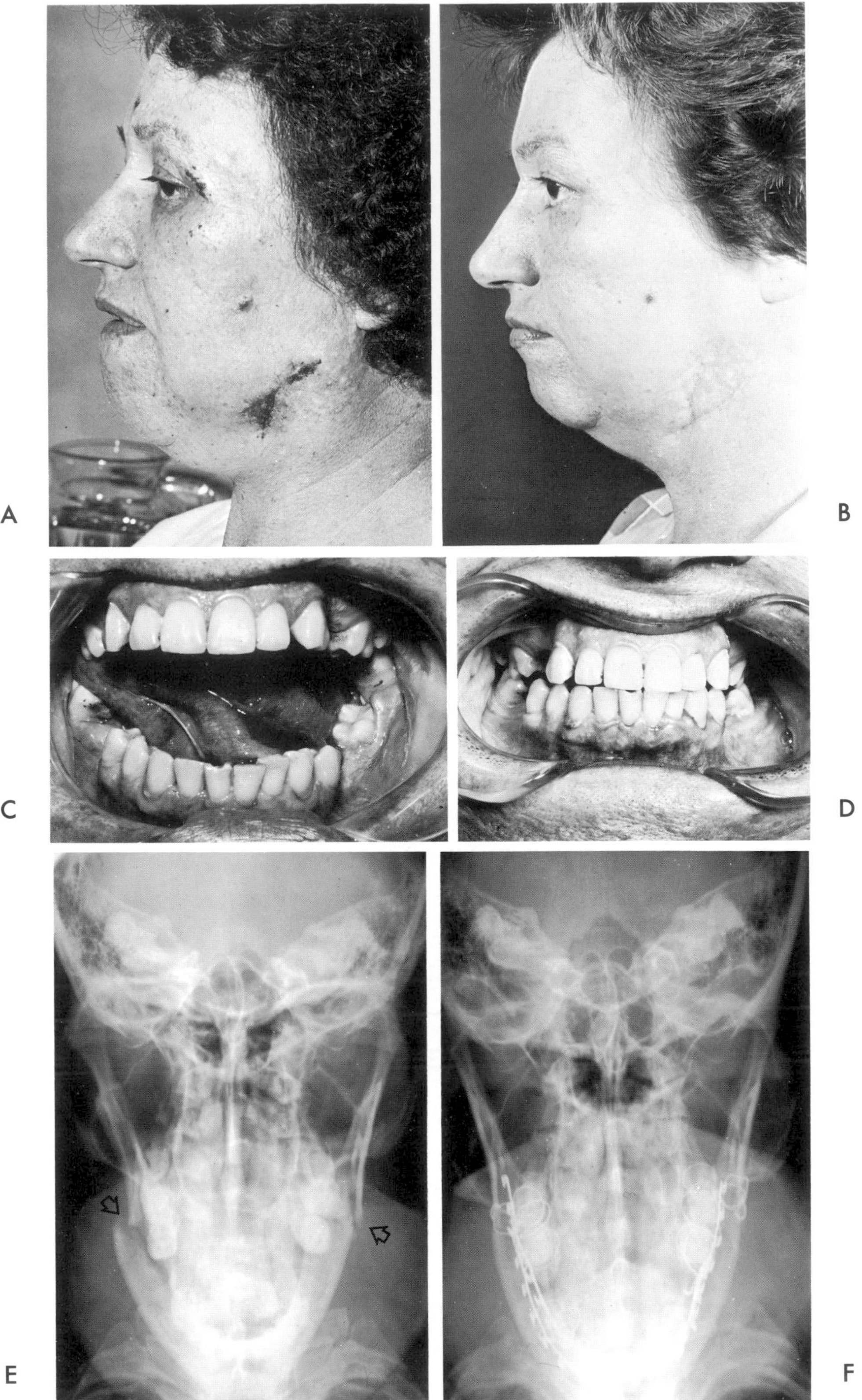

Fig. 144

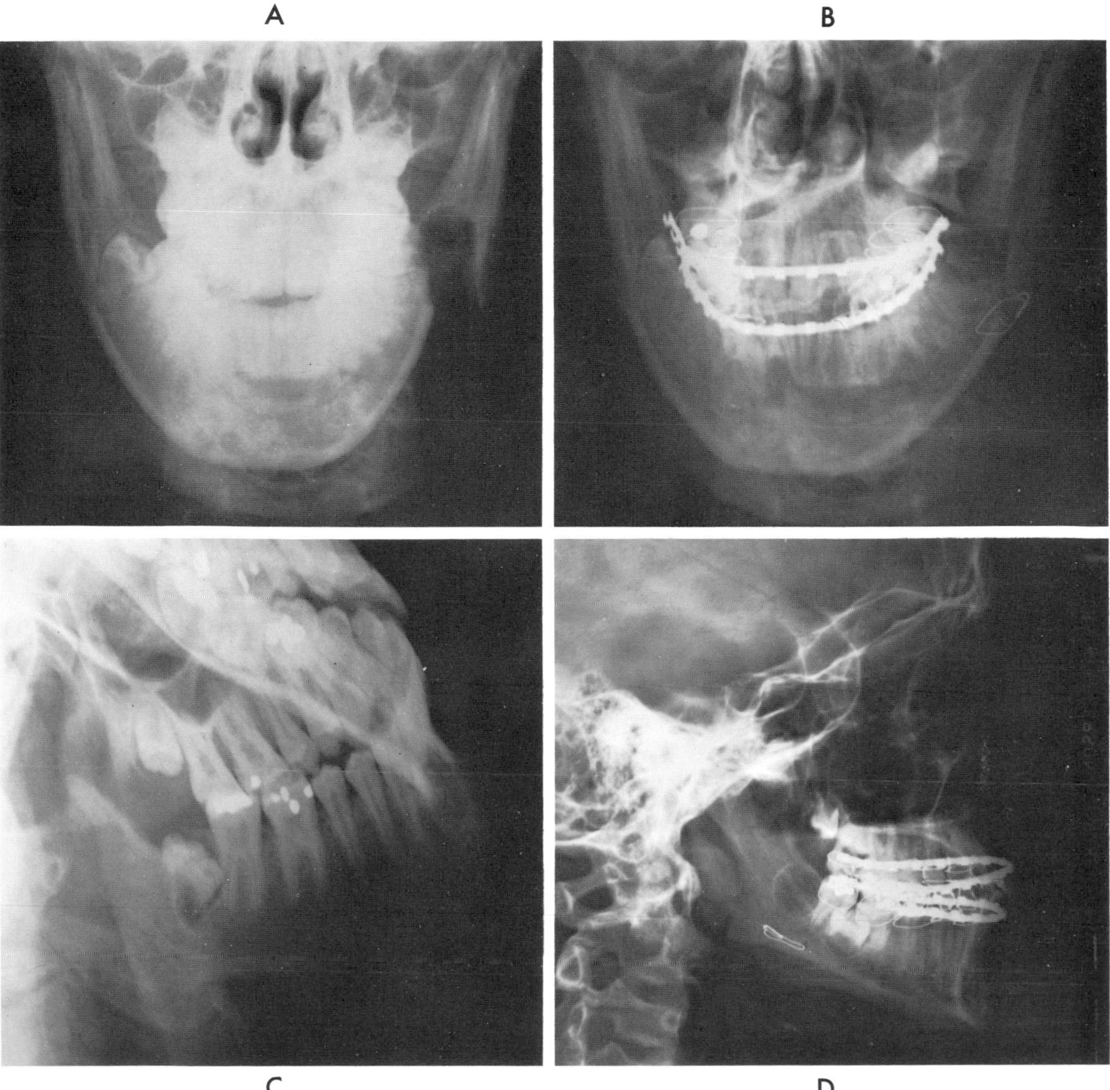

Figure 145. Fracture of the angle of the mandible on the left, extending through the socket of the unerupted third molar tooth. The tooth was removed and open reduction with interosseous wire fixation was performed. *A*. Preoperative view showing displacement of the proximal segment. *B*. Postoperative view showing reduction and fixation. *C*. Lateral view of the mandible showing fracture through the third molar region. *D*. Lateral view showing fixation with interosseous wire.

Figure 144. Bilateral compound fracture of the mandible with open bite deformity treated by bilateral open reduction and interosseous wire fixation supplemented with intermaxillary arch bar fixation. *A*. Preoperative lateral view. *B*. Postoperative lateral view. *C*. Preoperative occlusion. The patient is unable to close her mouth owing to premature contact of the left molar teeth. *D*. Postoperative occlusion. *E*. Preoperative roentgenogram showing bilateral fractures through the region of the angle of the mandible. *F*. Postoperative roentgenogram showing wires used for interosseous fixation and upper and lower arch bar attachments.

ble to avoid loosening of the wire and incarceration of soft tissues. The wires are cut, and the end of the wire is bent and inserted into one of the drill holes. A twisting motion while bending the wire prevents the ligature from loosening. If a single wire gives insecure fixation, additional holes are drilled at a higher level, one on each side of the fracture, and a crossed or figure-of-eight wire is used to give support at the fracture site.

When reduction and fixation are complete, the wound is closed in layers utilizing 000 or 0000 chromic catgut for approximating the periosteum and repositioning the masseter muscle. The muscle should be replaced in its original position by suturing the tissues on the lateral surface to those on the medial surface under the angle of the mandible. The deep fascia and the platysma muscle are closed in separate layers and 0000 catgut is used to close the subcutaneous tissues; the skin is closed with 00000 nylon sutures. If bleeding is persistent, or if there is a possibility of gross contamination, a rubber drain should be placed in the wound.

If the fracture is through the third molar tooth socket, the tooth may interfere with reduction of the fragments. The tooth may be extracted through the area of exposure (Fig. 145 *A–D*). Usually a developing tooth in the line of fracture does not interfere with reduction or fixation and need not be removed. Removal adds trauma and exposes more of the bone. If it seems advisable to remove the tooth through an oral incision, the alveolar bone may be trimmed with a rongeur and the mucosa sutured to cover the bone and close the oral wound.

If the angle fracture is associated with a fracture of the body of the bone on the opposite side, open reduction for fixation of the angle fracture is done because of its tendency for displacement. On the opposite side, intermaxillary fixation may be done for stabilization of the fracture in the body of the mandible. The intermaxillary fixation provides stability for the fragments on both sides.

If the mandible is edentulous with a fracture of the angle on one side and the body of the bone on the opposite side, bilateral open reduction is the treatment method of choice.

Region of the Ramus

Clinically the ramus of the mandible lies between an oblique line extending from the distal portion of the third molar to the superior posterior attachment of the masseter muscle; it is bounded above by two nearly equal lines which form a 90° apex at the midpoint of the mandibular notch (see Fig. 117 *A*). The ramus is fractured infrequently, for it is protected laterally by the heavy overlying masseter muscle, medially by the medial pterygoid muscle, and anteriorly by the lowermost fibers of the temporal muscle. Fractures of the ramus usually occur as the result of a direct lateral blow, a puncture wound, or a missile or gunshot wound (see Fig. 320 *A–C*). The ramus is thin and is weakened by the presence of the mandibular foramen. Fractures in this region may be extensions of fractures from the angle or from the coronoid or condylar process. Fractures of the ramus usually are associated with fractures of the angle or body of the mandible on the opposite side. The protective musculature of the ramus forms an excellent splint and tends to prevent displacement of the fragments.

Fractures in this region generally are treated by closed reduction and intermaxillary fixation. Gunshot wounds with destruction of segments of bone are treated by closure of soft tissues and conservation of any remaining viable bone fragments. Other treatment may consist of bone grafts after any infection has cleared and the tissues have healed completely.

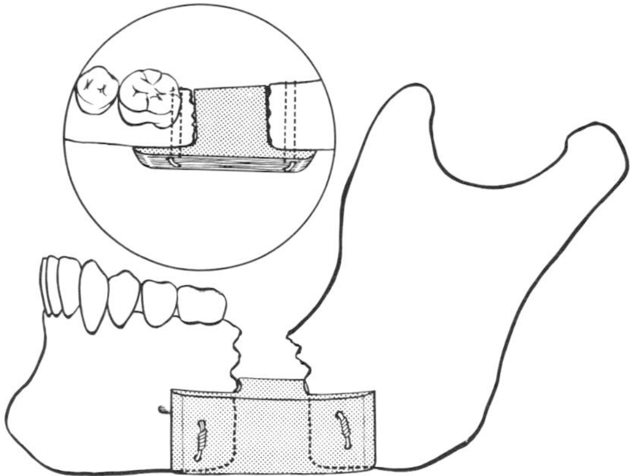

Figure 146. Use of immediate iliac bone graft for stabilization of bone fragments in the case of traumatic loss of bone. This method is applicable only if sufficient soft tissue is available for the covering of the bone graft.

REGION OF THE CONDYLAR PROCESS

Clinically the condylar process of the mandible is above and behind a line beginning at the depth of the sigmoid notch of the mandible and running downward and backward to the posterior border of the bone. The region includes the neck and the articular head of the condylar process. The condylar process is seldom fractured by direct force, but is fractured frequently by indirect force. The condyle is protected by the zygomatic process of the temporal bone and by ligaments and muscles about the joint. Occasionally open reduction is indicated for the treatment of fractures of the condylar process, but in most cases fractures in this region respond to simple, conservative management. Usually intermaxillary fixation for four to six weeks is sufficient for clinical healing in fractures of the condylar process.

Classification of Fractures

Fractures of the condylar process are classified according to the levels at which the fractures occur: *high fractures*—fractures above the level of insertion of the lateral pterygoid muscle; *middle fractures*—fractures immediately below the lateral pterygoid muscle attachment; and *low fractures*—fractures at the base of the condylar process.

Surgical Anatomy of the Condylar Process of the Mandible

The condylar process of the mandible consists of a rather thin mandibular neck, compressed from the front backward, which carries the mandibular head or condyle. The condyle is a semicylindrical bone whose long axis is oblique. If extended, the axes of the condyles would intersect at the anterior border of the foramen magnum. The lateral pterygoid muscle attaches to a rough depression on the anterior surface of the mandibular neck. Some fiber bundles of the upper head attach to the anterior surface of the disc. The resultant force of the muscle exerts on the condylar process a pull forward, downward, and medially. The capsule of the temporomandibular joint attaches in front, mainly above the insertion of the lateral pterygoid, while it reaches farther down to the lower area of the neck posteriorly.

The neck of the mandible is the thinnest portion of the mandible and the part most likely to be fractured from anterior or lateral blows. Violent force on the symphysial region may result in bilateral subcondylar fracture, and a blow to the side of the mandible may cause a fracture at the point of impact, with fracture of the mandibular neck on the opposite side. Fracture of the thin neck of the condylar process is the lesser evil. If an impact fails to fracture it, the head of the mandible may be driven into the middle cranial fossa or through the always-thin roof of the articular fossa. But fortunately, in most cases, the force of the impact is dissipated by a fracture of the neck of the mandible, and it is rare to find the condyle within the middle cranial fossa (Fig. 147).

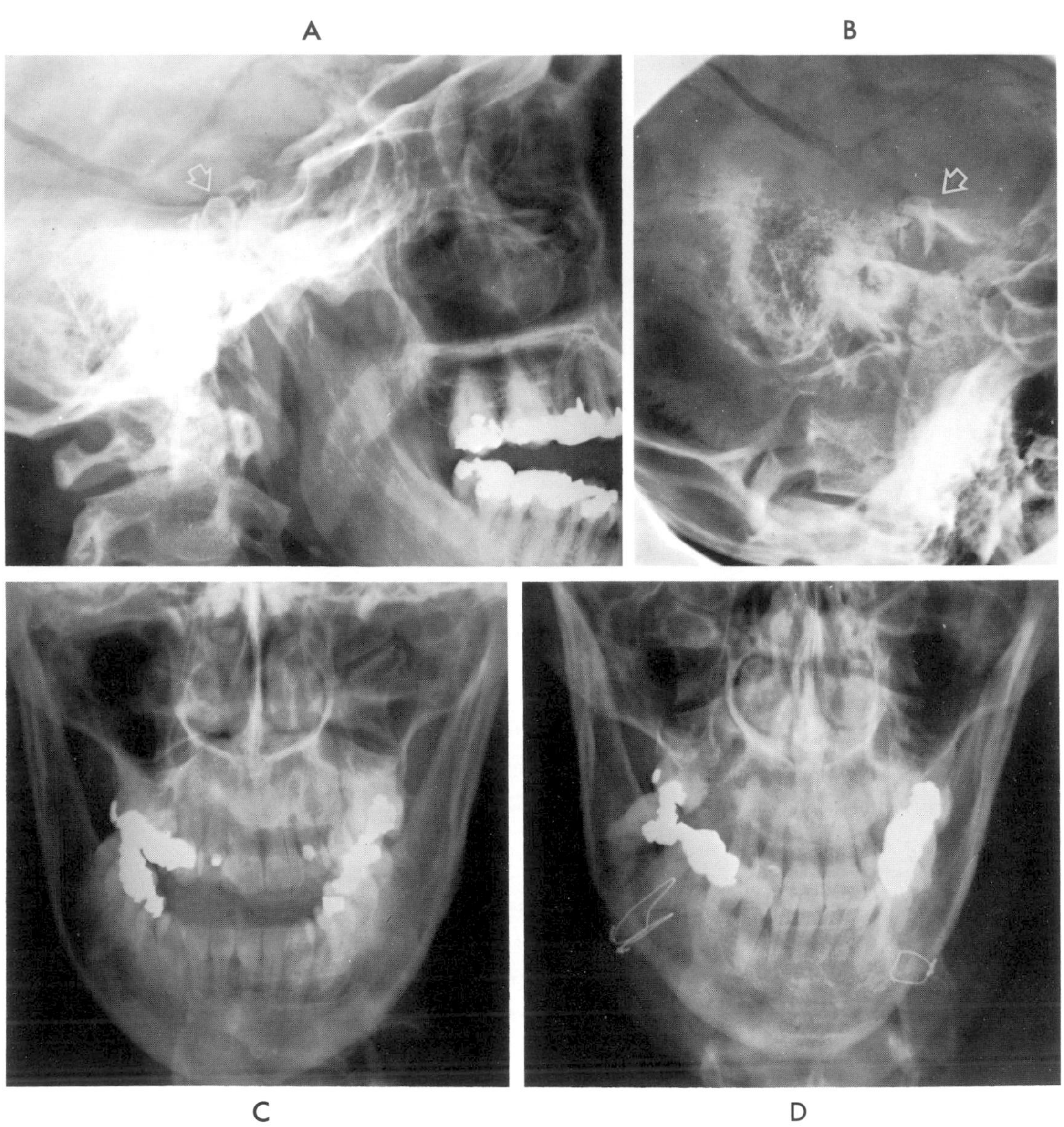

Figure 147. Dislocation of right condylar process into the middle cranial fossa. The patient was involved in an automobile accident with injury to the mandible, which drove the condyle through the glenoid fossa into the middle cranial fossa. The surgeon was fearful of reducing this dislocation in view of possible intracranial complications. The condyle was cut off and permitted to remain in its intracranial location. *A*. View showing intracranial dislocation of the condyle. *B*. Detail of temporomandibular joint showing the condyle in the cranial fossa. Note skull fracture. *C*. Malocclusion and open bite deformity of four years' duration following injury. *D*. Restored occlusal relationship following bilateral osteotomy of the mandible.

Fractures above the level of the insertion of the lateral pterygoid muscle may be totally or partially within the capsule of the joint. The articular surface may be completely detached within the joint, or the break may extend from above downward and backward to include most of the condyle. Fractures at this level show little displacement because they are located above the attachment of the lateral pterygoid muscle.

Fractures may occur immediately below the lowermost attachments of the lateral pterygoid muscle, and displacement of the condyle is forward and medially and downward owing to the lateral pterygoid pull. The fractured segment may be pulled out of position, even though it may still remain within the capsule. The mandibular head is usually displaced forward, but can also be rotated.

Diagnosis of Fractures of the Condylar Process

Diagnosis of fracture of the mandibular condyle and neck usually is made on the basis of clinical examination and confirmed by roentgenographic findings. Asymmetry of the face, caused by shifting of the mandible posteriorly and laterally, may be a prominent feature (Fig. 148). Premature contact of the teeth on the involved side is caused by the upward pull of the closing muscles of the mandible. Premature contact in the molar region creates a lever of Class I. This leaves the bite open in the front and on the opposite side (Fig. 149). Edema over the joint, ecchymosis, and sometimes hemorrhage into the external auditory canal may occur. Tenderness on palpation over the temporomandibular joint or the external auditory canal are usual findings.

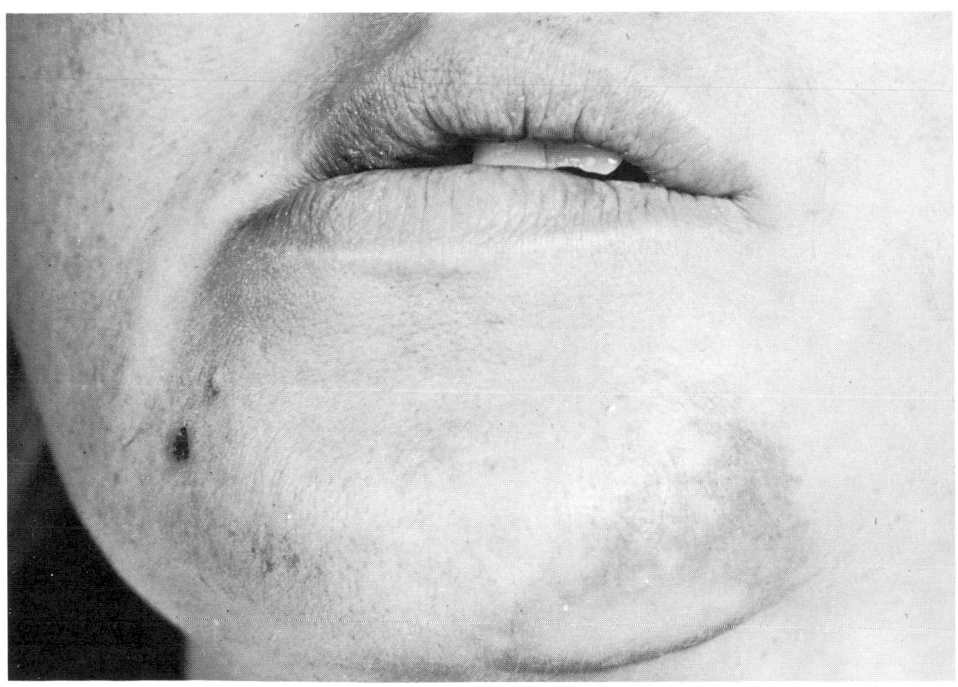

Figure 148. Fracture of the mandible with shift to the right side. Notice ecchymosis at the point of impact on the left side of the chin. The fracture was in the subcondylar region on the right.

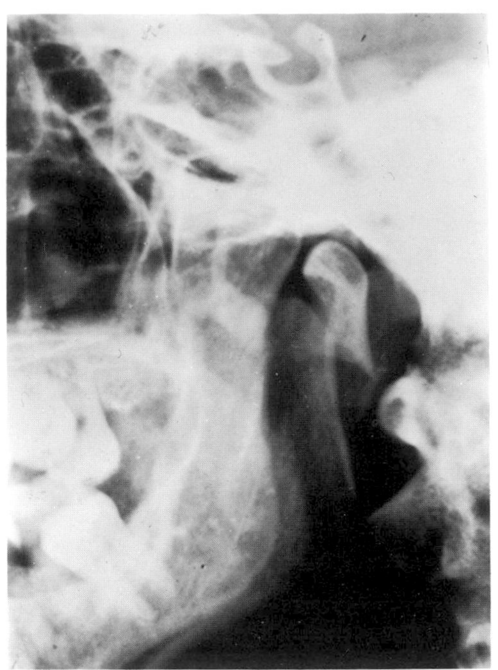

Figure 149. Fracture of the condylar process of the mandible with posterior displacement. In such fractures the patient may have forward displacement of the mandible with open bite deformity on the opposite side.

In bilateral fractures, the patient with teeth will exhibit an open bite deformity due to the overlapping of the fragments and premature contact of the posterior teeth (Fig. 150). The open bite deformity is caused by the contraction of the strong closing muscles of the mandible and upward displacement of its ramus with overlapping of the fractured segments. Inability to protrude the mandible is characteristic for bilateral fractures occurring below the level of the lateral pterygoid muscular insertions.

In unilateral fractures the patient is unable to protrude the mandible on the side involved, and the chin shifts to the affected side owing to the normal action of the lateral pterygoid muscle on the unaffected side and the loss of function on the injured side. Pain in the region of the ear and dysfunction on attempting to open the jaw are noted. The mandible actually may come to rest in a forward position. In such cases the upper end of the larger fragment may even contact the cranial base. One notes then an open bite with protrusion of the mandible.

Intracapsular fractures above the level of the insertion of the lateral pterygoid muscle do not exhibit displacement, because there are no muscles attached to the proximal fragment. The patients complain of pain in the temporomandibular joint and tenderness, on palpation, over the joint and in the external auditory canal. The teeth on the affected side cannot be brought into occlusion because intracapsular bleeding or edema has forced the condyle downward. Recovery may not be complete for several weeks. In children,

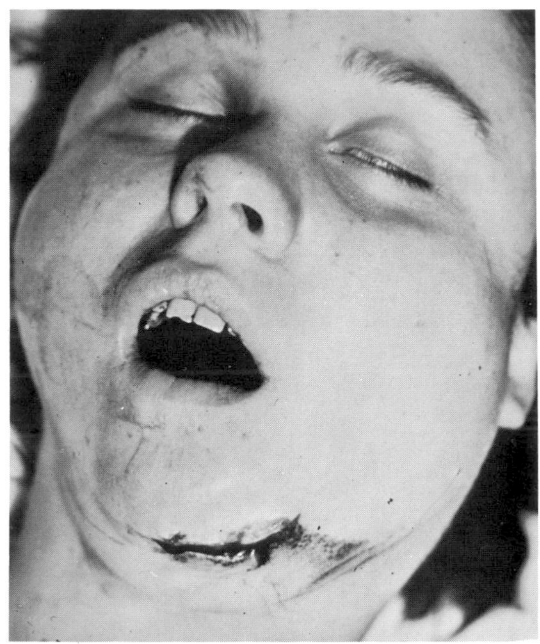

Figure 150. Patient with comminuted fractures of the body of the mandible and fractures of both condylar processes. Note retrusive position of the mandible and open bite deformity. The wound on the chin is at the point of impact.

this kind of injury may result in ankylosis of the mandible from aseptic necrosis of the condyle, organization of clots, formation of scars, and proliferation of bone (Fig. 334). Even though ankylosis does not occur, in some cases the growth centers of the condyle may be destroyed with subsequent failure of normal growth of the mandible (Fig. 335).

Fractures of the condylar process are difficult to demonstrate roentgenographically. Linear fractures or fractures with minimal displacement may be shown by laminographs but may be overlooked on the usual roentgenographic examination.

Most fractures of the condylar process show medial displacement. The condyle may remain within the articular capsule and the degree of the displacement may be minimal (Fig. 151). If dislocated, the condylar head may be completely evulsed from the joint and lie deep in the infratemporal fossa and as far anteriorly as the pterygoid plates.

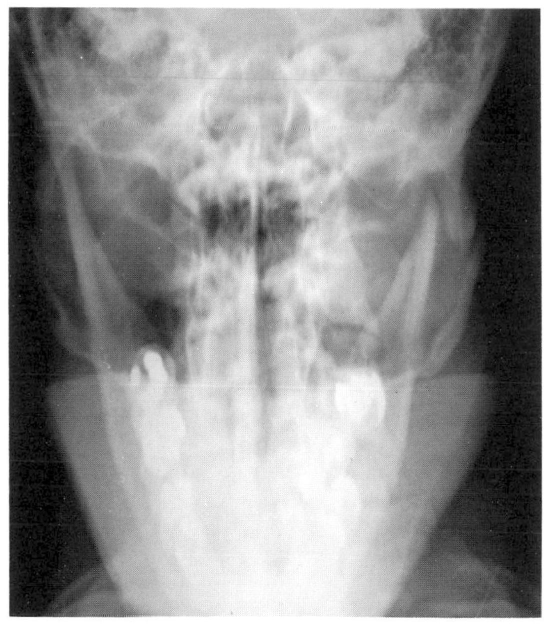

Figure 151. Fracture of the condylar process with lateral displacement of the neck. The head remains in the fossa, but the base of the fragment is displaced laterally.

Fractures that occur low on the condylar process may extend downward along the posterior border of the mandible, and roentgenographic examination will demonstrate medial displacement of the head and lateral displacement of the distal part of the fractured neck. Fracture of the tympanic plate is best shown by stereoscopic or laminographic views.

Treatment of Fractures of the Condylar Process

Fractures of the condylar process usually are treated by intermaxillary fixation, but occasionally open operation and direct wire fixation are indicated.

Nonoperative or closed treatment for fractures of the condylar process is the generally accepted method of management. No attempt is made to reposition the displaced mandibular condyle. Fixation is accomplished by means of arch bars and intermaxillary rubber bands or by wire fixation of the teeth.

In 1947 the members of the Chalmers J. Lyons Academy of Oral Surgery joined in a study of 120 cases of fractures of the condylar process of the mandible treated by immobilization. Almost without exception the results were acceptable. In a few cases there was slight malfunction due to deviation of the mandible to one side on opening, but in general the clinical results were satisfactory.

Most surgeons with experience in this field endorse the method of closed treatment and intermaxillary fixation as the method of choice in the management of fractures of the condylar process. Attempts have been made to force the condyle head into the joint by manipulation with a

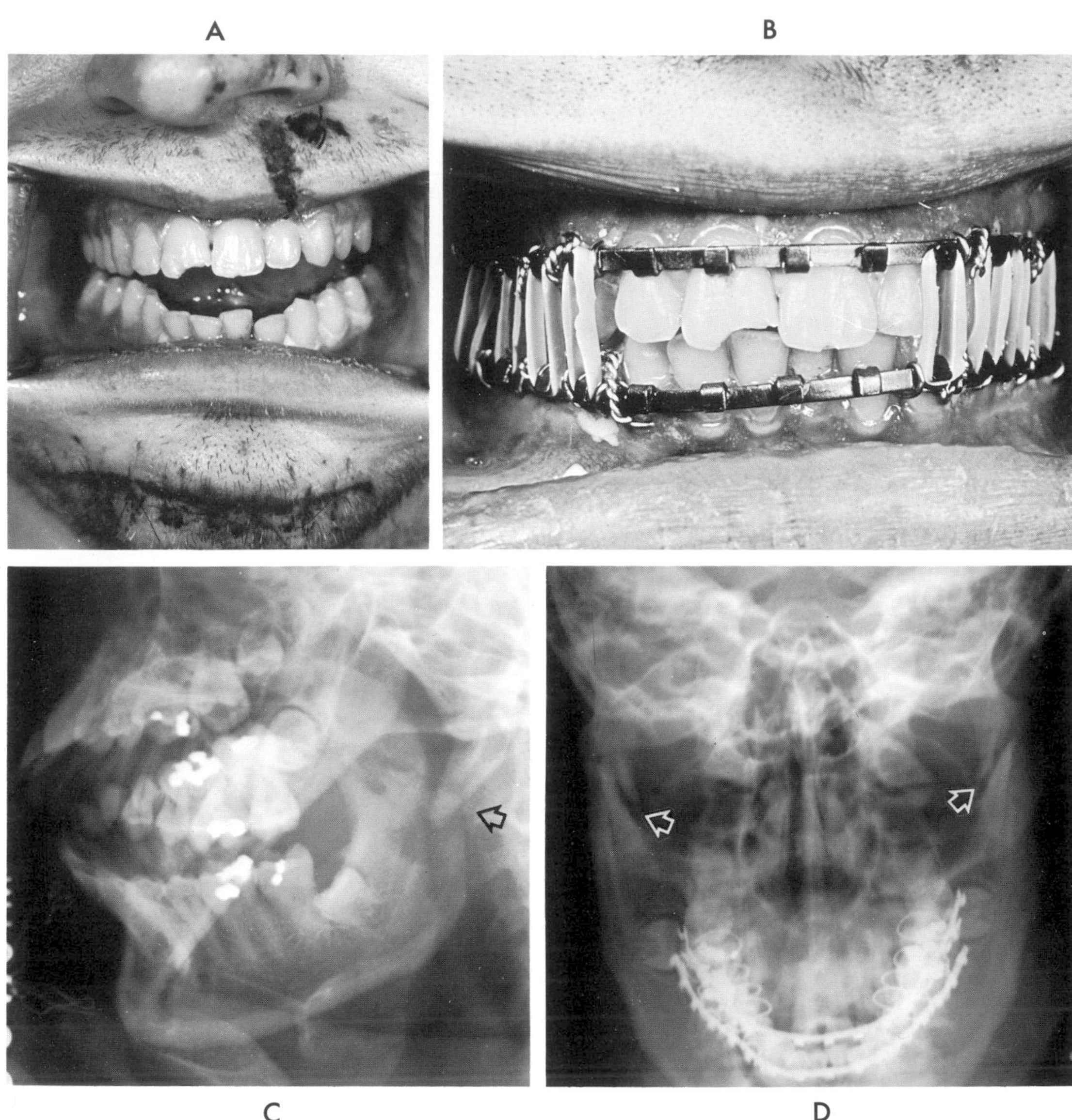

Figure 152. This patient received a blow upon the chin in an automobile accident and suffered a fracture in the region of the symphysis of the mandible and fractures of both condylar processes. *A.* Malocclusion, open bite deformity, and irregularity of the mandibular anterior teeth from displacement of mandibular fragments. *B.* Occlusion restored and secure fixation maintained by Erich arch bars and intermaxillary rubber band traction. *C.* Roentgenogram showing ramus of the mandible with fracture dislocation of the condylar process. *D.* Roentgenogram demonstrating fractures of both condylar processes treated by intermaxillary rubber band traction fixation. Most fractures of the condylar processes can be treated by simple immobilization with the teeth in occlusion.

pointed instrument passed through the soft tissues intraorally or through the skin anterior to the joint. Blind manipulations of this type may be damaging to the tissues and generally are unsuccessful. It is impossible to overcome the strong pull of the lateral pterygoid muscles in this manner. Roentgenograms following attempted reduction by this method fail to show improvement in the position of the fragments.

Intermaxillary fixation for a period of four to six weeks by any method that will hold the teeth in occlusion will give a satisfactory functional and cosmetic result. If sufficient teeth are present, arch bars ligated to the upper and lower teeth with intermaxillary rubber band fixation is the method of choice (Fig. 152 *A–D*). In cases of delayed treatment with development of an open bite, it may not be possible to replace the larger fragments manually, but traction with rubber bands attached to arch bars usually brings the teeth into functional occlusion in a matter of a few hours. In cases of long-standing condylar fractures, slow intermaxillary traction may be necessary over a period of several days or weeks before the teeth come into satisfactory alignment.

Condylar fractures associated with other fractures of the mandible may be treated concurrently by the same intermaxillary fixation used for treatment of fractures of the body or of the symphysial region (Fig. 153 *A, B*).

In the edentulous patient, bilateral subcondylar fractures may result in telescoping of the fragments and diminution of the

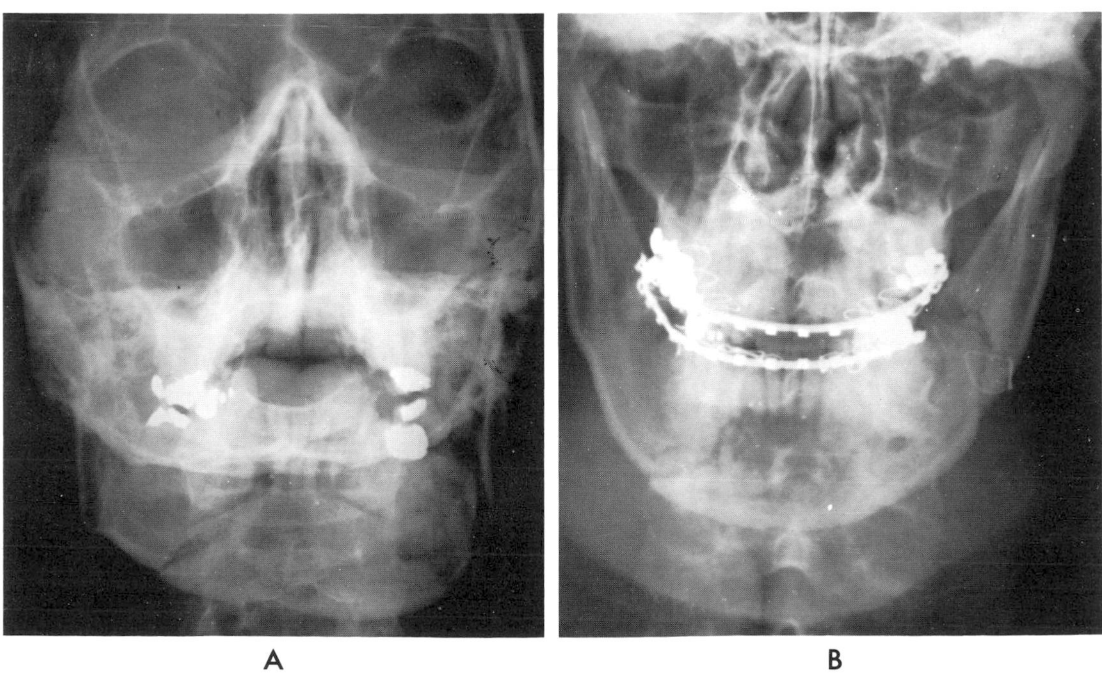

Figure 153. Multiple fractures of the mandible, including bilateral fractures of the condylar process and fracture of the body of the mandible on the right and of the angle of the mandible on the left. Treatment consisted of open reduction and fixation of the fracture at the left angle of the mandible and closed reduction of the mandibular body fracture on the right and of the two fractures of the condylar processes. Fixation by intermaxillary rubber bands and arch bars. *A.* Preoperative view. *B.* Postoperative view.

maxillary-mandibular distance. This closing of the bite may result in difficulty, or even the impossibility, of wearing dentures after healing takes place. The maxillary-mandibular distance may be maintained by fixation with the patient's artificial upper and lower dentures or by means of splints constructed for this purpose.

Open Reduction for Fractures of the Condylar Process

Because of the deep position of the condyle, the approach to the condylar process for open reduction is a formidable procedure. The overlying branches of the seventh nerve, the proximity to the (internal) maxillary artery and veins, and the insertion of the lateral pterygoid muscle make open reduction difficult and complications frequent. Open operation for treatment of fractures of the region of the condylar process have been used only in the last few years.

INDICATIONS. Open reduction may be indicated occasionally in children if the degree of separation at the fracture site has resulted in complete loss of continuity and probable loss of effectiveness of the growth center of the condyle. Without the growth center, the mandible will not grow properly and deformity will occur. In this type of case, an attempt should be made to reduce the condylar fracture.

Open operation may be indicated in the adult patient with an edentulous mandible and bilateral subcondylar fractures with telescoping of the fragments and shortening of the ramus and open bite deformity. With loss of vertical dimension posteriorly and open bite, open reduction may be advisable, because it may be impossible for the patient to wear artificial dentures if healing takes place in malposition.

The condylar region may be approached through a preauricular incision if the fracture is high on the process, or through an incision near the angle of the mandible if the fracture is low and the upper segment is long.

PREAURICULAR APPROACH TO THE CONDYLAR PROCESS. The temporomandibular joint is approached most often through a preauricular incision. The incision may extend from the hairline in the temporal region along the anterior margin of the ear to the lobule. Or an approach may be made through an angular incision that starts over the zygomatic arch and is carried posteriorly to the ear and downward anterior to the tragus (Dingman and Moorman, 1951). Care must be exercised to avoid injury to the branches of the seventh nerve in the preauricular area. The branches of the facial nerve are identified and retracted out of the field. The fascia overlying the temporomandibular joint is divided and the periosteum is elevated from the fractured segments. Identification may not be difficult if the head is within the confines of the temporomandibular joint. If the condyle has been evulsed from the joint and lies forward and medially, it may be difficult to find. It may be necessary to sever the attachments of lateral pterygoid muscle in order to reduce the fracture. Fixation is attained by a wire passed through drill holes in the bone on each side of the fracture site.

Hendrix, Sanders, and Green (1959) advocated the removal of the condylar process in cases in which the process had been evulsed from the joint and recommended its use as a bone graft (which has been separated from its blood supply) by reinserting and fixing it in the glenoid fossa after wires have been placed through drill holes. Georgaide has questioned the advisability of this method because of the separation of the lateral pterygoid muscle from the condylar process and the possibility of aseptic necrosis of the condyle.

Cases have been reported in which roentgenographic examination showed serious displacement of the fragments of the condylar process and in which roentgenograms made two or three years later showed that the head of the mandible had regained a fairly normal position spontaneously (Gregory, 1957). In one of Gregory's cases there was a right subcondylar fracture with severe medial angulation. The fracture was treated by intermaxillary fixation continued for several weeks. Roentgenograms made a few months later showed that the angulation between the fragments was persisting. But roentgenograms made three years later showed the condylar process in a fairly normal vertical position in the glenoid fossa. This phenomenon has been seen by other surgeons. One might assume that forces exerted by the muscles of mastication, which have been inactive during the weeks of fixation, afterward have favored a reconstruction of the condylar process by apposition and resorption to a fairly normal position and shape.

Subcondylar fractures of the mandible in children usually respond well to treatment with intermaxillary fixation. However, it must not be forgotten that, in children, a fracture wholly or partially within the capsule of the joint may be complicated by aseptic necrosis of the head, by fibro-osseous ankylosis of the temporomandibular joint, or even by destruction of the condylar growth center. Periodic observation is required following management of fracture of the condyle in children.

Risdon approach for open reduction of fractures of the condylar process. Risdon (1934) described an approach for operative procedures upon the ramus of the mandible. The approach is useful for reduction and fixation of a subcondylar fracture if the proximal fragment is long and extends downward along the posterior border of the mandible from its notch. A 5 cm. incision is made 1 cm. behind and below the angle of the mandible, taking the usual precautions to avoid damage to the ramus mandibularis of the seventh nerve. The skin, subcutaneous tissues, and platysma muscle are incised, and the layer immediately below the platysma is inspected for the presence of branches of the seventh nerve. If such are found, they are mobilized and retracted to prevent injury.

Dissection is carried up along the deep cervical fascia to the angle of the mandible where the incision is carried through the periosteum to expose the attachments of the masseter muscle at the inferior and posterior border of the angle of the mandible. The fibers connecting the periosteum to the mandible are incised, and the periosteum and muscle are elevated from the lateral surface of the mandible. The masseter muscle and the periosteum of the mandible are elevated to expose the site of the fracture. The elevator should be passed around the posterior border of the mandible, below and slightly above the site of the fracture. A 6 inch length of 25 gauge stainless steel wire is passed through a small drill hole at the angle of the mandible and is used for pulling the ramus in a downward direction; this helps in identifying the proximal segment. The displaced condyle is reduced by manipulation with a periosteal elevator. A right-angle retractor elevates the tissues so that the fracture site can be seen.

A stab wound is made in the tissues of the cheek overlying the site of the fracture, and the drill point is punctured through the tissue to the precise site at which the hole is to be made. This permits the drilling of holes perpendicular to the lateral surface of the fragments. The fragments are fixed with a section of 25 gauge stainless steel wire whose ends are twisted tightly, cut short, and flattened against the bone. The wound is closed without drainage, and fixation is supplemented by intermaxillary rubber bands or wires for four to six weeks.

Comminuted Compound Condylar Fractures

Gunshot wounds or missiles which penetrate into the region of the temporomandibular joint may result in compound comminuted fractures. Treatment consists in management of the soft tissue wounds and immobilization of the remaining portion of the mandible. If the joint is destroyed completely, or if necrosis is imminent as a result of loss of blood supply to the condylar process, it is advisable to remove the dislodged segments of bone to prevent fibro-osseous ankylosis. Even though the condylar process, or a part of it, is removed, function may still be satisfactory.

Region of the Coronoid Process

The coronoid process of the mandible is the upper portion of the ramus and is bounded by the ramus region below; it is the area above a line extending downward and forward from the depth of the sigmoid notch to the anterior border of the ramus. Isolated fractures of the coronoid process of the mandible are uncommon, and fractures in this region usually occur in conjunction with fractures of other parts of the mandible. The tip of the coronoid process is well protected by the overlying zygomatic arch and the fibers of the masseter muscle, and is well splinted by the tendinous attachment of the temporal muscle.

Severe traumatic force to the lateral surface of the face may result in fracture of the zygoma as well as the coronoid process of the mandible. In one of our cases, trauma suffered in an automobile accident resulted

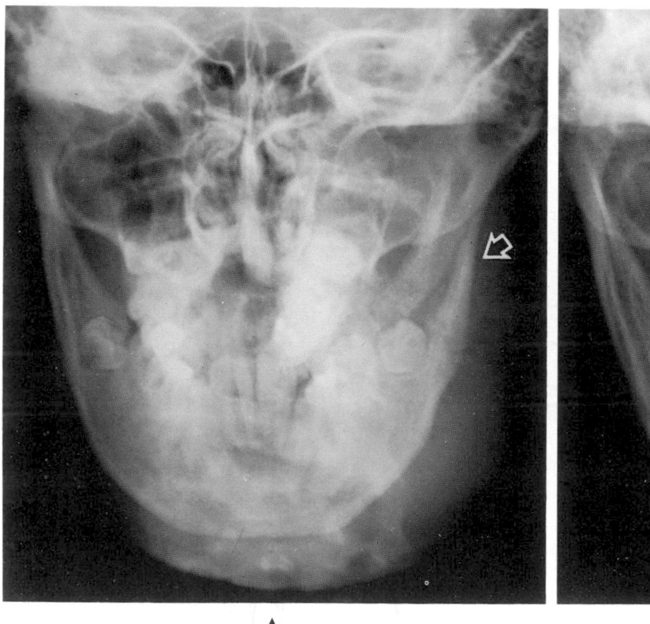
A

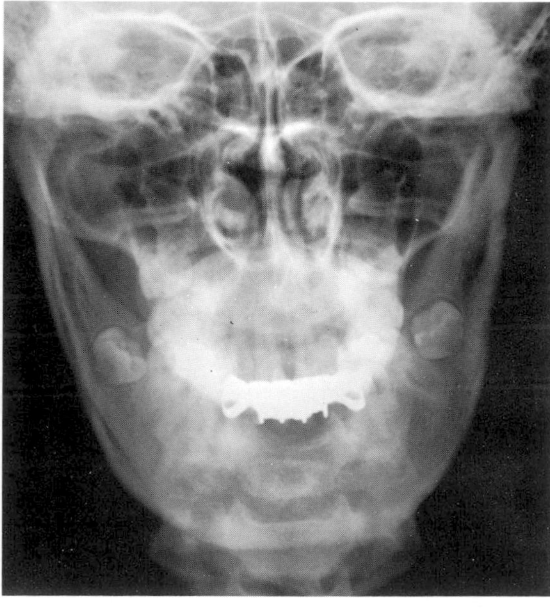
B

Figure 154. *A*. Fracture extending from the mandibular left third molar region through the lower part of the coronoid process into the base of the sigmoid notch. Fractures in this region are splinted well by the fascia and the attachments of the masseter, temporal, and medial pterygoid muscle. *B*. Result following healing after treatment by intermaxillary fixation (see Figure 203).

in avulsion of the skin and soft tissues of the side of the face with fracture of the zygoma, the coronoid process, and the temporal bone. In another case, multiple comminuted fractures of the coronoid process of the mandible, the zygoma, and the temporal bone occurred from a gunshot injury.

Fractures of the coronoid process usually are characterized by minimal displacement, and surgical intervention is unnecessary in isolated fractures. The splinting of the masseter and temporal muscles gives adequate support to the fractured segments so that other splinting is generally unnecessary (Fig. 154 *A, B*). The teeth may be placed in occlusion and secured with arch bars and rubber band traction, which, along with the natural muscle splinting, will allow for rapid healing.

Alveolar Fractures of the Mandible

The alveolar process of the mandible extends from the upper portion of the body of the mandible and provides support to the teeth.

Following extraction of the permanent teeth, the alveolar process no longer has a function and usually disappears owing to the atrophy of disuse. Atrophy of the alveolar process in areas of isolated extraction leaves weakened areas of the mandible which are liable to fracture. Following extraction of all the permanent teeth, atrophy of the alveolar process and part of the body may reduce the mandible to extreme thinness, which predisposes to fracture from minor injuries.

Fracture of the alveolar process may occur independently of complete fracture of the mandible. This usually occurs as the result of force sustained by the teeth, but may be due to direct blows to the alveolar process. Large tooth-bearing segments of alveolar bone may be fractured with total avulsion or displacement from the attached mucous membrane. Fractures of this kind are not uncommon in the mandibular anterior region where segments of bone may be fractured, with four to six teeth solidly attached to the alveolar fragment (Fig. 155). In some cases the fractured segments may contain roots or severely damaged or fractured teeth.

Treatment consists of removal of the smaller fragments of bone that do not have adequate soft tissue attachment or those segments that contain only roots of teeth or teeth that cannot be salvaged. Large segments of alveolar bone that still have satisfactory soft tissue attachment can be salvaged many times by stabilization in contact with the main portion of the bone. This may be done by wiring the teeth of the fractured segment to the arch bar or to the adjacent teeth. In some cases, recovery will take place if the soft tissue is sutured securely over the fractured alveolar segment so that it is re-

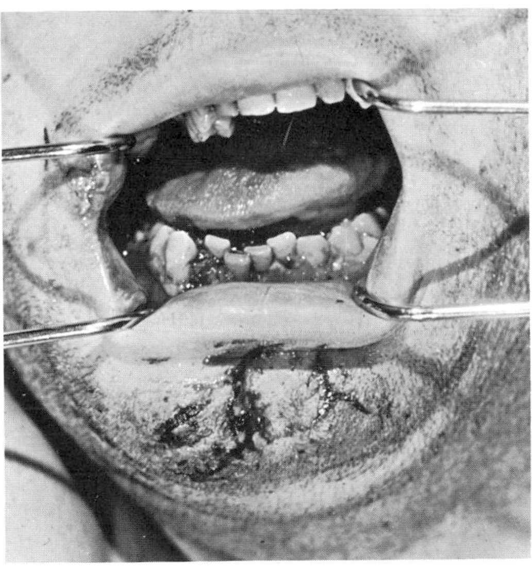

Figure 155. Compound comminuted fracture of the mandible with associated alveolar fractures and loosening of the teeth. Note edema of the tongue and ecchymosis of the floor of the mouth.

tained in position. If possible, the teeth should be fixed to an arch bar, or an orthodontic appliance should be made to provide stabilization of the teeth.

In severe injuries, segments of alveolar bone containing teeth may be dislodged completely and driven into the soft tissues of the tongue or floor of the mouth. Puncture wounds of the mouth following injury should be inspected carefully for segments of tooth, bone, or foreign materials.

DISLOCATION OF THE TEMPOROMANDIBULAR JOINT

Dislocation of the temporomandibular joint without fracture may be acute, chronic, or recurrent. Sicher (1960) stated: "The temporomandibular articulation is the only joint of the human body which can be dislocated without the action of an external force." Dislocation is a condition in which the mandibular condyle is displaced out of the glenoid fossa, usually anteriorly to the articular eminence, but generally remains within the confines of the joint capsule. Spontaneous dislocation is due to a break in the timing of the muscle action in the first phase of closing. In closing from maximal opening, the sequence of muscle action is the following: (1) relaxation of the protracting lateral pterygoid muscles, (2) retraction of the mandible, and (3) elevation of the mandible. If the lateral pterygoid muscles fail to relax at the right time, the elevators dislocate the mandible.

Traumatic dislocation is due to violence which forces the condyle out of the fossa. Dislocation of the temporomandibular joint may be unilateral or bilateral. It may be unilateral and associated with fracture dislocation of the joint on the opposite side.

Acute Dislocation of the Condyle of the Mandible

Acute dislocation, for the first time, seldom occurs during the act of eating, speaking, or laughing because all these movements are quite restricted. However, this may occur during yawning. Dislocation without fracture occurs only in the anterior direction. More violent forces may cause medial or lateral dislocation, but dislocation in these directions is always associated with fracture or severe injury to the temporomandibular joint.

Spontaneous dislocation of the condyle may be very distressing to the patient, especially if it is the first occurrence. In unilateral dislocation, the chin shifts toward the opposite side. The mandible on the involved side is in a protrusive relation and in an anterior open bite position. Dislocation usually is associated with muscle spasm which holds the condyle anterior to the articular eminence. In bilateral mandibular dislocation, the entire mandible is in anterior position with open bite bilaterally.

Failure to replace the condyle results in permanent dislocation with deformity and malfunction of the mandible. Reduction of dislocation of several months' to several years' duration has been reported. Gottlieb (1952), in a review of the literature, reported three cases of long-standing dislocation of the jaw that had been reduced by manual methods. Müller (1946) reported manual reduction of a dislocation that had been present for three months. Berg (1926) reported a case in which the dislocation had been present for two months, and Bouisson (1853) reported one of two months' duration in which the dislocation had been reduced manually. Ginestet, Desorthes, and Houessou (1948) reported ankylosis of the mandibular condyle three years after forceful reduction of a dislocated mandibular condyle.

Gottlieb (1952) treated three cases of long-standing dislocation successfully by resection of the condyle. Litzow and Royer (1962) reported a case of unilateral dislocation of six months' duration which was successfully treated by condylectomy; they removed the mandibular condyle with bone burs and chisels, through a Risdon (1934) approach (Fig. 186), from the angle of the mandible. Litzow and Royer stated that the direct approach to the temporomandibular joint through an incision in the preauricular or zygomatic area is hazardous because of the possibility of complete paralysis following injury to the seventh nerve. In one of our cases, a dislocation of two years' standing was reduced by manipulation and slow rubber band traction between maxillary-mandibular arch bars for one week.

Treatment by Manipulation

Treatment for acute dislocation is manipulation of the mandible to reposition the displaced condyle. This is best accomplished under moderate sedation to relax the musculature and allay apprehension in the patient. With the patient in the sitting position and the head supported, the operator stands in front of the patient, facing him, with the thumbs placed inside the mouth on the occlusal surfaces of the teeth, or on the alveolar ridges if no teeth are present, and the lower border of the mandible is grasped with the fingers. By pressing down firmly in the posterior area, while at the same time elevating the anterior area and pushing backward on the mandible, the condyle will slip over the articular eminence and back into position behind the eminence. If the muscle spasm is unusually severe, the operation cannot be accomplished without general anesthesia. Muscle-relaxing drugs and general anesthesia usually permit reduction.

Johnson's Method of Treatment Without Manipulation

W. Basil Johnson (1958) reported a method for reduction of acute dislocations of the temporomandibular articulation. In the three years prior to 1958, he reduced successfully 17 acute dislocations of the temporomandibular articulation, all of which were bilateral and nontraumatic with anterior displacement.

Johnson prepared the preauricular area of the face with a skin antiseptic, either on the right or left, this is to be used as the site of injection. Even though the dislocation is bilateral, it is only necessary to inject the local anesthetic unilaterally. The gloved index finger palpates the depression of the glenoid fossa, and this is easily accomplished inasmuch as the heads of the condylar processes are locked anterior to the eminences. Johnson reported the following: "A 1.8 cc. Carpule of lidocaine hydrochloride is loaded into the breech of a syringe equipped with a 25 gauge, 1⅞ inch needle—the usual length and gauge for intraoral injections. The needle is inserted into the subcutaneous tissue of the depression of the glenoid fossa, while directing the needle inward and slightly anterior toward the head of the condyloid process. The anesthetic solution is injected slowly as the needle progresses into the tissues. When the posterior slope of the eminence or the head of the condyloid process is contacted, the needle is slightly withdrawn and the remaining anesthetizing solution is injected into the tissues surrounding the glenoid fossa. The needle then is withdrawn" (Fig. 156).

Johnson reported that in all 17 patients the dislocations were reduced spontaneously without manual manipulation and in approximately one minute. In one of the cases, a dislocation of three days' duration, a bilateral injection was made because at the time

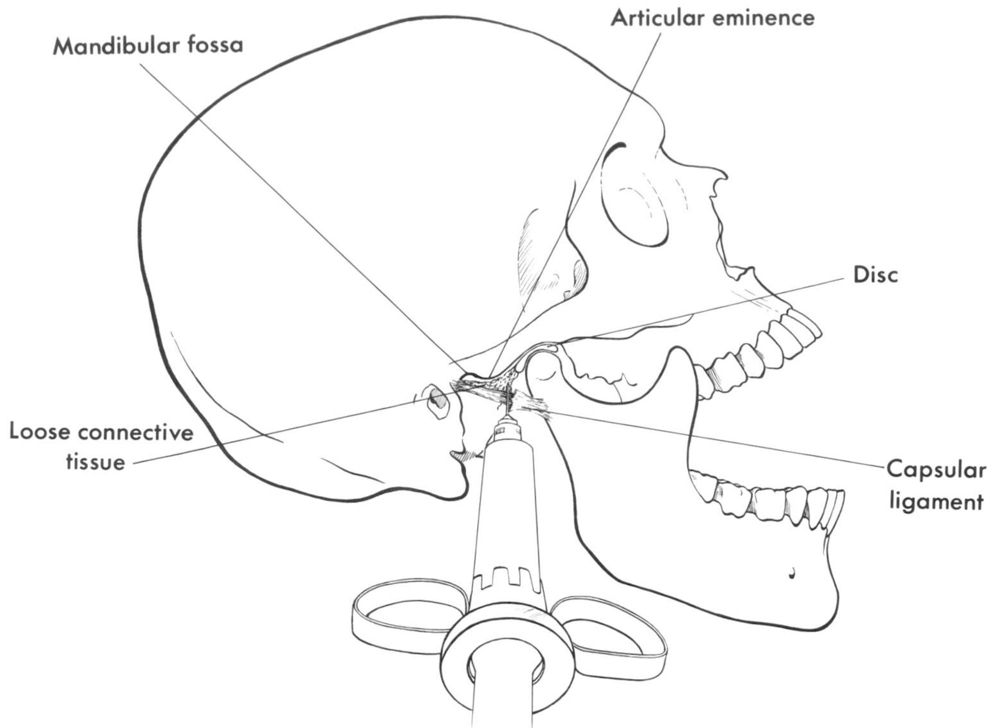

Figure 156. Johnson's method of injection of an anesthetic solution into the nerve-bearing loose connective tissue of the capsule following acute anterior dislocation. Note the attachment of the loose connective tissue to the disc.

it was not realized that the injection was required unilaterally only.

The explanation for the success of Johnson's method seems to lie in the fact that the injuries of the capsule maintain spasms of the masticatory muscles by neural reflexes. Since these reflexes stretch over the entire bilateral group of muscles, cutting the source of muscular disturbance by injection of one side only will spread its effect over all members of the group of mandibular muscles. Once the spasms are released, the patient is able to close his mouth and to retract the mandible into its normal position.

Postreduction

Acute dislocation is usually associated with some injury to the capsule and even to the articulating surfaces within the joint. This results in an inflammatory reaction and accumulation of fluid within the joint. The joint may be painful for several days after reduction. The patient may be unable to occlude the posterior teeth on the affected side for several days to two weeks because of the capsular and intra-articular edema which forces the condyle in a downward direction. The jaws should be placed at rest for a few weeks to permit the joint structures to recover without the additional trauma of function. The patient must be extremely cautious about overextending the joint for several months. Continued insults to the joint may cause permanent damage to the joint structures and result in a recurrent or chronic dislocation.

Habitual Dislocation of the Temporomandibular Joint

After the first episode, the capsule is torn or ligaments overstretched to cause habitual dislocation. The patient usually learns how to reposition the condyle and becomes quite expert in reducing his own dislocation. In some cases the patient is unable to reposition the condyle, but this can be done easily without anesthesia by the physician. Re-education of the patient in his eating and yawning habits, teaching him to avoid a wide opening of the jaws whenever possible, seems to be very helpful.

The Mandible

PART 2

OPERATIVE TECHNIQUE

Because of the mandible's contribution to speech, efficient mastication, deglutition, and to the form of the lower portion of the face, fractures of this structure must receive careful consideration.

The following section illustrates direct operative methods of reduction and positive fixation of mandibular fractures. Advances in techniques and therapeutics have made the direct approach both practical and desirable from the standpoint of accuracy of reduction, expediency, comfort to the patient, and the best results.

As the student peruses the methods described in the following pages he will note that certain artistic liberties have been taken in some of the illustrations—e.g., the hair has not been shaved in some instances and surgical drapes are not included in others. In some sketches only the skeletal structures are shown; in others, soft tissues are superimposed upon the skeletal. Artistic license was necessitated by limitations of the printed page; it was used for the sake of clarity and to give the reader the best possible view of the techniques illustrated.

REGION OF THE SYMPHYSIS

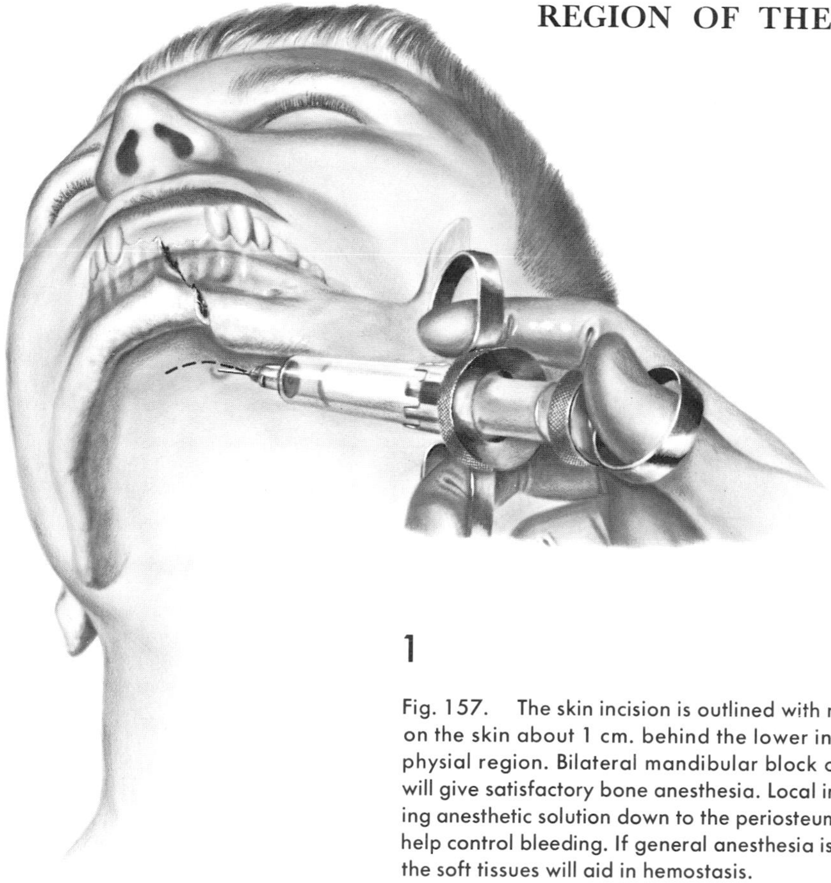

1

Fig. 157. The skin incision is outlined with marking ink. A curved line is marked on the skin about 1 cm. behind the lower inner margin of the bone of the symphysial region. Bilateral mandibular block or injection into the mental foramen will give satisfactory bone anesthesia. Local infiltration of an epinephrine-containing anesthetic solution down to the periosteum will anesthetize the soft tissues and help control bleeding. If general anesthesia is used, local injection of solution into the soft tissues will aid in hemostasis.

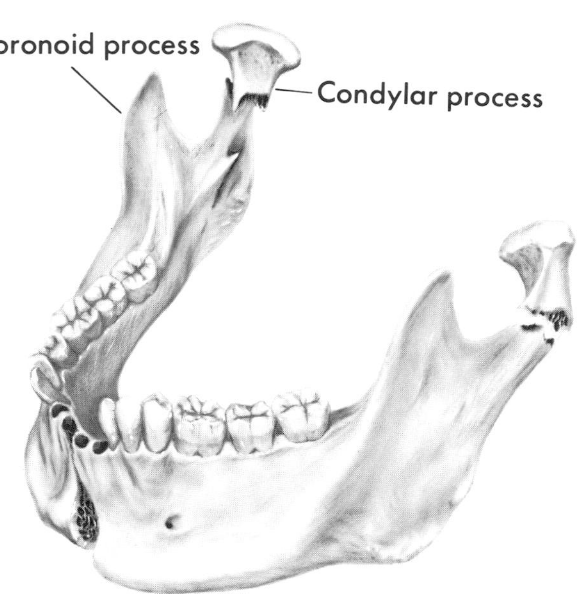

2

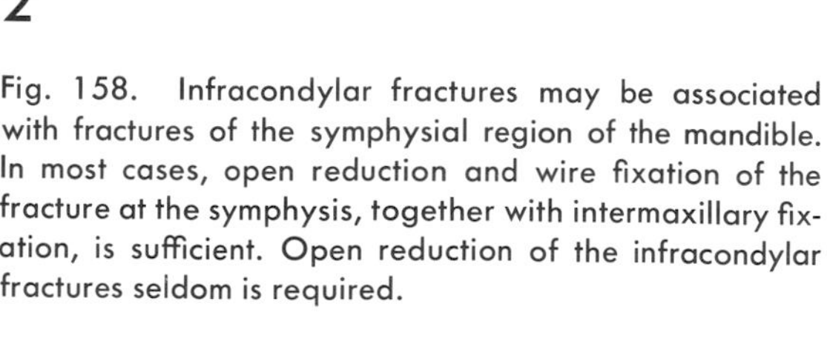

Fig. 158. Infracondylar fractures may be associated with fractures of the symphysial region of the mandible. In most cases, open reduction and wire fixation of the fracture at the symphysis, together with intermaxillary fixation, is sufficient. Open reduction of the infracondylar fractures seldom is required.

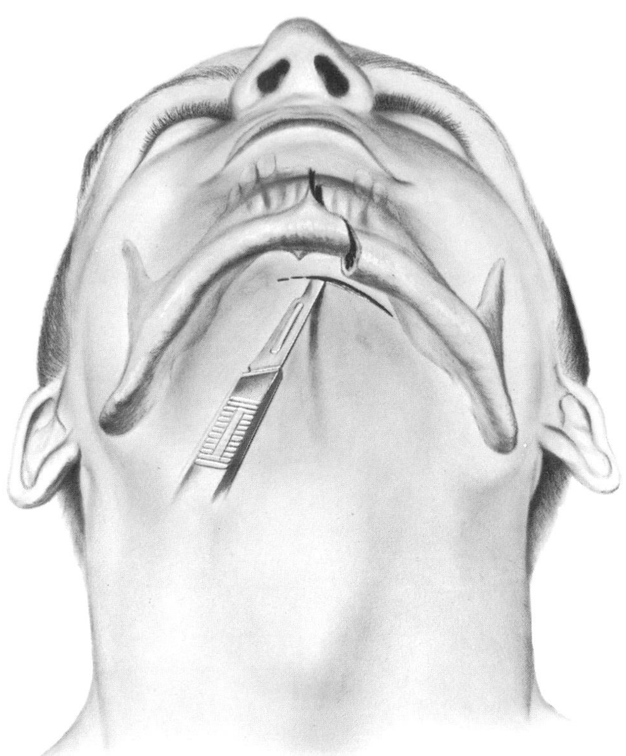

3

Fig. 159. An incision 4 or 5 cm. in length is made through the skin about 2 cm. behind the chin. The center of the incision should correspond with the site of the fracture, at the inferior border of the mandible. Most fractures in the symphysial region are oblique, with telescoping displacement of the fragments. Extension of the planned incision may be necessary to give adequate exposure.

4

Fig. 160. The dissection is carried through the platysma muscle to the inferior border of the mandible. The fracture usually can be identified through the tissues as an irregularity at the inferior margin of the mandible. Hemostasis is obtained by clamping bleeding vessels and twisting, ligation, or electrodesiccation. Careful electrocoagulation with low current gives effective hemostasis and may speed the procedure.

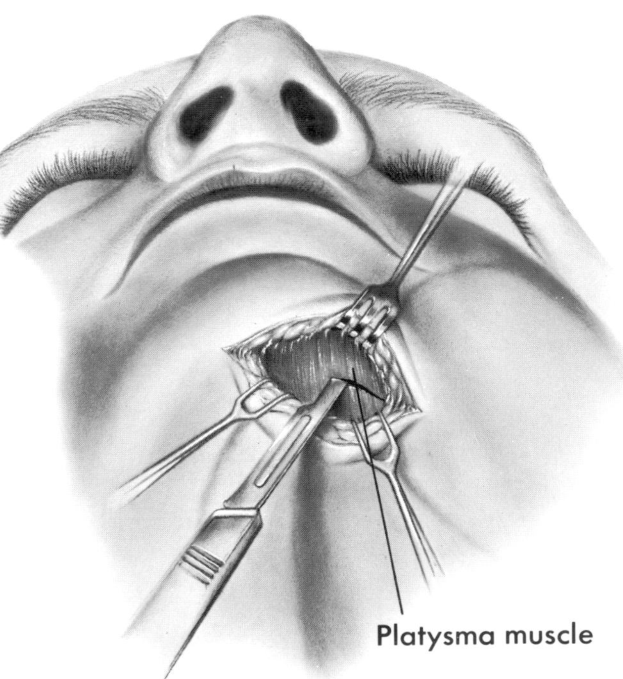

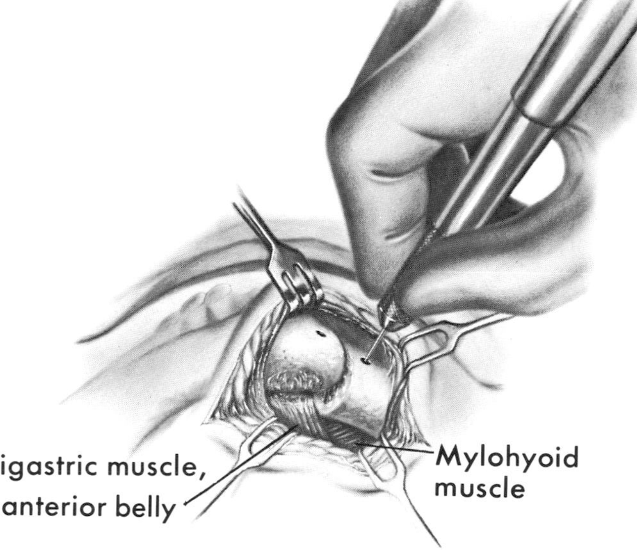

5

Fig. 161. The periosteum has been dissected with elevators to give adequate exposure of the bone for the drilling of bur holes about 5 to 7 mm. from the inferior margin of the mandible.

Dissection is more difficult on the inner surface of the mandible because the digastric muscle fibers are attached intimately to the bone in the digastric fossa. Separation may require dissection with a scalpel or sharp elevator next to the bone.

Irrigation helps to prevent overheating of the bone during the drilling of the holes. Suction is useful for the removal of excess solution and to provide a clear field of vision.

6

Fig. 162. A length of No. 25 gauge stainless steel wire is passed through one bur hole to the inner surface of the mandible and then back through the hole in the other fragment.

The fracture is reduced and the wire ends twisted together and cut. The joined tip is inserted into one of the bur holes (see inset). To prevent loosening of the wire ligature while bending, the wire should be twisted while it is being bent for insertion in the hole.

The wire-and-knot assembly is flattened against the bone by pressure made with a forceps as shown in Fig. 180.

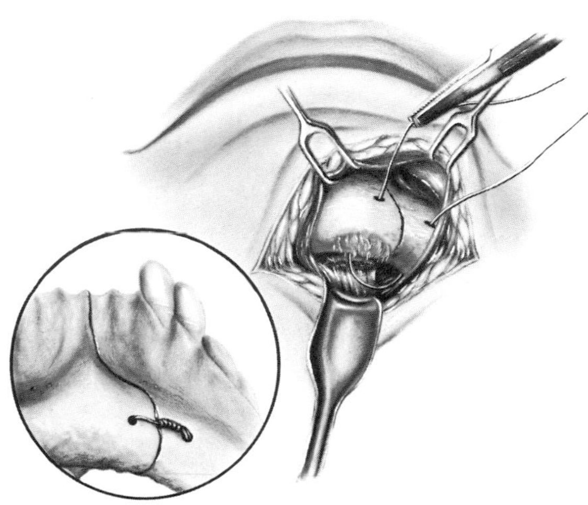

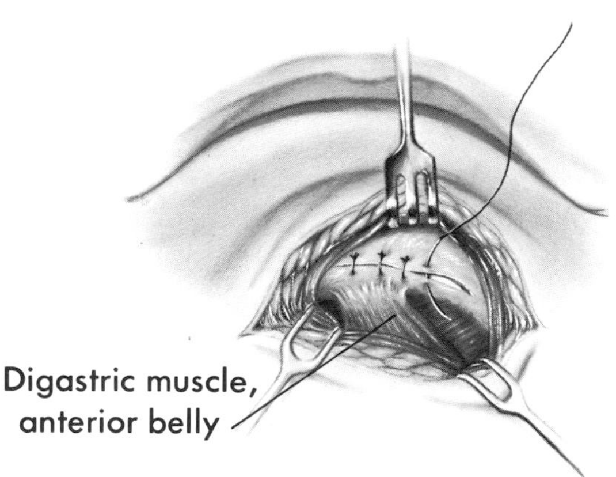

7

Fig. 163. The periosteum is sutured into place with interrupted catgut sutures. In most cases the incised end of the diagastric muscle with the periosteum can be sutured to the periosteum of the anterior surface. Periosteum stimulates callus formation and bone proliferation; therefore it should be replaced carefully.

8

Fig. 164. After the periosteum has been replaced, and after the digastric muscle has been reattached, the subcutaneous layers are closed with interrupted 0000 catgut or nylon suture. The skin is closed with interrupted 00000 nonabsorbable sutures. A small piece of fine-mesh petrolatum gauze is placed over the sutured wound, and a light compression dressing is applied.

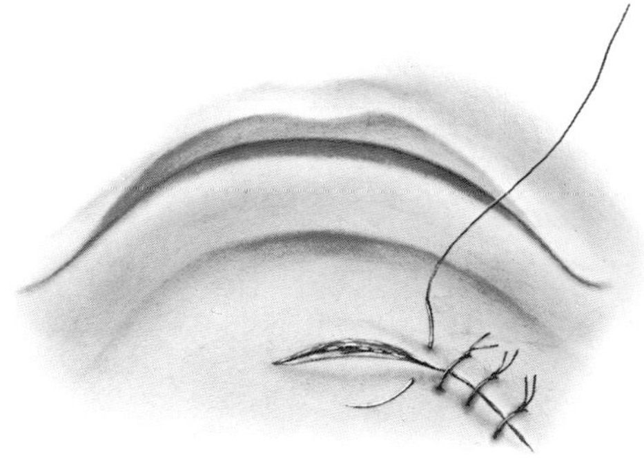

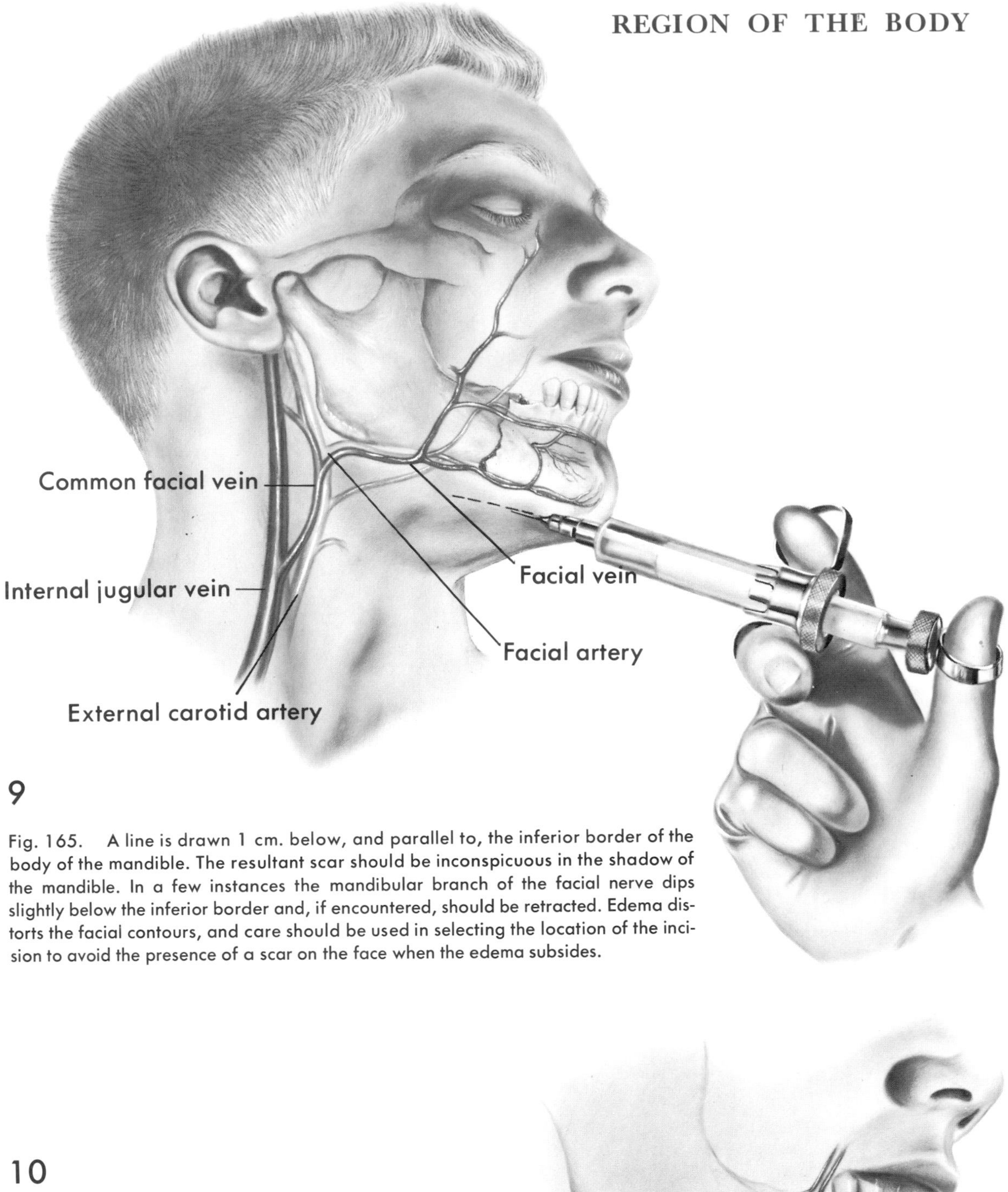

Common facial vein
Internal jugular vein
External carotid artery
Facial vein
Facial artery

9

Fig. 165. A line is drawn 1 cm. below, and parallel to, the inferior border of the body of the mandible. The resultant scar should be inconspicuous in the shadow of the mandible. In a few instances the mandibular branch of the facial nerve dips slightly below the inferior border and, if encountered, should be retracted. Edema distorts the facial contours, and care should be used in selecting the location of the incision to avoid the presence of a scar on the face when the edema subsides.

10

Fig. 166. The facial vein and artery may lie directly over fractures through the midsection of the body of the mandible. The vessels may be clamped and ligated safely if they cannot be retracted. Absorbable suture is preferable for ligatures, since this is potentially a contaminated region. Careful retraction of tissues is important to prevent damage to the ramus mandibularis of the seventh nerve.

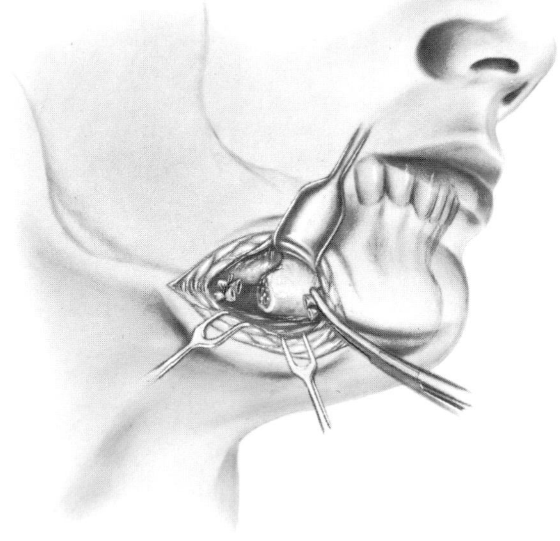

11

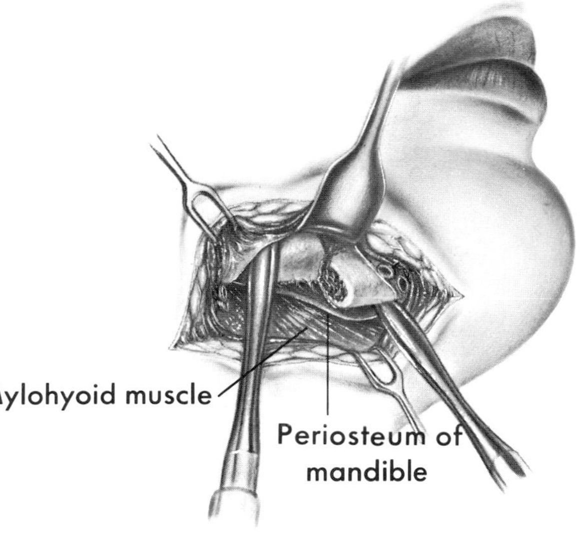

Fig. 167. Sharp periosteal elevators have been used to elevate the periosteum from the bone. Blood clots, tissue debris, and loose bone spicules have been removed from the region between the fragments. The loose tissue through which the approach is made permits easy shifting for adequate access to the fractured bone.

12

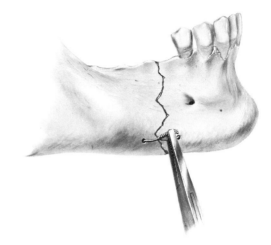

Fig. 168. When the fractured bone has been reduced and the wire twisted securely, the wire is cut to the correct length. The twisted tip is bent at right angles and inserted into a bur hole. The wire is flattened against the bone. This eliminates the possibility of irritation from the wire's tip projecting into the overlying soft tissues.

13

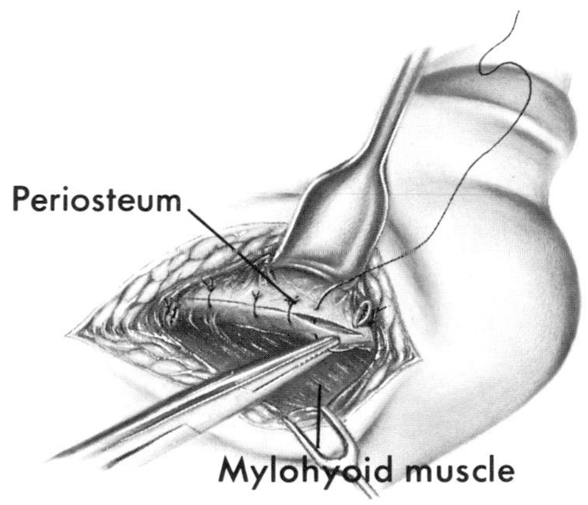

Fig. 169. The periosteum is closed carefully with 0000 absorbable sutures cut at the knot.

To minimize the possibility of adhesions of the skin to bone with an immovable depressed scar, accuracy in replacement and suture of the periosteum, musculature, and subcutaneous layers is important.

If gross contamination is suspected, or if hemorrhage cannot be controlled adequately, a small rubber drain should be placed in the wound; it may be removed in 24 to 48 hours.

14

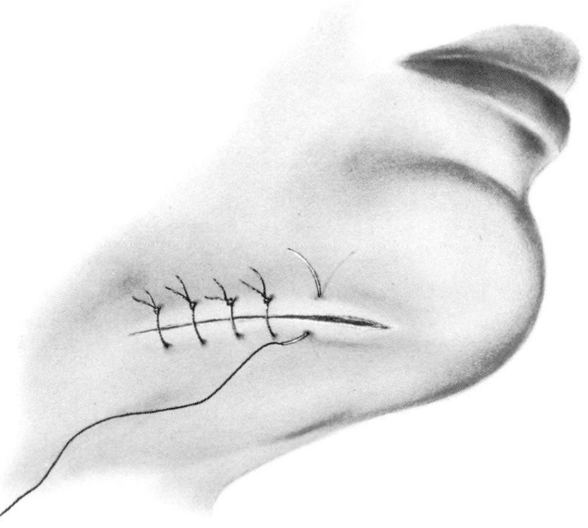

Fig. 170. Notice the location of the knots made in suturing the skin. It is important that these knots be kept at the side of the wound to avoid further scarring, for small pits caused by knots being placed in the incision area may persist.

To keep the scar as narrow as possible, sutures should be removed in 4 or 5 days and the scar line should receive good postoperative mechanical support, as is described on page 343.

To avoid small punctate scars near the incision line, interrupted, single strand synthetic sutures are used. Sutures should be tied loosely and removed in 3 or 4 days. Subcuticular closure is preferable if the wound needs support for 2 or 3 weeks.

Scars usually result when sutures that are too large are tied too tightly and retained too long.

REGION OF THE ANGLE

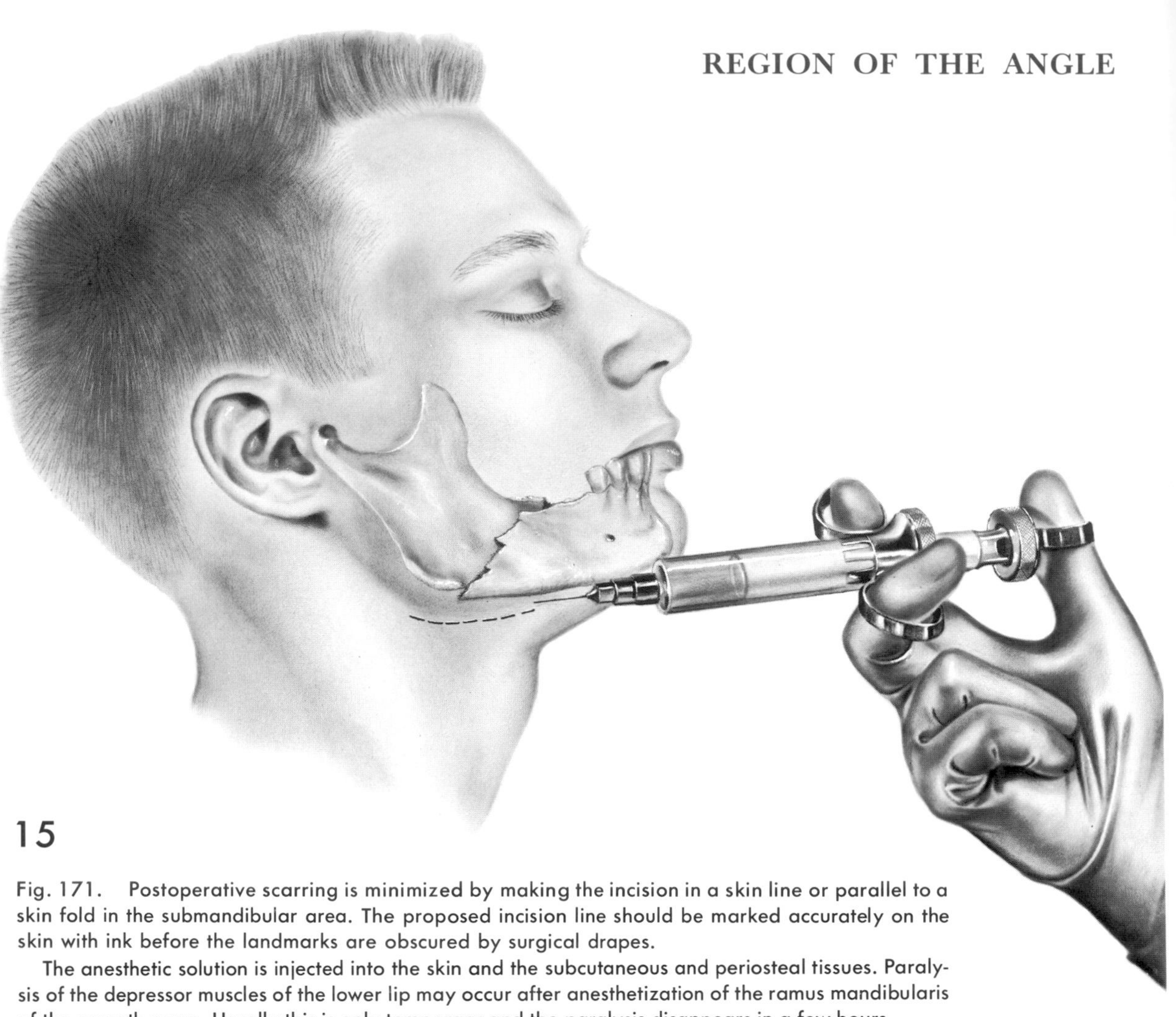

15

Fig. 171. Postoperative scarring is minimized by making the incision in a skin line or parallel to a skin fold in the submandibular area. The proposed incision line should be marked accurately on the skin with ink before the landmarks are obscured by surgical drapes.

The anesthetic solution is injected into the skin and the subcutaneous and periosteal tissues. Paralysis of the depressor muscles of the lower lip may occur after anesthetization of the ramus mandibularis of the seventh nerve. Usually this is only temporary and the paralysis disappears in a few hours.

16

Fig. 172. Fracture of the mandible may occur through the molar area with lateral displacement of the proximal segment. Lateral displacement is uncommon and is caused by the forces which caused the fracture. All tooth sockets are regions of weakness in the mandible, and so it happens that fractures of the tooth-bearing parts of the bone usually occur through a socket.

17

Fig. 173. If the teeth are loose or severely damaged, or if they interfere with reduction, they should be removed. In some cases a firm tooth, or a part of a tooth, in the line of fracture may be useful in maintaining reduction and should be spared. The ramus may be displaced medially or laterally, depending upon the nature of the fracturing force, the direction of the fracture, and the pull of the musculature adjacent. In most fractures occurring in this region the proximal fragment is displaced medially because of muscle action.

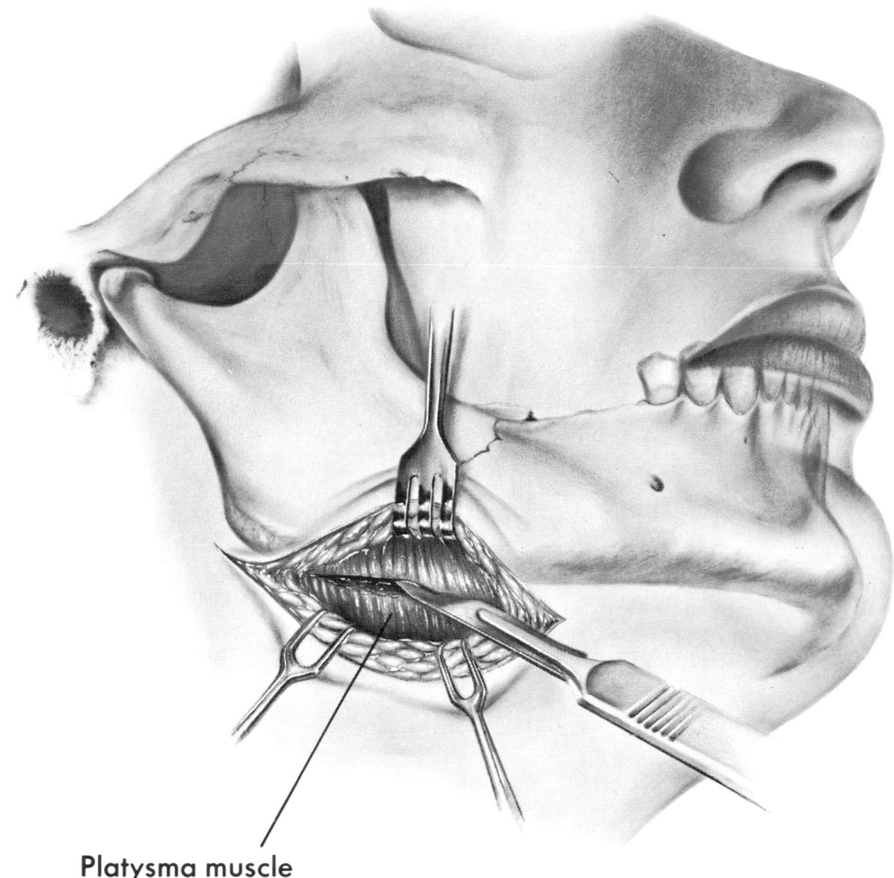

18

Fig. 174. The approach is similar to that used for fractures of the body of the mandible except that it is farther posterior. The ramus mandibularis of the seventh nerve dips below the border of the mandible in about 20 per cent of cases. After the platysma muscle is incised, the nerve may be seen in the immediately underlying fascia. A nerve stimulator is useful in identifying the nerve. Although the nerve usually recovers if cut, disability is annoying for a year or more.

19

Fig. 175. To gain access to a fracture in the region of the angle, the masseter muscle must be incised at the inferior border of the mandible. The muscle and periosteum are separated easily from the mandible, except over the thickened portion of the angle where fibers of the muscle insert directly into bone. These attachments resist elevation and must be divided with a scalpel. Then the periosteum can be separated from the bone readily, by using an elevator.

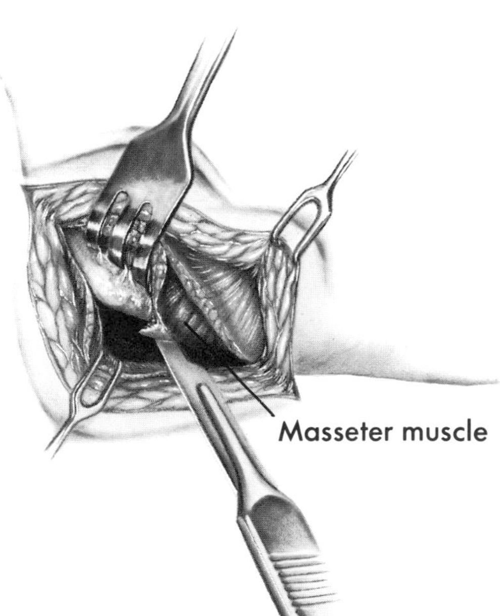

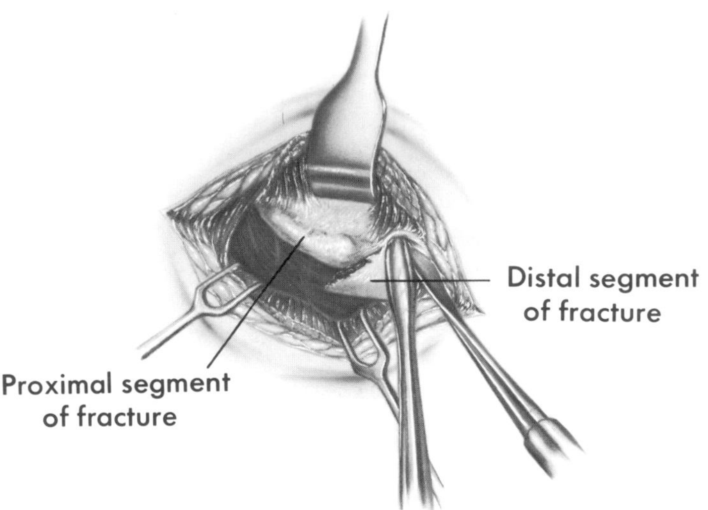

20

Fig. 176. Elevators are used to separate the periosteum from the bone on the lateral and medial surfaces of the mandible adjacent to the fracture. This simplifies reduction and provides access for the drilling of holes. Debris and organized tissue should be removed from the region to permit anatomic reduction of the fragments.

21

Fig. 177. The bone is grasped on both sides of the fracture with a forceps, and the fragments are manipulated into anatomic position. The bone forceps maintains reduction of the fragments and supports the bone while a bur hole is made through each fracture segment. Irrigation of the region with normal saline solution during the making of the holes prevents overheating of the bone.

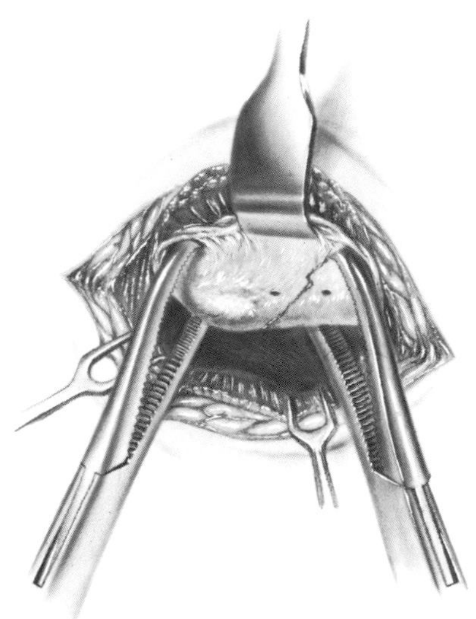

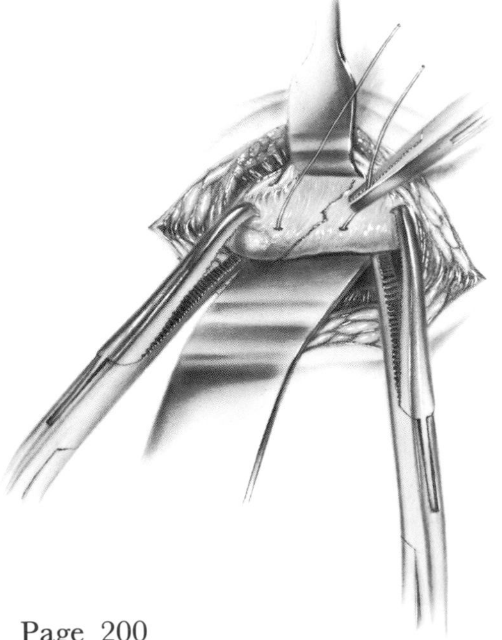

22

Fig. 178. A 6 inch length of 25 gauge stainless steel wire is inserted through the bur holes with both ends of the wire brought out upon the lateral surface. The wire is twisted securely against the bone with a wire-twisting forceps. A ribbon retractor is useful to provide exposure and to prevent damage to the medial soft tissues. A bone-holding forceps keeps the fragments in anatomic position while the assistant tightens the wire.

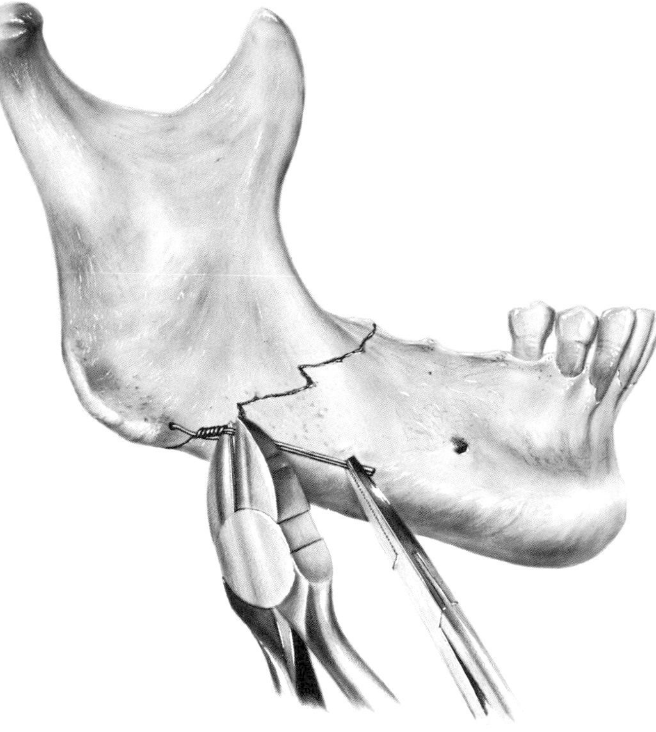

23

Fig. 179. It is rarely necessary to remove the stainless steel wire used in fracture fixation unless there is irritation of overlying soft tissues. The wire is inert and causes no reaction if cut short and pressed against the bone. The wire selected should provide completely adequate fixation and yet be as delicate as possible. Specially designed wire-handling instruments facilitate the operative procedure.

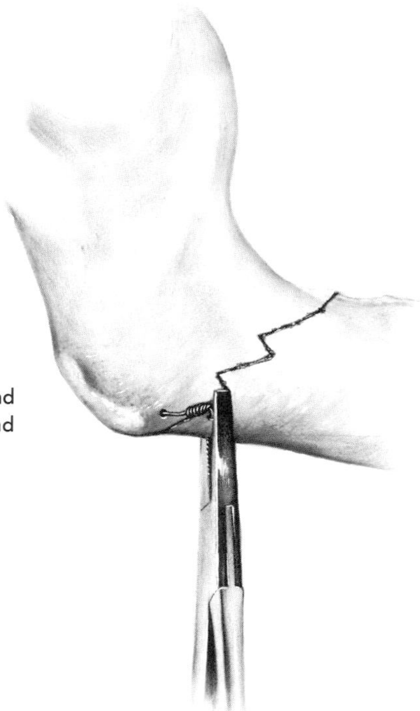

24

Fig. 180. A stainless steel wire placed carefully, twisted neatly, and flattened against the bone produces minimal foreign body reaction and remains permanently in the tissues without discomfort.

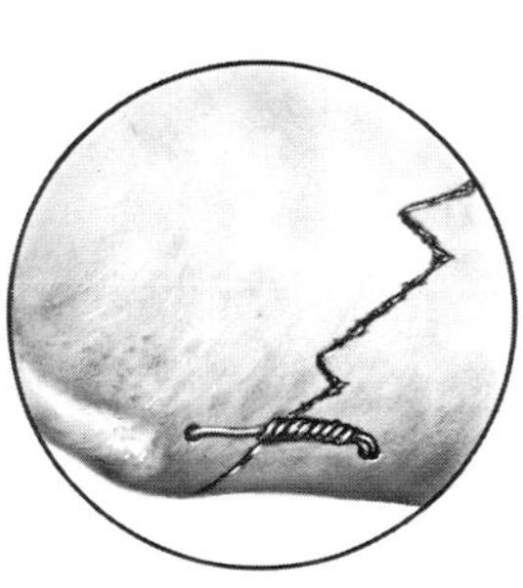

25

Fig. 181. After cutting and bending, the end of the wire is inserted into one of the holes and the wire mass is flattened against the bone by pressure with a wire-twisting forceps with one blade on each side of the bone.

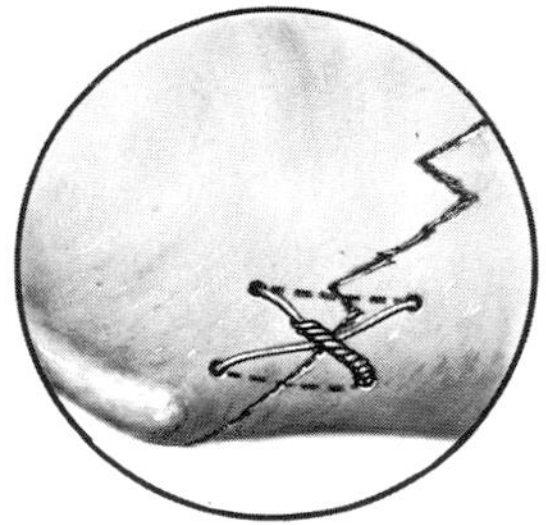

26

Fig. 182. If fixation is to be dependent wholly upon the interosseous wire without intermaxillary fixation as an adjunct, it may be necessary to use figure-of-eight or cross-wire fixation, as shown, for better stability. In drilling holes for this type of fixation, the nerve canal should be avoided.

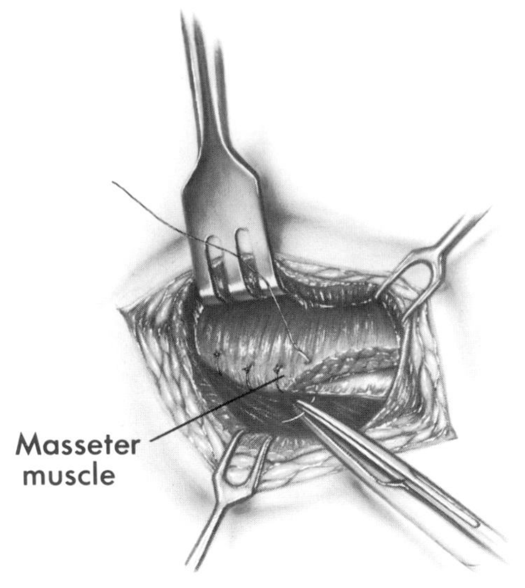

27

Fig. 183. The periosteum and the masseter and medial pterygoid muscles are approximated over the inferior edge of the bone in a slinglike fashion to ensure proper soft tissue coverage of the fracture site. Such coverage enhances the restoration of the blood supply to the fractured bone, which is important in uncomplicated repair.

28

Fig. 184. The platysma muscle is repaired with interrupted 0000 plain catgut sutures. If the soft tissues have been injured severely in the fracture, and there is a probability of tissue necrosis, seroma, or hematoma, a small rubber drain should be placed in contact with the bone at the lower end of the incision. The drain should be secured to the skin with a suture.

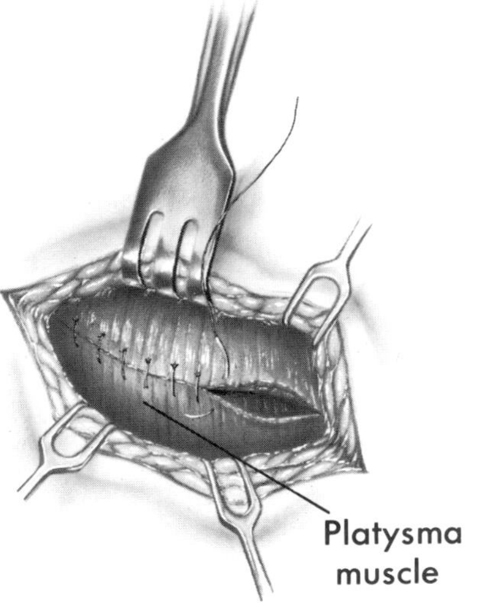

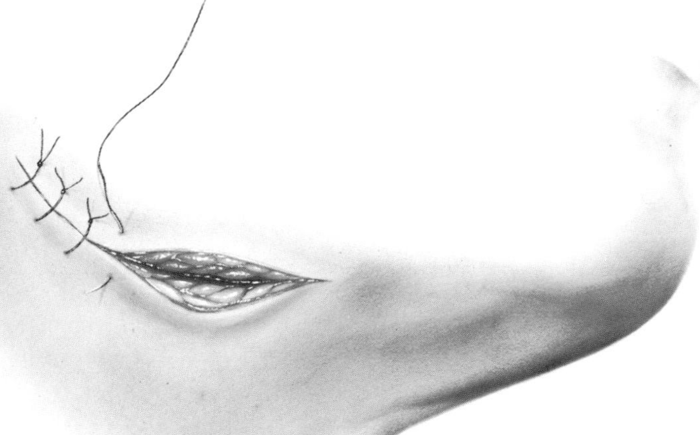

29

Fig. 185. Careful approximation of the subcutaneous tissues and meticulous suturing of the skin to produce a slight eversion at the wound margin will result in uncomplicated healing and an inconspicuous, fine scar. Stitch scars can be avoided by carefully tying the sutures with just enough tension to close the wound. Tight sutures cause necrosis and scarring of the skin. Most of the sutures can be removed on the second or third day and the remainder on the fifth day.

Submandibular Approach

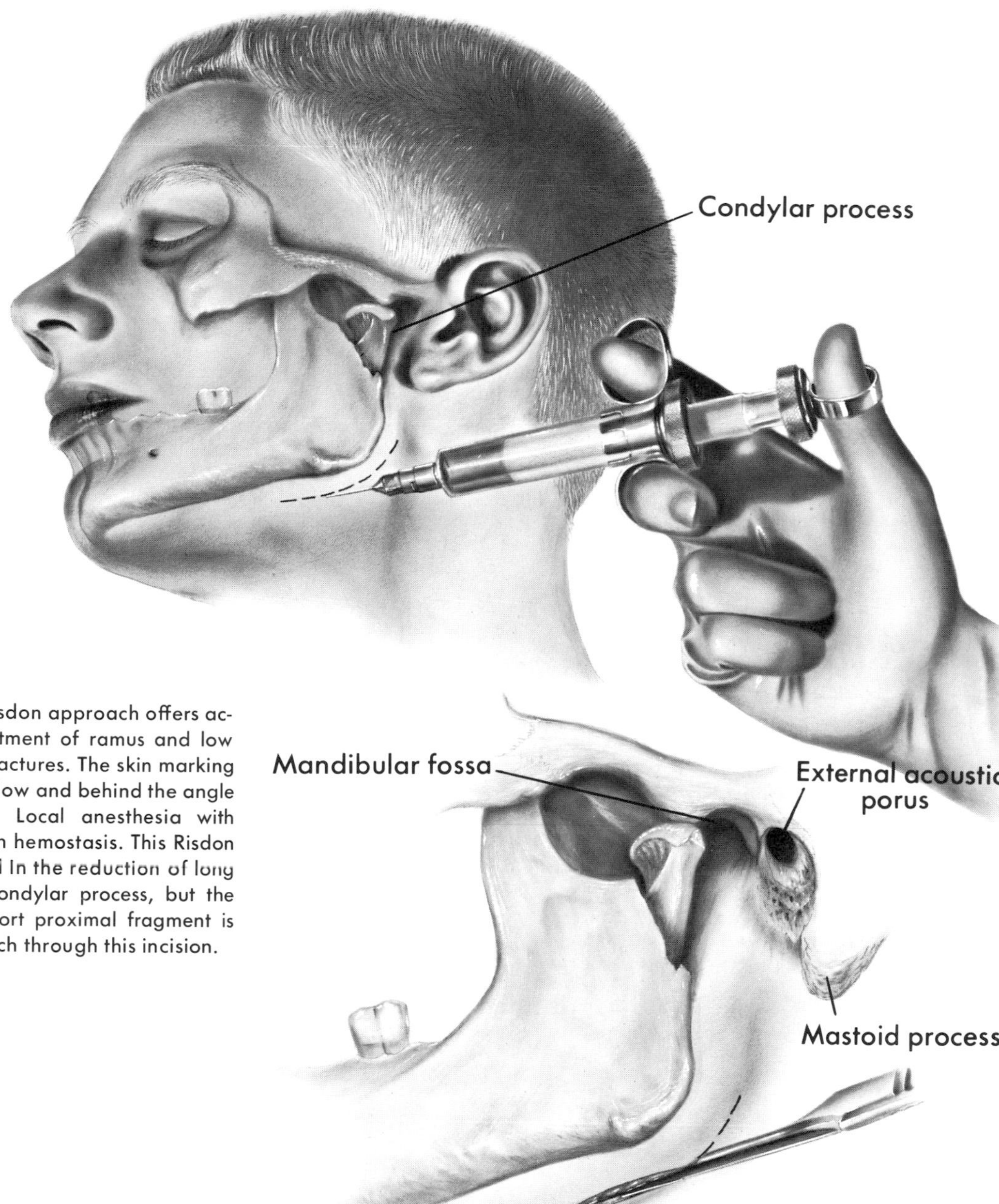

30

Fig. 186. The Risdon approach offers accessibility for treatment of ramus and low condylar region fractures. The skin marking is placed 1 cm. below and behind the angle of the mandible. Local anesthesia with epinephrine aids in hemostasis. This Risdon approach is useful in the reduction of long fractures of the condylar process, but the fracture with a short proximal fragment is difficult to approach through this incision.

31

Fig. 187. The dissection is carried through the skin, subcutaneous fascia, and platysma to the underlying fascia. At this level the cervical branch of the seventh nerve may be present in the wound. Cutting of this branch of the seventh nerve may be done without significant loss of function. It is advisable, if possible, to retract the nerve out of the field. The posterior facial vein may be troublesome and should be identified and ligated.

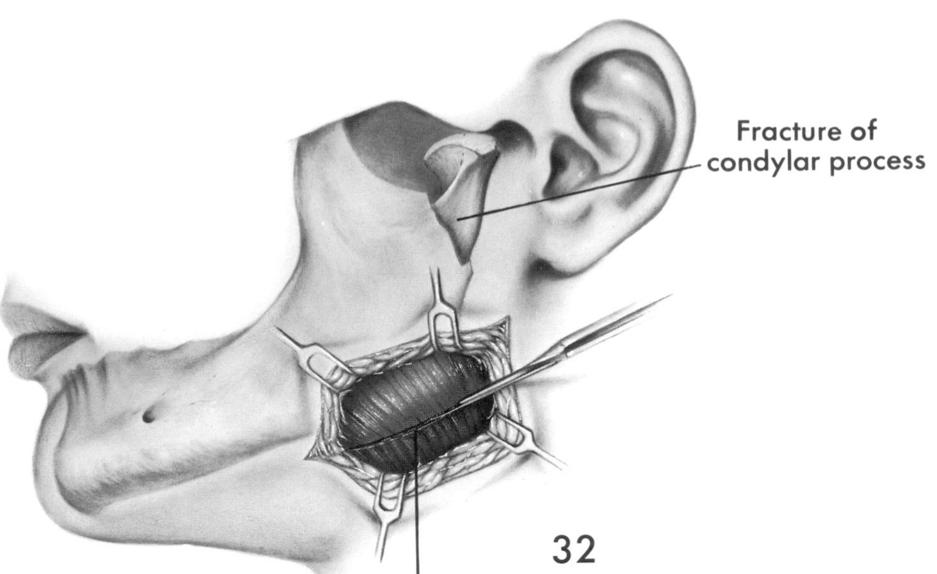

32

Fig. 188. In the retraction, the position of the tissues may be distorted so that an incision through the platysma may lie directly over the descending loop of the ramus mandibularis of the seventh nerve. A stimulator is helpful in locating the nerve so that it will not be injured. If identified, the nerve should be tagged with a fine, loose suture and pulled to the edge of the field with a smooth retractor.

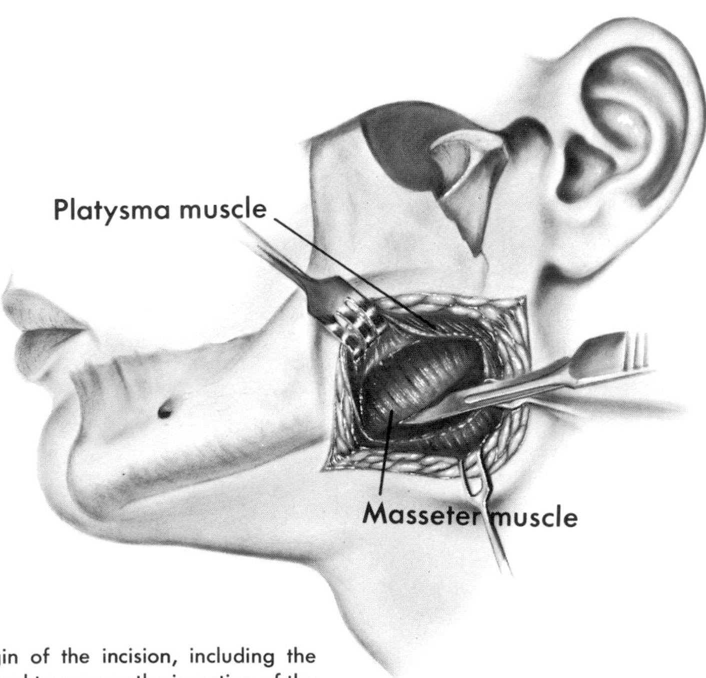

33

Fig. 189. The tissues along the upper margin of the incision, including the branches of the seventh nerve, are drawn upward to expose the insertion of the masseter muscle. The incision is made through the periosteum along the inferior border to the angle and upward along the posterior border for 2 cm. above the angle.

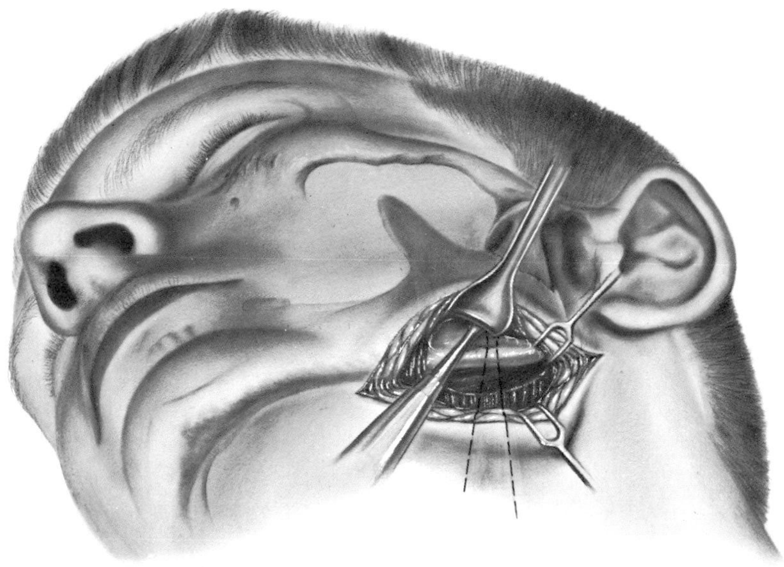

34

Fig. 190. The muscle insertion and the periosteum over the lateral aspect of the ramus are raised from the bone with a sharp periosteal elevator. The dissection is carried upward to the site of the fracture. A few densely adherent masseter fibers may be incised at the angle to facilitate elevation of the soft tissues from the bone. Visualization in this region is difficult unless the patient's neck is extended and his head rotated. An adjustable head rest is helpful in maintaining the head in a satisfactory position.

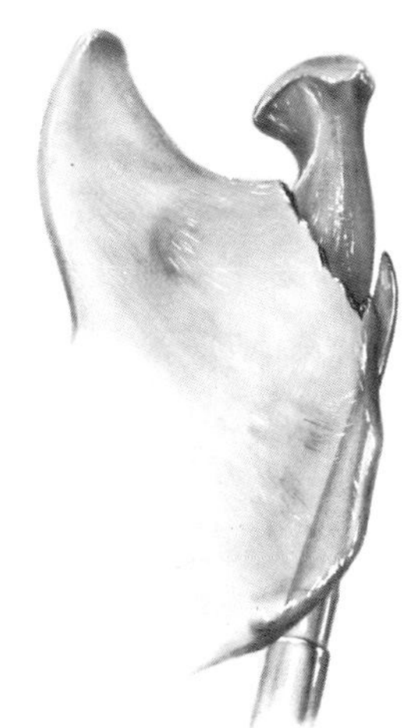

35

Fig. 191. A periosteal elevator is carefully slipped around the posterior border of the mandible below the periosteum to immobilize the fracture segments and permit reduction. The (internal) maxillary artery and a venous plexus near the condyle may give troublesome hemorrhage unless the dissection is performed with care.

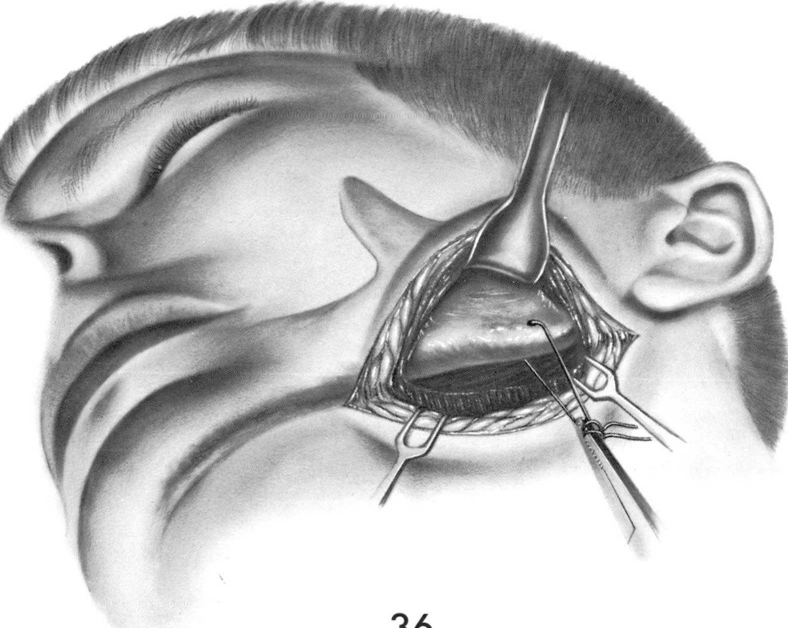

36

Fig. 192. A hole is drilled through the angle of the mandible to receive a stainless steel wire. The ends of the wire are left long and grasped with a wire-twisting forceps to pull the mandible downward and to aid in the reduction of the condylar fracture. A long, right-angled retractor is necessary to disclose the fracture site.

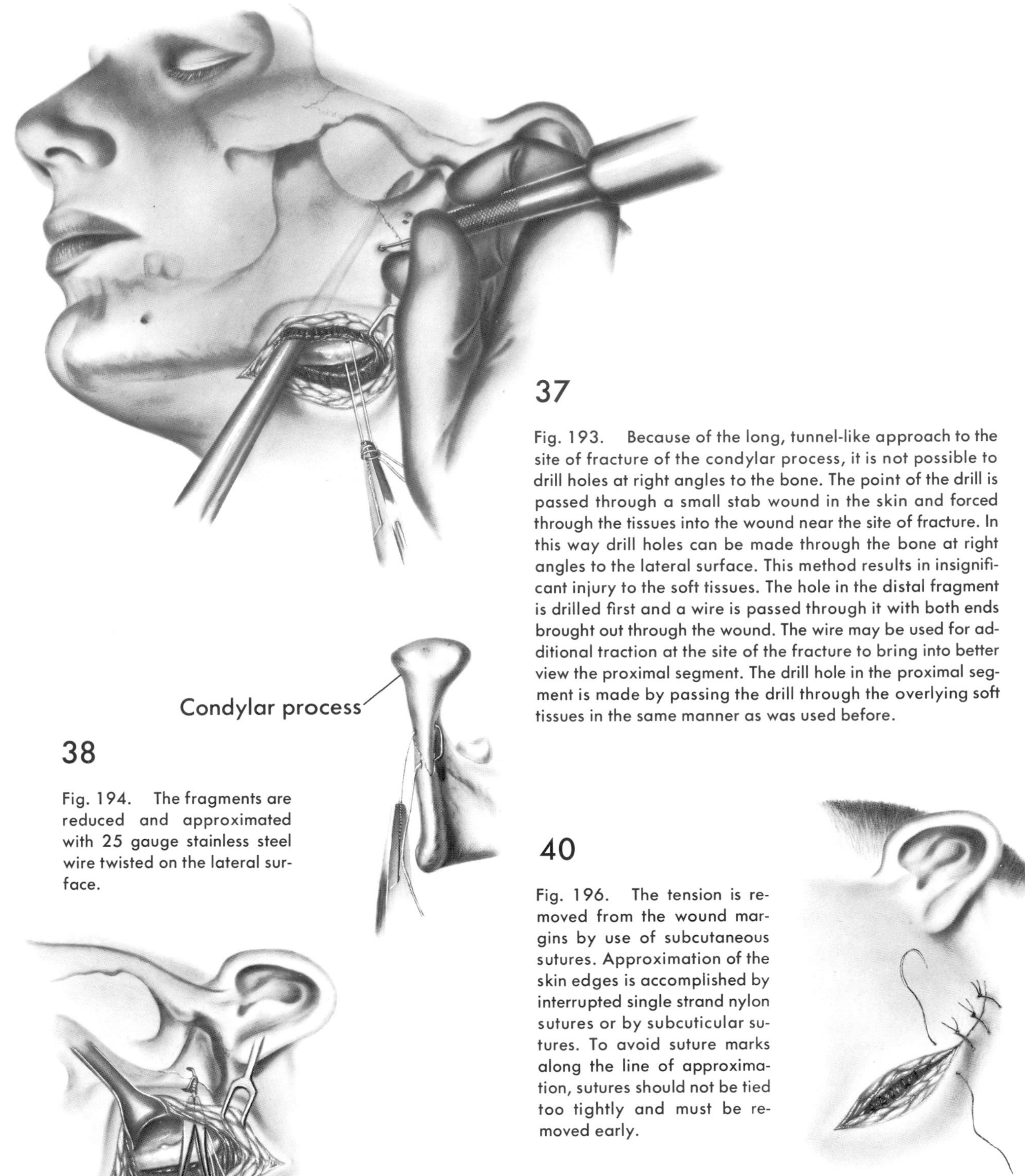

37

Fig. 193. Because of the long, tunnel-like approach to the site of fracture of the condylar process, it is not possible to drill holes at right angles to the bone. The point of the drill is passed through a small stab wound in the skin and forced through the tissues into the wound near the site of fracture. In this way drill holes can be made through the bone at right angles to the lateral surface. This method results in insignificant injury to the soft tissues. The hole in the distal fragment is drilled first and a wire is passed through it with both ends brought out through the wound. The wire may be used for additional traction at the site of the fracture to bring into better view the proximal segment. The drill hole in the proximal segment is made by passing the drill through the overlying soft tissues in the same manner as was used before.

38

Fig. 194. The fragments are reduced and approximated with 25 gauge stainless steel wire twisted on the lateral surface.

40

Fig. 196. The tension is removed from the wound margins by use of subcutaneous sutures. Approximation of the skin edges is accomplished by interrupted single strand nylon sutures or by subcuticular sutures. To avoid suture marks along the line of approximation, sutures should not be tied too tightly and must be removed early.

39

Fig. 195. The wire is twisted securely by means of a wire-twisting forceps. The twisted wire is cut sufficiently short to permit it to be bent and inserted into one of the drill holes or flattened against the bone. The fascia of the masseter muscle is sutured to the fascia of the medial pterygoid muscle at the inferior border of the mandible. This assures anatomic repositioning of the musculature. The wound is closed in layers with catgut sutures for the deep structures and single strand nylon sutures for approximation of the skin. Drainage is unnecessary if hemostasis is complete.

41 Fig. 197. The hair in the temporal area is shaved to provide adequate access through the preauricular incision. Infiltration of procaine, 1 per cent, with 1:100,000 epinephrine into the preauricular region and the region of the temporomandibular joint will provide adequate anesthesia and give hemostasis. The auriculotemporal branches of the fifth cranial nerve, and the branches of the great auricular nerve from the cervical plexus are sensory to this area. The use of epinephrine provides a relatively dry field unless one of the major arteries or veins is severed.

REGION OF THE CONDYLAR PROCESS

Preauricular Approach

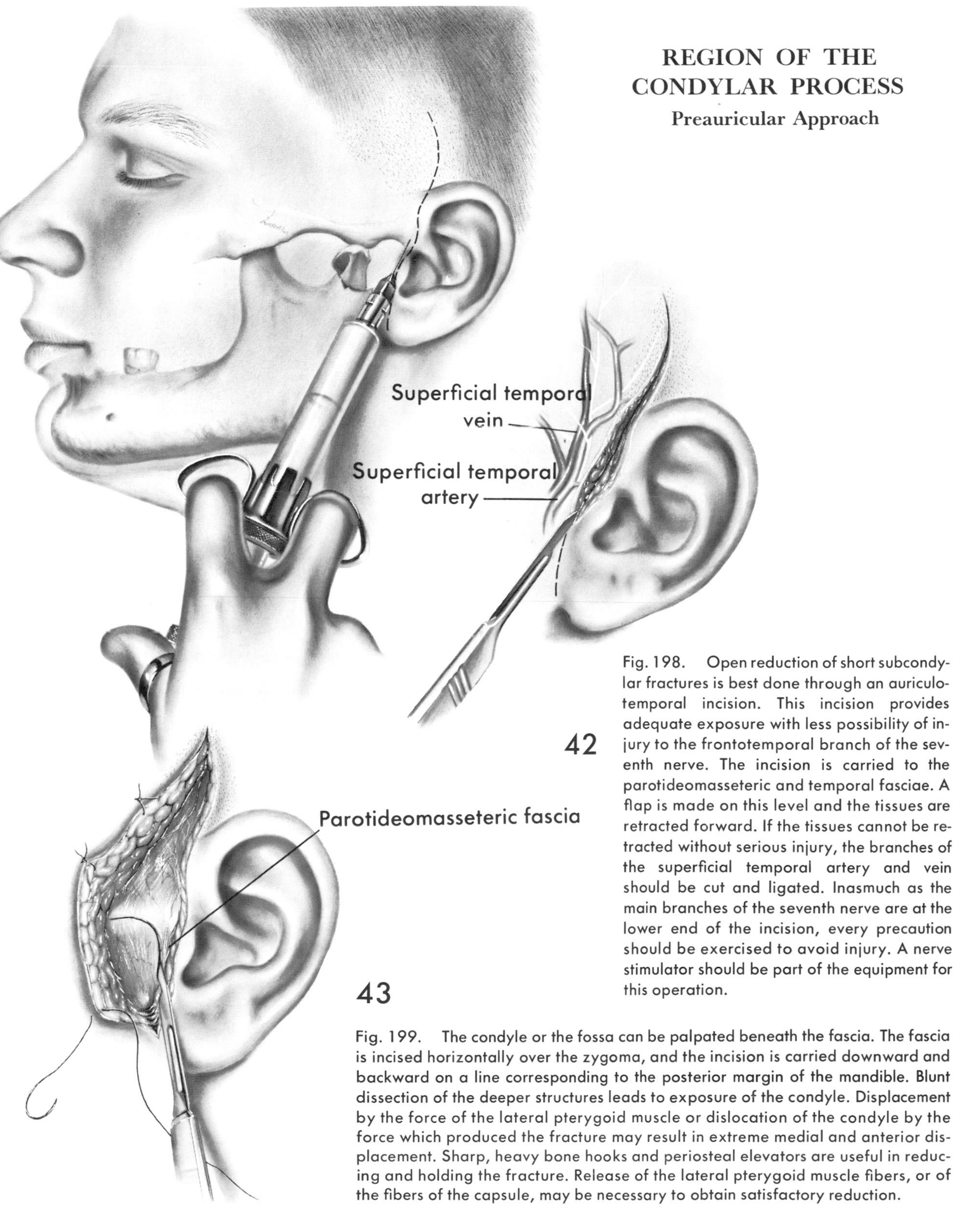

42 Fig. 198. Open reduction of short subcondylar fractures is best done through an auriculotemporal incision. This incision provides adequate exposure with less possibility of injury to the frontotemporal branch of the seventh nerve. The incision is carried to the parotideomasseteric and temporal fasciae. A flap is made on this level and the tissues are retracted forward. If the tissues cannot be retracted without serious injury, the branches of the superficial temporal artery and vein should be cut and ligated. Inasmuch as the main branches of the seventh nerve are at the lower end of the incision, every precaution should be exercised to avoid injury. A nerve stimulator should be part of the equipment for this operation.

43 Fig. 199. The condyle or the fossa can be palpated beneath the fascia. The fascia is incised horizontally over the zygoma, and the incision is carried downward and backward on a line corresponding to the posterior margin of the mandible. Blunt dissection of the deeper structures leads to exposure of the condyle. Displacement by the force of the lateral pterygoid muscle or dislocation of the condyle by the force which produced the fracture may result in extreme medial and anterior displacement. Sharp, heavy bone hooks and periosteal elevators are useful in reducing and holding the fracture. Release of the lateral pterygoid muscle fibers, or of the fibers of the capsule, may be necessary to obtain satisfactory reduction.

44

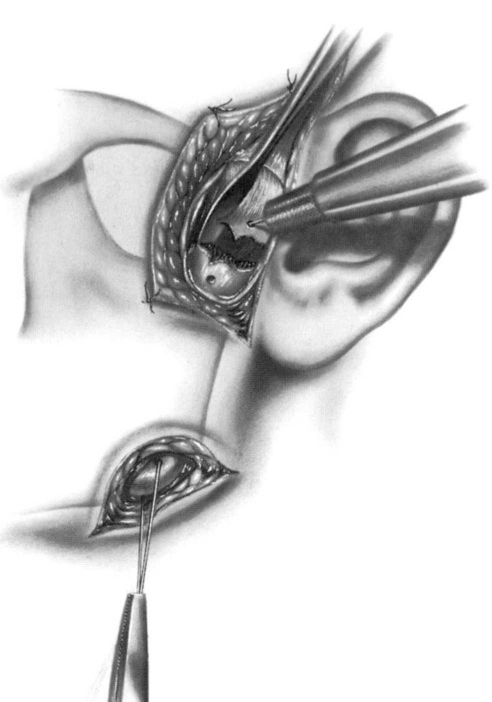

Fig. 200. A completely detached condyle may be used as a free bone graft, and will survive if reduced adequately and covered with soft tissue to ensure good blood supply. The neck of the condylar process is composed of very thin bone. The drill holes should be made far enough from the fracture to prevent the tightened wire from cutting through. A venous plexus and the (internal) maxillary artery are present on the medial side of the condyle, and troublesome bleeding may occur if these vessels are not protected with a periosteal elevator when the drill holes are made. The relation of the (internal) maxillary artery medial to the condyle should be kept in mind; damage to this vessel can result in serious hemorrhage.

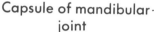

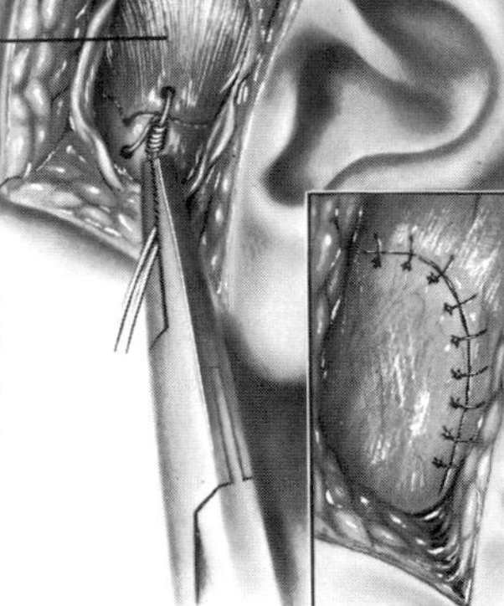

45

Fig. 201. One should use 25 gauge stainless steel wire to approximate the fractured segments. The wire is twisted tightly, cut short, and pressed firmly against the bone so that the sharp end does not cause irritation to the overlying soft tissues. The parotideomasseteric fascia is closed accurately with interrupted sutures.

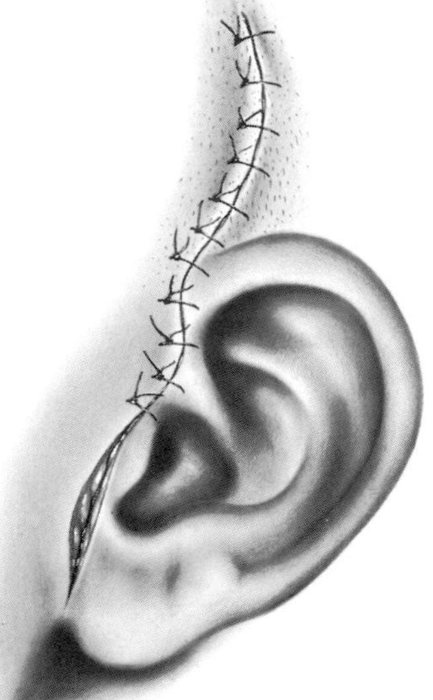

46

Fig. 202. After approximating accurately the underlying fascia and subcutaneous tissues to relieve all tension from the wound, the skin is approximated with nonabsorbable sutures. Single strand nylon on atraumatic needles is preferable because it causes minimal reaction. Sutures in the non-hair bearing area are removed in two or three days and the wounds are supported with collodion gauze strips. In the hair bearing area, the sutures should be removed in five to seven days.

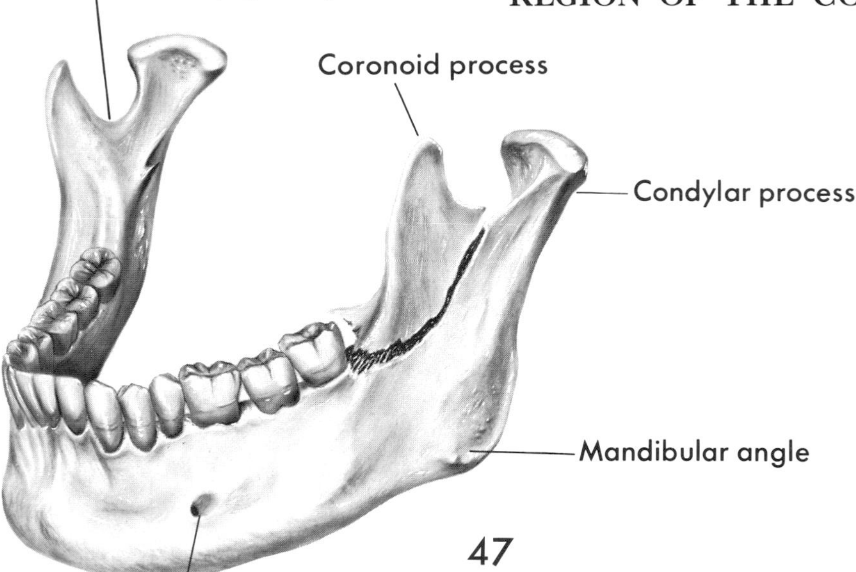

47

Fig. 203. Isolated fractures of the coronoid region are rare. Single fractures in this region sometimes are seen, usually caused by piercing or puncture. These fractures usually show minimal displacement because they are well splinted by the dense muscle and fascia.

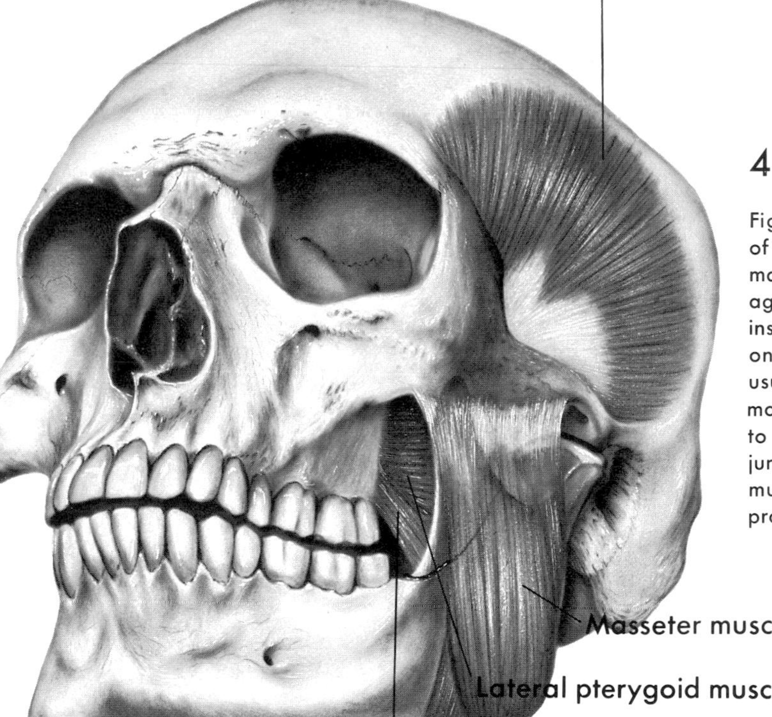

48

Fig. 204. Fractures of the coronoid process of the mandible are treated generally by intermaxillary fixation concomitantly with the management of associated fractures. In rare instances the coronoid fracture may be the only fracture of the mandible. The patient usually is more comfortable and will recover more quickly if the teeth are fixed in occlusion to provide immobilization and rest for the injured tissues. Intermaxillary fixation prevents muscle pull which might interfere with the processes of repair.

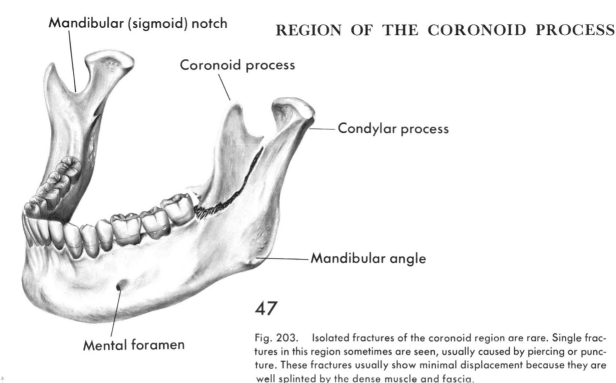

CHAPTER

7

THE ZYGOMA

PART 1

GENERAL CONSIDERATIONS

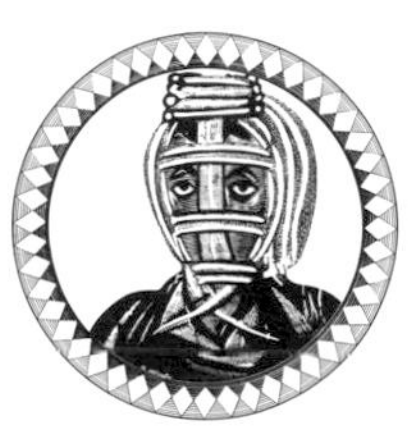

The position and contour of the zygomatic bone render it highly susceptible to injury. The zygoma, sometimes known as the malar bone, is quadrilateral with an outer, roughly convex surface, an inner concave surface, and four processes which articulate with the frontal, maxillary, and temporal bones and with the great wing of the sphenoid. Through its articulations it provides a strong buttress between the maxilla and the cranium. Its outer convex surface forms the prominence of the cheek. Its inner concave surface participates in the formation of the temporal fossa. The bone has a broad, strong articulation with the maxilla, weak attachments to the sphenoid and to the thin zygomatic process of the temporal bone, and a strong attachment to the zygomatic process of the frontal bone. It participates in the formation of the greater portion of the lateral floor of the orbit and, in some individuals, forms the lateral superior wall of the maxillary sinus (Fig. 205). Its surfaces provide attachments for the masseter, temporalis, and greater and lesser zygomaticus. The bone has small foramina through which pass the

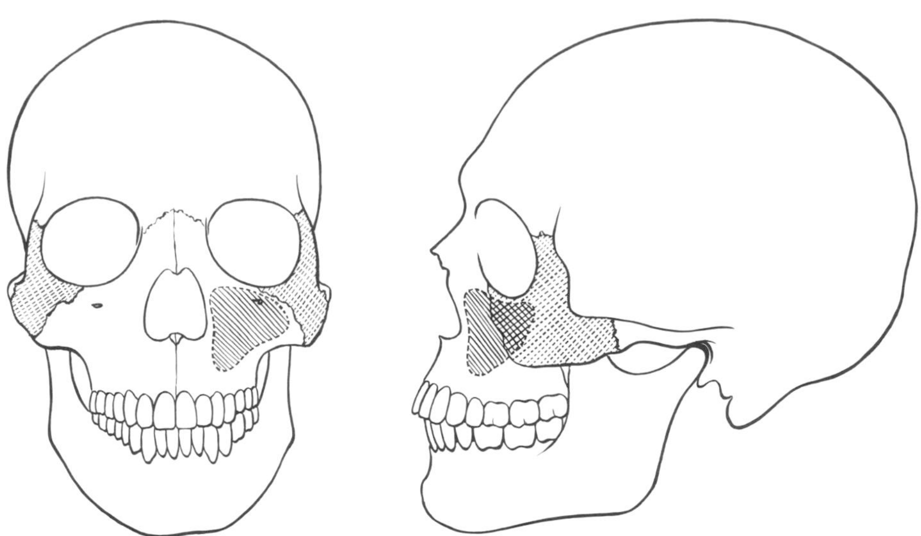

Figure 205. The zygoma and its articulations with the maxilla, the frontal bone, and the temporal bone. Shaded areas illustrate the position of the maxillary sinus in the maxilla.

zygomaticotemporal and zygomaticofrontal nerves, which provide sensory innervation to the soft tissues and skin of the cheek overlying the zygomatic prominence and the most anterior area of the temporal region.

THE ZYGOMATIC FRACTURE—A CLINICAL ENTITY

In considering the "zygomatic fracture," the clinician finds himself confronted with more than just the fracture of a single anatomic structure. Fractures of the zygomatic bone per se do occur, but in nearly all instances the fracture involves disruption of the adjacent articulating bones. Rarely does separation occur exactly within the lines of suture, but most often it extends to involve the zygomatic portion, or the lateral wall and thin orbital plates of the maxilla, or the zygomatic portion of the temporal bone and the thin plates of the sphenoid bone that help to make up the lateral wall of the orbit. Gerrie and Lindsay (1953) recognized how complicated these injuries may be in fractures of the zygomatic region and discussed fractures of the zygomaticomaxillary compound.

Knight and North (1961) recognized fractures of this region as a clinical entity and referred to them as "malar fractures." These observers noted that in fractures of the zygomatic region, the separation medially was usually by fracture of the maxilla through the floor of the orbit and the anterior and lateral walls of the maxillary antrum, laterally by fracture of the zygomatic process of the temporal bone, and above and behind by separation at the zygomaticofrontal and zygomaticosphenoid sutures. Fractures of the zygomatic arch involve both the temporal process of the zygoma and the zygomatic process of the temporal bone. From their study of 120 cases of zygomatic fractures, Knight and North developed a classification into six groups, as follows (Fig. 206):

Group I. No significant displacement. In this group, which made up 6 per cent of the cases, roentgenographic findings indicated fracture, but no clinical evidence of displacement was found. Treatment in this group was unnecessary.

Group II. Zygomatic arch fractures comprised 10 per cent of the cases studied. In this group, in which fracture was caused by a direct blow over the zygomatic arch, the arch was buckled inward without involving the walls of the antrum or the orbit. This buckling resulted in a typical angular deformity with three fracture lines (middle and each end of the arch) and two fragments. Most of the patients had trismus but no diplopia.

Group III. Unrotated body fractures comprised 33 per cent of the group. This was the largest segment of the series, and the injuries were caused by a direct blow over the prominence of the body of the zygoma with fracture and displacement of the bone directly into the antrum. The bone usually was driven directly backward, inward, and slightly downward, resulting in flattening of the cheek with a palpable step-deformity at the infraorbital margin. On radiographic examination, the displacement appeared to be downward at the infraorbital margin and inward at the zygomatic prominence with slight displacement at the zygomaticofrontal suture.

Group IV. Medially rotated body fractures comprised 11 per cent of the group studied. The fracture and displacement appeared to be caused by a blow on the prominence of the zygoma above its horizontal axis; thus the fractured bone was displaced backward, inward, and downward. The bones seemed to be rotated counterclockwise on the left when viewed from the front, and clockwise or toward the midline on the right. Roentgenographic examination in the Waters' position showed downward displacement at the infraorbital margin and displacement either outward at the zygomatic prominence (Type A) or inward at the zygomaticofrontal suture (Type B). These variations provided two subdivisions of the Group IV, types A and B.

Group V. Laterally rotated body fractures. This group comprised 22 per cent of the 120 cases studied. Fractures in this group appeared to be caused by blows below the horizontal axis of the bone, the bone being driven inward and backward. The bones seemed to be rotated clockwise on the left when viewed from the front and counterclockwise or away from the midline on the right. Radiographic examination showed displacement inward at the zygomatic prominence, and either upward at the infraorbital margin (Type A) or outward at the zygomaticofrontal suture (Type B). There were thus two subdivisions in this group, Type A and Type B.

Group VI. Complex fractures accounted for 18 per cent of the total. Included here were all cases in which there were additional fracture lines across the main fragment; minor degrees of comminution at the main fracture sites were disregarded.

SURGICAL PATHOLOGY OF THE ZYGOMA

Because of its prominent location, this sturdy bone is subjected to injury frequently. It will absorb moderately severe blows through its buttressing attachments. But separation of the zygoma from its articulating bones may be caused by severe blows such as may be received in a fall or from a fist. With moderately severe blows, the bone may separate at the zygomaticofrontal su-

(Text continued on page 216.)

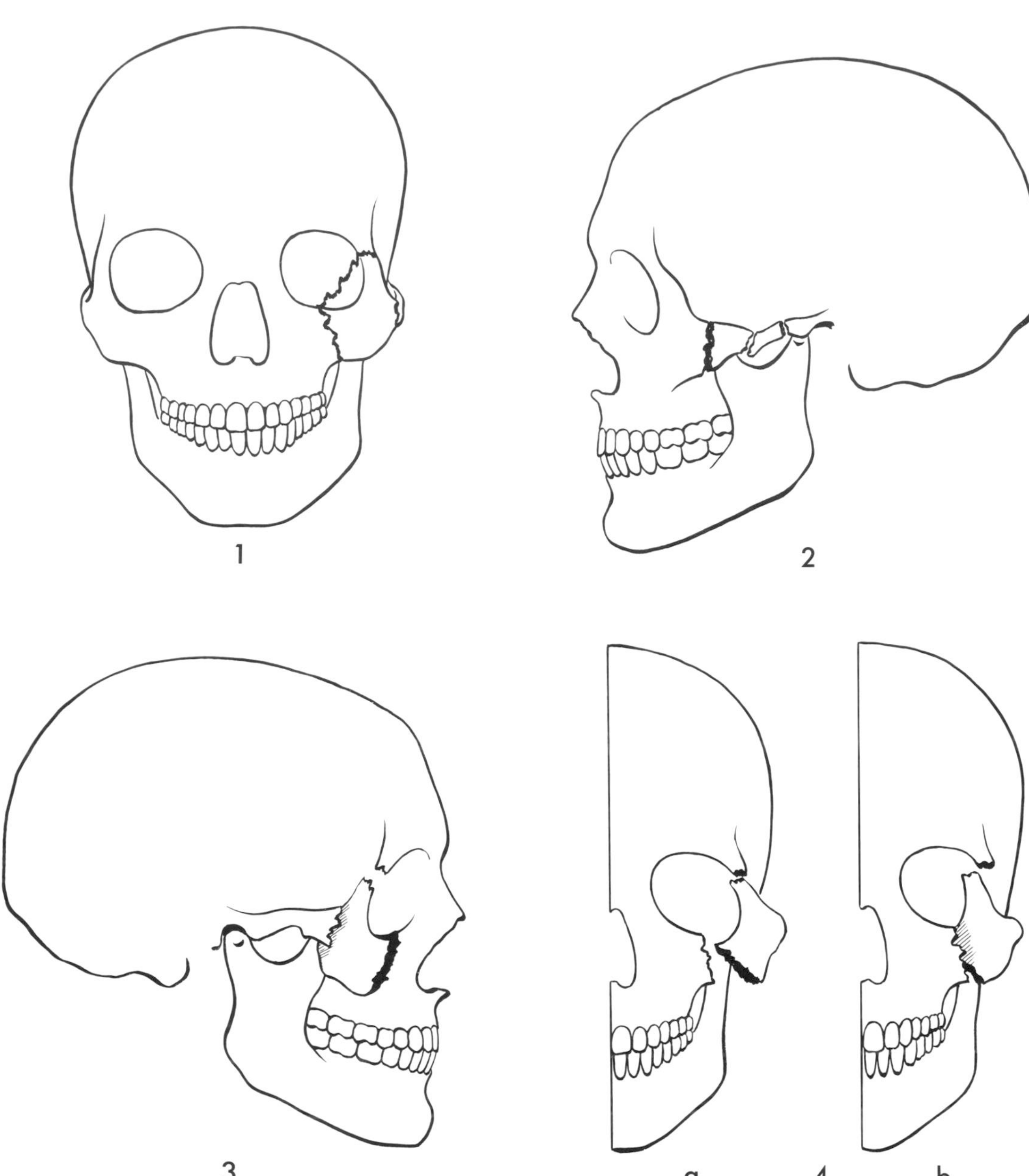

Figure 206. Fractures of the zygoma.
1. Group I. No significant displacement
2. Group II. Zygomatic arch fractures
3. Group III. Unrotated body fractures
4. Group IV. Medially rotated body fractures
    a. Outward at zygomatic prominence
    b. Inward at zygomaticofrontal suture

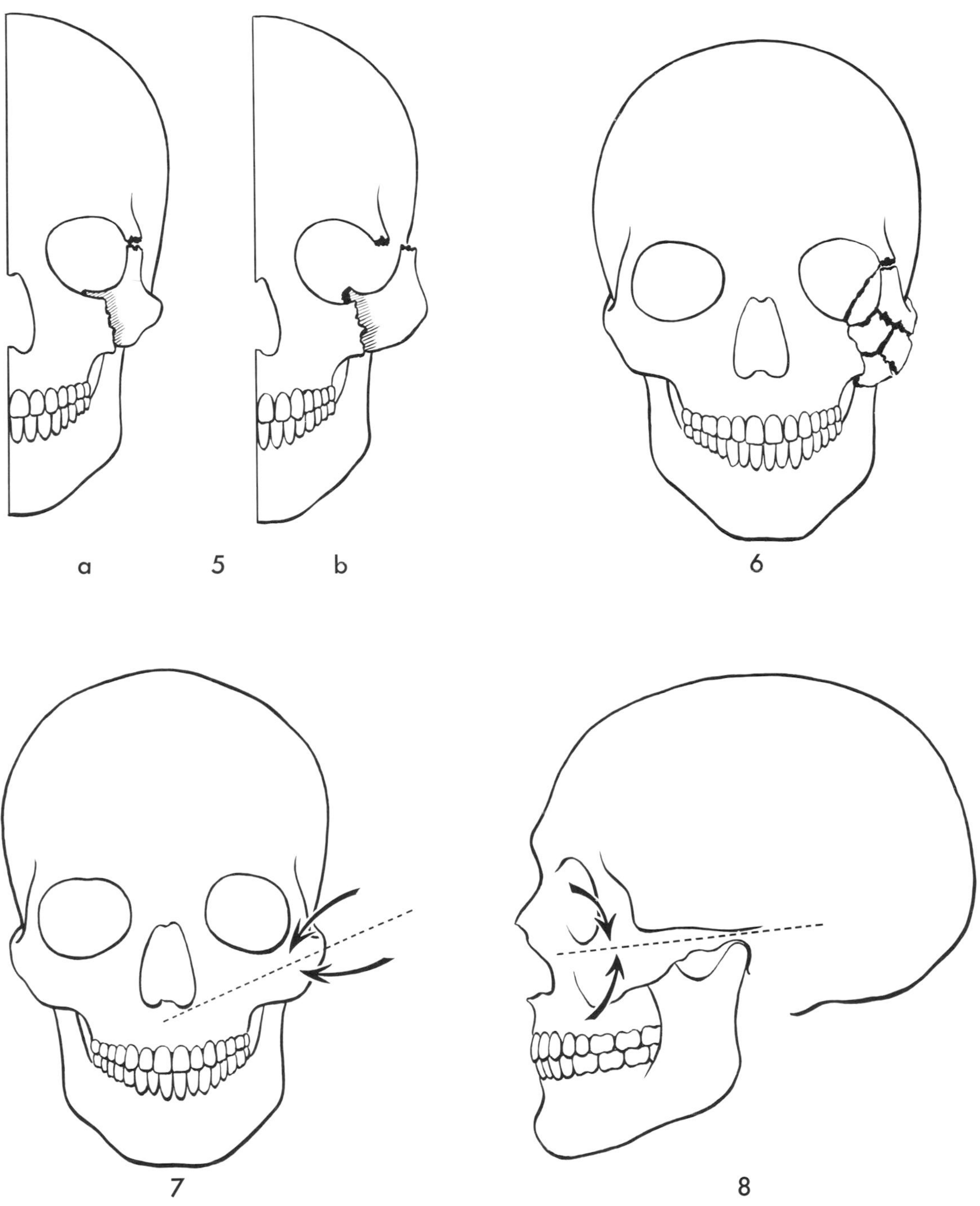

5. Group V. Laterally rotated body fractures
   a. Upward at infraorbital margin
   b. Outward at zygomaticofrontal suture
6. Complex fractures
7 and 8. Directions of force

ture and at its articulation with the sphenoid bone. At the same time the injury may be complicated by fractures of the anterior and lateral surface of the maxilla and the thin orbital portions of the zygoma. Fractures in the region of the zygomatic arch usually include a portion of the zygomatic process of the temporal bone. Violent shattering forces at the region of the zygoma may result in extensive comminution with separation at the sutures or extension into other bones. The broad buttressing surface which articulates with the maxilla tends to transmit forces that cause fracture of the thinner bone of the maxilla near the suture.

The zygoma is one of the principal buttresses between the maxilla and the cranium. Fractures of the zygoma combined with multiple fractures of the middle third of the face contribute to the instability of the maxilla. Fractures usually involve the infraorbital rim, portions of the zygoma being forced into the maxillary sinus. Tearing of the lining of the sinus causes hematoma or the extravasation of blood into the sinus and into the tissues underlying the cheek and lateral canthus of the eye. Unilateral epistaxis, hematoma, and ecchymosis are usual findings. The zygomatic compound may be depressed in the direction of the force, which is, in most cases, in a posterior, downward, and medial direction. Severe fracture with medial displacement of the zygomatic arch results in impingement of the bone fragments against the temporal muscle and the coronoid process of the mandible (Fig. 207). Severe trismus is nearly always associated with fractures of the arch, for the displaced segments interfere with the forward and downward movement of the coronoid process of the mandible when the patient attempts to open his mouth. If unreduced fragments penetrate the soft tissues and remain in contact with the coronoid process, their organization may result in fibro-osseous ankylosis with complete fixation of the mandible. This complication may necessitate excision of the coronoid process. In fracture-displacement of the zygomatic compound, a steplike deformity may be palpable through the skin in the region of the zygomaticofrontal suture or along the inferior orbital margin.

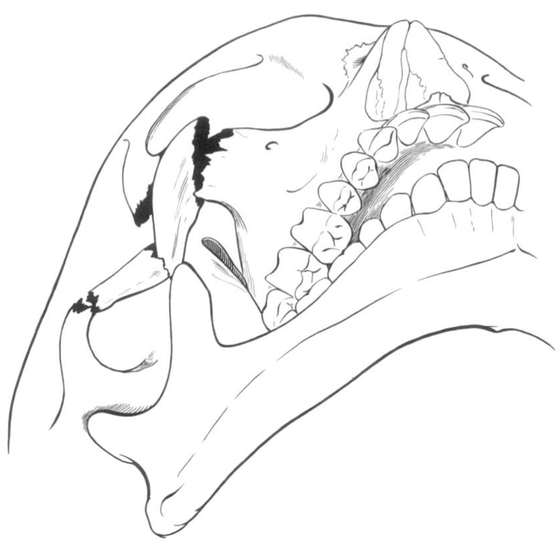

Figure 207. Fracture of the zygomatic arch causing impingement of the coronoid process of the mandible.

A visible deformity may be noted in fracture-displacement of the lateral orbital rim. The lateral palpebral ligament is attached to the zygomatic portion of the orbital rim, and displacement of the bone carries the lateral palpebral attachment with it, producing a dramatic, visible deformity (Fig. 208).

Disruption of the floor and lateral wall of the orbit results in dysfunction of the globe of the eye. The orbital septum of the lower lid, which attaches to the inferior orbital margin, is displaced in fracture-displacement of the infraorbital ridge, with a resulting retraction and shortening of the lid. The loss of bony support in the orbital

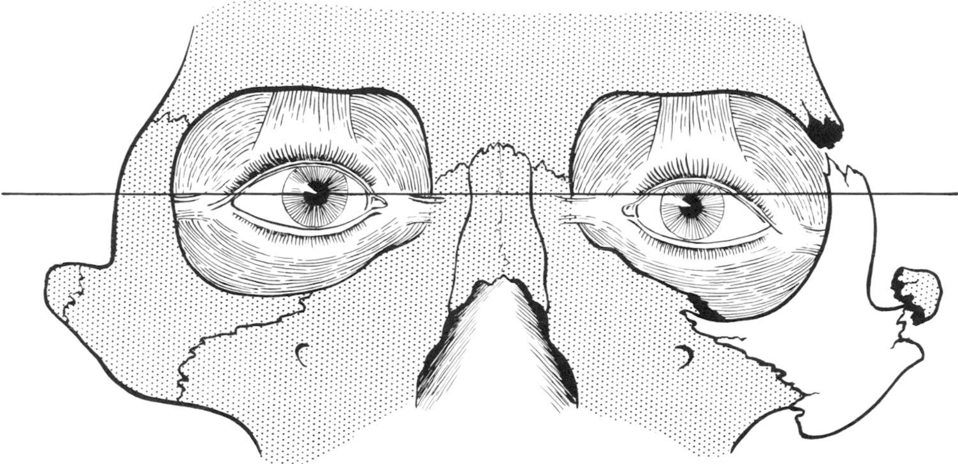

Figure 208. The lateral palpebral ligament is attached to the frontal process of the zygoma. In fracture-dislocation of the lateral orbital rim, the palpebral ligament is displaced with the bone fragment. *A*. The normal anatomic relations of the palpebral ligaments. *B*. Downward displacement of the eye and the palpebral ligament, with displaced bone fragments.

floor causes displacement of the globe and orbital contents, the result of downward displacement of Tenon's capsule and the lateral palpebral ligament.

Fractures may be complicated by fragmentation and the blow-out phenomenon of the floor of the orbit. Tearing of the periorbita and sinus lining, with fragmentation and displacement of the bone segments, produces an opening into the maxillary sinus. The orbital contents may herniate partially into the maxillary sinus where fat, periosteum, and muscle become incarcerated between the fractured bone segments. Failure to recognize and treat this herniation will cause permanent diplopia due to incarceration of the inferior oblique and, possibly, inferior rectus muscle. The trapped muscles cannot rotate the eye downward and outward and act as a check, for instance, against the function of the superior rectus in upward rotation.

Loss of sensation in the region supplied by the infraorbital nerve is a common finding in fractures of the zygomaticomaxillary compound. The infraorbital nerve emerges below the infraorbital rim from a canal which passes through the roof of the maxilla but which is in close proximity to the zygoma. Fractures in this region usually damage the nerve by tearing it or by the impingement of bone fragments against it in its course through the canal. Laceration of the nerve within the canal from impacted fragments of bone may result in permanent anesthesia. In most cases, infraorbital nerve anesthesia disappears within 12 or 18 months. Anesthesia persisting longer than 18 to 24 months is an indication for exploration of the nerve canal.

DIAGNOSIS OF FRACTURES OF THE ZYGOMATIC COMPOUND

A detailed history may be helpful in arriving at a diagnosis. From knowledge of the kind of injury and the direction of the force of application, the degree and extent of deformity may be predicted. A blow from a fist, a fall against a hard object, or a shattering wound to the side of the face in most cases will produce a fracture of the zygoma. If the patient is seen immediately after the injury, before the clinical picture has become obscured by edema and hematoma, the classic signs of fracture in this region may be seen. Flatness of the face may be noted with depression of the globe, displacement of the lateral palpebral ligament, retraction of the lower lid with flattening of the malar prominence, and ecchymosis of the lids, conjunctiva, and sclera with unilateral epistaxis. Pain on motion of the mandible and trismus is suggestive of fractures involving the zygomatic arch. Anesthesia in the distribution of the infraorbital nerve (that is, the upper lip, the lower eyelid, and the lateral nasal area) indicates fracture of the adjacent maxilla with injury to the infraorbital nerve. Severe fracture-displacement produces immediate diplopia; however, in some patients this may not be evident until the edema of the orbit subsides.

Bimanual comparative palpation of the bone structures of the face may suggest fracture. Both sides of the face are palpated simultaneously, and as the fingers pass around the orbital rim, fractures of, or near, the zygomaticofrontal or zygomaticomaxillary sutures may be palpated. Zygomatic arch fractures usually can be determined by irregularity or indentation over the arch. Fractures of the lateral and anterior wall of the maxilla at the junction of the zygomatic process will be revealed intraorally as definite irregularities under the mucosa as the finger palpates the anterior and lateral maxillary wall. The normal intraoral zygomatic prominence may be missing, and a deep groove may be felt from medial displacement of the maxillary process of the zygoma.

Roentgenographic Findings in Fracture of the Zygomatic Region

The most useful roentgenographic view for evaluating fractures of the zygomaticomaxillary compound is the posterior-anterior oblique projection of the face, known as the Waters' position (see Fig. 52). This view shows the structure of the bone and outlines the irregular contour of the zygoma with minimal superimposition of other structures. The roentgenograms should be made by the stereoscopic method. If there is a possibility of fragments displaced from the orbital floor, planograms may be of value. The zygomatic arches can be demonstrated well by the submental-vertical projection of the zygomatic arches (Fig. 56).

The roentgenographic findings depend upon the location of the fracture sites and the degree of displacement. The usual findings are deformity at the infraorbital margin and separation at the zygomaticofrontal suture. Irregularities of the lateral wall of the maxilla show well in the Waters' position. Opacity or clouding of the maxillary sinus, from blood, is seen in almost all zygomaticomaxillary fractures.

TREATMENT OF FRACTURES OF THE ZYGOMATIC COMPOUND

The plan of treatment is to be determined by the clinical and roentgenographic findings. The kind of fracture, the degree of fragmentation, and the direction and degree of displacement of the bone fragments dictate the management of zygomatic fractures. The objective in management is, of course, to place the fragments in normal position and to provide active support during the course of healing.

Numerous effective methods have been described for the reduction of fractures in this region. In the less severe cases, fixation may be obtained from the normal muscular and fascial attachments of the bone, or by impacting the fragments against adjacent bones. Fixation with interosseous wiring under direct vision or the use of gauze packing in the maxillary sinus and in the infratemporal region, or of extraskeletal appliances, all have a place in the management of zygomatic fractures. Some fractures can be reduced and managed by conservative procedures, whereas others with greater comminution and displacement require aggressive open operative procedures to obtain a satisfactory result.

Knight and North (1961) found that certain kinds of fracture were unstable and that the fragments would not remain in position following reduction. They noted that 100 per cent of fractures in Group II were stable and needed no fixation after reduction. Forty-five per cent were unstable in Group III, 100 per cent unstable in Group IV, all were stable in Group V, and 70 per cent were unstable in Group VI. This indicates that all fractures with displacement and medial rotation (Group IV) require supplementary fixation following reduction and that 70 per cent of those in Group VI require supplementary fixation. Fixation may be obtained by packing the maxillary sinus, by pin fixation, and by direct interosseous wiring.

For years occasional disappointment was encountered by these authors in their treatment of zygomatic fractures when the usual closed methods of reduction were used. In many patients treated by the closed technique, reduction was accomplished easily but late complications occurred: diplopia, malunion, and facial deformity. Either the reduction had not been complete or a new dislocation of the fracture occurred in the postoperative period.

The present authors determined to test the effectiveness of the method of closed reduction. In a number of patients treated by the usual closed methods of elevation of the zygoma, in whom an immediate satisfactory clinical result seemed to have been achieved, the fracture sites were exposed later through brow or lower lid incisions so that the position of the fragments could be seen directly. Careful evaluation of a number of these patients demonstrated, interestingly enough, that the fracture-dislocation usually was more severe than it had appeared to be from clinical and roentgenographic evaluation. In a number of instances the true condition had been obscured by edema and hematoma. Exploration of the orbit indicated that intraorbital edema was masking comminuted displaced and blow-out fractures. Some depressed fractures of the orbital floor, with herniation of the orbital contents into the maxillary sinus, went unrecognized. These fractures were being overlooked and became evident only after the orbital edema had subsided and diplopia had ensued. After the surgeon had thought that he had reduced the fractured zygoma satisfactorily by one of the closed techniques, direct inspection by means of an incision showed that, in many cases, the fracture had been reduced but that displacement had recurred afterward. The displacement recurring after the closed reduction was caused by the pull of the masseter muscle. This re-displacement would have been much greater had it not been for the resistance offered by the inelastic temporal fascia, which acts as a suspensory bracing of the zygomatic arch.

On the basis of this clinical study, it is our opinion that most displaced fractures of the zygoma should be treated by open reduction and direct wire fixation. Our practical application of this principle has given us great satisfaction and excellent results. We are convinced that this method is by far the preferred method of satisfactorily reducing a fracture of the zygoma.

Methods of Reduction of Fractures in the Zygomatic Region

Keen (1909) advocated the use of a sharp, curved elevator passed up through the buccal mucosa behind the tuberosity of the maxilla and the application of a forward, upward, and outward force. This is an effective method in some cases but displacement may result from contraction of the masseter muscle. The method is not effective in reduction of fractures of the zygomatic arch.

Lothrop (1906) described reduction of zygomatic fractures through an antrostomy under the inferior turbinate. A large, curved trocar was passed into the maxillary sinus, and force was applied to the lateral and anterior sinus wall in an upward and outward direction to rotate the depressed fragments into position.

Gillies Method

The approach of Gillies, Kilner, and Stone (1927) is popular for reduction of fractures of the zygoma. The temporal approach is used, with a heavy elevator passing under the medial surface of the zygoma and the application of upward, forward, and lateral force. This method is especially useful for reduction of impacted fractures or those of several weeks' standing with partial organization. It is possible to exert strong leverage against the medial or temporal surface of the zygoma with this approach.

The Gillies operation is accomplished by shaving the hair from the temporal region and making a vertical incision about 2 cm. long in the direction of the skin lines and above and behind the hairline. The incision is carried through the skin, subcutaneous tissues, and the two layers of the temporal fascia to the temporal muscle. A heavy elevator is slipped between temporal fascia and the muscle, and readily passes into the temporal fossa on the under surface of the zygoma. Strong leverage is exerted against a rolled towel, which acts as a fulcrum, and the zygoma is guided into position by the opposite hand, which palpates the structures through the skin. The wound is sutured together in layers. The subsequent scar is in the hair-bearing scalp and is insignificant.

Open Reduction and Internal Wire Fixation of Fractures of the Zygomaticomaxillary Compound

When fractures of the zygomatic region are seen and diagnosed within the first two or three hours after injury, reduction and fixation should be done early. This early treatment depends, however, upon the patient's general condition, and operation should not be done until the patient is a satisfactory risk for surgery. After a few hours, edema and hematoma in the periorbital region complicate the operative procedure, and it may be advisable to defer the operation for two or three days until the tissues return to a more nearly normal condition. Zygomatic fractures never need be considered as acute surgical emergencies. Reduction and fixation may be carried out effectively as late as 10 to 14 days after injury with satisfactory results. After a delay of several days, organization at the site of in-

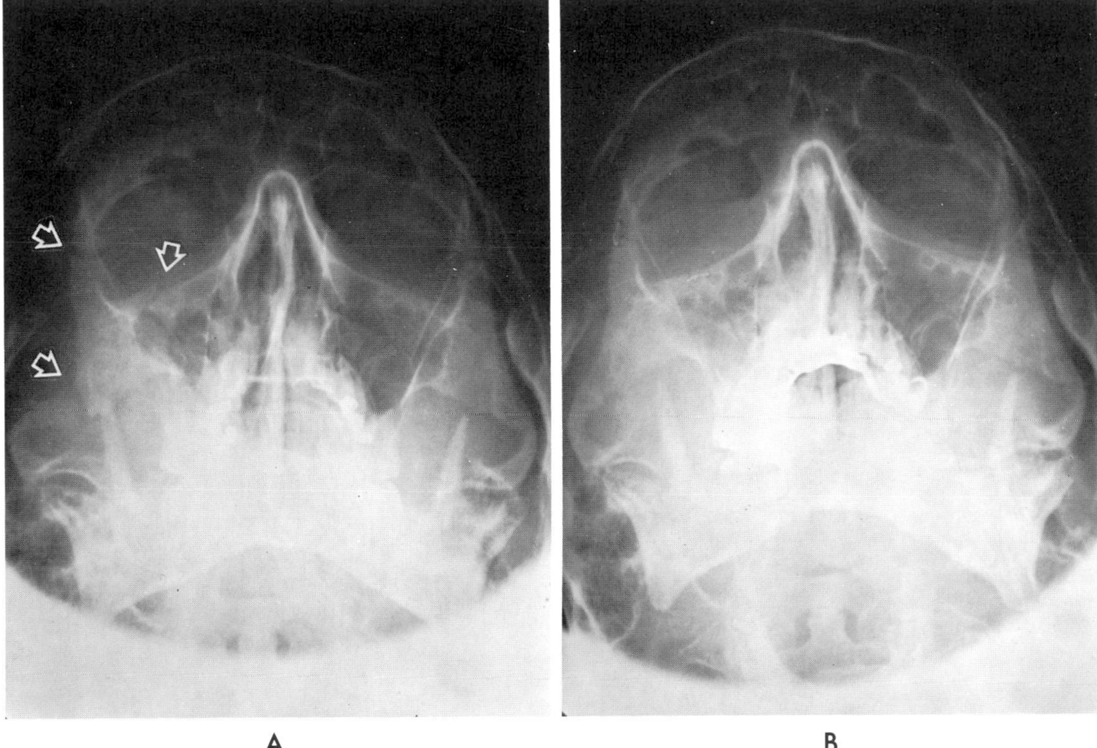

Figure 209. A. Depressed fracture of the right zygomaticomaxillary compound. Note depression of the body of the zygoma, depression of the right zygomatic arch, and medial displacement of the zygoma with encroachment upon the maxillary sinus. There is a step deformity of the infraorbital margin and fracture of the right maxillary sinus wall. *B.* Postoperative roentgenogram following elevation and fixation of zygomatic fracture.

jury may fix the bones somewhat, necessitating the application of greater force to mobilize the fragments.

In most cases open reduction can be accomplished by two incisions: one in the lateral end of the brow and the other at the inferior margin of the lower lid. If made in the direction of the skin lines, incisions here can be generous without danger of encountering structures of significance or resulting in objectionable scars. The brow incision provides excellent access to the zygomaticofrontal suture line, and the infraorbital incision permits exposure and inspection of the infraorbital margin and the floor of the orbit. By stretching the tissue laterally, the entire lateral orbital margin can be explored. It is undesirable and unnecessary to shave eyebrows or cut eyelashes in preparing for any operation upon the facial bones.

The incisions are outlined with marking ink in the lateral brow and in the skin folds of the lower lid. The incision in the lower lid should be placed in a location convenient for the approach to the fracture itself. The brow incision, even though not made directly over the zygomaticofrontal suture, permits exposure of the injured area by allowing a shifting of the tissue sufficient to gain access to the site of the fracture. Preoperative injection with a local anesthetic solution containing epinephrine helps reduce operative hemorrhage. A few minutes should elapse following the injection for maximum vasoconstriction to be established.

After marking the line of incision in the brow, the tissues are supported firmly over the ridge between the palpating fingers and a bold cut is made through all the layers of the skin and subcutaneous tissues down to the bone. A few small blood vessels may be severed; they should be clamped and ligated. The periosteum is elevated with two sharply pointed elevators and the fracture site in the zygomaticofrontal region exposed. Before attempting to elevate the zygoma, the lower lid incision should be made and the fracture site identified. The heavy zygoma elevator is then passed downward through the brow incision on the medial surface of the zygomatic bone and placed so that it securely engages the temporal surface of the zygoma. With the palpating hand placed over the prominence of the zygoma, and with one of the fingers in the inferior wound, the zygoma is manipulated upward, anteriorly, and laterally into position. This may require the application of considerable force, especially if the fracture is impacted or is of several days' standing. Depressed fractures of the zygomatic arch can be elevated through the brow incision by passing the elevator posteriorly underneath the zygomatic arch.

After the fracture has been reduced, drill holes are made through the bone on each side of the fracture with a small bur, and stainless steel wire of appropriate size is passed through the holes; 24 to 28 gauge wire usually suffices to support the fragments. In most cases, the fragments will remain in position without separation until the wire is twisted securely against the bone. In some cases, it is necessary to use heavy bone hooks to elevate and hold the fragments until they are properly wired.

In cases in which there is comminution of the arch of the zygoma, a slightly curved horizontal incision can be made over the arch. This allows the surgeon to reduce the bony fragments and fix them with wire (Fig. 210 *A–H*).

When one is treating a comminuted fracture, wiring should be done in an orderly direction from the more fixed fragments toward the looser ones. By using a periosteal elevator or a flat ribbon retractor, the floor of the orbit is exposed and explored. In a severely injured patient, several fragments may be noted in the orbital floor. Some of these may have been forced downward into the maxillary sinus, and the orbital fat and contents may be herniated partially into the maxillary sinus. The bone of the orbital floor is so thin that efforts to retrieve the fragments and secure them in proper relation are ineffective.

To reconstruct the orbital floor for support of the orbital contents a small, thin bone graft, or a thin wafer of preserved or fresh cartilage, placed in the floor may be effective. Converse (1962) advocated the use of a thin sheet of collagen to bridge the defect in the orbital floor and to support the orbital structures until organization has taken place. Collagen has been used effectively by the authors, who have found it satisfactory in reconstruction of the floor of the orbit. The use of thin layers of plastic materials has been suggested by some authors, even though the incidence of complications is higher with the use of nonbiologic materials. Freeman (1962) reviewed a large series of cases in which he reconstructed the floor of the orbit with thin sheets of plastic material at the time of fracture reduction.

McCoy et al. (1962) advocated the use of fresh bone or cartilage as the material of choice in reconstruction of the floor.

Packing of the Maxillary Sinus for Treatment of Fractures of the Zygomaticomaxillary Compound

For reducing and fixing fractured osseous parts of the zygomatic compound, an approach through the maxillary antrum may be useful. The Caldwell-Luc method gives access to the antrum through the canine fossa of the maxilla (Fig. 211). If there is a fracture of the anterior wall of the maxilla, the opening caused by the fracture may be enlarged by using bone drills or biting forceps. If no fracture exists, a surgical opening can be made. Through the Caldwell-Luc approach it is possible to reduce displaced fragments of the zygoma by upward and outward pressure. Fragments that may have herniated into the maxillary sinus are elevated into position and held by packing the sinus with selvage gauze permeated with petrolatum. An antrostomy is performed beneath the inferior turbinate bone, and the end of the packing is brought out into the nasal cavity. The oral wound is closed. Adequate drainage is obtained through the nasal opening. The packing is removed after it has accomplished its purpose, in a week to ten days. Sinus infection is not a common complication incident to this method. McCoy et al. (1962), however, reported a case in which packing of the maxillary sinus caused fragments of bone to be forced against the optic nerve to produce blindness. He condemned this method as dangerous, archaic, and ineffective.

In one of our patients, in whom the zygomatic arch would not stay in position after reduction, the bone was supported by a Penrose drain packed against the medial surface of the arch itself. The packing was removed in five days and the arch remained in excellent position (Fig. 212).

Kazanjian Suspension Method

Kazanjian (1933) advocated the use of extraskeletal fixation for support of the fractured zygomatic compound. A small hole is drilled through the infraorbital rim, and a stainless steel wire is inserted with both ends brought out through the wound, where they are twisted together into a loop or hook. Rubber band traction between the suspension wire and an outrigger on a head cap provides support for the zygomatic fragments (Fig. 213). Upward and outward traction is maintained for two to three weeks, after which time the bone usually remains in position without support. This method is reserved for patients in whom complete stabilization by open reduction and wire fixation cannot be accomplished. If, in spite of what appears to be adequate immobilization by open reduction and interosseous wire fixation, the fragments are still unstable, the suspension method is useful as supplemental fixation.

Management of Compound Comminuted Fractures of the Zygomatic Region

Fractures in the zygomatic region may be compounded intraorally or extraorally when the overlying soft tissues are crushed or lacerated by the traumatic force. Management of the wound requires the removal of foreign bodies, debris, blood clots, and loose fragments of bone that have no residual blood supply and serve no useful purpose. Viable fragments of bone may be replaced and the contour of the area may be reconstructed by interosseous wiring through the open wound (Fig. 214). The wound should be extended, if necessary, to gain good access to the region. Careful debridement and closure of the soft tissues over the comminuted fragments generally results in healing without infection.

(*Text continued on page 227.*)

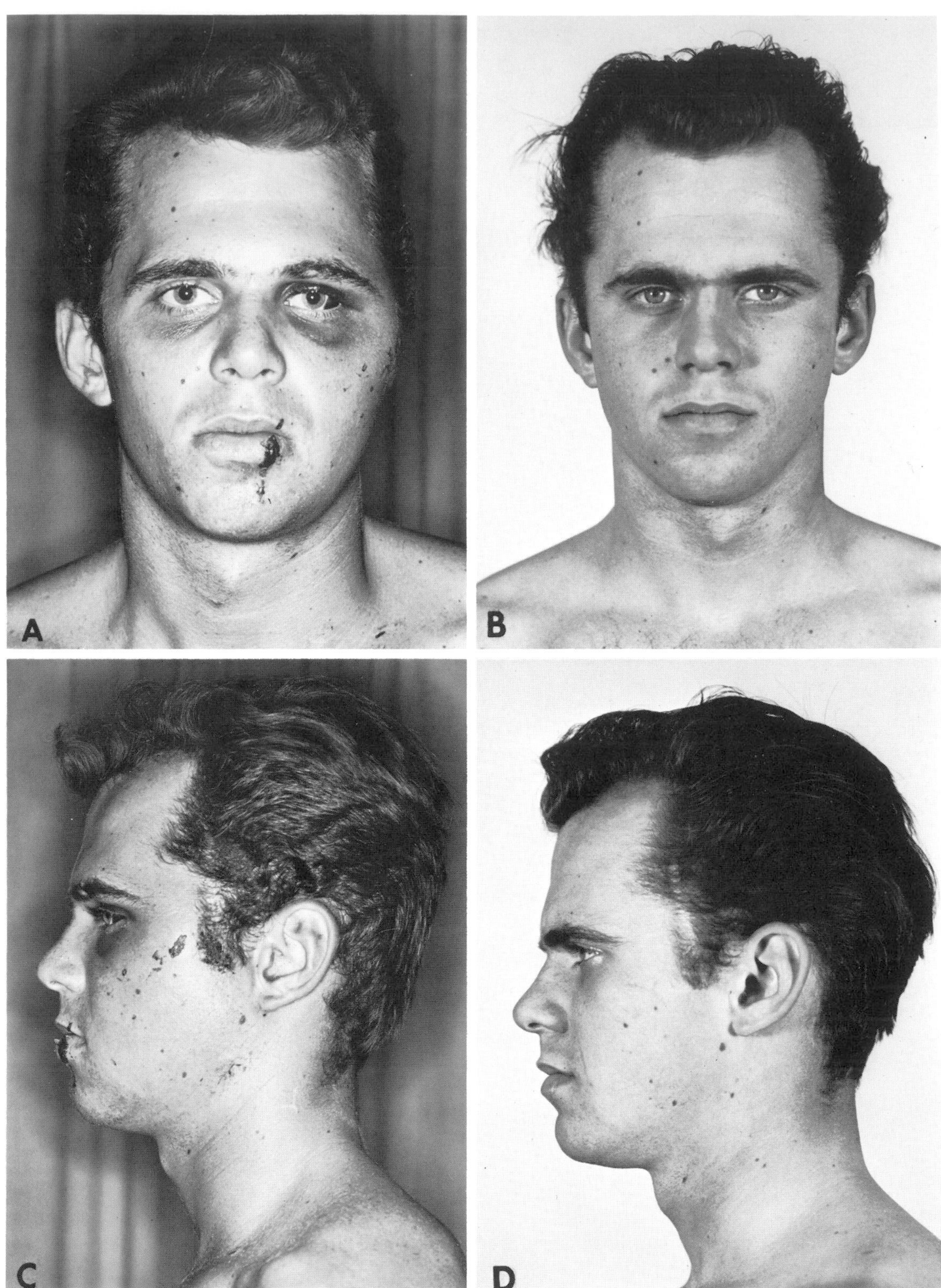

Figure 210. Comminuted fracture of the left zygomatic arch treated by open reduction and multiple interosseous wire fixation through a horizontal incision over the zygomatic arch. *A* and *B*. Preoperative and postoperative frontal views of unstable comminuted fractures of the zygomatic arch. *C* and *D*. Preoperative and postoperative views from the left side. Note minimal operative scar over the zygomatic

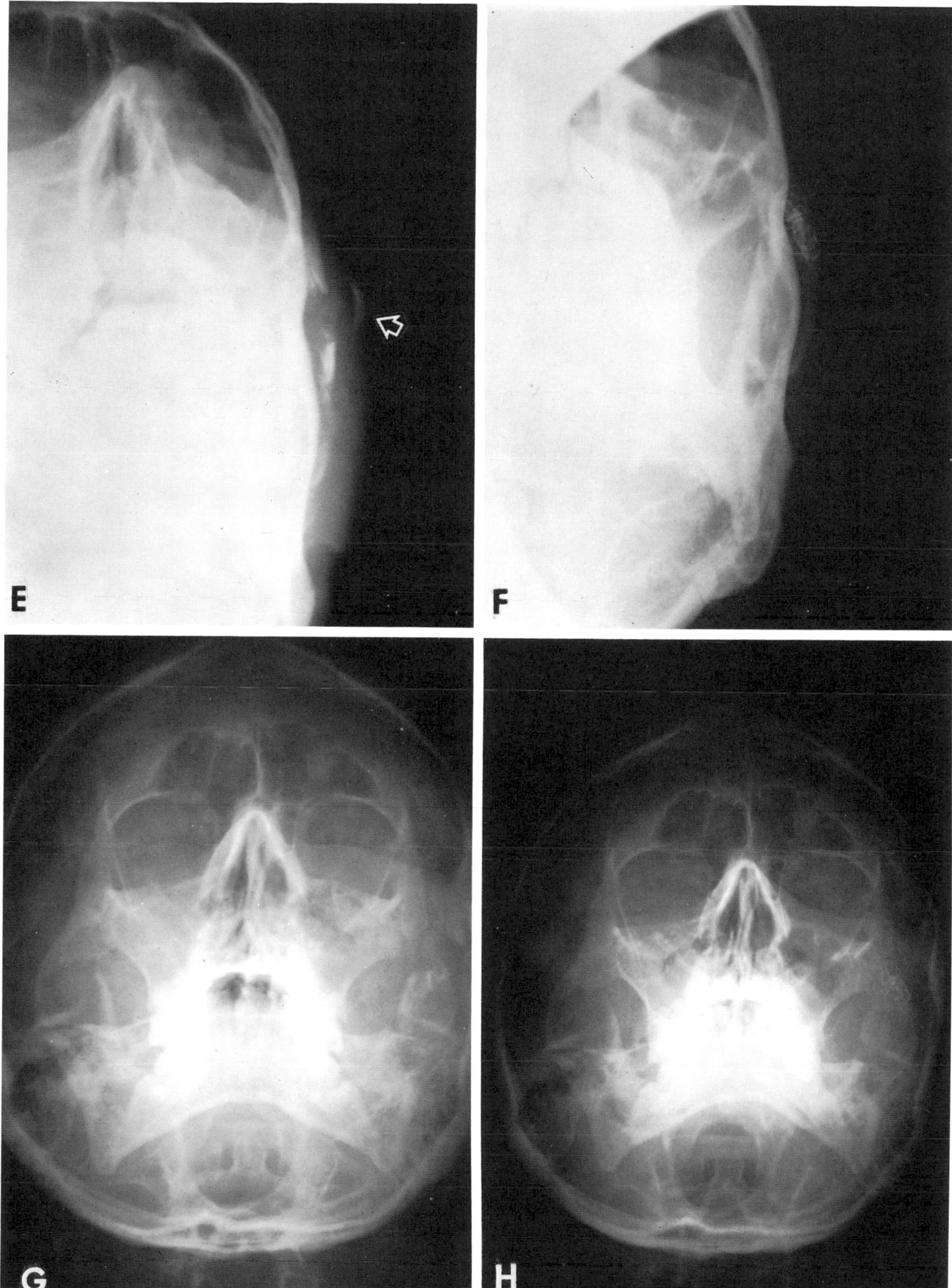

prominence; scar in the left temporal region is from previous surgery. *E*. Comminuted displaced unstable fracture of the left zygoma. *F*. Reconstructed zygomatic arch. Note multiple small stainless steel wire ligatures. *G*. Preoperative Waters' view showing comminuted displaced fracture of the left zygoma. *H*. Postoperative Waters' view showing reconstruction of zygomatic arch.

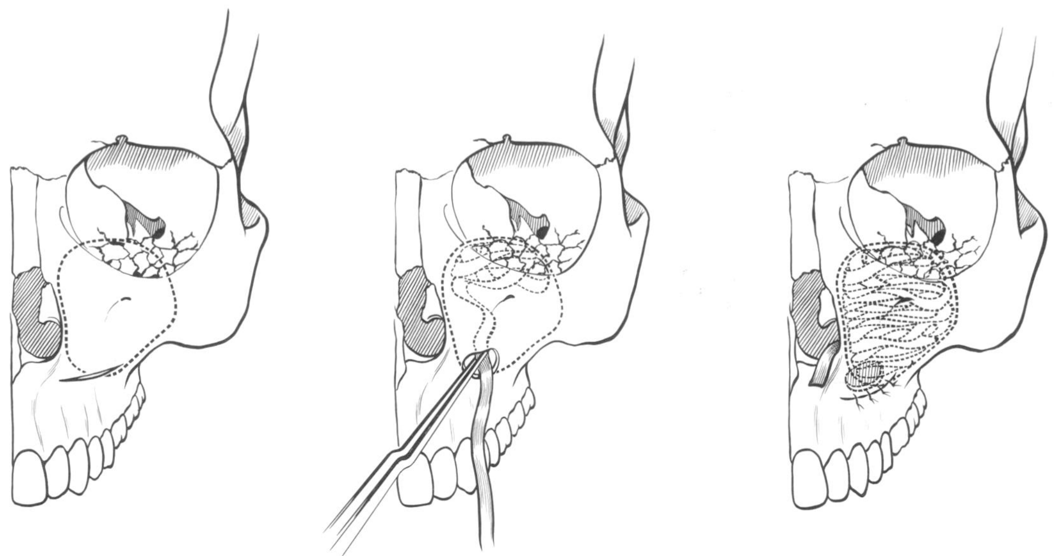

Figure 211. Support of multiple comminuted fractures of the floor of the orbit can be obtained by packing the maxillary sinus through the canine fossa. The packing may be removed in 7 to 10 days through a nasal antrostomy. The Caldwell-Luc incision is closed to prevent contamination of the maxillary sinus.

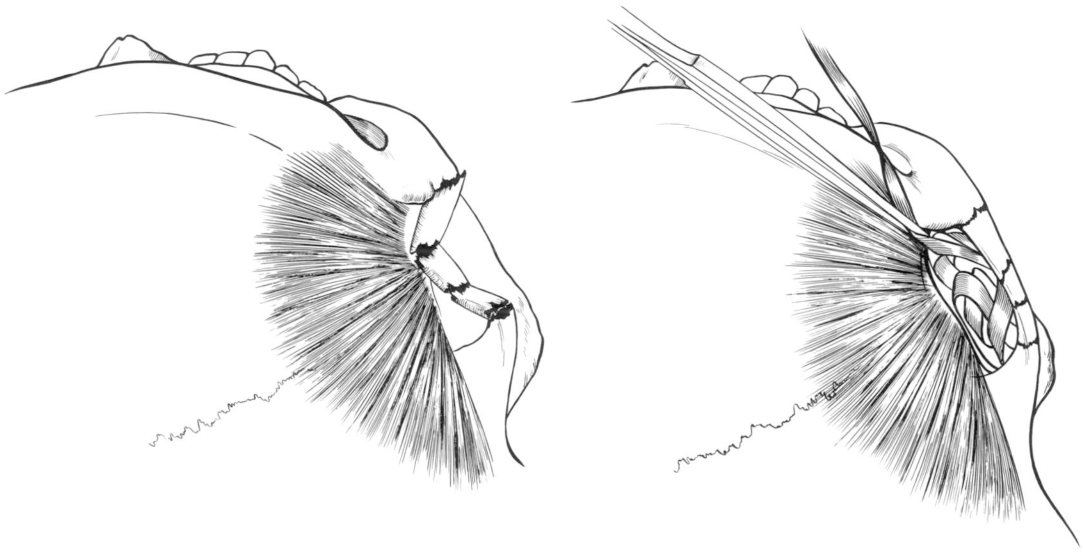

Figure 212. Comminuted unstable fractures of the zygomatic arch may be supported by rubber dam packing in the temporal fossa. Support for 5 to 7 days permits organization and healing of the tissues in normal position.

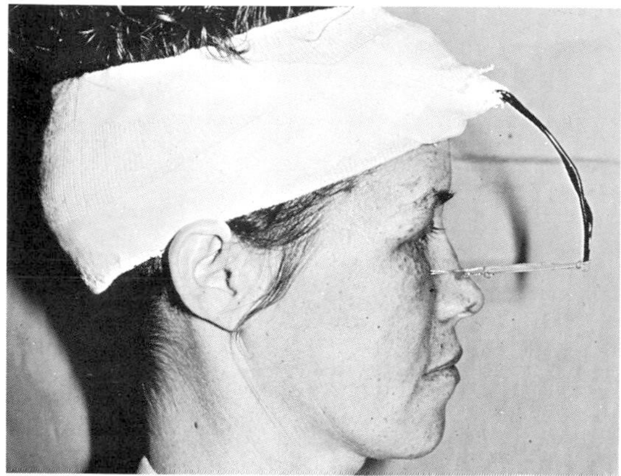

Figure 213. The suspension method of supporting a fracture of the zygoma in which there is a tendency for recurrent dislocation following reduction of zygomatic fracture. A head cap with an outrigger constructed of coat hanger wire provides forward support to the zygomaticomaxillary compound.

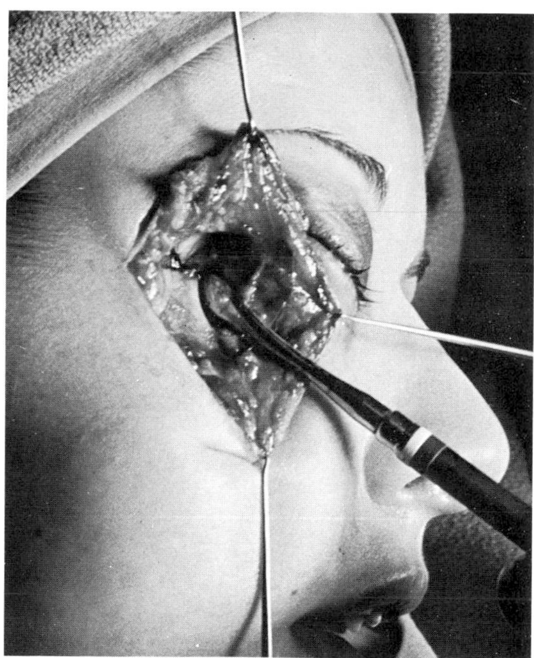

Figure 214. Traumatic fracture of the right zygoma. Note separation at the zygomaticofrontal suture. The fracture was reduced and fixed by means of interosseous wiring applied through the lacerated soft tissues. Whenever possible, bone should be repaired before soft tissue wounds are closed.

Open Reduction and Wire Fixation of Compound Comminuted Fractures of the Zygoma

New methods of anesthesia, improved surgical techniques, antibiotics, and blood replacement make it possible to do open operations with interosseous wire fixation quickly, safely, and effectively. Open reduction is supplanting methods that depend upon closed or blind operations and complicated appliances for fixation.

Wire Pin Fixation of Zygomatic Fractures

Brown, Fryer, and McDowell (1952) made a valuable contribution to the treatment of facial fractures by their introduction of the stainless steel pin method of fixation. After reduction, stainless steel pins are driven through the skin and fractured zygomatic bone segments in a transverse direction, and then into the solid parts of the maxilla and zygoma on the opposite side. The pins are cut off at skin level and are retained for four to six weeks. This is an expedient and effective method only in the hands of experienced surgeons. Complications in the form of osteomyelitis, malunion, nonunion, and facial deformity have been seen following attempts by inexperienced surgeons to use this method of treatment.

Late Reduction of Zygomatic Fractures

When the condition of the patient does not permit operation within the first week or ten days, the facial bones may heal in malposition. Some acute zygomatic fractures are not recognized, and weeks or months later, after the edema has subsided, deformity, diplopia, and malfunction may be noted. In some cases malunion occurs because the patient or his relatives refuse to consent to treatment. Malunion in the zygomatic region is sometimes seen a few months to several years after injury.

The process of organization and repair begins immediately after the injury, and the processes of fibrous and bony union may render the reduction of the fracture difficult. If correction is done within six weeks to three months, the bone may be moved satisfactorily by the usual methods, which have already been described. After three or four months, open operation may be necessary with dissection of the organized tissues from the line of fracture. The fracture often can be mobilized by the use of sharp periosteal elevators, but in some patients who have not been treated for several months or years, osteotomy will be required. Late procedures can be done with the same surgical approaches as have been described for open reduction of zygomatic fractures.

Great force may be necessary to refracture the bone, even after elevators have been used to break up the callous or bony union. A broad, heavy instrument, passed through the Gillies or brow incision, offers an opportunity to apply considerable force to the deep surface of the zygomatic arch without damage to the bone or to adjacent soft tissues. The late reduction of fractures in this region may be a formidable procedure, and one cannot stress too strongly that the earliest possible treatment be undertaken.

Although the later operation usually gives a satisfactory result, it may be less than optimal. In planning the late definitive procedure the surgeon should be prepared to utilize a graft to reconstruct the floor of the orbit, if repositioning of the bones does not appear to give adequate elevation of the floor. Even though the bones are replaced accurately, in some cases enophthalmos and depression of the eyeball may be disturbing factors. These complications are thought to be caused by atrophy of the orbital fat or shrinking of the fascia surrounding the muscles and the bulb, or both. This usually makes correction of enophthalmos unsatisfactory.

Function and appearance may be improved, however, by elevation of the bulb, which in many cases corrects the diplopia. The eyeball may be elevated by the insertion of a bone or cartilage graft under the periorbita. If supplemental grafts are used at the time of mobilization and elevation of the zygoma, the desired thickness of the graft may be determined at the operating table by noting the difference in measurement between the defect and the amount of elevation obtained by repositioning the bone. When it is planned to elevate the eyeball without attempting to reposition the bone, an accurate preoperative measurement can be made. Ophthalmologic consultation is desirable in determining the amount of depression of the globe. The graft can be cut to the measurement represented by the discrepancy in level between the two globes. When iliac bone is used for reconstruction of the orbital floor, overcorrection by 25 per cent is advisable as there is often partial resorption of the graft. Irradiated costal cartilage is excellent for reconstruction of the orbital floor and there is little tendency for the graft to become resorbed. One should avoid placing the graft too far back in the orbit, as it may interfere with the infraorbital and zygomatic nerves and vessels passing through the inferior orbital fissure. In cases of long-standing comminuted malunion of the zygoma, in which the bone has lost all semblance of its normal form, attempt at osteotomy and repositioning is inadvisable. In such cases the orbital margin may be built up with overlying grafts of bone or cartilage to improve the contour and give a more satisfactory result than might be attained by attempting to reduce healed comminuted fractures (Fig. 215 *A–D*).

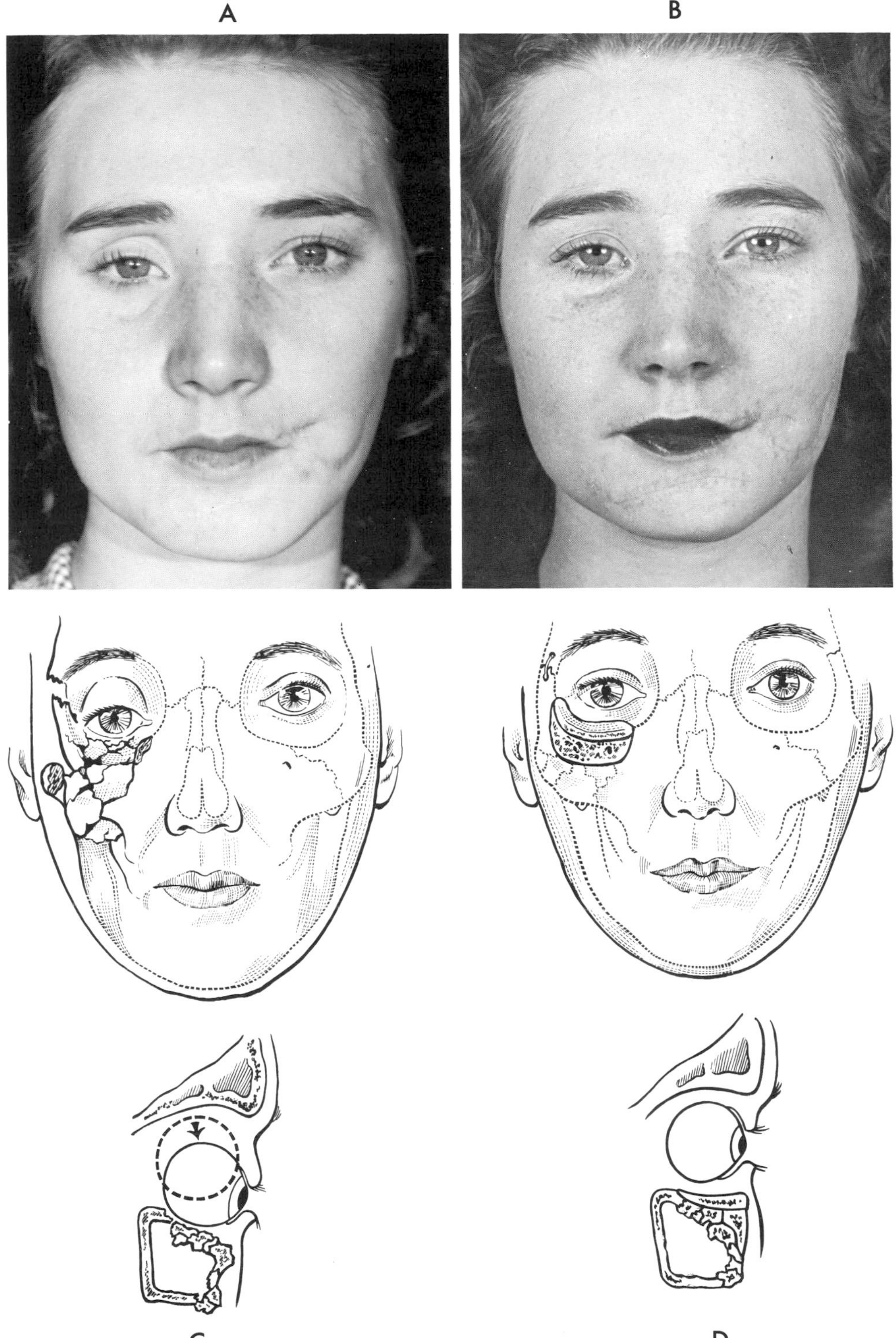

Figure 215. *A*. Five years after multiple facial injuries as a result of an automobile accident. *B*. Six months after bone graft to the right orbital region; one month after correction of facial scars. *C* and *D*. Method of reconstruction of infraorbital margin and orbital floor with autogenous iliac bone. (From Dingman, R. O.: Symposium: malunited fractures of zygoma; repair of deformity. Tr. Am. Acad. Ophth., *57*:889–896, Nov.–Dec., 1953.)

Fractures of the Floor of the Orbit Without Fractures of the Infraorbital Rim (Blow-out and Blow-in Fractures)

The term blow-out fracture, widely used today for a fracture of the orbital floor which is displaced downward into the maxillary sinus, and conversely the term blow-in fracture in which the orbital floor is displaced upward into the orbit, do seem to us equivocal and are better replaced by precise terms. We would suggest the terms *depressed* and *elevated* to refer to fractures of the orbital floor (Fig. 216 *A, B*).

Depressed (Blow-out) Fracture of the Orbital Floor

The detection and diagnosis of a depressed fracture of the orbital floor may be masked and difficult to discover because of the presence of orbital and periorbital edema, hematoma, and hematoantrum. Clinically the intact infraorbital ridge, and radiographically the opacity of the sinus due to the accumulation of blood, may result in missing the diagnosis of a depressed fracture of the floor of the orbit. When the history and kind of injury are suggestive of such a fracture, careful inspection should be made for its detection.

Clinically the infraorbital ridge may be intact and without palpable deformity. On roentgenographic examination in the Waters' projection, malposition of the fragments of the orbital floor may be overlooked. Because of lack of density, the fracture may be obscured by overlying bone or by the presence of blood in the maxillary sinus. The diagnosis may be made either by the use of planograms, which show frag-

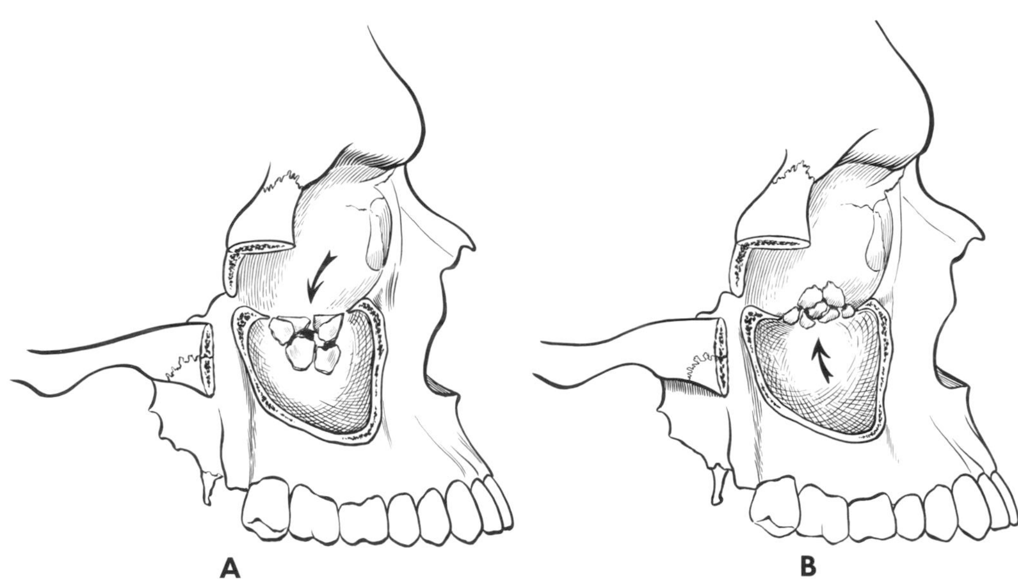

Figure 216. *A.* Depressed fracture of the floor of the orbit (blow-out fracture) with displacement into the maxillary sinus. *B.* Elevated fracture of the floor of the orbit (blow-in fracture) with displacement into the orbital cavity.

ments of bone or of soft tissue herniated into the maxillary sinus through the orbital floor, or by inspection of the orbital floor upon open exploration. The floor of the orbit may be inspected through an incision in the lower lid and exposure of the infraorbital margin with dissection of the periorbita. The orbital floor also may be inspected from the maxillary sinus through an opening in the canine fossa, but this does not permit as accurate an inspection as does the orbital approach.

Depressed fracture of the floor of the orbit probably was described first by William Lang in 1889 in an article entitled "Traumatic Enophthalmos with Retention of Perfect Acuity of Vision" (Fig. 217). Lang reported that on December 18, 1888, Hugh S., age 13, was struck on the right eyebrow, as he was running in the street, by the shaft of a cart driven at a trot. He was knocked down but immediately got up and ran home. The lid wound was sutured. For 12 hours after the injury he bled profusely, and blood dripped heavily from the right nostril. The child was not unconscious at any time. Within a short time the lids were swollen and closed. When the edema subsided it was noticed that the right eye was sunken in its orbit. One month later the patient came under the care of Dr. Lang and it looked as if he had a small artificial eye in the right orbit. He had a scar in the upper lid, and the palpebral fissure was 4 mm. shorter and 4 mm. narrower vertically than the left. He had difficulty in overcoming the narrowing except when he opened his lids as widely as he could by exertion.

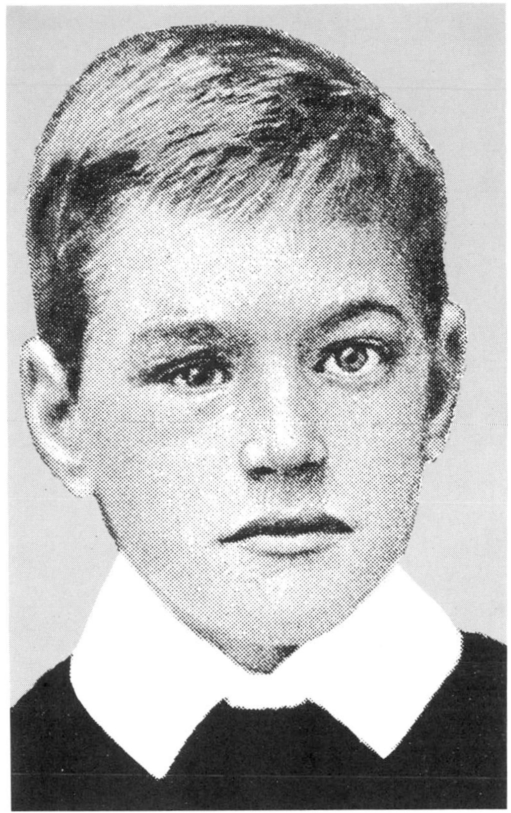

Figure 217. Photograph of patient (Hugh S.) with the first recorded depressed (blow-out) fracture of the orbit, December 18, 1888. (Lang, W.: Traumatic enophthalmos with retention of perfect acuity of vision. Trans. Ophth. Soc. United Kingdom, *9*:43, 1889.)

"The R. pupil measured 7.5 mm., and was somewhat pear-shaped, with the narrow end downwards. The iris acted very slightly to light and convergence, with the exception of the lower part, which was immovable. The L. pupil measured 5.5 mm."

Ocular movements on the right were limited in every direction, but least when the patient looked inward. Consequently there was diplopia in every direction, with the single exception that when he was looking horizontally forward with his head thrown back slightly, he saw binocularly. The right globe was displaced downward and the right cornea was 8 mm. behind the level of the left. There was doubtful anesthesia over the right cheek and forehead. He had no difficulty in breathing through his nose. Sensation of olfaction was not as good on the right as on the left. The orbital margins showed no abnormality and there was no pain elicited on pressing the orbital margin. The teeth were normal, and although the inner canthus and caruncle were in a plane anterior to that of the cornea, there was no epiphora.

Lang called the condition traumatic enophthalmos in contradistinction to symptomatic enophthalmos caused by wasting disease or paralysis of the cervical sympathetic chain. He described the traumatic varieties of enophthalmos as being divided into two groups, one in which the eye is entirely lost to view, and the other in which the cornea is quite visible though situated at a level much posterior to its normal position, giving the appearance of an artificial eye. He cited two recorded cases, one by von Becker of Helsingfors and the other by Tweedy. In each case the accident was caused by a cow's horn driving the globe into the antrum through a perforation of the lower orbital wall. In von Becker's case the sight was retained but the eye was useless as the cornea was directed upward and the globe was firmly fixed by adhesions. In Tweedy's case the eye was removed because it was blind. The operation was accomplished with considerable difficulty, however, since adhesions were very firm and numerous.

In the second variety, four cases were recorded by Professor Nieden and his assistant, Dr. Gessner. In each case the injury occurred to a miner when a mass of coal fell on the head or face. Only one eye was affected in each patient and the sinking varied from 2 and 3 to 4 mm. The vision was normal and binocular in three of these cases; in the fourth it was one-eighth normal with but slight changes in the fundus. The palpebral fissure was narrowed by 2 mm. and there was a scar over the eyebrow in three of the four cases. Movement of the upper lid, as well as that of the globe upward, was limited, but in the downward direction the movement was increased while the lateral movement was somewhat limited. In two of the cases, pain was produced on pressing the orbit. Nieden considered that the sinking of the globe was due to atrophy of the orbital fat, while Gessner thought that the globe was drawn back by shrinking of the connective tissue and the orbital fat. Lang said, "Meanwhile I would suggest that the injury may have produced a fracture and depression of a portion of the orbital wall; the orbital fat would then be no longer sufficient in quantity to fill this enlarged postocular area without a sinking-in of the globe from atmospheric pressure and the resulting limitation in the ocular movements. These cases might then be considered as less exaggerated but similar to those of von Becker and Tweedy."

Lang continued: "The apparent increase in the downward movement of the globe is, I think, to be explained by the anatomical arrangement of the inferior rectus, which, as was shown in a paper in our 'Transactions' by Lang and Fitzgerald, 'On the Movements of the Lids,' acts as the depressor of the lower lid. As the two points of insertion of the inferior rectus (the direct into the globe, the indirect into the lower lid) are separated more widely than normal by the sinking of the globe away from the lower lid, the action on the lid is more exaggerated, thus giving rise to the appearance of a greater power of depression than normal.

"That a fracture took place in my case is, I think, very probable, as the patient bled very freely at the nose, and the accommodation was paralyzed. (*January 31st*, 1889.)

"The president [of the society] thought the retrogression of the eyeball immediately on receipt of an injury could only be explained by fracture with displacement of the walls of the orbit. An instance of such fracture with displacement of the floor of the orbit is mentioned by C. Hyrtl in his 'Topogr. Anat.'"

Although Lang in 1889 did not have access to roentgenographic study, it is undoubtedly true that Hugh S. had a depressed fracture of the floor of the orbit.

This clinical entity was rediscovered and described by Converse and Smith (1950). It also was discussed by Pfeiffer (1943). Converse and Smith coined the term "blow-out fracture" and were instrumental in bringing this important entity to the attention of the medical profession.

If a depressed fracture of the floor of the orbit is present, orbital fat and contents will be seen herniating into the upper portion of the maxillary sinus. In some cases it is possible that such a fracture may not be associated with a severe tear of the periosteum of the orbital floor, but there may be a saucer-like depression of the bony roof of the maxillary sinus which, in effect, enlarges the size of the orbit, permitting downward displacement of the globe and enophthalmos (Fig. 218 *A, B*). The fracture is detected by roentgenographic evaluation or by exploration.

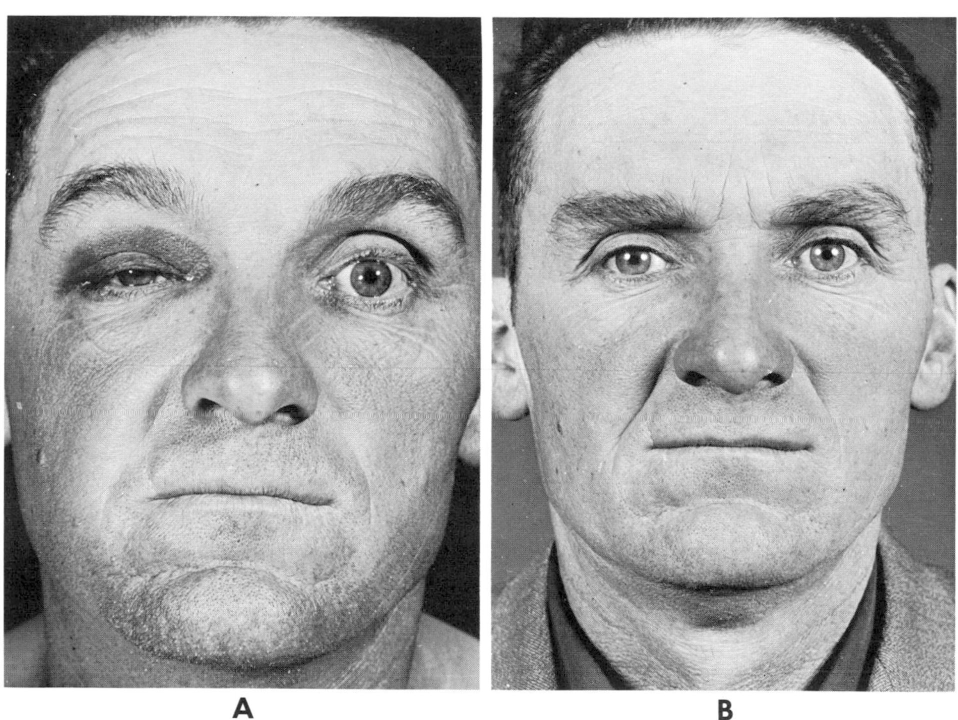

Figure 218. Fracture of the right zygoma with depressed (blow-out) fracture of the orbital floor. Correction was accomplished by open reduction through brow and infraorbital incisions, direct wire fixation of the fragments, and reconstruction of the orbital floor with a preserved costal cartilage graft. *A*. 24 hours following injury. *B*. One year following open operation and cartilage graft to the orbital floor.

Treatment of Depressed (Blow-out) Fracture of the Floor of the Orbit

The fractured segments may be replaced and supported by antral packing. If there is severe tearing in the periosteum, with displacement of the fragments and orbital contents into the maxillary sinus, packing may not give support sufficient to ensure healing of the bones in their proper relations. In such cases a thin layer of autogenous iliac bone or cartilage, preserved homologous cartilage, plastic material, or collagen may be placed on the orbital floor for reconstruction. These grafts give adequate support and provide an excellent method of reconstruction. The herniated orbital contents are elevated into the orbit and the graft placed across the defect (Fig. 219 *A, B*). Some surgeons suggest antral packing in addition to grafts to the orbital floor, to ensure better positioning to the fragments. If the antrum is packed through a Caldwell-Luc approach, the end of the dressing should be brought out through an antrostomy under the inferior turbinate bone, and the oral wound should be closed securely with sutures.

Treatment of Elevated (Blow-in) Fracture of the Orbital Floor

One of our patients received a severe blow to the anterior wall of the maxillary sinus and the infraorbital rim. Clinical and x-ray examination failed to show a fracture of the infraorbital rim, but a radiograph showed clearly an upward bulging of the orbital floor (Fig. 221). The patient had edema of the lids and slight exophthalmos of the right eye.

The diagnosis was confirmed by exploration of the orbital floor. In treatment the elevated fragments were depressed. There did not appear to be an opening into the maxillary sinus, and the bone fragments retained their position without fixation. The postoperative course was uneventful. We elected to diagnose the fracture in this sin-

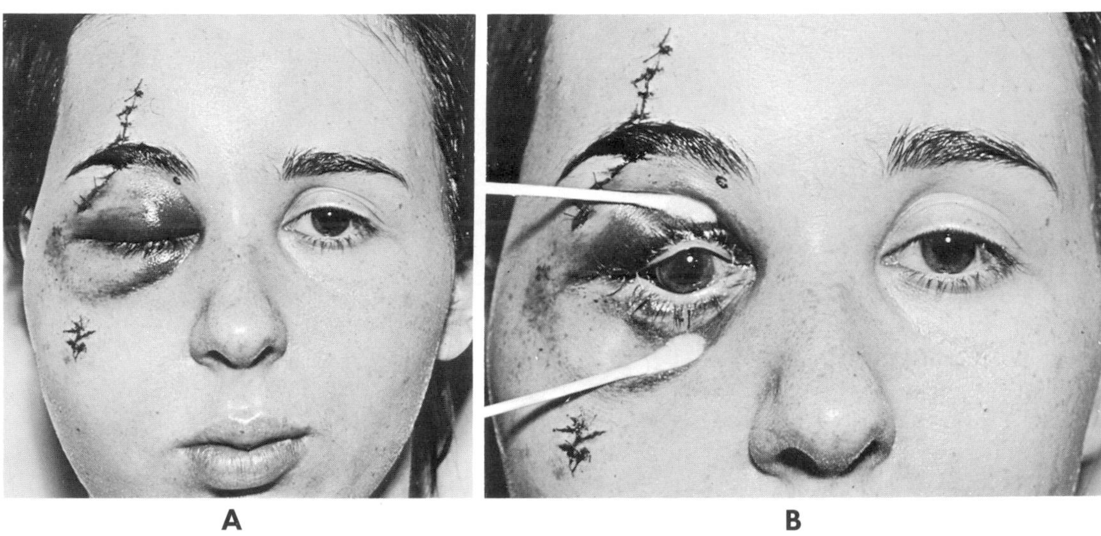

Figure 219. Comminuted fracture of the right zygoma associated with depressed (blow-out) fracture of the floor of the right orbit, corrected by open reduction, interosseous wire fixation, and preserved costal cartilage homograft to the orbital floor. *A*. Appearance of the patient four days after injury. *B*. Note depression of the right eye.

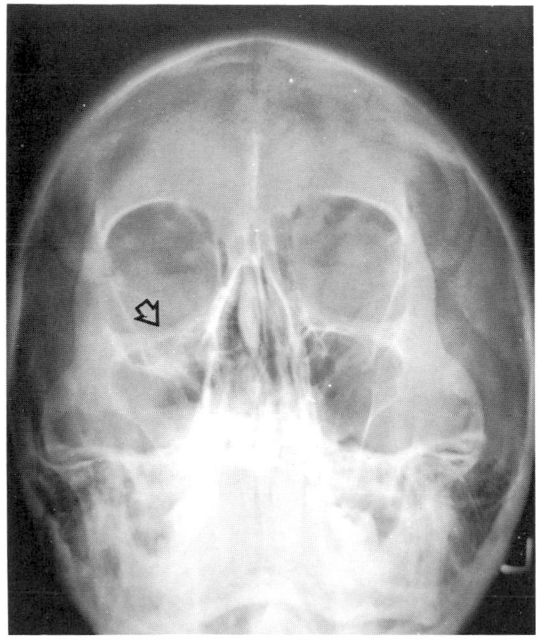

Figure 220. Roentgenogram of a depressed (blow-out) fracture of the floor of the right orbit. Note fragments of bone driven from the orbital floor into the maxillary sinus. This type of fracture may be overlooked easily in the presence of blood in the sinus and edema of overlying tissues. Laminographic technique may be utilized if a depressed fracture is suspected.

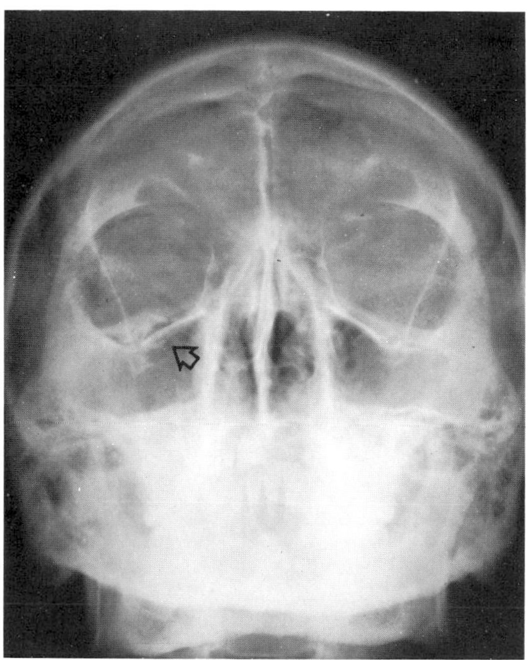

Figure 221. Elevated (blow-in) fracture of the orbital floor. This fracture was caused by a force directed upward and backward against the anterior maxillary wall and infraorbital margin. Segments of the floor are driven or buckled upward to encroach upon the orbital space. The location of the elevated (blow-in) fracture may be demonstrated by laminographic technique.

gle case as an elevated fracture of the floor of the orbit (blow-in fracture) in contrast to the depressed fracture (blow-out fracture).

LATE COMPLICATIONS OF FRACTURES OF THE ZYGOMATIC REGION

Late complications result primarily from malunion. Many of these can be corrected by osteotomy and replacement of the zygoma with direct wire fixation (Fig. 222 *A–E*). In some cases osteotomy for restoration of the contour of the face, and elevation of the orbital floor, can be complemented by bony or cartilaginous grafts (Dingman and Harding, 1951). Fibro-osseous ankylosis of the coronoid process of the mandible may result from the impingement of fractured segments of the zygomatic arch against the coronoid processes of the mandible. If it is impossible to reposition the zygomatic arch, excision of the coronoid process through the intraoral route usually will permit freedom of mandibular movement. Traumatic enophthalmos associated with shortening of the fascia, vessels, mus-

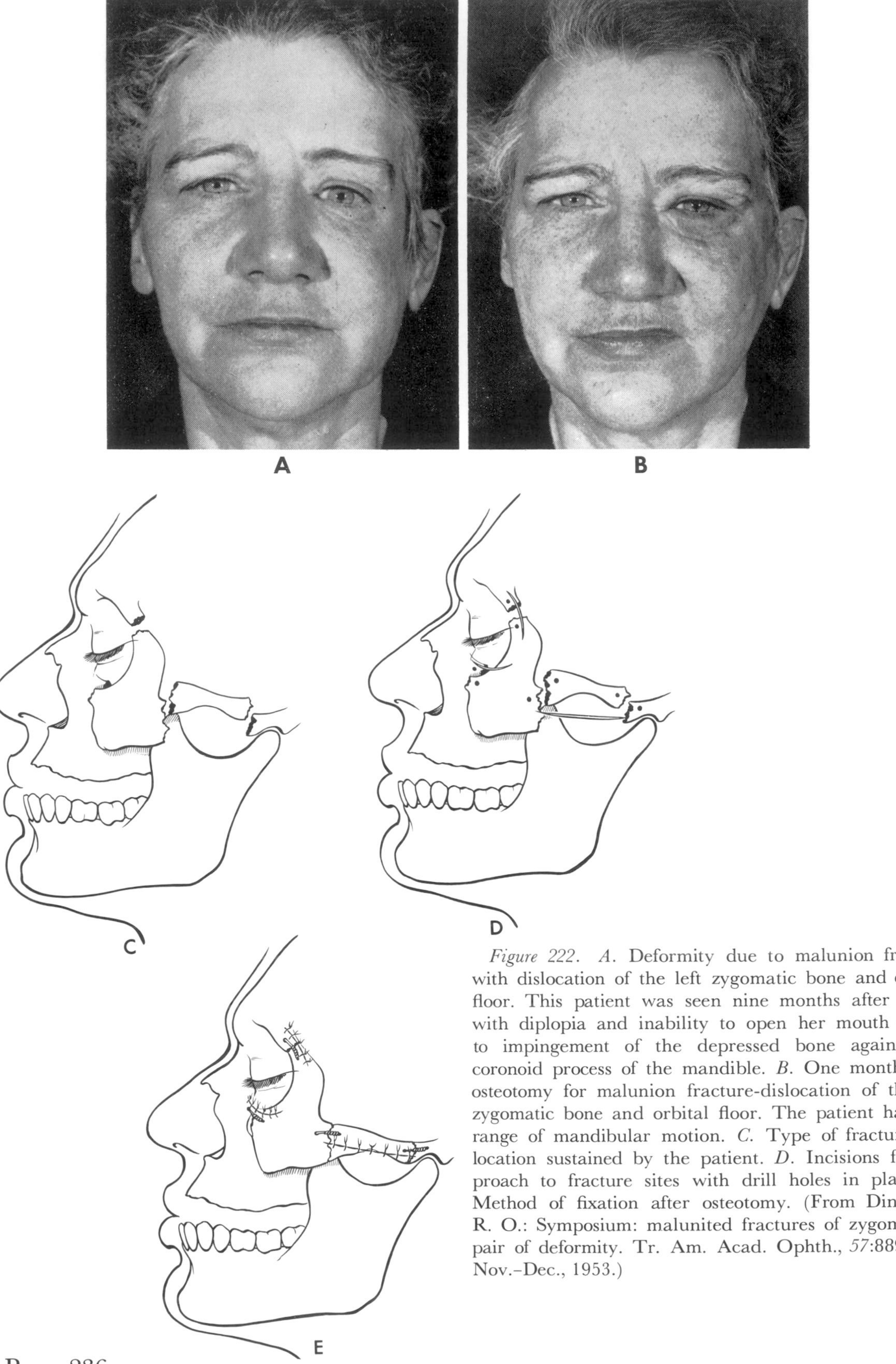

Figure 222. *A.* Deformity due to malunion fractur with dislocation of the left zygomatic bone and orbita floor. This patient was seen nine months after injur with diplopia and inability to open her mouth owin to impingement of the depressed bone against th coronoid process of the mandible. *B.* One month afte osteotomy for malunion fracture-dislocation of the lef zygomatic bone and orbital floor. The patient had ful range of mandibular motion. *C.* Type of fracture-dis location sustained by the patient. *D.* Incisions for ap proach to fracture sites with drill holes in place. *E* Method of fixation after osteotomy. (From Dingman R. O.: Symposium: malunited fractures of zygoma; re pair of deformity. Tr. Am. Acad. Ophth., *57*:889–896 Nov.–Dec., 1953.)

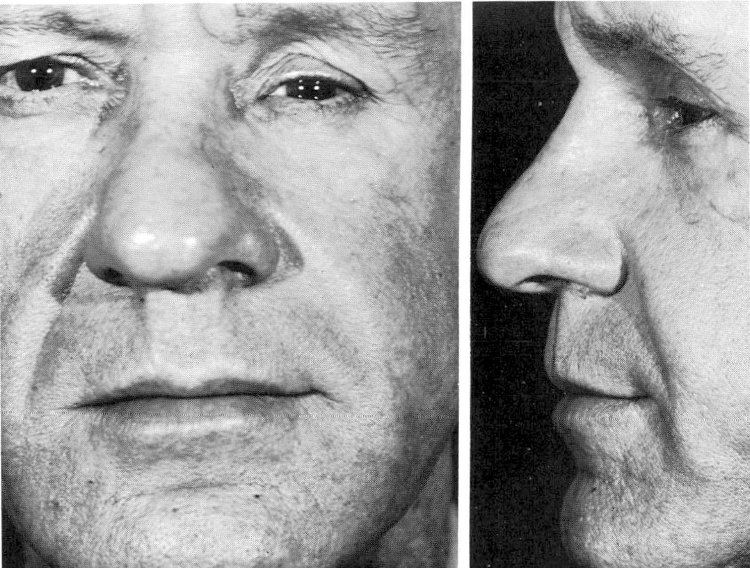

Figure 223. Depression of the left eye with enophthalmos due to fracture of the left zygoma with malunion.

cles and nerves and with atrophy of the orbital fat is impossible to correct completely. Some improvement can be obtained by elevation of the orbital contents and reconstruction of the orbital floor with grafts of cartilage or bone. Insertion of the grafts has the effect of increasing the volume of the orbital contents, thus forcing the globe forward and upward. The degree of improvement by use of this method is difficult to predict.

Early recognition and reconstruction of the orbital floor by use of grafts of bone or cartilage is the best method for preventing these deformities (Fig. 223).

Anesthesia persisting for 18 to 24 months is an indication for exploration of the infraorbital canal. Bone splinters or constricting portions of the canal should be removed so that the nerve will have an opportunity for regeneration. In some cases anesthesia is permanent, and although it is temporarily annoying, the patient becomes accustomed to it after a few months.

The Zygoma

PART 2

OPERATIVE TECHNIQUE

The zygoma gives prominence to the cheek, takes part in the formation of the orbit as well as of the maxillary sinus, and acts as a strong buttress for stabilization and support of the face. Because of its prominent position in the face, this bone is frequently subjected to fractures and dislocation.

Inadequate management of injuries to the zygomatic compound can result in serious esthetic and functional disability. While closed reduction techniques are popular and attractive in the management of fractures in this region, the experienced surgeon will be quick to see, in many cases, the limitations that closed methods impose.

The open methods outlined on the following pages take into account the accessibility of the fractured region and the opportunity for accurate repositioning and positive fixation. Open methods make it possible to explore and examine the orbital floor for displaced segments whose displacement, if uncorrected, may cause ocular, functional, and cosmetic disability. The open approach permits direct reconstruction of the orbital floor.

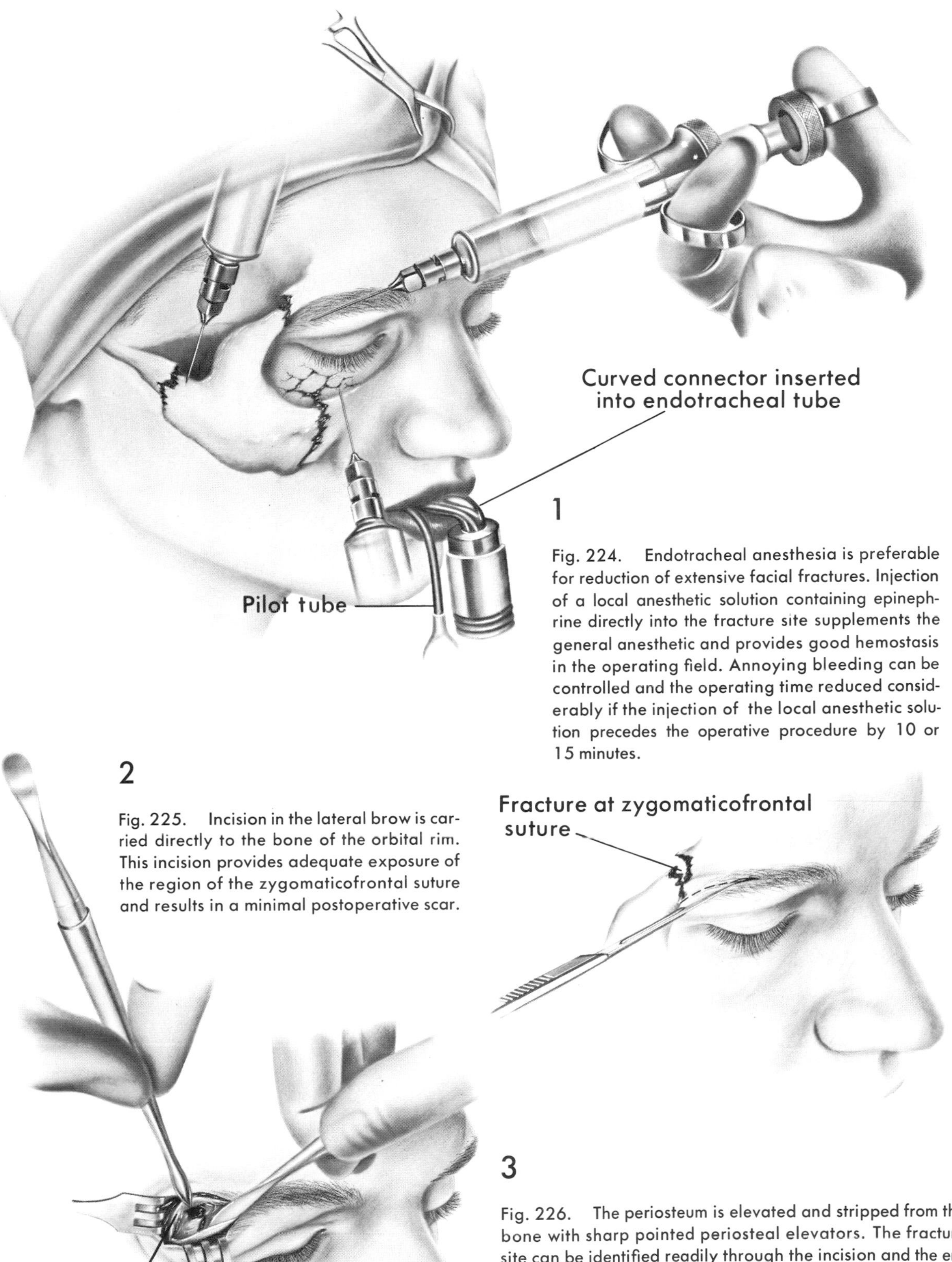

Fig. 224. Endotracheal anesthesia is preferable for reduction of extensive facial fractures. Injection of a local anesthetic solution containing epinephrine directly into the fracture site supplements the general anesthetic and provides good hemostasis in the operating field. Annoying bleeding can be controlled and the operating time reduced considerably if the injection of the local anesthetic solution precedes the operative procedure by 10 or 15 minutes.

Fig. 225. Incision in the lateral brow is carried directly to the bone of the orbital rim. This incision provides adequate exposure of the region of the zygomaticofrontal suture and results in a minimal postoperative scar.

Fig. 226. The periosteum is elevated and stripped from the bone with sharp pointed periosteal elevators. The fracture site can be identified readily through the incision and the entire lateral orbital rim can be explored through the brow incision, if necessary.

4

Fig. 227. The infraorbital margin is exposed through a skin incision, following the wrinkle lines of the lower lid. Dissection is carried down carefully to the level of the periosteum. The periosteum is incised along the crest of the infraorbital ridge.

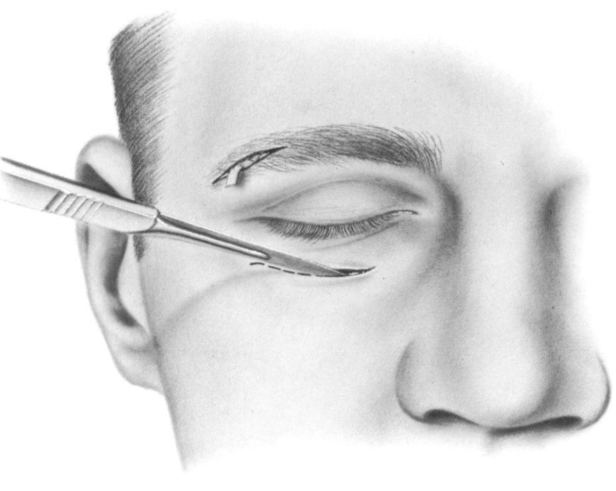

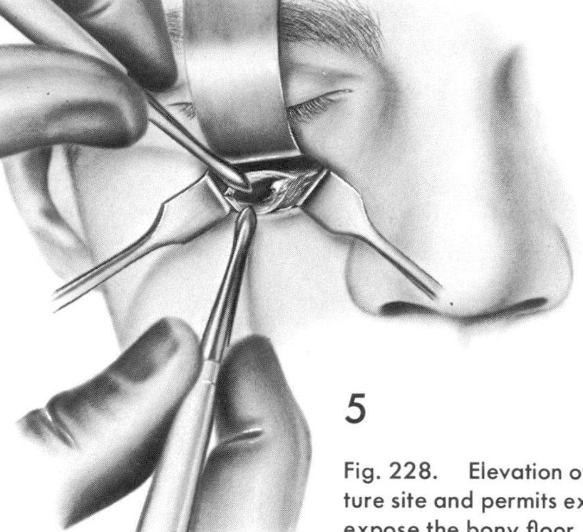

5

Fig. 228. Elevation of the periosteum from the infraorbital rim exposes the fracture site and permits exploration of the orbital floor. The periorbita is elevated to expose the bony floor, to demonstrate any fractures, and to detect herniation of orbital contents into the maxillary sinus.

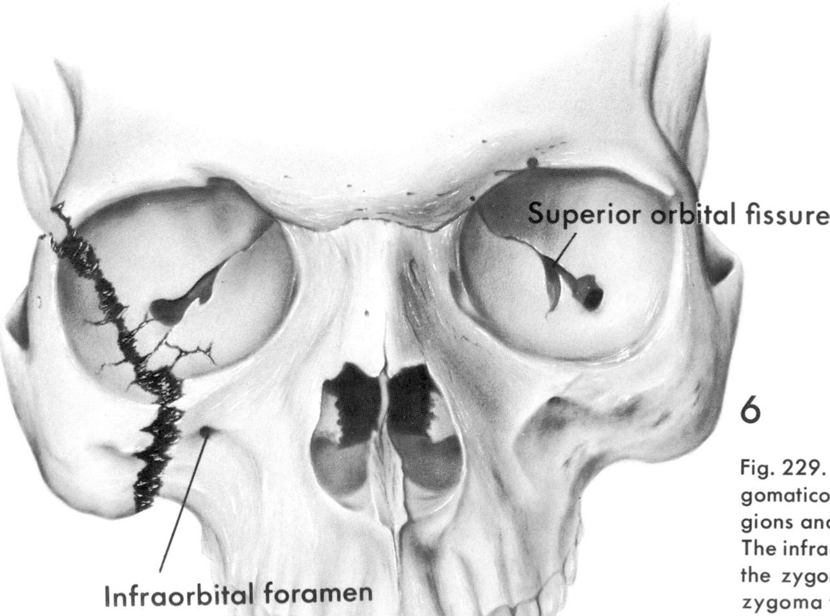

6

Fig. 229. Fractures may occur through the zygomaticofrontal and zygomaticomaxillary regions and extend across the floor of the orbit. The infraorbital canal in the maxilla is close to the zygoma. In most cases of fracture of the zygoma the infraorbital nerve is torn or damaged at the time of injury. Anesthesia of the upper lip, tip of the nose, and lower lid is the usual finding.

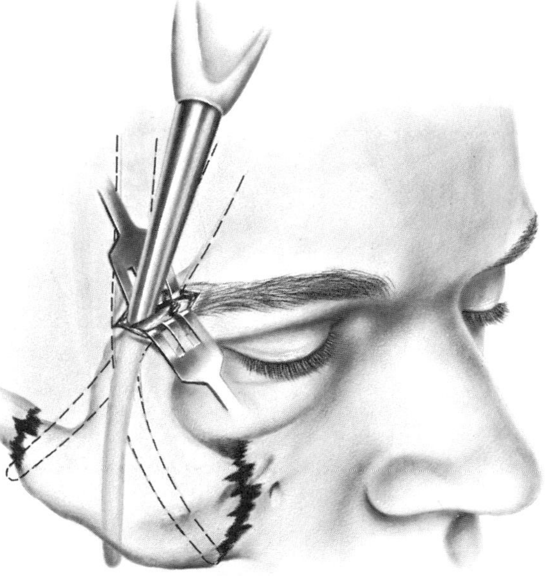

7

Fig. 230. A heavy elevator, shaped like a urethral sound, is passed through the brow incision on the temporal side of the zygoma into the temporal fossa. This approach may be used for elevation of the body of the zygoma or the zygomatic arch. Great leverage against the inner surface of the zygoma is possible through this approach.

8

Fig. 231. A depressed fracture of the zygomatic arch usually consists of two segments. The bone fragments are supported by the heavy temporal fascia and usually remain in place without fixation when elevated into position. The elevator is passed through the brow incision or through a temporal incision (Gillies approach for reduction of fracture of the zygoma).

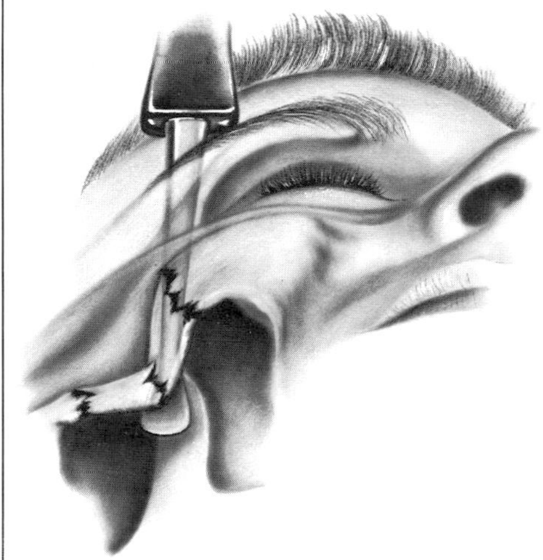

9

Fig. 232. Many fractures of the zygoma are unstable when elevated into position and must be supported by adequate fixation. Direct interosseous wire fixation through small drill holes provides excellent support. The drill holes are made on each side of the fragment and are directed from the anterolateral surface backward into the temporal fossa.

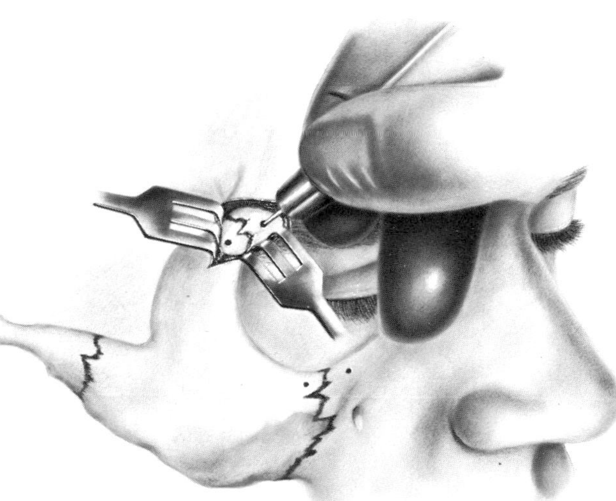

10

Fig. 233. The wire is passed through the drill holes on each side of the fracture with both ends of the wire directed toward the temporal side of the zygoma. The wire is twisted tightly to fix the bone securely in position. The twisted wire is cut to about 1 cm. in length, and the end is pressed against the temporal side of the bone so that it cannot irritate the adjacent soft tissues.

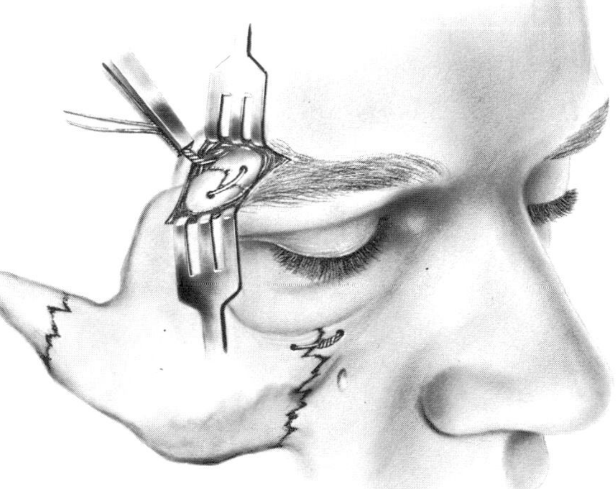

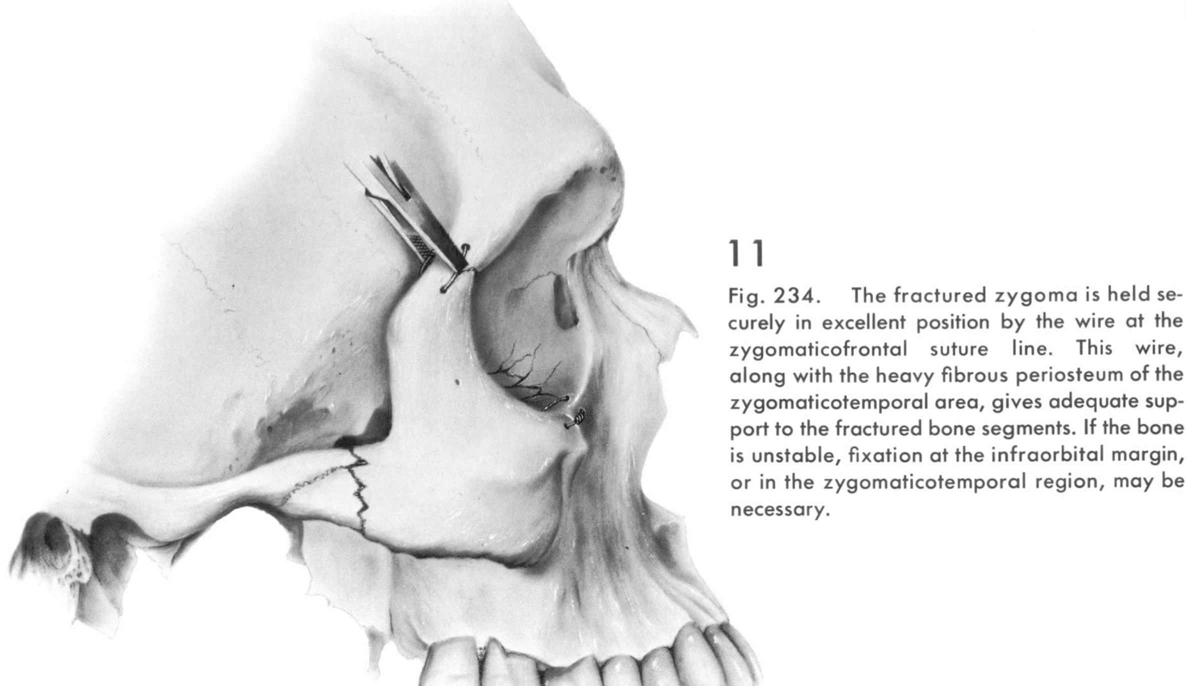

11

Fig. 234. The fractured zygoma is held securely in excellent position by the wire at the zygomaticofrontal suture line. This wire, along with the heavy fibrous periosteum of the zygomaticotemporal area, gives adequate support to the fractured bone segments. If the bone is unstable, fixation at the infraorbital margin, or in the zygomaticotemporal region, may be necessary.

12

Fig. 235. The maxillary sinus is in close relation with the body of the zygoma. Fractures of the zygoma in adults almost invariably are associated with fractures of the anterior and superior walls of the sinus. The sketch shows the location of the sinus in the maxilla.

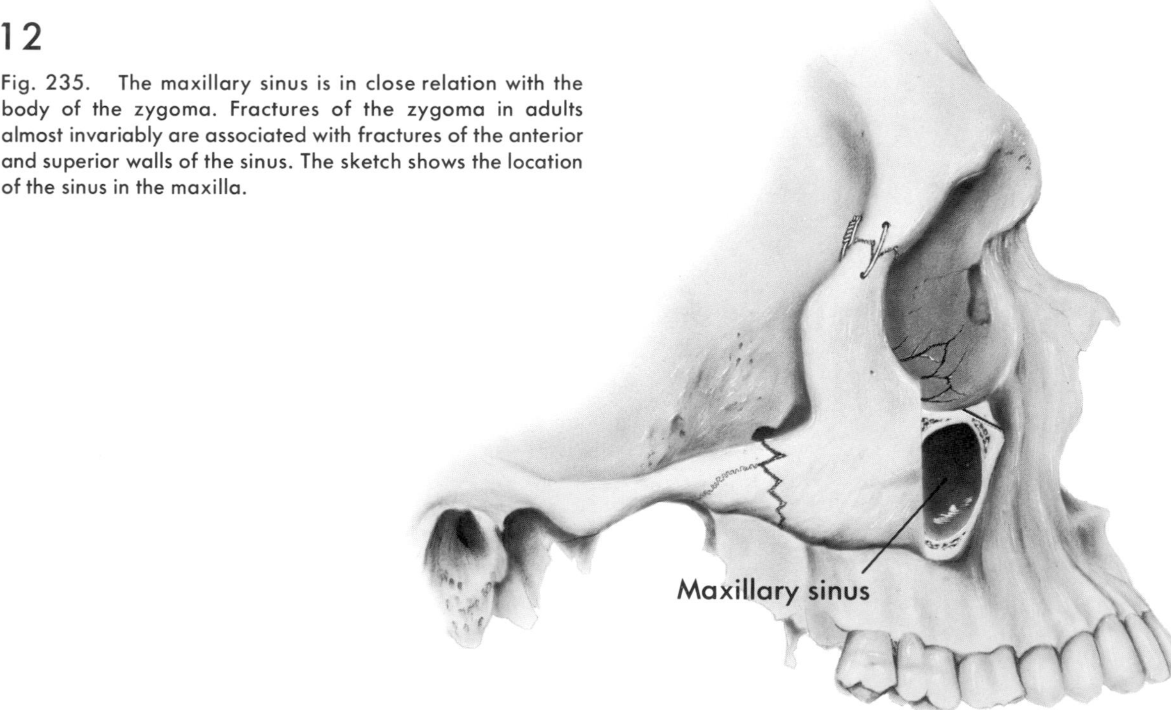

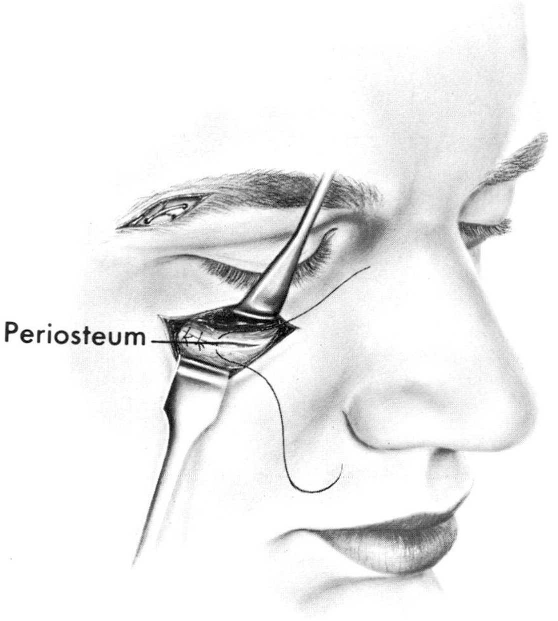

13

Fig. 236. After reduction, the fragments of the infraorbital margin and the anterior wall of the maxilla may be stabilized by direct wiring. The bones will heal more quickly and will be less liable to infection or other complications if the periosteum is sutured securely over the place of the fracture. Accurate approximation of the deeper structures and the skin will result in better closure with less probability of a depressed scar.

14

Fig. 237. The wound edges are carefully coapted with fine silk or nylon sutures tied with just enough tension to bring the tissues together. The final scar is barely noticeable if the skin incision is properly placed and if the tissues are handled carefully and closed with fine sutures, which are removed in three to four days. The brow and infraorbital incisions may be left without dressings if covered with a thin layer of petrolatum.

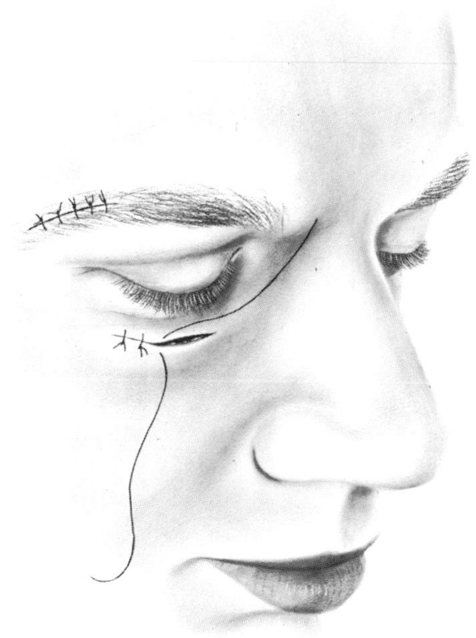

CHAPTER
8

THE MAXILLA

PART 1

GENERAL CONSIDERATIONS

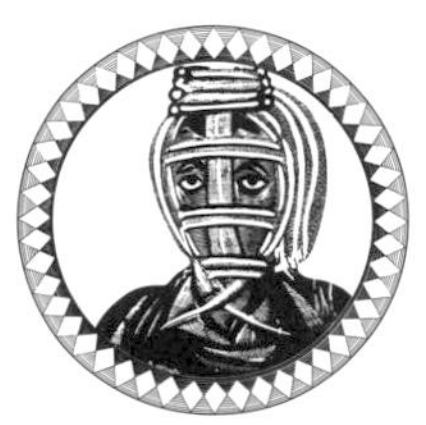

From a functional and clinical point of view the upper jaw should be regarded as a composite of four bones, the two maxillae and the two palatine bones. This concept describes the upper jaw as the antagonist of the lower jaw, the mandible (Sicher, 1963). Commonly in fractures of the upper jaw all four bones are involved.

In the following section the terms upper jaw and maxilla are used synonymously.

Fractures of the maxilla are seen less frequently than fractures of the mandible. The ratio of 1 to 4 as stated by Rowe and Killey (1955), and Kazanjian and Converse (1959), however, seems to be increasing in favor of fractures of the upper jaw, incident to an increase in facial injuries from high speed transportation accidents. A more recent series by McCoy et al. (1962) indicates a higher incidence of maxillary fractures in relation to mandibular fractures. The greater portion of the middle third of the face is made up of the maxilla, which is attached to the cranium and supported by a strong system of buttresses. Violent forces to the head are dissipated or absorbed by fractures of the maxilla and other facial bones, and thus offer protection to the brain and spinal cord. Fractures of the maxilla occur in conjunction with the guest passenger injury, or the facial smash injury, sustained in automobile and plane crashes. The maxilla is capable of absorbing considerable force by transmission of the force to the adjacent articulating bones. By absorbing the energy of the forces transmitted to the face, these bones are highly protective to the cranium.

ANATOMIC CONSIDERATIONS

The maxilla, the composite of the maxillary and palatine bones, forms the largest part of the middle third of the face and contributes to the formation of the orbit, the nasal cavities, and the hard palate. The body of each maxillary bone is hollowed by the maxillary sinus.

The body of each maxilla has four processes—frontal, zygomatic, palatine, and alveolar. In the child the maxillary sinuses occupy only a small portion of the maxilla, but they enlarge with advancing age, and in the adult they occupy most of the interior of the bone, being covered only by a very thin lamina of bone (Fig. 238). The alveolar process of the maxilla contains the teeth.

Following removal of the teeth there is atrophy of the alveolar process with thinning of the bone. In the aged patient, the alveolar portion of the bone may have receded completely back to the level of the nasal spine with only a thin layer of bone separating the floor of the sinuses from the oral cavity. The middle face receives its nerve supply from the second division of the fifth nerve. Branches to the teeth pass through the outer wall of the bone. The infraorbital nerve passes through the infraorbital canal below the floor of the orbit to innervate the soft tissues of the lower lid, the cheek, the lateral aspect of the nose, and the upper lip. The palatine branches innervate the mucosa of the palate. The nasopalatine nerve passes anteriorly in the mucosa of the septum bilaterally and through the incisive

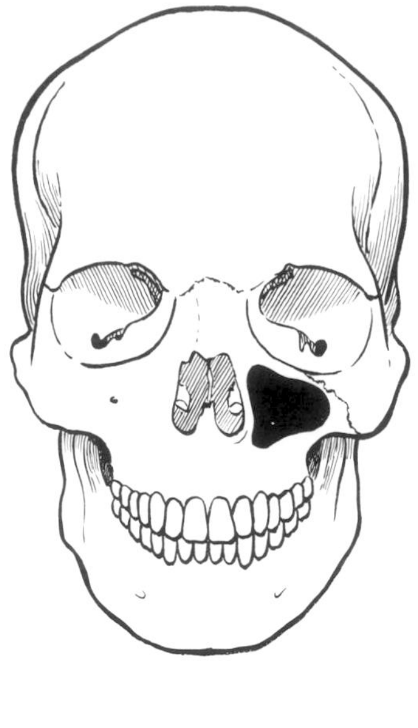

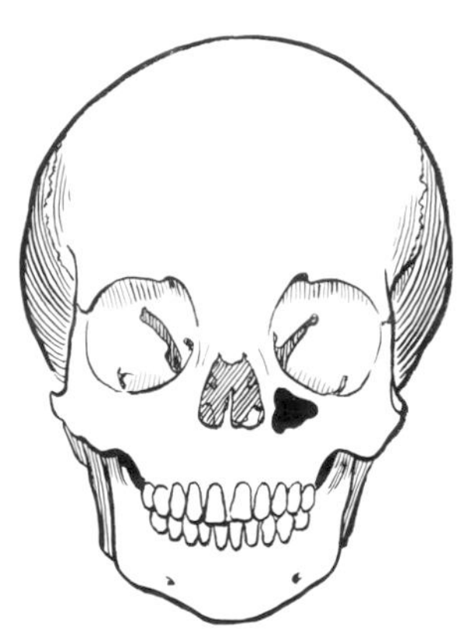

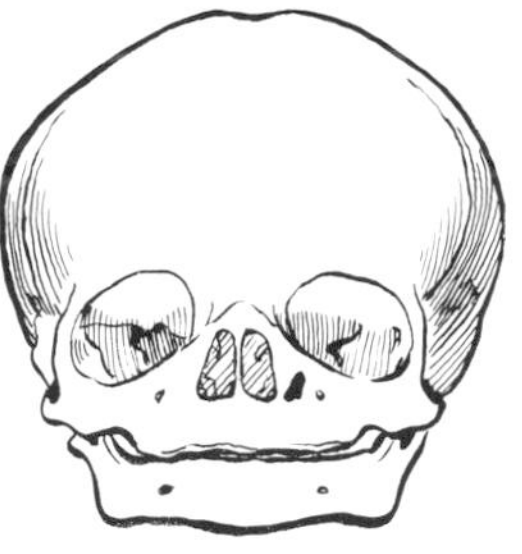

Figure 238. The skull in the adult, and at five years and six months. At birth the maxillary sinus is small, but gradually increases in size to occupy a large portion of the maxilla.

foramen to innervate the mucosa of the anterior palatine area. The stability of the maxilla is obtained by bracing against the anterior part of the cranial base.

On either side one finds three pillars or buttresses—anterior, middle, and posterior (Fig. 239). The anterior or the canine pillar starts in the region of the alveolar process of the canine, forms the lateral boundary of the anterior nasal aperature, and continues as the frontal process of the maxilla to the frontal bone. The middle or zygomatic pillar starts in the region of the first molar, bends upward and outward as the zygomaticoalveolar crest and the zygomatic process of the maxilla, to continue in the plate and the frontal process of the zygoma to end at the zygomatic process of the frontal bone. The posterior or pterygoid pillar is the pterygoid process of the sphenoid bone to which the pyramidal process of the palatine bone is anchored.

These roughly vertical pillars are braced against each other by the superior and inferior orbital rims and the zygomatic arch (Sicher, 1963).

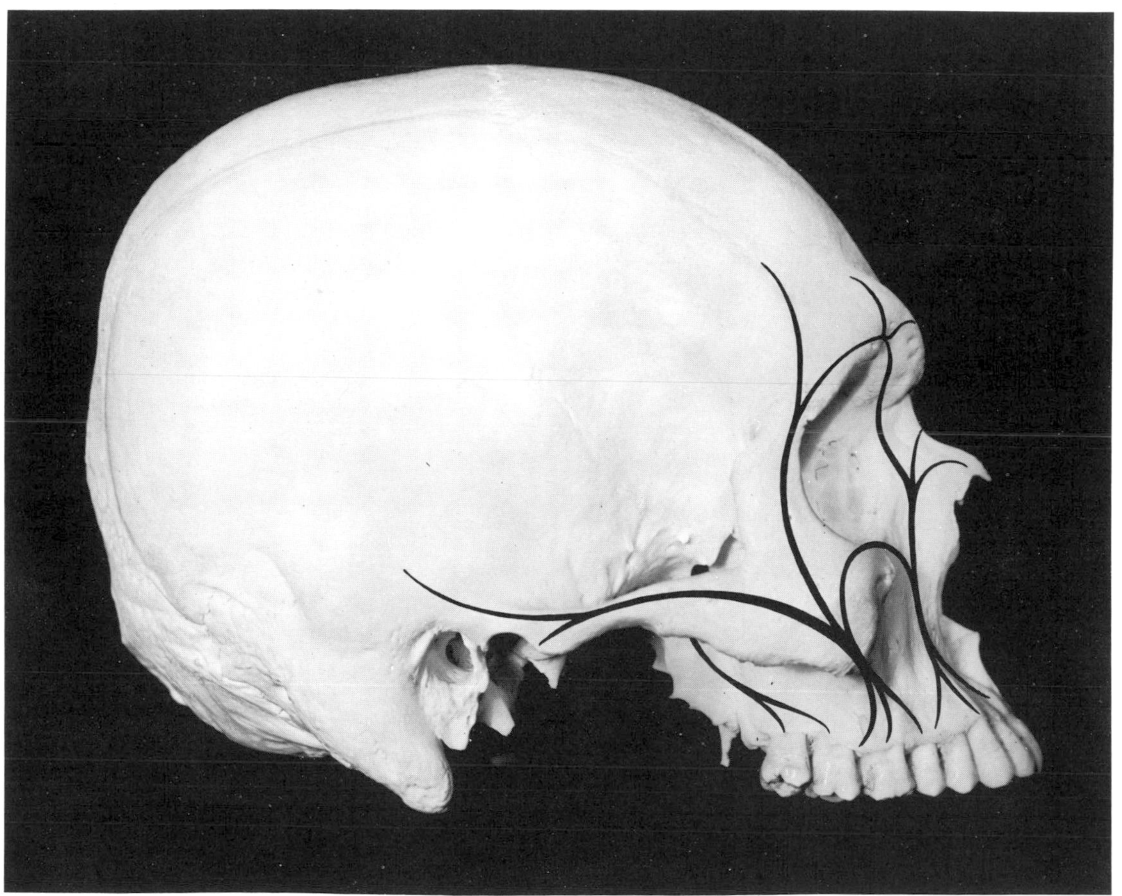

Figure 239. The supporting pillars of the maxillary skeleton. (After Sicher: *Oral Anatomy.* 3d ed. St. Louis, The C. V. Mosby Company, 1960.)

Surgical Anatomy

Fractures of the maxilla are usually the result of direct force to the bone, and range from simple alveolar fractures and fractures involving only the maxillary bone to extensive injuries including the bones of the nose, sinuses, orbit, palate, and indeed any of the bones of the face and skull with which the maxilla is associated so intimately.

Displacement is usually entirely the result of the traumatic force. Muscle contraction plays an unimportant role in displacement of maxillary fractures, except in those extending into the region of the pterygoid plates, in which displacement of the maxilla may be in a downward and posterior direction because of the action of the pterygoid muscles. In complete craniofacial separa-

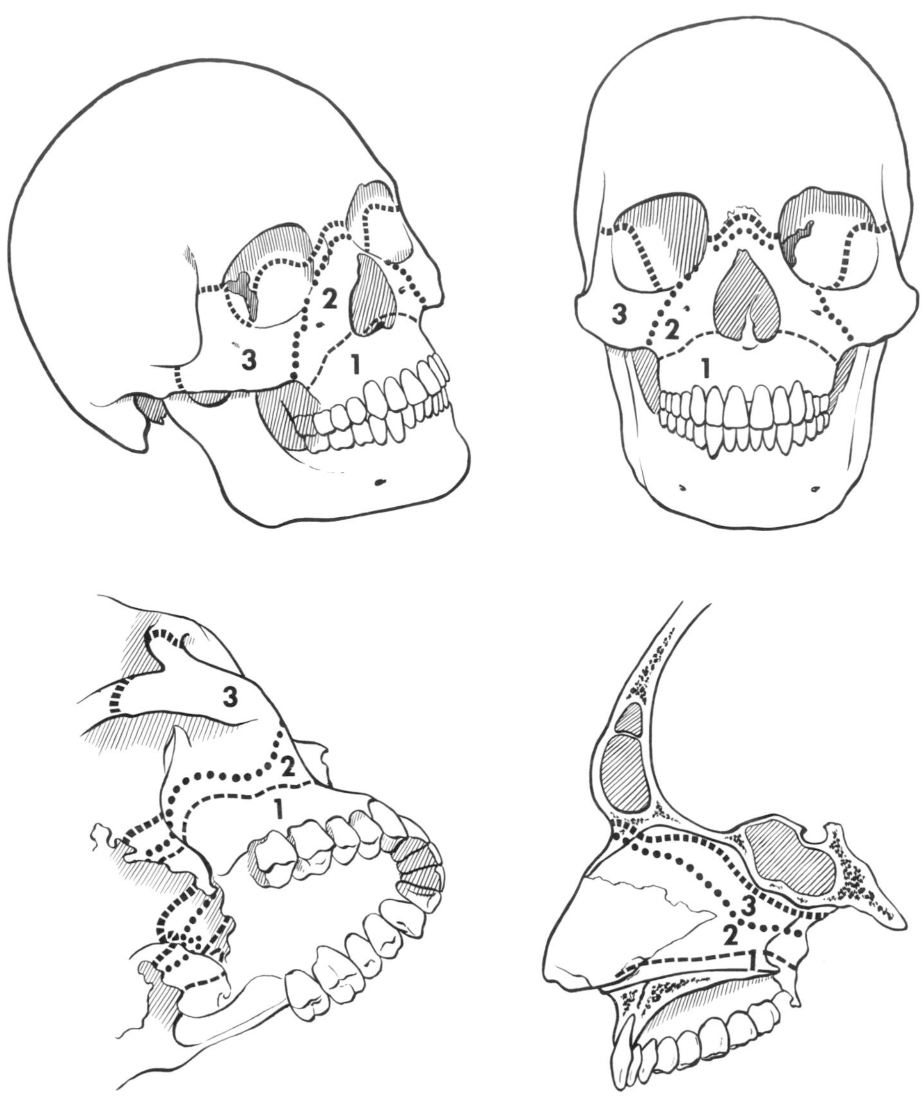

Figure 240. Fractures of the maxilla. 1. Le Fort I (transverse or Guérin fracture). 2. Le Fort II (pyramidal fracture). 3. Le Fort III (craniofacial disjunction).

tion associated with fractures of the zygoma, action of the masseter muscle may be a factor in displacement. The small muscles of expression attached to the maxilla are insignificant in causing displacement of fragments.

The lacrimal fossa is formed partially by the maxilla, and injuries to the nasolacrimal duct may be associated with fractures of the maxilla. The ethmoidal air cells and the cribriform plate are associated intimately with the maxilla. Severe fractures with dislocation may result in dural laceration and brain damage caused by impaction of the maxillary or nasal bone structures into the interorbital space and cranium. The heavier portions of the maxilla give strength to the bone and fractures are most likely to occur through the thinner parts. The experiments of Le Fort (1900, 1901) demonstrated the regions of greatest structural weakness and led to the Le Fort classification of fractures of the maxilla (Fig. 240).

CLASSIFICATION OF FRACTURES OF THE MAXILLA

Transverse maxillary, Le Fort I, or Guérin fracture. This fracture occurs transversely through the maxilla above the level of the teeth. The fractured segment contains the alveolar process, portions of the walls of the maxillary sinuses, the palate, and lower portions of the pterygoid processes of the sphenoid bone.

Pyramidal or Le Fort II fracture of the maxilla. This is caused by blows to the upper maxillary region, which produce fractures of the nasal bones and of the frontal processes of the maxilla. The fractures then pass laterally through the lacrimal bones, through the inferior rim of the orbit, through the floor of the orbit, and near or through the zygomaticomaxillary suture. The fractures continue backward along the lateral wall of the maxilla, through the pterygoid plates, and into the pterygomaxillary fossa. This fracture, because of its general shape, has been termed the pyramidal fracture. In severe injuries with comminution, there may be great displacement with damage to the ethmoidal and lacrimal regions, with a sideward spreading, which produces a widening of the interorbital space.

Craniofacial disjunction, Le Fort III. Craniofacial disjunction occurs when the traumatic force is sufficient to cause complete separation of the facial bones from their cranial attachments. The fractures usually occur through the zygomaticofrontal, maxillofrontal, and nasofrontal sutures; through the floors of the orbits; and through the ethmoid and the sphenoid with complete separation of all the structures of the middle facial skeleton from their attachments. In some of these fractures, the maxilla may remain attached to its nasal and zygomatic articulations, but the entire middle third of the face may be detached completely from the skull and be suspended only by soft tissues. Such injuries are almost always associated with multiple fractures of the facial bones (Fig. 241 *A–C*).

Other Fractures of the Maxilla

Alveolar fractures of the maxilla. The alveolar process may be fractured by direct force applied in an anterior or lateral direction or by a force from an upward blow against the mandible. The mandible may be driven forcibly against the maxilla, with an upward and outward force against the maxillary teeth, which results in fracture of the alveolar process and lateral displacement. Such an injury may occur when the chin is forced sharply against the chest. Alveolar fractures may involve bone contain-

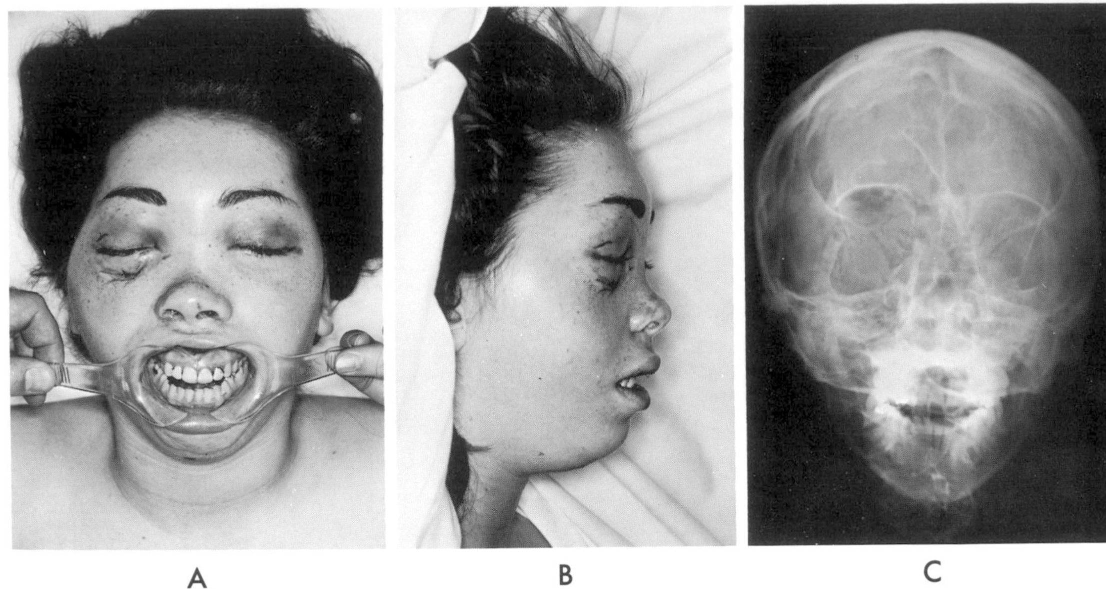

Figure 241. Facial smash injury resulting in multiple facial fractures (Le Fort III). *A*. Front view showing elongation of the face and malocclusion. *B*. Profile view showing dish-face deformity. *C*. Radiograph showing loss of all architectural detail of facial bones.

ing one or more teeth. If the force is severe, complete avulsion of the fragments may occur, but in most cases the fractured alveolar bone is supported by attachments of the adjacent soft tissue.

Vertical fractures of the maxilla. This fracture may result in separation of the two halves of the maxilla. The fracture usually passes to one or the other side of the nasal septum through the thinner portions of the palatine processes of the maxilla and palatine bones, and through the lateral part of the nasal fossa. Such vertical fractures are often associated with fractures of the frontal process of the maxilla and of the nasal bones of the same side. Vertical fractures are caused by a force directed from the side against the anterior portion of the maxilla or the palate.

ETIOLOGY OF FRACTURES OF THE MAXILLA

The increase in incidence of fractures of the maxilla is accounted for by an increase in automobile, airplane, and other high speed transportation accidents. The so-called "guest-passenger" injury occurs when an automobile passenger is thrown forward against the instrument panel or the back of the front seat and strikes the middle third of his face.

The kind of injury sustained depends upon the force, direction, and location of the blow. Fracture of the alveolar process or a transverse fracture of the maxilla may occur if the impact is low on the maxilla. Forces applied at higher levels may result in a comminuted fracture of the maxilla, or the pyramidal fracture. More violent forces at a higher level may result in extensive comminution and craniofacial dislocation. Most forces are directed from before backward, but sidewise or upward forces that strike the anterior part of the maxilla are frequent. Maxillary displacement usually is downward and backward; this gives the appearance of a sunken middle third of the face with elongation. Forces from the side may result in partial fracture of the maxilla or in an alveolar fracture in which the segments of the bone are driven into the maxillary sinus or into the palate. Shattering of the alveolar process, or unilateral maxillary fracture, may be caused by forces from below upward and outward or by force against the mandible transmitted through the teeth outward in all directions.

Impacted fractures of the maxilla are infrequent, but the entire maxilla may be driven upward and backward into the interorbital space, or into the pharyngeal region, and may be firmly impacted. Indeed, the impaction may be so firm that no motion between the fragments can be elicited upon clinical examination, and thus even severe fractures of this kind may be missed. With great displacement, even though no movement can be elicited, the fracture, of course, is discovered easily.

DIAGNOSIS OF FRACTURES OF THE MAXILLA

The diagnosis of fractures of the maxilla is made on the basis of the history, the clinical examination, and the roentgenographic evaluation.

A history of the details of the accident, including the kind, direction, and velocity of the force which caused the injury, may be helpful in establishing a diagnosis. The less severe injuries, which are caused by short falls, blows from fists, and other less traumatic forces, may cause fracture with minimal separation of the fragments and little comminution. Intense forces such as are met, for example, in high speed transportation accidents suggest the probability of severe comminution and displacement of fragments.

Inspection

Evidence of severe soft tissue injury to the facial region is highly suggestive of underlying fractures. Bleeding from the nose, periorbita, and conjunctiva and scleral ecchymosis, or edema and subcutaneous hematoma, are highly suggestive of fractures of the maxillary and nasal regions. Fracture with dislocation results in a "dish-face" deformity, with a long, donkey-like appearance in the middle third of the face (Fig. 242). Malocclusion, open bite with

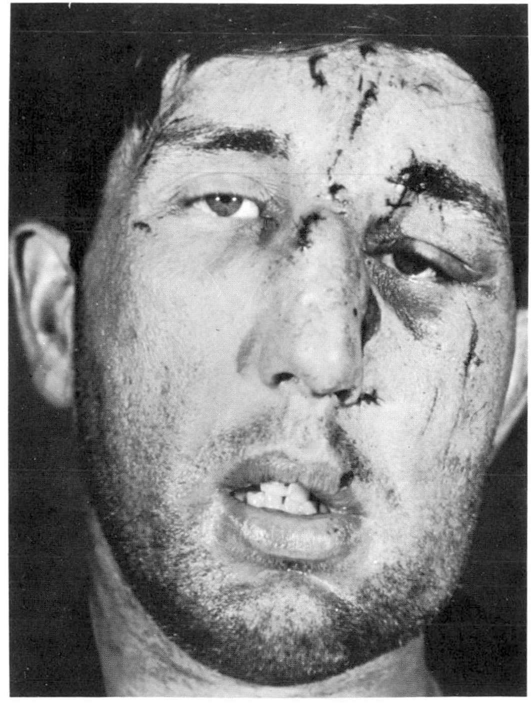

Figure 242. Elongation of the face and depression of left eye in a patient who suffered extensive multiple fractures of the bones in the middle third of the face. The entire nasomaxillary structure and the left zygoma have been displaced downward.

premature contact of the posterior teeth, and posterior displacement of the maxilla may be prominent features. Tearing of the soft tissues of the labial vestibule or of the palate suggests underlying fractures.

Palpation

Simultaneous bilateral bimanual palpation of the orbital margins, the nasal bony processes, the prominences of the zygoma, and the intraoral prominences of the maxilla may indicate irregularities from fractures. Palpation may reveal fractures of the alveolar process with displaced fragments. Steplike defects in the region of the zygomaticomaxillary suture suggest fractures of the infraorbital rim and, probably, pyramidal fractures of the maxilla. Crepitation or movement of the nasal bony processes on palpation indicates that nasal fractures may also have occurred.

DIGITAL MANIPULATION. Mobility of the maxilla may be detected by grasping the anterior portion of the bone between the thumb and index finger. If movement can be elicited, it is suggestive of fracture of the zygomaticomaxillary compound. Alveolar segments containing teeth move easily upon manipulation. One cannot rely, however, only upon movement as a sign for detection of fractures, for some fractures may be impacted and no movement can be elicited on manipulation. Impacted fractures may be overlooked if the occlusion has been only partially impaired. Manipulation of the anterior part of the maxilla may cause movement of the entire middle third of the face, including the dorsum of the nose. Such movement indicates a pyramidal fracture (Le Fort II) or a craniofacial dislocation (Le Fort III). Crepitation may be elicited in some, but not all, cases of anterior maxillary fracture; its absence is no guarantee that the maxilla has not been fractured.

Inspection of the Teeth for Occlusion

Inspection of the teeth for occlusion may help a great deal in establishing a diagnosis. Malocclusion, when the mandible is intact, is highly suggestive of fracture-displacement of the maxilla. Absence of malocclusion, however, is not always significant, for it is possible to have a craniofacial separation and still have fair occlusion. Complete disruption of occlusion occurs in patients in whom the fragments have been rotated or severely displaced.

Detection of Cerebrospinal Rhinorrhea

Severe maxillary fractures with craniofacial dislocation and cribriform plate injury may be associated with the drainage of a clear fluid from the nostrils or from the pharynx. It may be difficult to determine whether this discharge is cerebrospinal fluid or simply mucus from the nose. Chemical examination of the fluid, the continuing appearance of the fluid at the nostrils or in the pharynx, and perhaps the patient's noticing that the fluid tastes salty should suggest to the surgeon that the fluid in question actually is cerebrospinal fluid.

Roentgenographic Findings

The most reliable method of diagnosis of maxillary fracture is by clinical examination, but such examination should be complemented with roentgenography. Because of the superimposition of structures, roentgenographic examination of fractures of the maxilla may be difficult. Stereoscopic roentgenograms in Waters' position are excellent for demonstrating fractures of the maxilla and its associated structures. Fractures of the maxilla without displacement may be difficult to demonstrate. The Waters' projection gives a view with the least possible superimposition of the structures. It shows the lateral walls of the maxillary sinus, the sinuses themselves, the infraorbital margins, and the nasal structures without distortion and with little superimposition from other structures.

Opacity of the roentgenographic image of the maxillary sinus usually means that the sinus is filled, wholly or partially, with blood through a tear of its lining mucous membrane. Fracture of the maxilla may be indicated by disruption of the frontomaxillary or nasofrontal region. Steplike irregularities in the infraorbital regions may indicate zygomaticomaxillary fractures. A break in continuity, or irregularity, of the lateral wall of the sinus usually is present in transverse maxillary fractures. Alveolar fractures are best demonstrated by the occlusal roentgenographic technique. Midsagittal fractures are best demonstrated by the superior-inferior or superior-inferior oblique projection of the hard palate.

TREATMENT OF MAXILLARY FRACTURES

Emergency Treatment

The treatment of the acutely injured patient with a maxillary fracture should be directed toward establishment of a satisfactory airway and control of hemorrhage.

Establishment of the airway. With comminution and displacement of fractured segments of the maxilla, the airway may be impaired or blocked by fragments of bone, displaced soft tissues, blood clots, loose teeth, broken dentures, or extraneous foreign materials. The airway should be established by protraction of the tongue, removal of foreign material from the pharyngeal region, and control of nasal and oral bleeding. If edema of the pharyngeal tissues or lack of bony support prevents creation of an airway, tracheotomy should be done without delay.

Control of hemorrhage. Maxillary fractures associated with lacerations of the oral mucosa and overlying skin may cause severe hemorrhage. The greater palatine vessels or the (internal) maxillary artery may be damaged by the shearing force of displaced maxillary segments. Significant hemorrhage may occur from lacerations and tears of the mucosa of the nasal cavity and the maxillary sinuses. Tears of the larger vessels may result in exsanguinating hemorrhage. Bleeding may be controlled by pressure dressings, packing of the wounds, or posterior pharyngeal tamponade. Ligation of the external carotid artery should be done if less heroic measures cannot control bleeding.

Definitive Care

The definitive care of maxillary fractures, just as in other fractures of the facial skeleton, should be directed toward replacement of the bony fragments and teeth in proper anatomic relations and their support during the course of healing. The method of choice depends upon the degree of fragmentation and the presence or absence of teeth in the maxilla and mandible. Treatment varies from nonoperative procedures to open operation for reduction and fixation.

Treatment of Alveolar Fractures of the Maxilla

When the alveolar process of the maxilla is fractured, whether by an impact from outside or inside the mouth, a fragment which supports one tooth or several teeth may be dislodged. Simple fractures with minimal displacement respond to digital manipulation for reduction. Good splinting by the overlying soft tissues makes fixation unnecessary.

If the teeth are in good apposition, a fragment may be held reduced by ligating the teeth to an arch bar supported by the uninjured alveolar process (Fig. 243). If the fragments cannot be reduced, and if there is premature contact with the teeth of the mandible, traction may place the fragment in its normal position. This kind of reduction can be accomplished by the use of an upper and lower arch bar with intermaxillary rubber band traction. The pressure of the mandible against the fractured segment will reduce it within a few hours. If the traction does not reduce the fragment within 24 hours, it may be assumed that intervening bone or soft tissue prevents reduction. An operation may be necessary to remove the obstruction before the fracture can be reduced satisfactorily. Fixation of fractured alveolar segments should be maintained for three to four weeks.

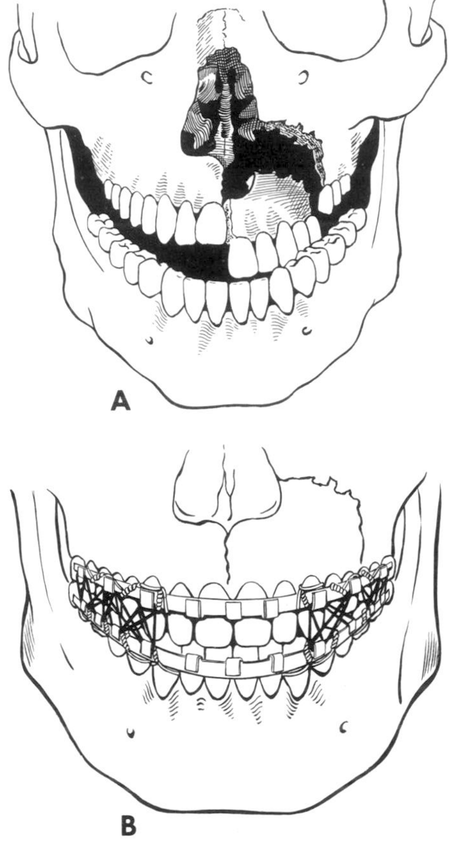

Figure 243. Segmental fracture of the maxilla, including the alveolar ridge and a portion of the palate. *A*. Fracture-dislocation of the anterior and lateral walls of the maxilla and a portion of the palate, with posterior and downward displacement. *B*. Upper and lower arch bars with rubber band traction force the fractured segment into position. The teeth in the fractured segments are ligated to the arch bar for stabilization until healing takes place. The usual period of fixation for such a fracture is three to four weeks.

Treatment of Le Fort I (Transverse, Guérin) Fracture

In the absence of complicating infection, transverse maxillary fractures heal rapidly. The transverse fracture (Le Fort I or Guérin fracture) in which there is a good complement of occluding teeth may be treated by intermaxillary fixation with arch bars and rubber bands as well as a head-cap that includes a chin support. The displacement of the maxilla may be backward or sideways or turned upon the vertical axis. The fractured segment may be loose and suspended only by soft tissues or impacted against the structures immediately above the line of fracture. Reduction usually is accomplished without difficulty in the early case, but in the case of impacted fractures and long-standing displaced maxillary fracture, reduction may be difficult and require extensive manipulative force or anterior traction.

The primary object of treatment in fractures of this kind is the re-establishment of functional dental occlusion, and this reestablishment should be accomplished before the maxilla is fixed. The maxilla is manipulated into a position in which the teeth are in a good occlusal relation, and upward traction is applied. The pressure of the mandible against the maxilla reduces the fracture and holds the fragment or fragments in position until healing occurs. However, head-caps for fixation usually are unreliable and uncomfortable. If prolonged pressure is applied to the chin to reduce the fracture effectively, pressure sores will occur. And, at any rate, more positive fixation can be obtained by internal wire suspension of the mandible and maxilla. Fixation is obtained by suspending the maxilla to the first solid structure above the fracture site. In the transverse maxillary fracture the pyriform margin, the infraorbital ridge, or the zygoma may be used for support.

Internal Wire Fixation for Transverse Fracture of the Maxilla (Le Fort I)

Utilizing the intact mandible and the dental occlusion as the guide for positioning of the maxilla, infraorbital fixation is carried through small incisions just below the bony margins of the orbit. Drill holes are made on both sides through the infraorbital rim lateral to the infraorbital foramen. The incision in the lower lid is the same as described for reduction of fractures of the zygoma (see Chapter 7, Part 2). One end of the long stainless steel wire, 24 or 25 gauge, is passed through the hole in the infraorbital ridge and is looped over the infraorbital margin. Both ends of the wire are directed through a passing needle into the mouth, where they are secured to the upper arch bar. The teeth are held in occlusion by intermaxillary rubber band traction, and while the assistant applies upward and slightly backward pressure against the chin to reduce the maxillary fracture, the wires are twisted securely around the upper arch bar. By this method the maxilla is guided into position by occlusion with the intact mandible and is supported by the wire from the infraorbital ridge to the upper arch bar. Care is taken to approximate the periosteum over the infraorbital ridge and the wound is closed in layers.

Accurate reduction and positive fixation by this method are possible with minimum effort and maximum comfort to the patient. The patient may return to productive activity very early because the arch bars and internal wires are concealed and there is little possibility of the appliance slipping or getting out of adjustment.

Treatment of Le Fort II (Pyramidal) Fracture

As in the lower level Le Fort I or transverse maxillary fracture, displacement depends upon the degree and direction of the fracturing force. If the fracture is displaced backward, reduction is obtained by forward traction until the teeth are brought into such apposition that normal occlusion can be obtained. After reduction of the pyramidal fracture, the teeth are placed in normal occlusion and fixed by upper and lower arch bars with rubber band traction. With the intact mandible as a guide, the maxilla is brought into anatomic position.

Fixation may be attained by direct interosseous wiring in the infraorbital area on both sides if there has been little comminution at the orbital margins and if there is not an associated fracture of the zygoma. Fixation may be obtained also by craniomaxillary suspension wires passed from the zygomatic process of the frontal bone down through the soft tissues medial to the zygoma into the vestibule of the mouth in the region of the premolar teeth. One wire on each side is passed medially to the mandibular arch bar, the other laterally to it. The surgeon's assistant applies traction upward against the mandible to force the maxilla

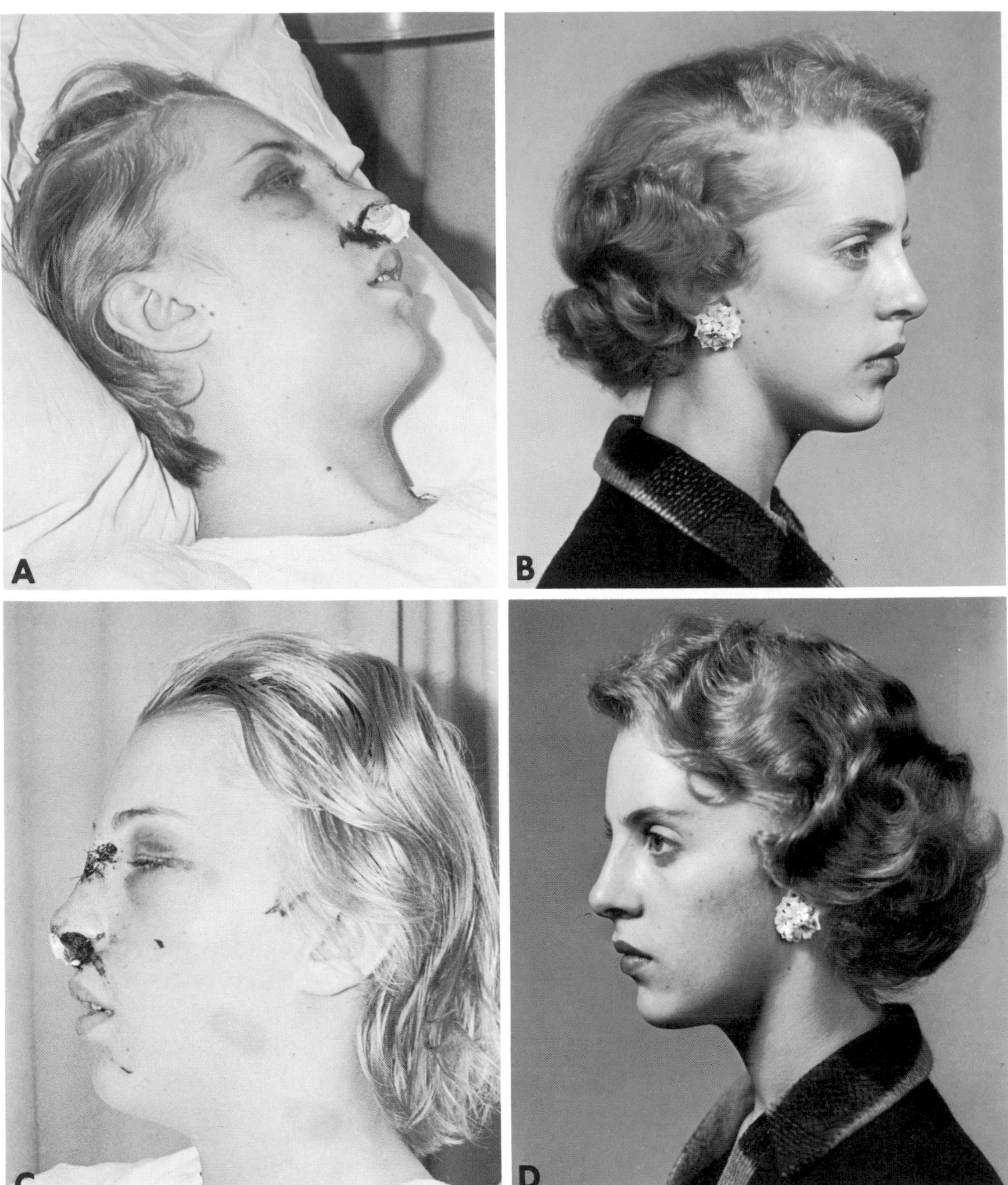

Figure 244. Compound comminuted pyramidal fracture of the maxilla involving the left zygoma with a smash fracture of the nasal bones and nasal septum. Treated by craniofacial internal wire suspension and interosseous fixation of multiple bone fragments. This operation was performed under general anesthesia administered through a tracheotomy tube. *A.* Right profile, preoperative view. *B.* Profile view one year after operation. *C.* Left profile, preoperative view. *D.* Left profile one year after surgery. *E.* Waters' view showing multiple facial fractures, including a pyramidal fracture of the maxilla and the left zygoma, and

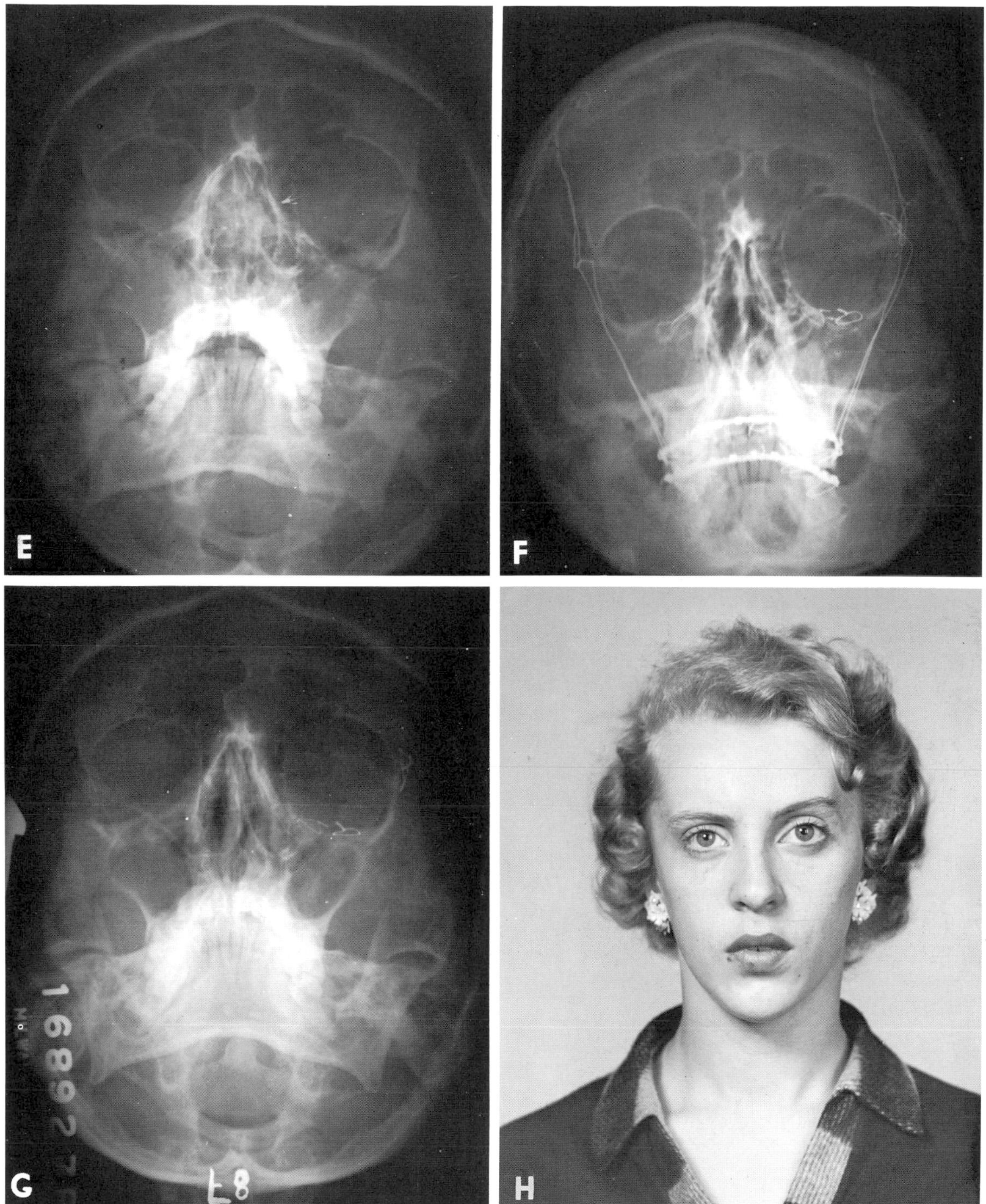

smash fracture of the nasal bones and septum. *F.* Waters' projection showing fixation appliances, cranial suspension, and interosseous wire fixation. *G.* Waters' view one year after operation. *H.* Front view one year after surgery. Note minimal scar from tracheotomy.

into position while the surgeon himself tightens the suspension wires about the mandibular arch bar. Forehead and infraorbital pull-out wires facilitate the removal of the suspension wires at the termination of treatment (Fig. 244 *A–H*).

Treatment of Le Fort III (Craniofacial Disjunction) Fracture

The Le Fort III fracture (craniofacial disjunction) of the maxilla is associated with fractures of the zygoma and nose. Its management will be considered in Chapter 10.

Management of Impacted or Partially Healed Fractures of the Maxilla in Malposition

Fractures of the maxilla heal rapidly, and those seen two or three weeks after injury may be difficult or impossible to reduce manually or by the other usual methods. Early malunion and impacted fractures sometimes respond well to reduction by skeletal traction.

Under most circumstances the use of head-caps and other appliances to provide external traction is unsatisfactory, but the head-cap may be useful in the treatment of some impacted or early malunion fractures of the maxilla. A plaster head-cap is constructed to include an outrigger which projects downward and forward in front of the face. An upper arch bar provides an attachment for a wire loop. Strong rubber band traction is applied between the projection on the head-cap and the upper arch bar.

Extraskeletal traction has been effective in cases in which it was impossible or impracticable to use a head-cap for skeletal traction. Traction on the maxilla is obtained by using a rope passed through pulleys attached to a bed frame. One end of the rope is attached by a hook to the upper arch bar and a moderate amount of weight is applied to the system, which must be watched carefully to prevent over-reduction. When the maxillary segment comes forward far enough to permit reasonable occlusion, as indicated by maxillary-mandibular tooth relations, additional intermaxillary fixation is applied.

The Edentulous Maxilla

Fractures of the edentulous maxilla are seen less frequently than fractures of the maxilla containing teeth, and they are usually associated with extensive fractures of the other bones of the middle third of the face. Fractures of the edentulous maxilla are seen infrequently because of the absence of teeth through which fracturing forces may be transmitted. Older patients are exposed less frequently to the hazards of youth; this undoubtedly reduces the incidence of maxillary fractures in the edentulous jaw. Artificial dentures give protection to the edentulous maxilla. Forces that would fracture teeth or the alveolar bone in the patient with teeth are absorbed or dissipated by breaking of the artificial denture. Fractures of the edentulous maxilla are caused by direct frontal or lateral blows to the bone in nearly all cases.

If displacement is minimal, with little or no facial deformity, the discrepancy between the maxilla and the mandible can be corrected by adjustment of the dentures, and treatment seldom is necessary. The fractures heal in two or three weeks without treatment. New dentures may be constructed as soon as the edema and hematomas have subsided.

If displacement of the fractured segments is significant and results in deformity of the middle third of the face, thus posing problems for the construction of new artificial dentures, an effort should be made to reduce and immobilize the bone fragments. If the fracture is transverse (Le Fort I) and the upper denture is usable, the fracture may be reduced manually and fixed by use of the denture (Fig. 245). The denture is applied to the maxilla and is brought into normal occlusal relations with the natural lower teeth or with the patient's lower artificial denture. A head-cap with a chin support used for a few days may be enough to hold the fragments in position without further fixation. Sufficient healing generally takes place in a matter of ten days to two weeks.

If the displacement is significant and the patient has no upper denture, open reduction of the fracture and direct wiring at the pyriform margin or at the zygomaticomaxillary suture line may be done. In the pyramidal (Le Fort II) fracture, the upper denture is wired to the fractured segments by a circumferential wire anteriorly and posteriorly. The denture then is brought into occlusion with the patient's own lower teeth or his lower denture. With the mandible as a guide, the anatomic position of the maxillary fragments can be determined readily, and fixation may be maintained by internal wire suspension from the infra-orbital margins or from the zygomatic process of the frontal bone.

Comminuted displaced fractures of the anterior maxillary wall may be reduced by an open operation through an incision in the canine fossa. The sinus is packed with a rubber drain or gauze strips to hold the fractured segments in position. The end of the gauze is brought out through a nasal antrostomy under the inferior turbinate. Fixation for 8 to 10 days permits the fracture segments to heal in normal position (see Fig. 211).

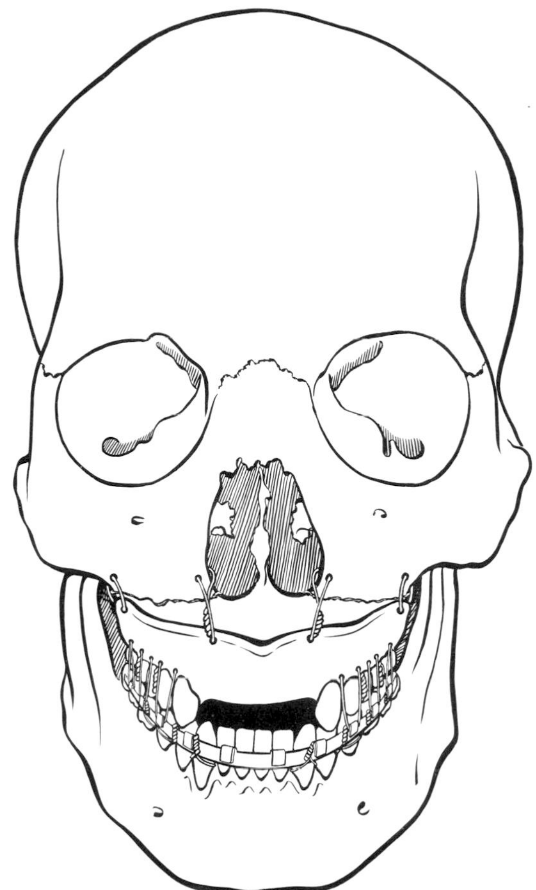

Figure 245. Fixation of a transverse maxillary fracture (Le Fort I) in an edentulous maxilla by supporting the maxilla with the patient's upper denture. Suspension wires are passed through drill holes in the pyriform margin of the nasal cavity and through the zygomatic process of the maxilla. Removal of four maxillary anterior teeth from the denture facilitates feeding the patient.

Postoperative Care of Maxillary Fractures

The postoperative management of fractures of the maxilla consists of the usual methods of blood and fluid replacement, adequate nutrition, and antibiotics when these are indicated. The local care of the wounds requires frequent cleansing of the mouth with irrigations or saline mouthwashes. The nasal cavity is involved frequently and may present problems in maintaining an adequate airway. Nosedrops containing vasoconstricting drugs and frequent suctioning of the nasal cavity usually will keep the airway open and provide adequate ventilation of the maxillary sinuses so that disintegrating clotted blood and mucus in the sinuses will drain adequately. Soft tissue wounds require frequent cleansing and early removal of sutures to avoid scarring along the line of closure.

COMPLICATIONS OF MAXILLARY FRACTURES

Early Complications

Hemorrhage. Extensive hemorrhage due to the acute trauma causing the fracture results from laceration of the soft tissues or tearing or shearing of major vessels by displaced fragments of bone. This may threaten exsanguination if not treated rapidly.

Airway obstruction. In fractures above the level of the teeth, the nasal cavity and the maxillary sinuses are involved. The margin of the nasal aperture is composed of the frontal processes of the maxilla, and fractures of these processes, with displacement, may encroach upon and compromise the airway. Blood clots, fragments of bone, and tooth structures should be removed from the nasal cavities and the pharyngeal area as soon as possible. An oral airway or a nasopharyngeal tube passed through one of the nostrils may help establish an airway. If these measures do not give a good airway, tracheotomy should be performed. The frequent use of constricting nosedrops and removal of blood and mucus by suction is helpful in the management of the complication of the obstructed upper airway.

Infection. Fractures of the maxilla may be complicated by infection introduced at the time of injury, by the presence of loose teeth or bone fragments in the soft tissues or in the maxillary sinuses, or by fractures through a sinus with a pre-existing chronic infection. Appropriate methods of management of local infection include opening and drainage of the maxillary sinus; removal of foreign bodies, bone fragments, or teeth from the sinuses or the nasal cavity; the insertion of drains where indicated; and the use of appropriate antibiotics. Maxillary fractures may be associated with fractures of the ethmoid or its cribriform plate with a leaking of cerebrospinal fluid from the nose or from the pharyngeal area. Prophylactic antibiotics should be given and the fractures reduced as soon as the patient is in satisfactory condition. The patient should be prohibited from blowing his nose. Antral packing and suction should be avoided in the presence of cerebrospinal rhinorrhea.

Late Complications

Malunion, nonunion, nasal obstruction, chronic sinusitis, malocclusion, deformity, interference with function of the lacrimal apparatus, loss of sense of smell, and anesthesia are all late complications of fracture of the maxilla.

The Maxilla

PART 2

OPERATIVE TECHNIQUE

The great importance of the maxilla becomes apparent if we regard the upper jaw as the antagonist of the mandible and keep in mind that it consists essentially of the two maxillary and two palatine bones and that it furthermore is linked by complicated buttresses to the cranial base. Forming the skeleton of the middle face, it also furnishes walls to the orbit, to some of the paranasal sinuses, and to the nasal and oral cavities.

This structural and functional complexity of the maxilla makes accurate repositioning of fractured maxillary fragments critical indeed. Accurate repositioning is essential to restoration of functional dental occlusion, establishment of an adequate airway, restoration of appearance of the middle facial area, and support of the contents of the orbit.

Open operations can be carried out safely upon the maxilla. The approach illustrated in the following pages has proved to be eminently effective in producing consistently excellent results both functionally and esthetically.

Meticulous attention to the details of this chapter should result in gratifying experiences to the surgeon and in safe and helpful procedures to his patients.

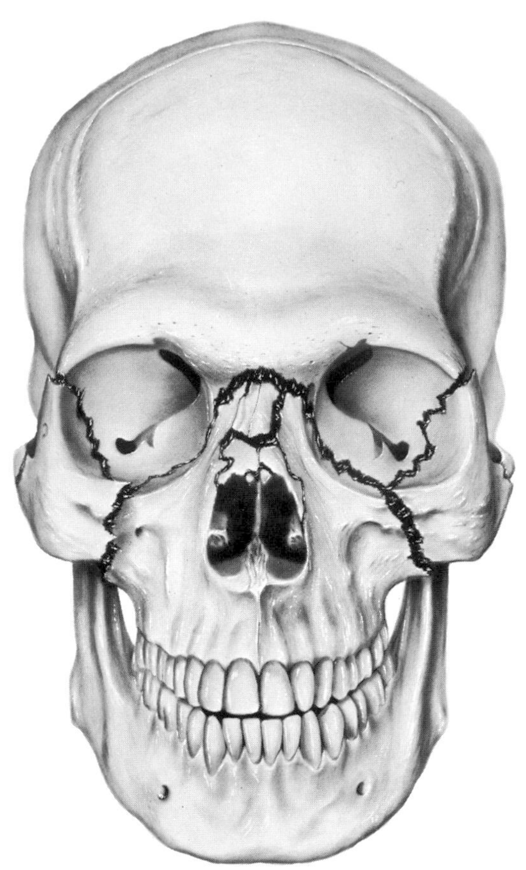

1

Fig. 246. Severe trauma to the middle third of the face may result in complete craniofacial dislocation. The facial bones are broken loose from their articulations at the base of the skull. This fracture with craniofacial disjunction is associated frequently with fractures of the cribriform plate, causing lacerations of the dura and cerebrospinal rhinorrhea. Many or all of the facial bones may be involved with comminution and downward and posterior displacement. The fractured segments may be supported only by soft tissue attachments.

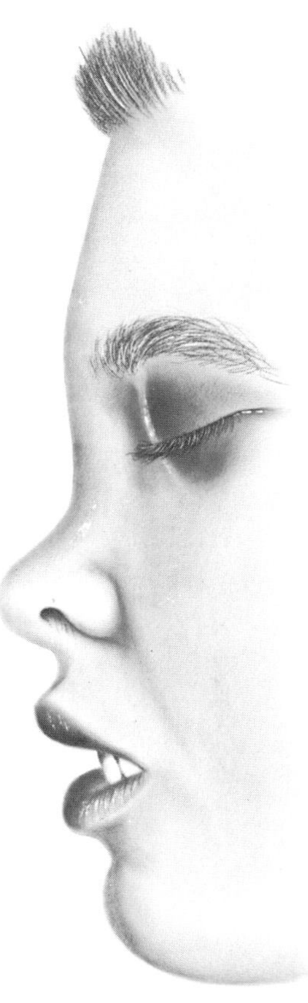

2

Fig. 247. Fractures due to trauma to the nasal region may result in craniofacial dislocation (Le Fort III fracture) with comminution of the nasal bones, septum, ethmoid, and sphenoid with a dish-face profile.

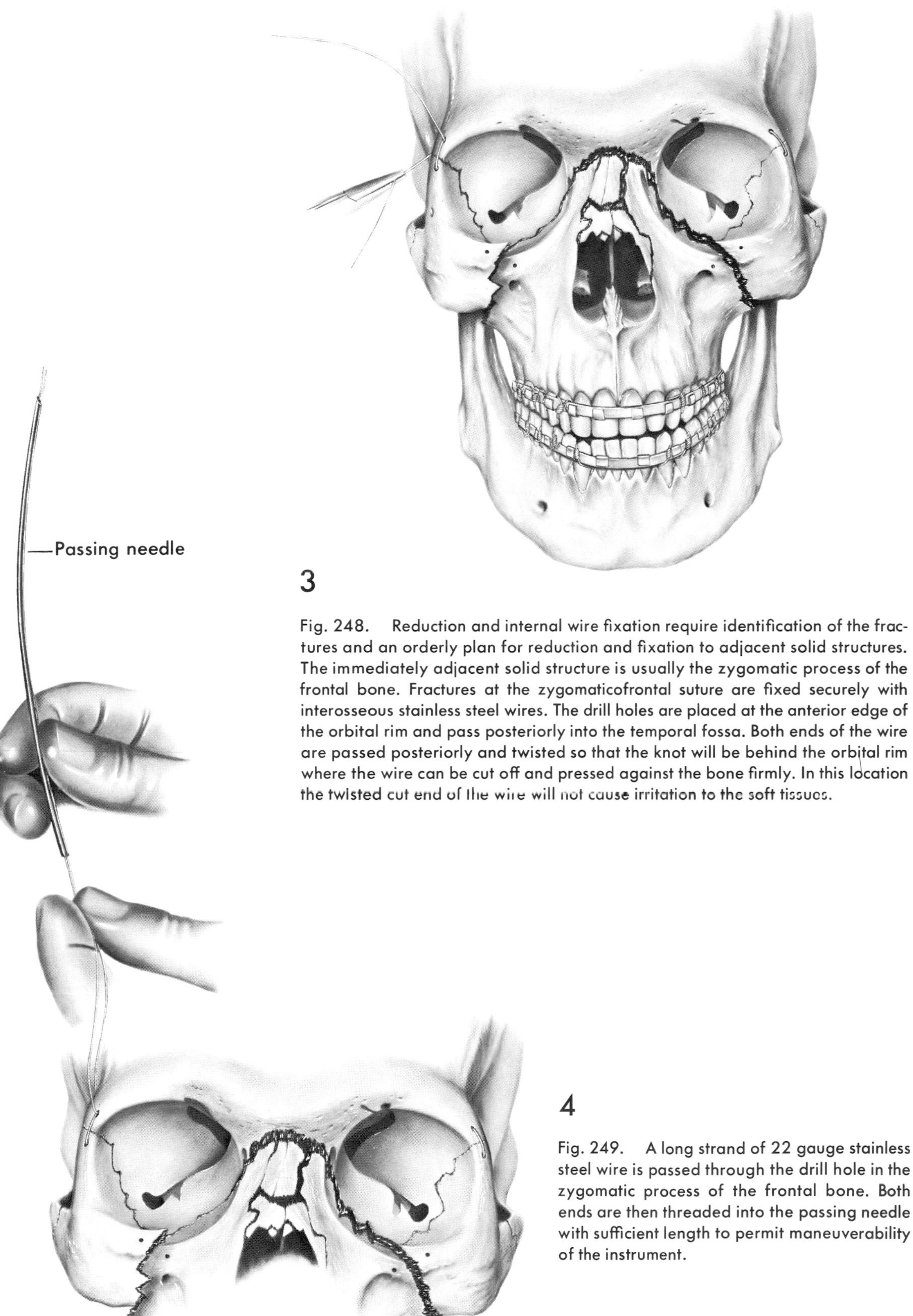

3

Fig. 248. Reduction and internal wire fixation require identification of the fractures and an orderly plan for reduction and fixation to adjacent solid structures. The immediately adjacent solid structure is usually the zygomatic process of the frontal bone. Fractures at the zygomaticofrontal suture are fixed securely with interosseous stainless steel wires. The drill holes are placed at the anterior edge of the orbital rim and pass posteriorly into the temporal fossa. Both ends of the wire are passed posteriorly and twisted so that the knot will be behind the orbital rim where the wire can be cut off and pressed against the bone firmly. In this location the twisted cut end of the wire will not cause irritation to the soft tissues.

4

Fig. 249. A long strand of 22 gauge stainless steel wire is passed through the drill hole in the zygomatic process of the frontal bone. Both ends are then threaded into the passing needle with sufficient length to permit maneuverability of the instrument.

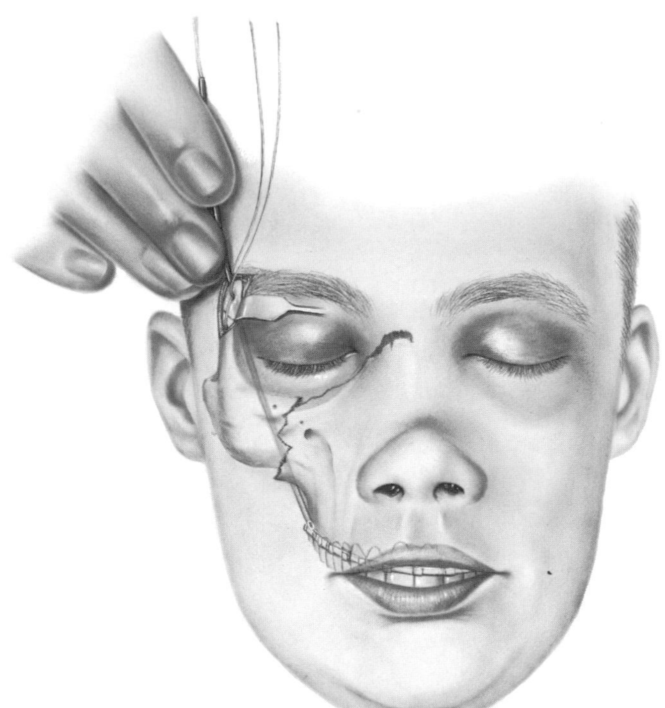

5

Fig. 250. The pointed end of the passing needle is placed in the brow incision and directed downward on the temporal side of the zygoma along the lateral wall of the maxilla into the mouth opposite the premolar or molar teeth.

6

Fig. 251. Proper curvature of the passing needle permits it to be guided easily into the buccal vestibule opposite the upper second premolar or first molar tooth.

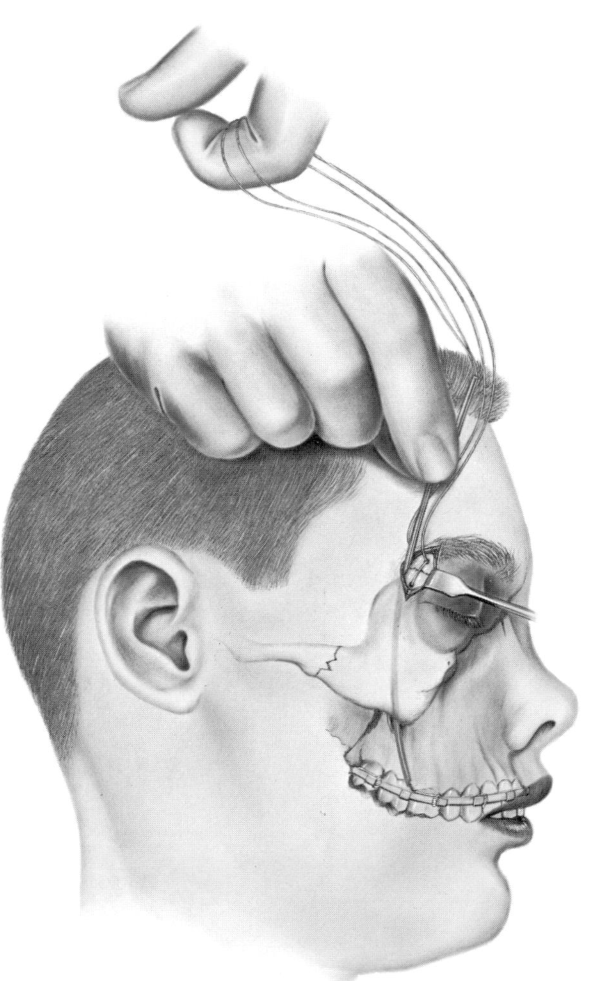

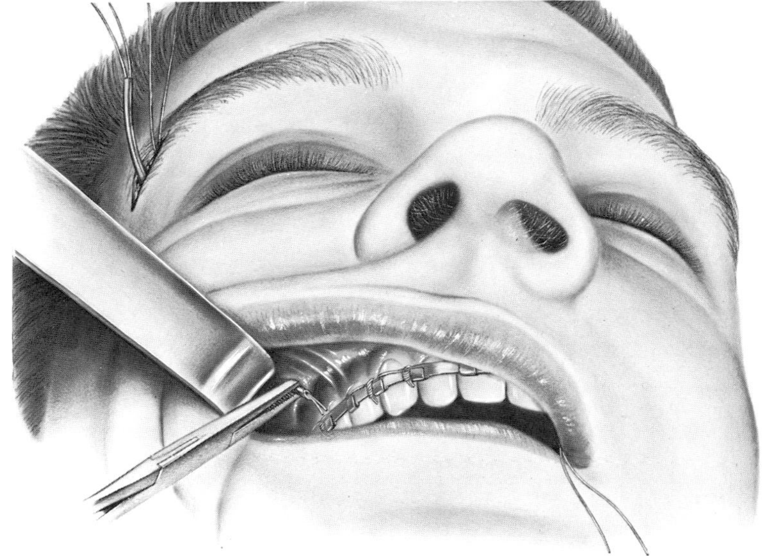

7

Fig. 252. As the beveled end of the passing needle comes into the mouth through the buccal mucosa, the end is grasped with a hemostat and pulled through into the mouth. The wires are pulled down and rest at the corner of the mouth. Precaution is taken to avoid buckling or bending of the wire at the site of the drill hole in the frontal bone. After the long wires, to be used for craniofacial suspension, have been brought out through the mouth, the teeth are brought into occlusion and fixed by intermaxillary rubber band traction.

8

Fig. 253. When the teeth are in occlusion, an assistant exerts firm traction against the inferior border of the mandible to produce upward force. Simultaneous traction on the anterior maxilla and on the nasal bone structures by means of an Asch forceps will permit the facial bones to come into proper position.

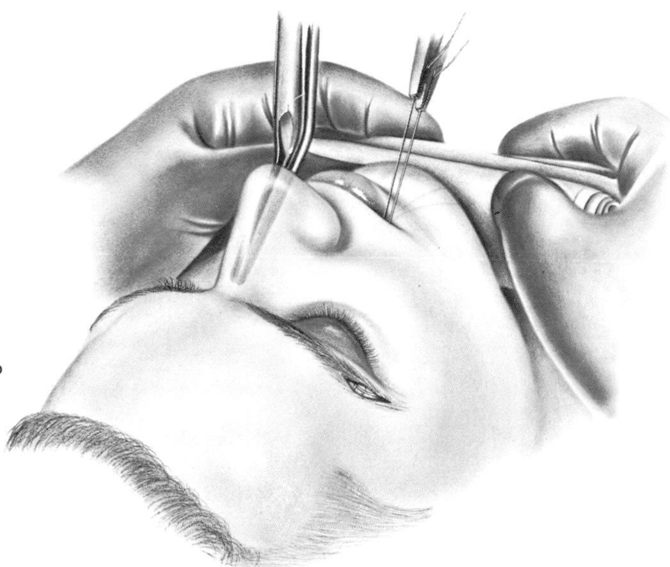

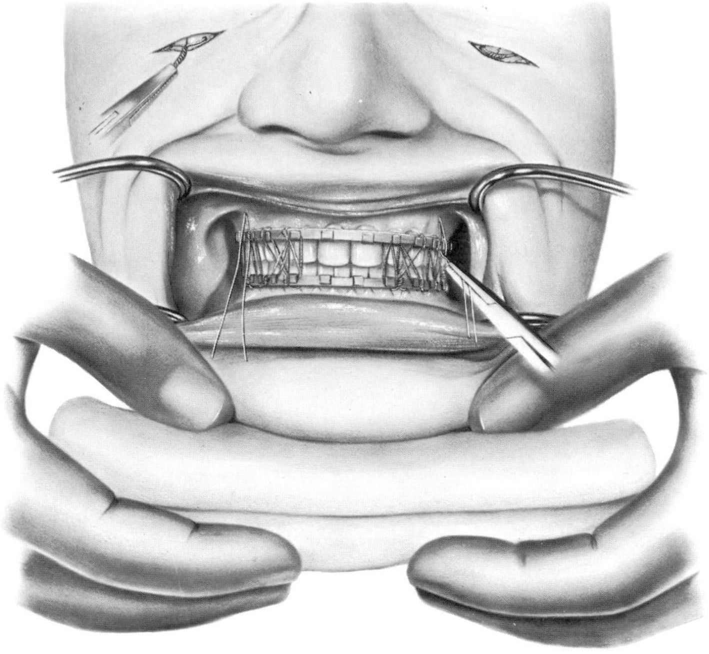

9

Fig. 254. One of the cranial suspension wires is passed on the inner surface of the upper arch bar in the premolar region, and the other is brought out on the outer surface of the bar. When satisfactory positioning of the total bony complex has been established, pressure is maintained against the mandible and the cranial suspension wires are twisted securely against the arch bar.

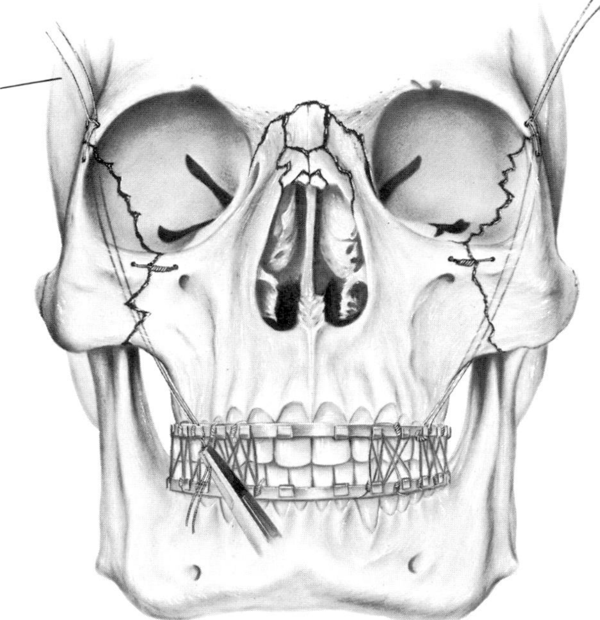

10

Fig. 255. Craniofacial suspension supplemented with interosseous wire fixation at the infraorbital areas and at the zygomaticofrontal sutures gives positive fixation at the fracture sites. The intact mandible and normal dental occlusal relations provide a guide for reduction of fractures in the middle third of the face. Pull-out wires in the forehead region simplify the removal of the cranial suspension wires. At the end of the period of fixation, which is usually four or five weeks, the long wires are cut as they emerge through the oral mucosa. Tension on the pull-out wires permits easy removal. The small interosseous wires cause no reaction and are not removed.

CHAPTER
9

THE NOSE

PART 1

GENERAL CONSIDERATIONS

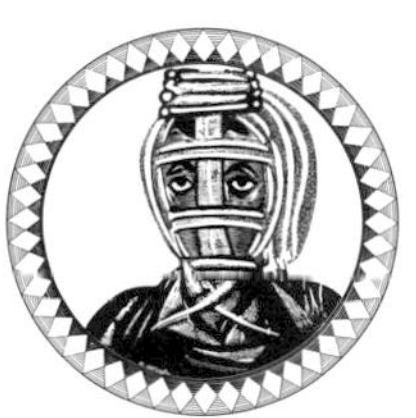

The prominent position of the nose subjects it frequently to trauma. Nasal fractures are secondary in occurrence only to fractures of the clavicle and wrist. Injury may result in esthetic and functional disability of great importance. In cases of acute injury, restoration of appearance and function is best attained by early management of cartilaginous and bony fractures and dislocations.

All severe blows to the nose should be suspected to have caused fractures or dislocations. Early treatment is relatively easy and usually satisfactory. Delay in treatment or neglect of nasal bone fractures may result in a deformity that is difficult or impossible to correct.

Any of the parts comprising the nasal framework may be damaged. One or both nasal bones may be fractured or detached from the maxilla, the septum, or the frontal bone; from each other; or from the cartilages. Complicating fractures of the cribriform plate or the perpendicular plate of the ethmoid, of the lacrimal bones, and of the vomer are not uncommon. The cartilages may be torn loose from their attachments to the septum, the nasal bones, or the maxilla. The cartilages may be torn or fractured and displaced. The septal cartilage is highly susceptible to fracture-displacement. It may be deviated to one side or, in a sigmoid fashion, to both sides. It may be dislodged from the maxilla or torn loose from its attachments to the perpendicular plate of the ethmoid and the vomer. The alar cartilages may be lacerated or separated by severe blows upon the tip of the nose.

SURGICAL ANATOMY OF THE NOSE

The external nose is pyramidal. It forms the anterior wall of the nasal fossae. Its free anterior surface is continuous at its root with the forehead, and its lateral surfaces join the cheeks and the movable alae. The nose terminates below at the tip or lobule where the base of the pyramid presents two openings, the nares, separated by a median structure, the columella and septum. Bones and cartilages support the thin subcutaneous layer and the skin on the outside and, similarly, the submucosa and mucosa on the inside of the nose. Muscular, nervous, and vascular structures pass between the mucosa and the overlying skin. Cartilaginous tissues support the lower two-thirds of the nose, while the upper third is supported by the nasal bones and the frontal processes of the maxilla. The skin overlying the upper two-thirds of the nose is thin, pliable, and freely movable on the underlying subcutaneous structures. The thick, immovable skin of the tip is rich in sebaceous glands and is tightly fixed to the perichondrium of the cartilaginous structures. The excellent blood supply of the skin and the mucosa of the nose permits early uncomplicated recovery from injury and extensive operative dissection. Lacerations and soft tissue injuries heal rapidly and usually with little scarring.

The cartilages are the triangular or upper lateral cartilages, which are continuous with the quadrilateral septal cartilage, and the alar or lower cartilages, which are supplemented by sesamoid and minor cartilages in the lateral alar regions. The bony structures include the paired nasal bones, the frontal processes of the maxilla, and the bones of the septum.

The Bones of the Nose

The paired nasal bones comprise the upper portion of the nasal framework. They articulate with the frontal processes of the maxilla laterally, and superiorly with the nasal spine of the frontal bone. The bones articulate with each other in the midline and are held in a viselike fashion between the frontal processes of the maxilla and the nasal process of the frontal bone. The nasal bones are thick at their articulations and in their upper two-thirds, but become thinner near the lower part of the organ where they are subjected frequently to trauma and fractures. The bony nasal septum articulates with the undersurface of the nasal bones and acts as a pillar to lend additional support of the nasal dorsum.

The Cartilages of the Nose

The cartilages give form to the lower half of the nose and support the skin externally and the mucosa and nasal lining internally. The upper lateral cartilages have semirigid attachments to their articulating bones but a less rigid membranous attachment to the alar cartilages. Movement of the alar cartilages by the musculature of the nose is important in facial expression. The lower boundaries of the nasal bones and the maxilla make up the pyriform opening of the nasal cavity.

The Nasal Septum

The partition of the cavity, the nasal septum, is a thin vertical structure made up of cartilage and bone. The nasal tip is supported by the quadrilateral cartilage of the septum, which in turn is supported below by the maxilla and vomer and behind and above by the perpendicular plate of the ethmoid. Its anterior portion is attached by fibrous tissues to the alar cartilages and continues into the triangular cartilages. The fibrous tissue between the anterior edge of the septal cartilage and the medial crura of the alar cartilages permits considerable movement of the nasal tip and is known as the false or the membranous septum.

The septum divides the nasal cavity into two chambers. It is made up of a cartilaginous and bony structure covered by perichondrium and periosteum, respectively, which, together with the mucosa form a continuous covering. The vomer and the perpendicular plate of the ethmoid, attached to the nasal crest of the palatine bone and nasal crest of the maxillae, make up the bony septum. Traumatic epistaxis, tears, or hematomas in the nasal mucosa are highly suggestive of fractures. These findings almost always are associated with fractures because of the intimate relations of the nasal lining with the supporting structures. Fractures and displacements of the cartilages may occur independently of bone injury, but usually are associated with fractures of the bony framework.

FRACTURES OF THE NOSE IN CHILDREN

Unrecognized, untreated fractures of the nose in children are of greatest importance. Normal growth and development of the facial structures may be impaired seriously. Nasal fractures in children frequently are overlooked. The small structures may be difficult to evaluate because of hematoma, edema, or tenderness following the injury. It can be assumed safely that any child who has epistaxis following an injury to the nose has sustained a fracture. If necessary, examination and reduction should be done under general anesthesia. The serious consequences of lack of treatment are manifested by external and internal nasal deformity in adult life. Examination and elevation of the nasal structures of children under anesthesia is warranted in order to avoid the possibility of overlooking fracture-displacement of the bone or cartilages. Operation is not indicated in every child who receives a blow to the nose, but if there is any suggestion of deformity, this may be the only way of making a positive diagnosis. For discussion in greater detail, see Chapter 11, Facial Fractures in Children.

NASAL FRACTURES IN THE ADULT

The kind and extent of fractures in the adult varies with the site of the impact and the direction and intensity of the force. Nasal fractures are caused by direct forces from the front, from the base, or from the side.

Violent, direct, frontal forces may result in smash fractures of the nasal bones, the frontal process of the maxilla, the lacrimal bones, and the septum. In this kind of fracture the structures are squashed, and comminuted fragments may be driven into the orbit or into the ethmoidal region. Lateral splaying of the fragments may result in severe soft tissue damage with lateral displacement of the lacrimal bones and medial palpebral ligaments. Splayed nasal fractures may be associated with damage to the nasolacrimal ducts, the perpendicular plate of the ethmoid, the ethmoidal sinuses, the cribriform plate, and the orbital parts of the frontal bone. There may be comminution with broadening and widening of the interorbital space, dacryocystitis, interference with drainage of the tears, permanent

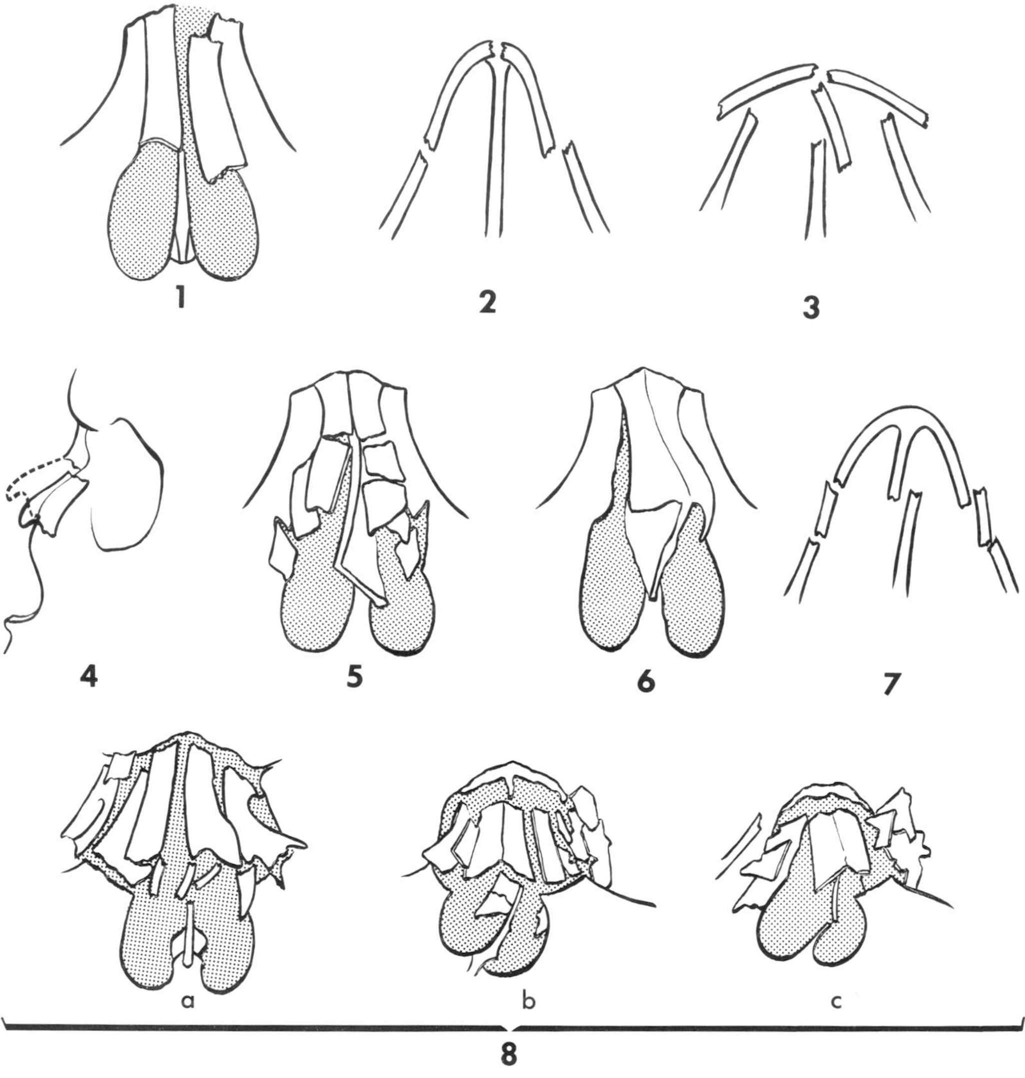

Figure 256. Fractures of the nasal bones. (1) Isolation of one nasal bone with inferolateral displacement. (2) Diagrammatic horizontal section showing separation of the nasal bones in the midline and from the frontal process of the maxilla; nasal septum intact. (3) Fracture of the septum permits a flattening and spreading of the nasal bones; open-book fracture. (4) Fracture of the two nasal bones with posteroinferior displacement. (5) Comminuted fracture of the nasal bones and the anterior parts of the frontal processes and the nasal septum; displacement mainly down and back. (6) Fracture of the nasal septum with separation of the nasal bones from the frontal process of the maxilla with elevation of the bridge of the nose. (7) Cross-sectional diagram of a fracture similar to that in 6. (8) Three examples of smash fracture of the nose with embarrassment of the interorbital space.

epiphora, and permanent pseudohypertelorism unless the displacements are corrected properly (Fig. 256).

Fractures of the nose from force applied to the side may involve only one nasal bone with medial displacement, but most commonly in adults a violent blow from the side results in fractures of both nasal bones and fracture of the nasal septum with lateral shifting of the entire bony framework. The bone on the side of the injury is displaced medially, the one on the opposite side laterally (Fig. 257). Early complete blocking of the airway by pieces of bone, cartilage, or mucosa, or by extensive edema and blood clots, usually is seen following severe nasal injuries. This obstruction makes complete evaluation of the injuries difficult, especially if the patient is seen a few hours after the accident. The septal cartilage or the triangular or alar cartilages, any or all, may be fractured independently or in conjunction with fractures of the nasal bones.

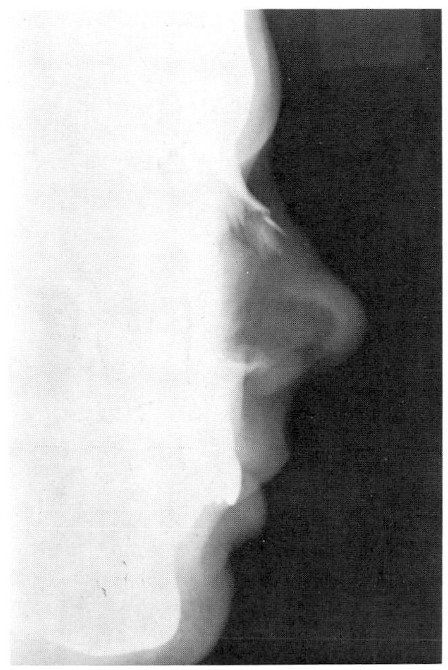

Figure 257. Lateral roentgenogram of nose, showing fracture of the left nasal bone.

The flexibility of the septal cartilage permits it to absorb injuries of moderate degree without fracture. In more severe injuries the septum may be fractured or displaced from the maxillary crest, from the vomerine groove, or from its attachment at the anterior nasal spine of the maxilla, with displacement into the adjacent airway. Fractures of the septum occur in the vertical plane. They may telescope and overlap. The anterior part of the septum, which is less securely attached than its posterior part, may be fractured and displaced posteriorly. Fracture of the quadrilateral cartilage at its junction with the perpendicular plate of the ethmoid and displacement backward result in shortening of the nose, retraction of the columella, and deepening of the nasolabial folds.

A common deformity seen in adults, undoubtedly caused by trauma in childhood, is the severe angulation of the septum about 1 cm. from the anterior edge, which angulation, partial or complete, obstructs one of the nostrils. The septal cartilage behind may deviate to obstruct the opposite naris. In such a deformity, the nasal dorsum is deviated and the tip is dragged laterally with the deviated cartilage. Lack of tip support in septal deformities is recognizable by separation of the alar cartilages with a flat, broad-tipped nose.

THE DIAGNOSIS OF NASAL FRACTURES

A history of the injury and roentgenographic studies are helpful in establishing a diagnosis of fractures of the nose, but clinical evaluation is the most important factor. Helpful points in the history are the direction, degree of severity, and kind of the injuring force, the presence of pre-existent nasal disease, the history of previous operations upon the nose, and the appearance of the nose before injury.

Roentgenographic examination may be helpful in diagnosis but often shows nothing in the usual views. Fractures may be demonstrated well by using a dental x-ray film held at the side of the nose and parallel to the sagittal plane, with exposure of the film from the side. The bony septum may be shown well by the Waters' or reverse Waters' projections (see Figs. 52 and 53), and the view for nasal bones, lateral projection, may demonstrate fractures of the nasal bone (see Fig. 257). If the bones are prominent and extend beyond the forehead-chin line, they may be demonstrated by using the superior-inferior projection of the nasal bones with occlusal films (see Fig. 58).

Clinical evaluation is the most reliable procedure in assessing the total injury. Exact diagnosis may be difficult because of edema, hematoma, and lacerations, especially if the patient is seen a few hours after the injury. Edema of the lids, periorbital ecchymosis, and subconjunctival hemorrhages are usually seen. Nasal obstruction may result from edema, blood clots, swelling of the mucosa of the turbinate bones, or dislocated bony, cartilaginous, and mucosal parts. Subcutaneous emphysema may be present because of the patient's repeated efforts to blow blood clots from his nose. Air passes through the torn mucoperiosteum and spreads in the subcutaneous tissues.

Movement of fragments with crepitation on palpation and with great tenderness may be prominent features. Movement, of course, is difficult to elicit in cases of displaced, impacted telescopic fractures. Edema and dislocation of tissues may make it difficult to detect lacerations and fractures of the intranasal structures. To evaluate the injury adequately, the mucosa should be shrunk with a cocaine-adrenalin solution and the intranasal structures examined carefully with a nasal speculum, a good light, and suction for the removal of mucus, clots, and debris. Lacerations of the mucosa occur frequently at the junction of the upper lateral cartilages and at their attachment to the bony margins. Fractured bone segments may act as secondary missiles and cause laceration of the intranasal mucosa, or the soft tissues may be forced upward and sheared off at the bone margin.

THE TREATMENT OF NASAL FRACTURES

The best opportunity for successful management of nasal fractures exists during the first two or three hours after the injury has been sustained and before the true state of injury has been obscured by edema, hematoma, and obstruction of the airway. Most simple fractures of the nose respond well to outpatient management in which the bones are elevated and the septum straightened with a rubber-covered forceps or specially designed septal forceps. Extensive comminuted compound fractures require special management. In all cases the best results are obtained under conditions that permit adequate anesthesia, a good light for intranasal illumination, suction equipment, and adequate surgical equipment.

Anesthesia

Accurate evaluation and manipulation of the fractured nose is not possible without good anesthesia. Children are best managed under general anesthesia, even if the procedure is brief. Endotracheal intubation is the technique of choice, because it gives the operator an opportunity to assess the damage accurately and to obtain good reduction and fixation in a methodical, careful manner.

Whether under local or general anesthesia, the operation is facilitated by inserting into the nostrils cotton pledgets soaked in a cocaine-epinephrine or xylocaine-epinephrine solution. These vasoconstricting anesthetic drugs give good anesthesia, reduce edema, and decrease the amount of bleeding that occurs when reduction is performed. Good vasoconstriction and anesthesia is obtained by using a quantity of 10 per cent solution of cocaine with an equal quantity of 1:1000 epinephrine. If edema of the mucosa is severe, changing of the packs two or three times over a period of 15 to 20 minutes will shrink the mucosa so that the intranasal structures can be carefully inspected.

For the adult patient, the use of intranasal topical anesthesia in conjunction with the injection of local anesthetic solutions containing epinephrine, such as those used in the preparation of the patient about to undergo rhinoplasty, gives an excellent result (Dingman, 1961). This kind of anesthesia makes it possible to reduce most nasal fractures with ease and with little discomfort to the patient. It is frustrating to have an uncomfortable patient squirming about on the operating room table under incomplete anesthesia, and under such circumstances the surgeon may have to be satisfied with a result that does not please him entirely.

Surgical Treatment

The rich vascular supply of the nasal region helps to promote early union of the tissues. Consequently, the best results are obtained by primary treatment. Secondary procedures are often difficult and unsuccessful. There are no muscular forces working upon the bone fragments to cause displacement, and reduction can be maintained with an external splint along with intranasal packs after the fragments have been returned to their normal position. There is little tendency for recurrent dislocation of the fragments except in cases in which extreme comminution has occurred, where the mere weight of the soft tissues might displace the small fragments.

Some fractures in which the entire nasal bony pyramid is shifted in the direction of the force that was applied can be replaced by simple digital manipulation. The nasal septum may be fractured but not greatly displaced, and the bones will literally snap back into position where they will remain without splinting or support. Fractures with somewhat greater displacement usually respond to simple upward and forward elevation; the elevation may be accomplished by an instrument manipulated under the nasal bones by one hand. At the same time the surgeon is using his other hand to mold the bones from the outside. A large Kelly forceps with rubber tubing on each of the blades is an excellent instrument for the reduction of nasal fractures. Or one may use a submucous elevator. It should be covered with rubber tubing or with twists of cotton which have been moistened with petrolatum.

The Walsham and the Asch forceps designed especially for treatment of nasal fractures are useful inasmuch as they permit the application of force through both nasal cavities at the same time, or one blade may be placed inside the nose and the other outside to manipulate the lateral bone structures. The instrument must be placed carefully under the fracture, not too high in the nose or it will impinge upon the undersurface of

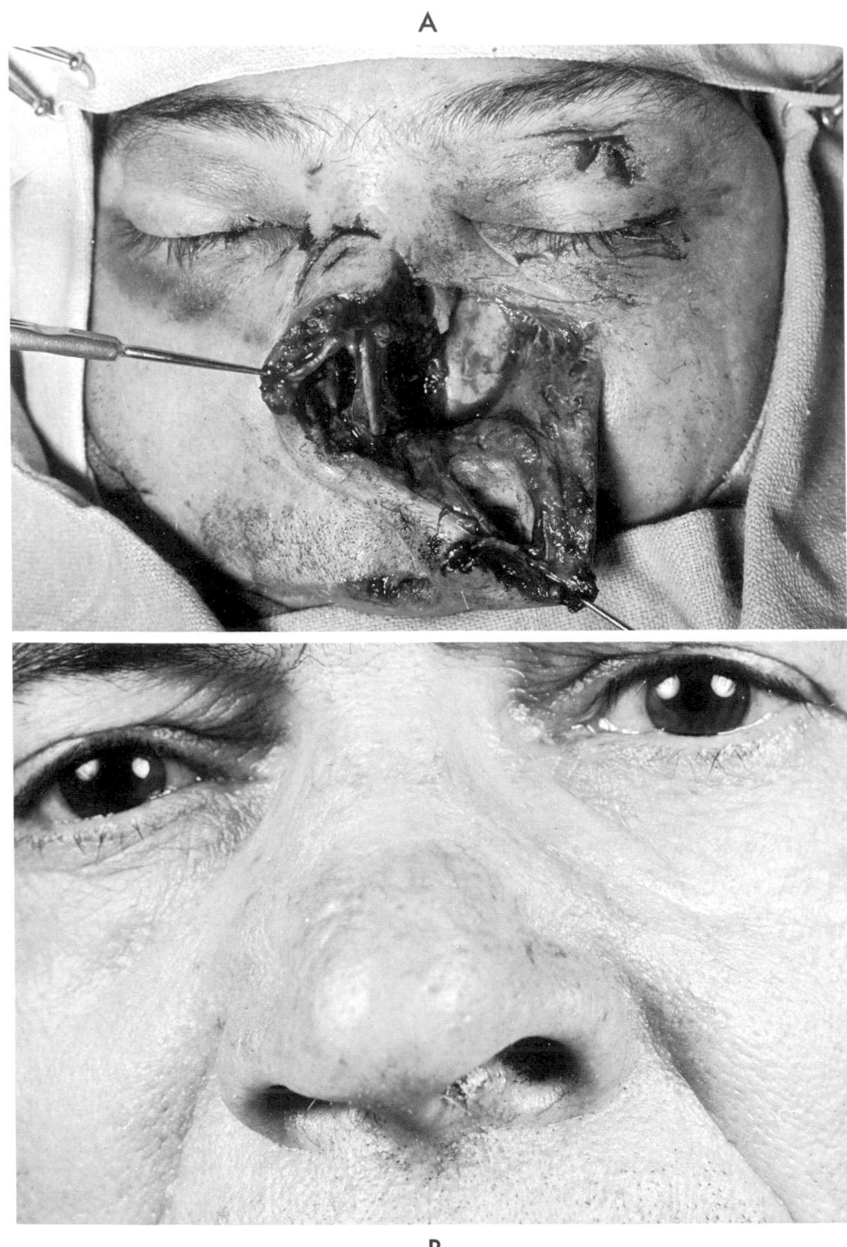

Figure 258. Laceration with compound fracture of the nasal bones and frontal process of the left maxilla, fracture of the nasal septum, and fracture of the anterior maxillary wall. *A.* The injury was managed by direct wiring of all bony and cartilaginous fragments, with closure of the lining of the nose, the subcutaneous tissues, and the skin. Intranasal packing gave support to the bony structures during the course of healing. *B.* Result one year following operation. Patient has excellent appearance and normal nasal cavities with straight septum.

the adjacent portion of the frontal bone and damage the mucosa without effectively reducing the fracture.

The fractured, dislocated nasal septum is often replaced by elevation of the nasal bones (Fig. 258 *A*, *B*). After such elevation, careful examination of the nasal cavity should be done with a good light and a nasal speculum with suction. If the septum is out of position, it may be elevated or replaced by use of the Asch forceps (Fig. 259). It may be difficult to determine whether septal deviation was caused by the injury or existed previously. Usually the acute deformity is associated with tears of the mucosa or with hematoma.

A long nasal speculum introduced deeply into the airway is helpful in the reduction of fractures of the septum and the nasal bones. Pressure against the septum is obtained by opening the blades of the speculum. Small, completely detached segments of bone

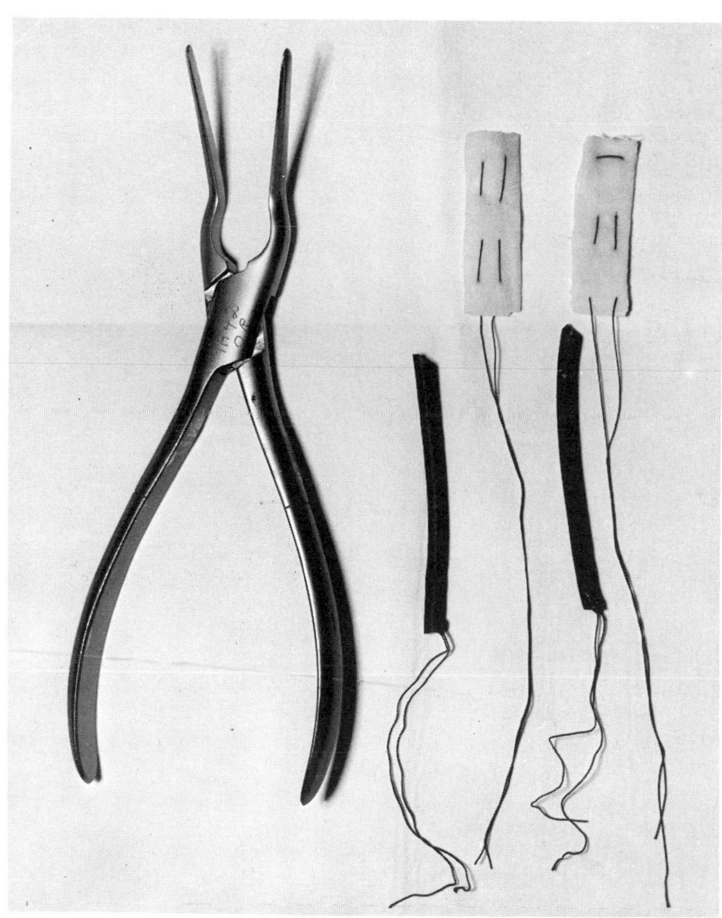

Figure 259. Asch septal straightening forceps for reduction of nasal fractures. Soft rubber intranasal tubing gives an added measure of comfort to the nose dressed with gauze packing. The prepared gauze packs are impregnated with a waxy, antiseptic, slightly anesthetic material.

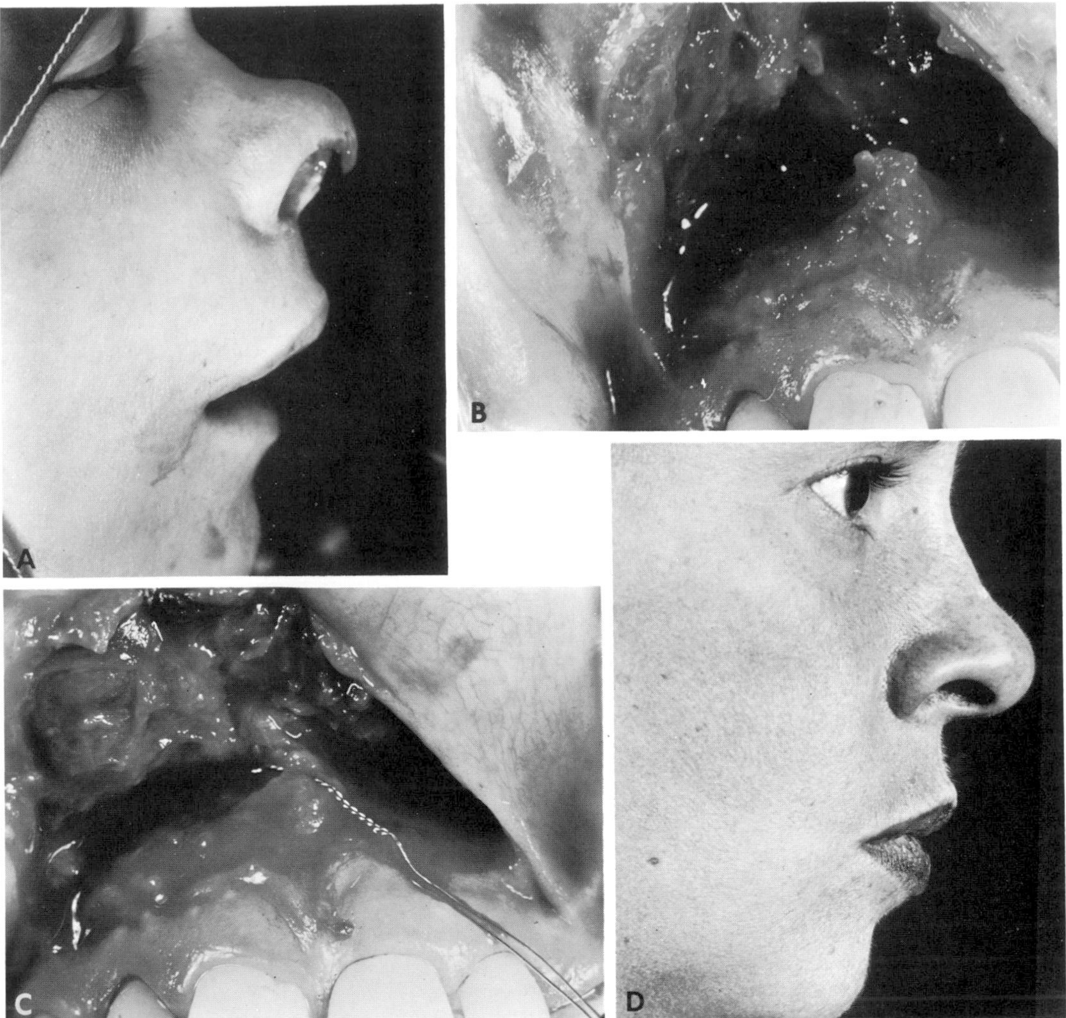

Figure 260. Telescoping fracture from a blow at the anterior edge of the septum at the base of the nose. *A*. Profile view showing upward and backward displacement of the nasal structures. *B*. View on the undersurface of the lip showing torn mucosa and separation of the nasal septum from the anterior nasal spine. *C*. The nasal septum has been replaced on the maxillary crest and wired to the anterior nasal spine. *D*. Result two years after operation.

should be removed and torn mucosa gently placed back into position where it can be held by intranasal packs. After elevating and molding the bones with the fingers, their position may be maintained by packing with prepared gauze packs impregnated with Carbozine* (see Fig. 259). The waxy Carbozine on the packs permits them to be molded into a cast which conforms to the anterior nasal cavity. The support is adequate without producing necrotizing pressures, and the packs remain in good position without shifting. They can be removed with little discomfort or bleeding, as the gauze does not adhere to the wound.

Ordinary petrolatum gauze strips may not maintain their position, because the gauze slips backward into the nasal space and often annoys the patient by dangling in the throat.

Treatment of fractures caused by an upward blow on the undersurface of the nose consists of reduction of the septal fracture and repositioning of the cartilages. Fractures may occur in the midportion of the quadrilateral cartilage or at the junction of the quadrilateral cartilage with the perpendicular plate of the ethmoid, with dislocation at the anterior nasal spine and vomer. In the early stages of the acute injury, reduction usually can be accomplished by digital molding and forward and downward traction with tissue hooks or a towel clip. Reduction of the structures when the injury has occurred 3 or 4 days earlier sometimes becomes difficult, and if the fracture occurred two weeks earlier or more, an approach through a septal incision and partial submucous resection may be necessary to reduce the anterior septal structures. Fixation may be obtained by wiring the septum to the anterior nasal spine, to an adjacent tooth, or to a drill hole made in the bony margin of the pyriform aperture. Intranasal packs and external nasal splints may be needed (Fig. 260).

* C. S. Ruckstuhl Co., St. Louis, Mo.

The Smashed Nose

This injury is caused by a force applied violently from the front. It presents, of course, more complex problems. Nevertheless, reduction can be maintained frequently by packing the nostrils and applying the usual external splint. However, when severe comminution of the bony and cartilaginous structures has occurred, reduction may be difficult to maintain. The tightness of the skin resulting from edema may cause the bony and cartilaginous fragments to recede, and possibly even to overlap in the nasal cavity.

The nasal bones are elevated and held in position by an assistant while the surgeon, using two pieces of 24 gauge stainless steel wire threaded on Keith straight surgical needles, fastens the sutures and splint. One needle is passed through the skin and lateral fracture line in the region of the frontal process of the maxilla, through the cartilaginous septum, and through the fracture line and skin on the opposite side. The other needle with its wire is passed similarly, but at a higher level, between the fragments and through the bony septum. If too much resistance is encountered to the penetration of the needle, a hole may be drilled through the septum. After penetrating the septum, the needle is carried between the fragments on the opposite side and through the skin. The parallel ends of the wires are passed, on each side, through holes in lead, aluminum, or copper plates; the ends are twisted against the plates and are cut short to avoid injury to the soft tissues (Fig. 261).

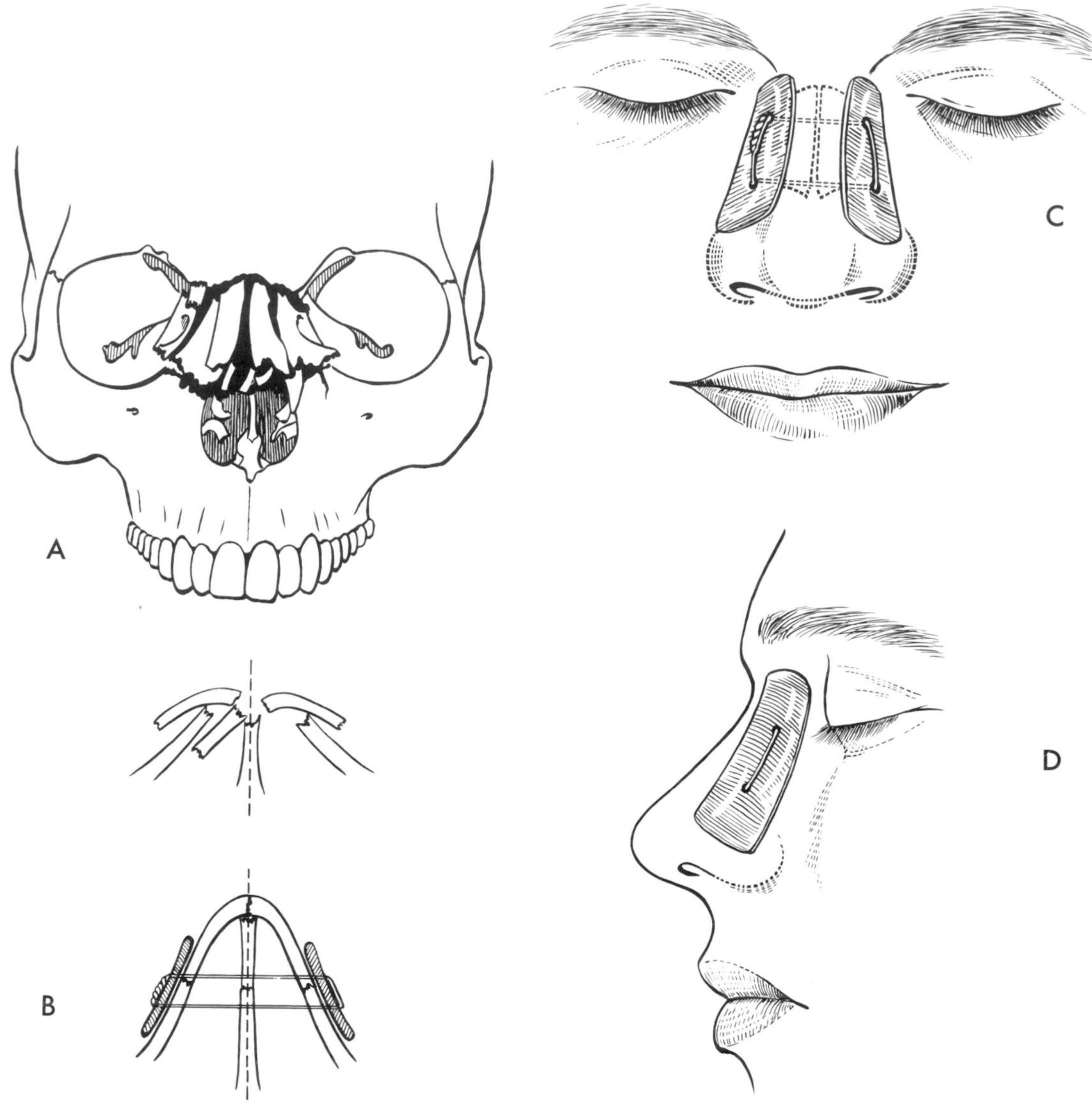

Figure 261. The use of through-and-through wires and metal plates for support of a comminuted nasal fracture. *A.* Complicated comminuted fracture of the nasal and adjacent bones. *B.* Diagram of a smash fracture and method of supporting fragments with through-and-through wires tied over lead plates. *C.* Through-and-through wires twisted over lead plates to give lateral support to comminuted fracture of the nasal and adjacent bones. *D.* Lateral view of lead plates and through-and-through wires.

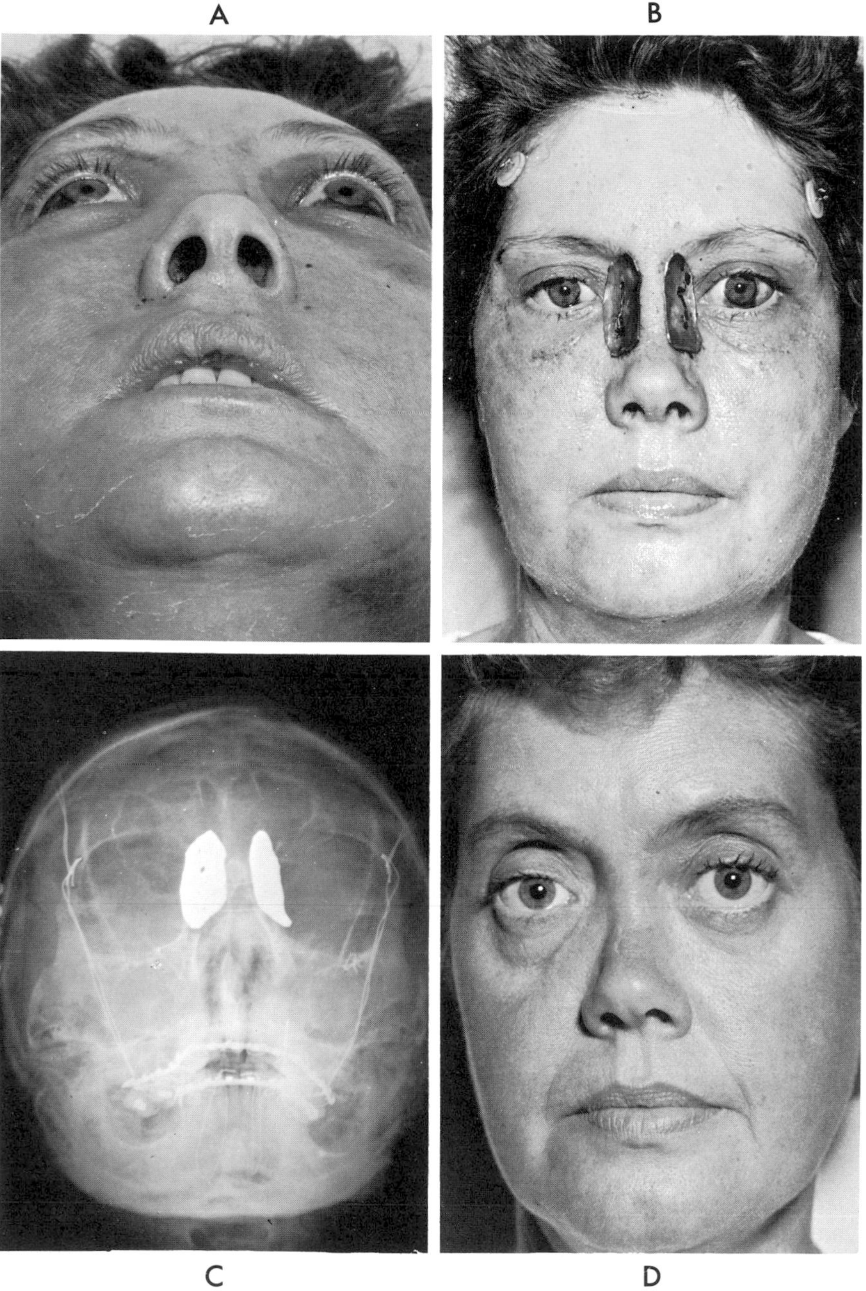

Figure 262. Pyramidal fracture of the maxilla and smash injury of the nose associated with fracture of the left zygoma treated by craniofacial internal wire suspension, interosseous fixation of zygomatic fractures, and through-and-through wire fixation over lead plates for support of nasal fractures. *A.* Depression of nasal structures and middle third of face at the time of admission five days following an automobile accident. *B.* Lead plate through-and-through fixation method for support of nasal fractures. *C.* Waters' projection roentgenogram showing interosseous wiring, craniofacial internal wire suspension, intermaxillary fixation, and through-and-through wire fixation for nasal fractures. Supplementary circumferential wiring of the mandible was done to give support to the mandibular arch bar. *D.* Postoperative result nine months following surgery.

In this kind of fracture, support may be obtained more simply by the use of a through-and-through wire suture tied over metal plates, one on each side of the nose. The loop of the suture rests on a metal plate applied to the external surface of one side of the nose. The loose ends of the wire are twisted against a similar plate placed against the opposite side of the nose. The soft edges of the plates are rolled outward to prevent irritation to the skin, and tape or any thin dressing material may be placed between the metal plates and the skin to prevent irritation. If additional support is required to keep the septum in place, gauze strips impregnated with Carbozine may be used. In practically all cases, the metal plate splint will give satisfactory support, but if additional support is needed, an external splint of plaster, dental compound, copper, or aluminum may be placed over the plates.

Immobilization with intranasal packing and nasal splints is maintained for 10 days or two weeks, depending upon the degree of comminution and the difficulty in maintaining position of the bone fragments (Fig. 264). Nasal splinting, which depends upon head-caps, head bands, or splints attached to the teeth, is usually unsatisfactory. Intranasal prong appliances that depend upon forward pressure usually result in pressure necrosis of the mucosa, cartilages, or nasal bones. The head-cap appliances usually are unstable, frequently get out of adjustment, and are ineffective in maintaining the structures in position.

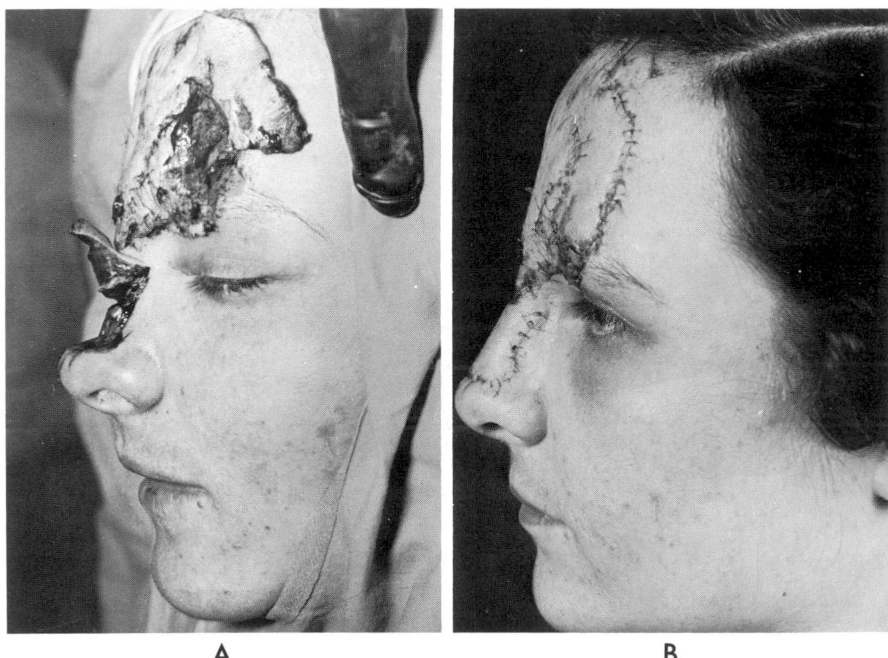

Figure 263. Compound fracture of the nasal bones due to a slicing injury from windshield glass. Deformity repaired by reduction of bone fragments, direct interosseous wiring for support, and meticulous closure of soft tissue wounds. *A.* Appearance of the patient upon admission to the hospital. *B.* Two days after operation.

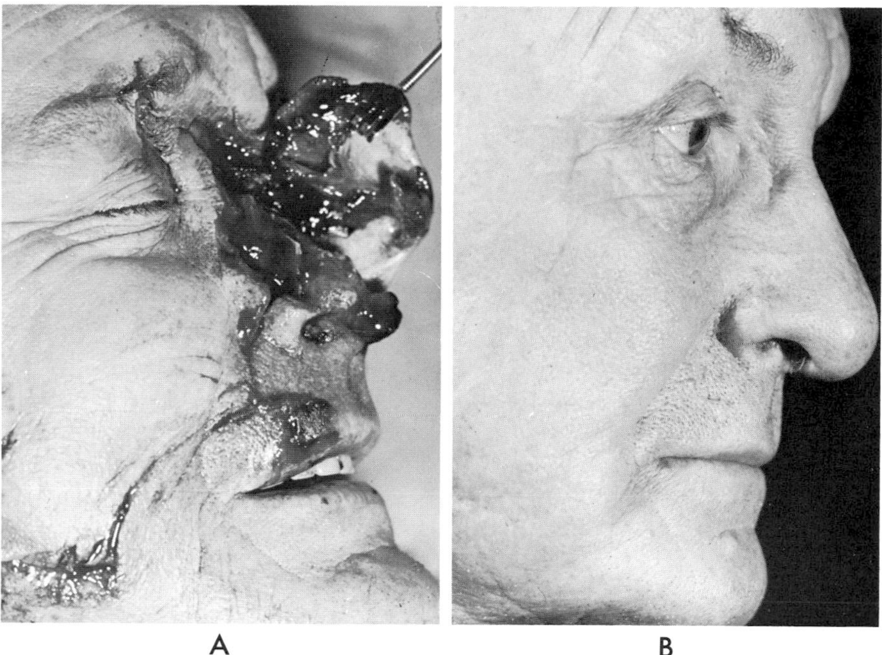

Figure 264. *A.* Laceration with compound fracture of all the nasal structures, repaired by meticulous repositioning and fixation of nasal structures, and gentle support with intranasal packing and external nasal splint. *B.* One year following operation.

External nasal splints may be constructed of plaster, lead, copper, aluminum, dental compound, or any one of the gauze plastic-impregnated materials. The simple soft sheet of aluminum or copper may be molded into a satisfactory splint and can be tailored to fit at the operating table.

Contusions of the nose may result in hematoma in the subcutaneous tissues or in the subperichondrial layer of the septum. These may make examination inconclusive, for it is difficult to determine whether or not fractures are present. Hematoma may be present without fracture, from rupture of subcutaneous or submucosal vessels. In the subcutaneous area hematomas usually are absorbed. In the region of the septum, secondary infection may occur with septic necrosis of the cartilaginous septum and septal perforation, and with subsequent collapse of the nasal dorsum.

Nasal Fractures Associated with Other Injuries

Severe nasal injuries may be complicated by fractures of adjacent bony structures, including the maxilla, zygoma, ethmoid, lacrimal, sphenoid, and bones of the nasal septum. One of the commonest injuries associated with nasal fractures is fracture of the infraorbital margin and floor of the orbit. Fractures of the frontal process of the maxilla may extend into the orbit or be associated with pyramidal (Le Fort II) fractures. Associated fractures of the zygoma may also be present with complete depression of the orbital floor. Roentgenograms taken in Waters' position show these fractures quite well (see Fig. 52). There is usually marked edema of the lids and nasal region; there may or may not be diplopia. Reduction of nasal fractures is done concomitantly with reduction of fractures of the zygoma and maxilla. (See Chapter 10 on Multiple Facial Fractures.) Injury to the eye may be a complication of nasal fractures, and ophthalmological consultation is recommended.

The lacrimal apparatus can be damaged by severe complicated comminuted splaying fractures of the nasal pyramid. A force on the nasal dorsum may splinter the nasal bones and the frontal processes of the maxillae, which are forced laterally into the nasolacrimal area, causing lacerations of the duct or fracture of the lacrimal bones. Fractures of the maxilla frequently are complicated with nasal fractures. A large portion of the nasal pyramid is made up of the frontal process of the maxilla, and displaced fractures of this structure may obstruct the nasal passages. In fractures of the maxilla, alveolar structures or teeth may be forced into the nasal cavity and impinge upon the nasal floors to reduce the airways on one side or both. Fragments of the hard palate may be driven into the nasal cavity in severe injuries. Fragments of bone which encroach upon the nasal cavity may be reduced by applying pressure with a nasal speculum, by downward pressure with a large sound, or by digital pressure with the little finger in the nasal cavity. Nasal fractures may be associated with severe injury to the ethmoidal structures; the nasal bones and septum may be driven into the region of the ethmoid with damage to the structures of the interorbital space.

Fractures of the nasal process of the frontal bone or the walls of the frontal sinuses occasionally accompany severe nasal injuries. Nasal injuries may be associated with fractures of the cribriform region or of the anterior cranial fossa with cerebrospinal rhinorrhea. Neurosurgical consultation is advisable in the management of patients with these injuries. Reduction of fractured facial bones is not contraindicated by cerebrospinal rhinorrhea. In some of our patients in whom this complication was of several days' duration, rhinorrhea subsided after replacement of the nasal and maxillary bones. If reduction of facial fractures is deferred until spinal fluid drainage subsides, the most favorable period for reduction may have passed. Some patients drain fluid for several weeks. After such a delay it is virtually impossible to reduce these fractures satisfactorily. Nasal packing and irrigation are contraindicated in the presence of cerebrospinal rhinorrhea.

If the fracture involves the frontal bone and passes through the inner plate of the frontal sinus with dural tear and cerebrospinal fluid leak, drainage of the frontal sinus into the nose is called for. A rubber tube can be placed into the fractured part through a nasal opening made into the frontal sinus.

In compound facial injuries with cerebrospinal fluid leakage from the ethmoid region, reduction of fractures is not contraindicated, but the patient should be well protected with broad-spectrum antibiotics given preoperatively and postoperatively. If nasal suction is used, it should be done with a sterile catheter each time the suction is used.

Septohematoma

Septohematoma may occur as the result of fractures with bleeding in the subperichondrial space. It shows as a unilateral or bilateral thickening of the mucosa overlying the septal cartilage. The hematoma must be evacuated through an incision, or permanent thickening and narrowing of the airway may ensue. Breakdown of parts of the nasal septum due to septic necrosis or abscess of the nasal septum may occur, with loss of bone and soft tissues if the hematoma is not treated.

Infected hematoma is a common cause of septal perforation. Treatment consists of incision through the mucoperichondrium and aspiration of the blood clots with a suction pipette. Usually packing will permit healing within a few days. The hematoma may recur, however, and the septum should be inspected from time to time to make certain that the hemorrhage is not continuing. Adequate drainage is obtained by making a horizontal incision through the mucoperiosteum on one side, along the floor of the nose. This also permits evacuation of the clots by suction.

COMPLICATIONS OF NASAL FRACTURE

Early Complications

Early complications, consisting of edema, ecchymosis of the skin of the nose and eyelids, scleral chemosis, epistaxis, hematoma of the nasal septum, and infection, seldom are serious. Edema usually disappears within a few days, and bleeding from the nose generally is of short duration; it ceases spontaneously or may be controlled with intranasal packs. Hematoma of the skin and the mucosa of the nose is controlled by evacuation, or incision and drainage. Infection is managed by adequate drainage, hot packs, and antibiotic therapy.

Delayed Complications

Untreated hematoma of the septum may organize and produce subperichondrial and subperiosteal fibrosis with increased thickness of the nasal septum and partial nasal obstruction. In cases of repeated trauma, the septum may be 1 cm. in thickness and be replaced largely with calcified material. Submucous resection with excision of the septum may be necessary to provide an adequate airway. Synechia between the septum and the turbinates may be encountered. Management consists of lysis with gauze packing between the cut surfaces for four or five days. The nasal passage may be blocked by malunion of fragments of bone or cartilage, or by contracture from loss of lining. These complications can be corrected by osteotomy, Z-plasty for the release of scar tissue contractures, with replacement of scar with skin grafts. Septic necrosis of the bony structures may be seen in cases of compound fracture of the nose, and from infected hematomas. Infection may have destroyed the entire nasal bony framework. Treatment consists of incision, adequate antibiotic therapy, and removal of sequestra from the wound. Comminuted fragments may have been driven into the interorbital space with damage to the lacrimal apparatus and fractures of the cribriform plate. Malunion fractures result in external nasal deformities and deformities of the septum, which may require late reconstructive procedures.

Even under the most expert management and the most meticulous care, some severe fractures require secondary procedures for definitive correction.

The Nose

PART 2

OPERATIVE TECHNIQUE

The importance of the nose in respect to function and cosmesis must not be underrated. When the nasal structures are injured, the critical need is for management that will restore function as well as normal appearance. Generally speaking, the nose restored to normal from the standpoint of function is restored also from the standpoint of appearance. While the prominent position of the nose makes restoration of appearance extremely important, it is equally important to bring the intranasal structures into such anatomic position as will provide an adequate airway passage. Under the most expert care, residual deformity may persist, however, and some patients will require secondary surgical correction.

A careful study of Part 1 of this chapter and of the following illustrated pages should enable the surgeon to treat nasal injuries with consistently excellent results from the points of view of function and appearance. A careful study of this and the preceding chapters should enable the surgeon who treats facial trauma to obtain excellent results in the treatment of fractures of the bones.

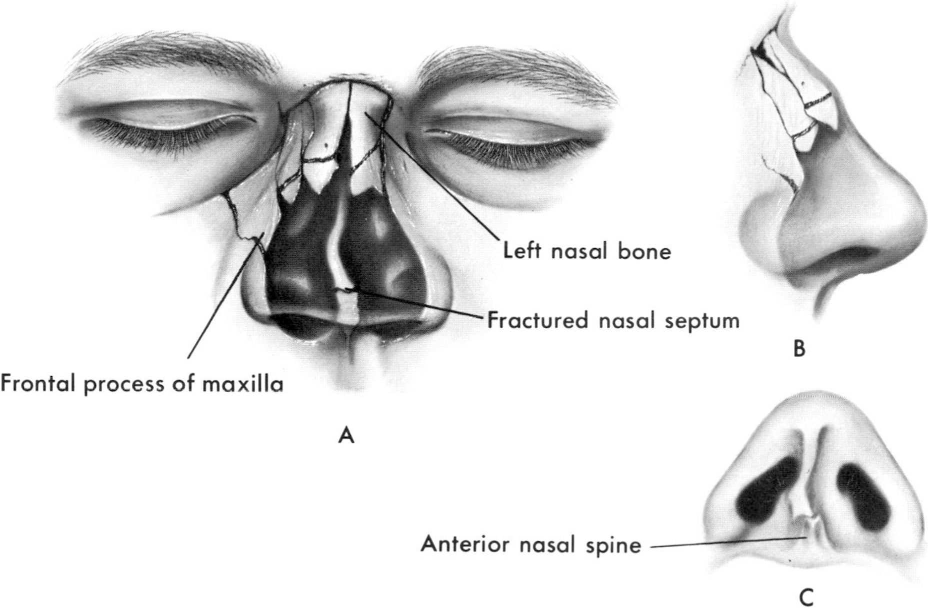

1

Fig. 265. *A.* Fracture of the nasal bony structures. The fracture involves the frontal process of the right maxillary bone, the nasal bones, and separation of the right nasal bone from the left. The nasal septum may be fractured in this type of injury. *B.* Lateral view of fractured nasal structures. C. Fracture with dislocation of the septal cartilage from the anterior spine of the maxilla and from the vomer crest is often associated with nasal bone fractures. Reduction is most effective when performed early. Late reconstruction is difficult and sometimes unsatisfactory.

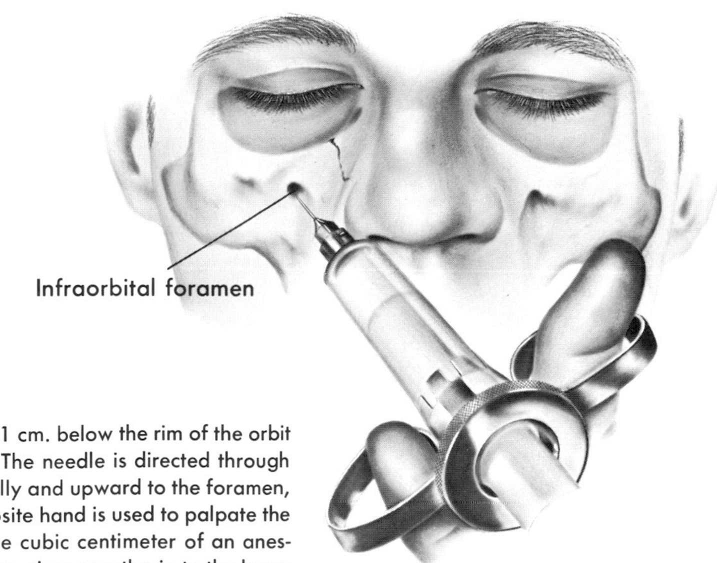

2

Fig. 266. The infraorbital foramen is located 1 cm. below the rim of the orbit at the medial third of the infraorbital margin. The needle is directed through the skin near the nasal ala and is passed laterally and upward to the foramen, which opens downward and medially. The opposite hand is used to palpate the bony margin while advancing the needle. One cubic centimeter of an anesthetic solution deposited near or into the foramen gives anesthesia to the lower eyelid, lateral nose, ala, and upper lip.

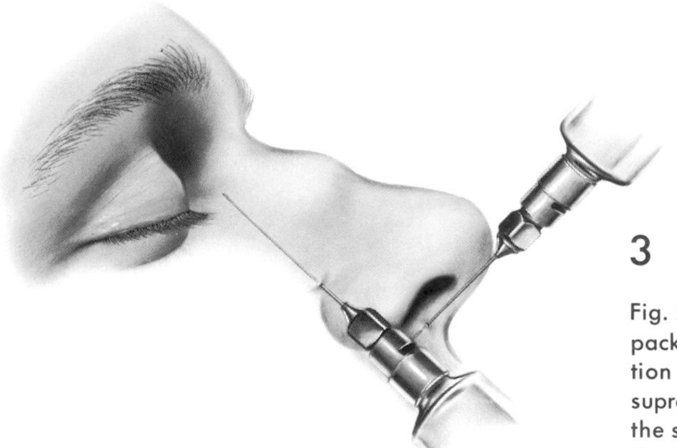

3

Fig. 267. Intranasal anesthesia with cocaine-epinephrine packs is supplemented by injection of a local anesthetic solution into the external nasal structures. The needle is passed supraperiosteally along the base of the nasal pyramid, and the solution is deposited from the region of the medial canthus to the nasolabial groove. Injection of the columella gives anesthesia for reduction and fixation of fractures of the anterior nasal spine and nasal floor.

4

Fig. 268. The tissues in the region of the anterior nasal spine and pyriform margins of the maxilla are anesthetized by depositing solution while passing the needle laterally through a puncture in the philtrum of the upper lip to the alar area.

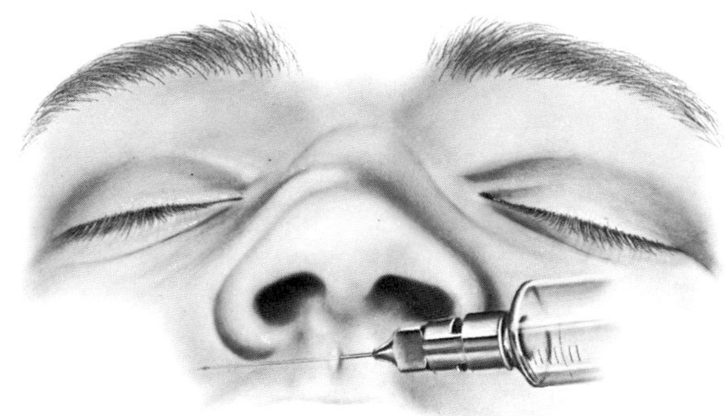

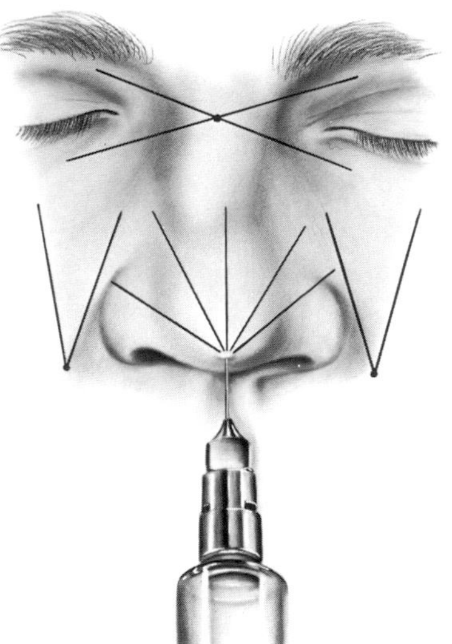

5

Fig. 269. The nose is anesthetized by the same technique that is used for routine rhinoplasty procedures. The tissues in the region of the glabella can be infiltrated as shown, with deposition of anesthetic solution in the lateral nasal and medial canthal areas on both sides. Through a single injection at the tip, the needle can be advanced in any direction for infiltration of the structures of the nasal tip. The infraorbital and lateral nasal injections are made through skin punctures in the region of the nasolabial groove on both sides.

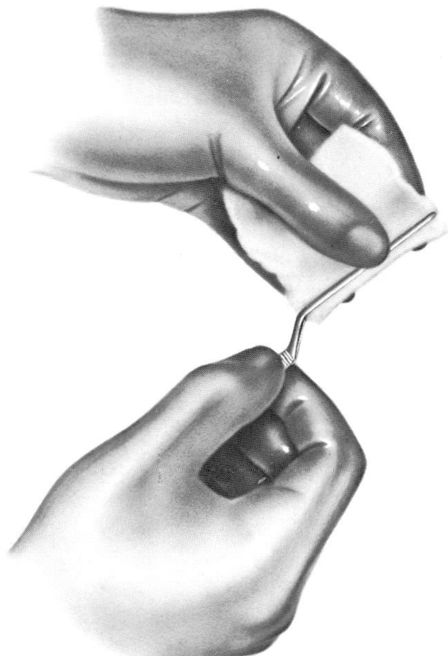

6

Fig. 270. A thin section of long fiber cotton, approximately 2 x 2 inches, is grasped at the margin with the long blades of a bayonet nasal forceps. A good grade of long fiber cotton is desirable to prevent fraying and irregularity of the nasal tampon. If pieces of short fiber cotton are used, they may be lost in the wound and cause a foreign body reaction and delayed healing.

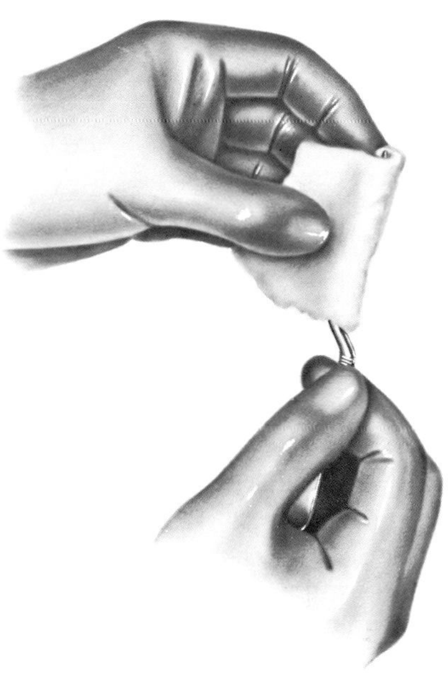

7

Fig. 271. The bayonet forceps is rotated between the thumb and index finger of the right hand and the cotton is then wound firmly onto the end of the forceps. A small amount of saline on the fingers helps to give continuity to the fiber cotton. The tampon should be wrapped to a size that will fit easily into the nasal cavity—about the diameter of a lead pencil.

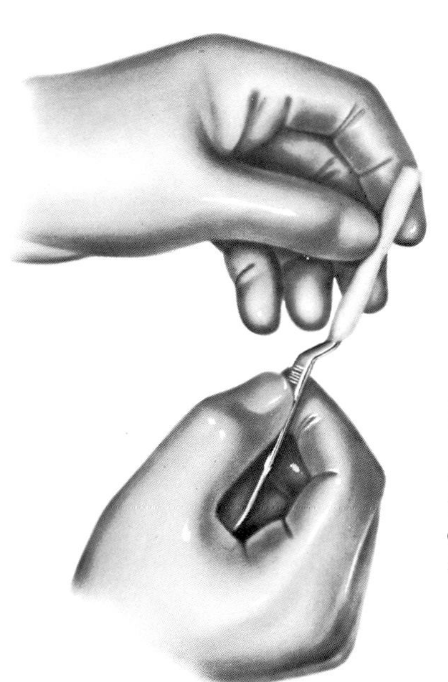

8

Fig. 272. While holding the twisted cotton in the left hand, the forceps is withdrawn from the interior of the cotton pledget. If made carefully, the tampon will be a firmly packed, 2 inch long, pencil-like section of cotton without loose or frayed ends.

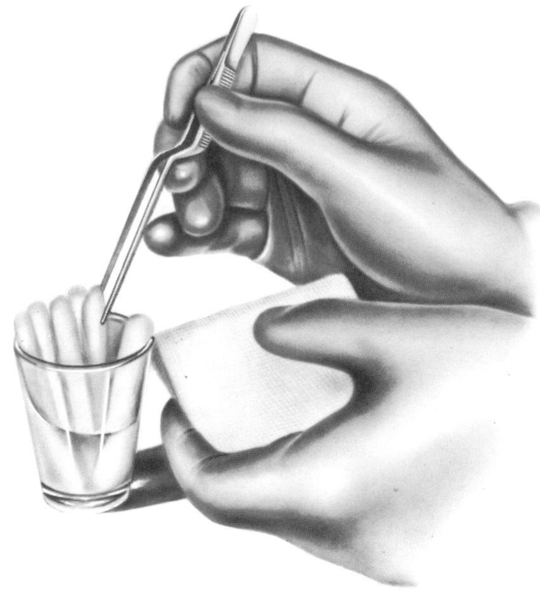

9

Fig. 273. Six cotton pledgets are placed into a medicine glass containing 15 cc. of 10 per cent cocaine or other topical anesthetic solution mixed with an equal amount of 1:1000 epinephrine solution. For identification, to avoid accidentally injecting the solution with a syringe, it is recommended that one drop of methylene blue dye be placed into the container holding the anesthetic solution. Then it cannot be mistaken for other clear solutions such as procaine or adrenalin.

10

Fig. 274. The cotton pledgets are removed from the container, squeezed firmly between the fingers, and placed upon a thin gauze sponge.

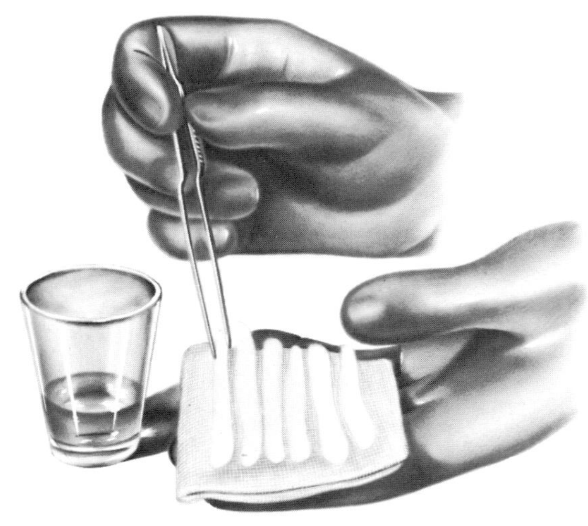

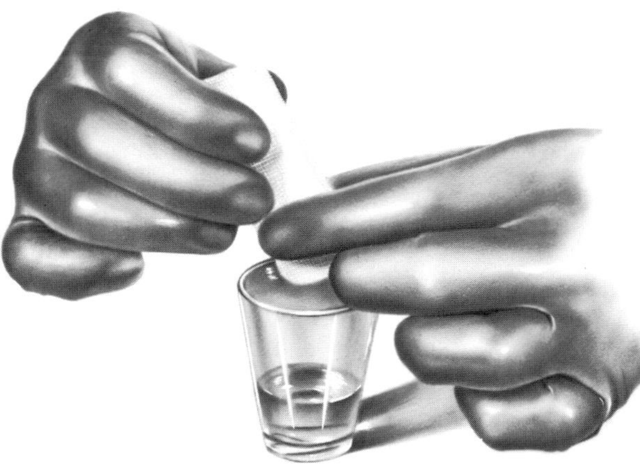

11

Fig. 275. The gauze sponge is folded over carefully to contain the cotton pledgets, and the excess anesthetic solution is squeezed out between the fingers. The cotton pledgets should be moist but not saturated or dripping with the anesthetic solution, which can be absorbed in excess amounts by the nasal mucosa and cause toxicity. A moist nasal pack is sufficient to give good topical anesthesia.

12

Fig. 276. The cotton pledgets, with the excess topical anesthetic solution expressed, are prepared for insertion into the nasal cavity. If the nose has been sprayed with an atomizer containing a topical anesthetic solution a few minutes prior to insertion of the nasal cotton pledgets, the nose can be packed with minimal discomfort to the patient.

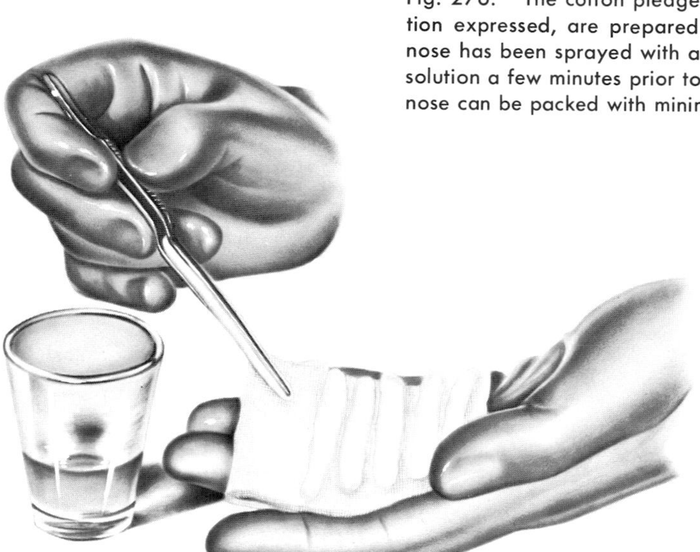

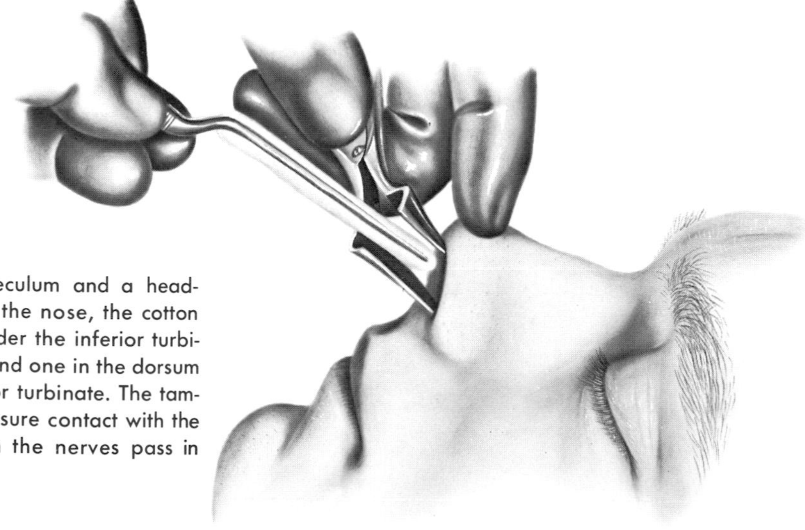

13

Fig. 277. By using a long-blade speculum and a headlight for illumination of the interior of the nose, the cotton tampons are placed carefully—one under the inferior turbinate, one under the middle turbinate, and one in the dorsum of the nose in the region of the superior turbinate. The tampons are placed back in the nose to assure contact with the mucosa in the regions through which the nerves pass in a downward and forward direction.

14

Fig. 278. It may not be possible to place the cotton tampons to the desired depth in the nasal cavity on the first attempt owing to deformity of the septum or enlargement of the turbinates. The tampons should be placed with care to prevent injury to the nasal mucosa. In 5 minutes the cotton tampons should be removed and fresh ones inserted. After this elapse of time the nasal mucosa will have shrunken considerably and the second application of the tampons will be easier and placement more favorable. The tampons should be left in the nose for 5 to 10 minutes before starting the operation.

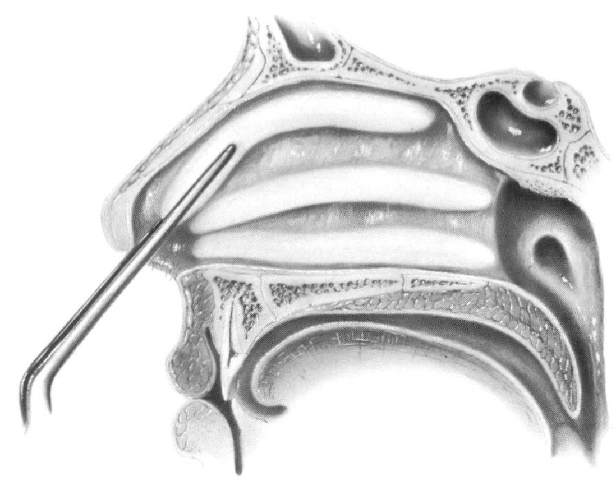

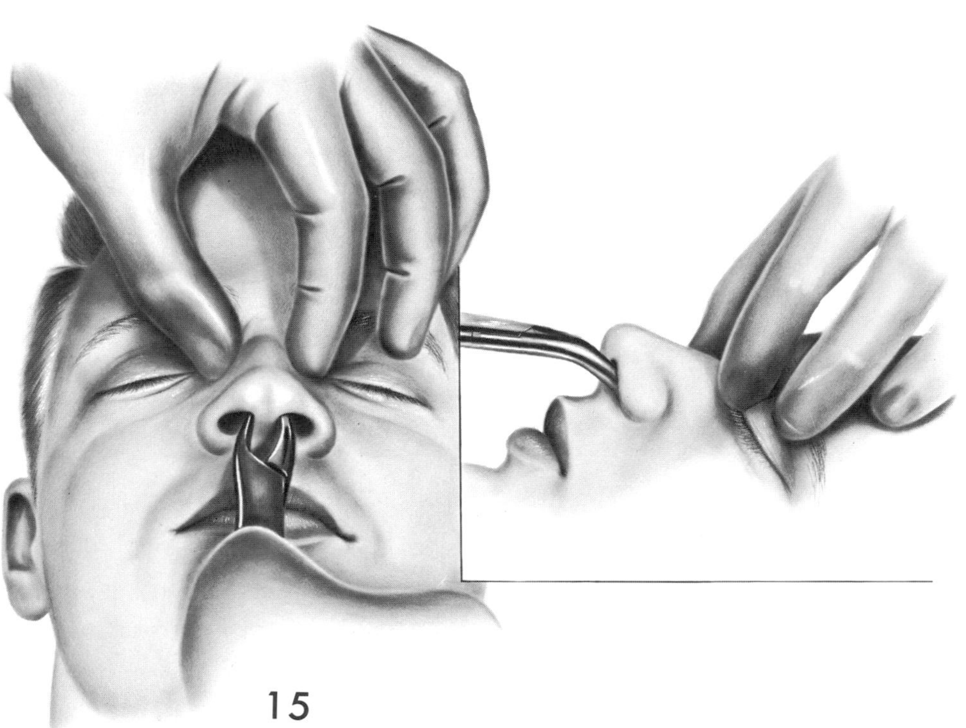

15

Fig. 279. The Asch forceps is inserted carefully into the nose, one blade on each side of the septum. By upward and anterior force with the forceps and with digital manipulation on the external portion of the nose, the fractured segments can be guided accurately into position. Usually the septum cannot be repositioned until the nasal bones have been elevated into position to relieve impinging structures from the dorsal nasal septum. After the bony and cartilaginous framework has been manipulated into position, the intranasal structures are examined. A septum that has buckled can be straightened with the Asch forceps by applying pressure against the two sides of the septum. In some cases of injury of several days' standing it is necessary to approach the fractured dislocated segments of the septum by open operation. A submucous resection type of incision is made and the fractured segments identified and reduced.

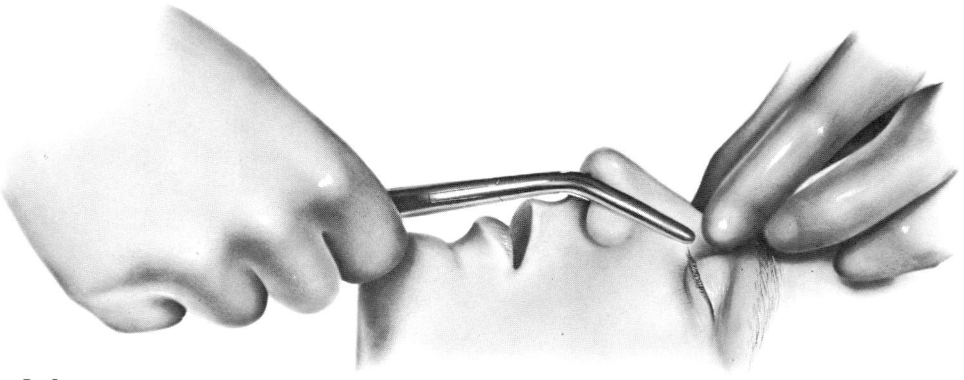

16

Fig. 280 Unilateral nasal fractures or fractures with displacement can be manipulated by using one blade of the Asch forceps intranasally with the other blade on the external surface of the nose. Manipulative force applied to the instrument plus digital molding pressure will usually reduce fractures of the lateral nasal wall.

17

Fig. 281. Anterior and upward force is applied to the undersurface of the nasal bony processes, and at the same time the opposite hand is used to apply digital pressure and manipulate the external nasal structures. Except in cases of extreme comminution, the bones and cartilages will remain in reduction so that packs can be inserted for support.

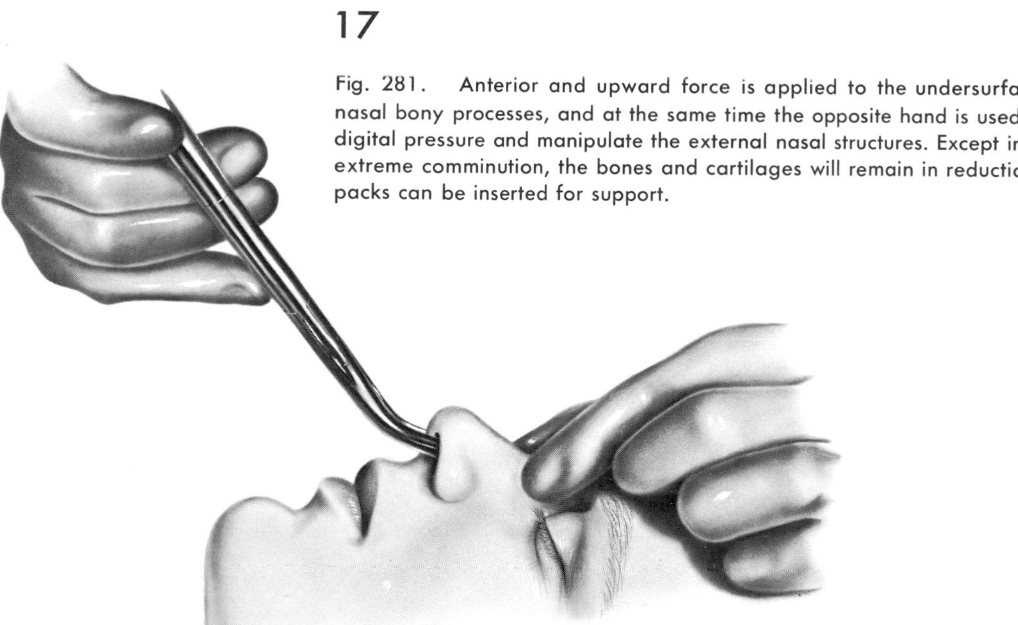

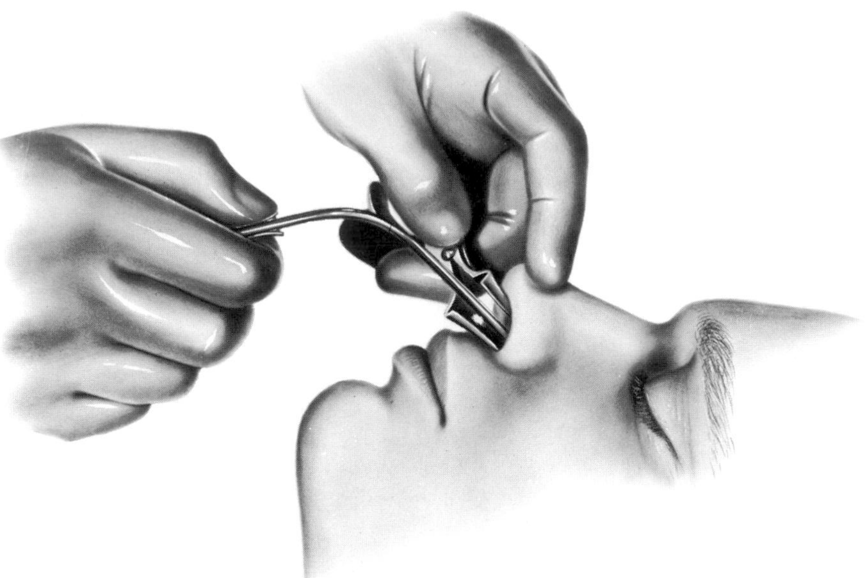

18

Fig. 282. After reduction of all displaced bones and soft tissues, the interior of the nose should be inspected under direct illumination to be certain that the septum is in anatomic position. Suction for removal of clots and mucus and a nasal speculum to spread the nostrils permit careful inspection of the reduction of the structures. Flaps of torn mucosa are replaced in preparation for support by the nasal packs.

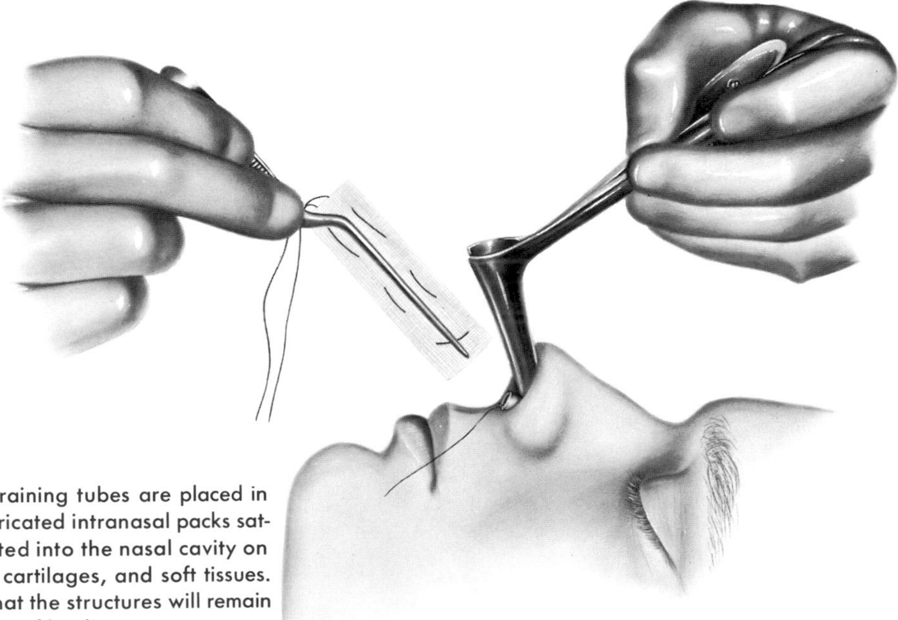

19

Fig. 283. Small, soft rubber draining tubes are placed in the floor of the nose, and prefabricated intranasal packs saturated with Carbozine are inserted into the nasal cavity on each side to support the bones, cartilages, and soft tissues. The packs are placed firmly so that the structures will remain in fixed position during the course of healing.

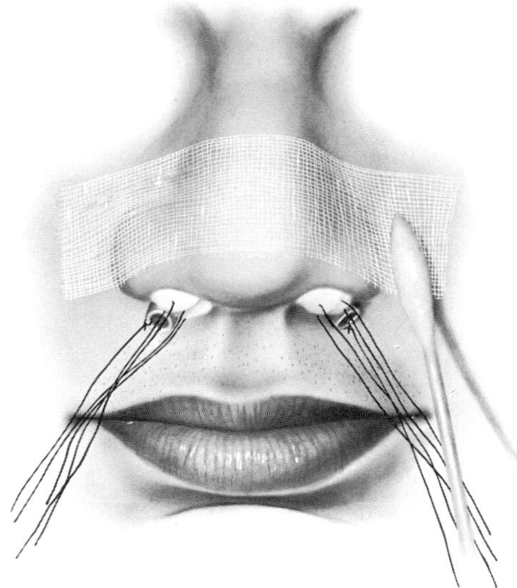

20

Fig. 284. The rubber tubing is cleansed once or twice a day by suction to prevent plugging with mucus. The tubing provides aeration of the nasopharynx and helps to equalize pressures in the region of the eustachian tubes. The rubber tubes give added comfort. However, they are not intended to provide an airway adequate for breathing. A layer of coarse mesh gauze placed over the nasal tip and fixed with nonflexible collodion gives support to the tip of the nose.

21

Fig. 285. The strings attached to the rubber tubing and intranasal packs are folded up over the gauze strip and are secured by a second collodion gauze strip across the tip of the nose. This fixation prevents loss and makes removal easy. The packs and tubing are left in place for 7 to 14 days, depending upon the degree of comminution and displacement. Nosedrops passed through the tubes two to three times daily with a medicine dropper help irrigate the tubes; some solution may reach the mucosa and give relief from congestion.

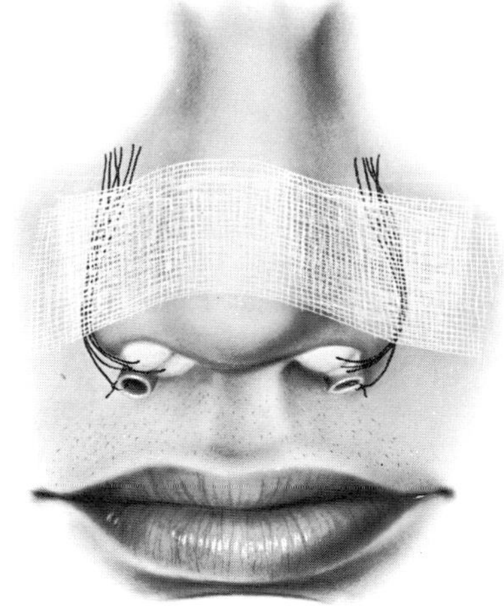

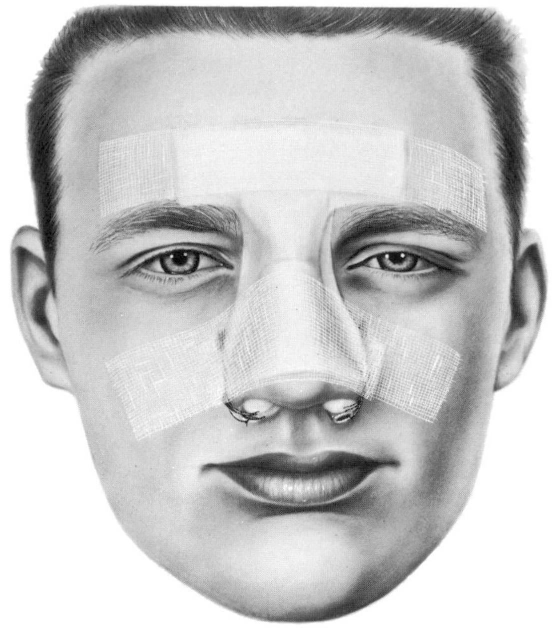

22

Fig. 286. Nasal splints may be constructed of metal, dental compound, plaster, or synthetic resins. Synthetic acrylic plaster is easily molded, sets readily, and has the advantages of impermeability, hardness, and strength. It can be molded readily over the skin to which it fits closely. The splint provides support for the nasal bones and prevents hematoma and edema of the nasal structures.

23

Fig. 287. A small section of folded gauze is placed over the nasal tubing and held with adhesive tape to absorb blood or mucus that may come from the nasal tubing or the nasal vestibular openings. The snuffer is changed as often as necessary by the nurse and after a few days can be changed as necessary by the patient. Frequent change of dressing and cleansing of the nose add to the comfort of the patient.

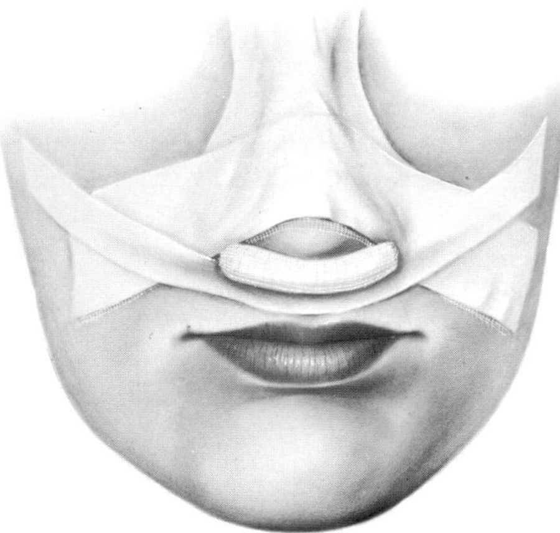

CHAPTER

10

MULTIPLE FACIAL FRACTURES

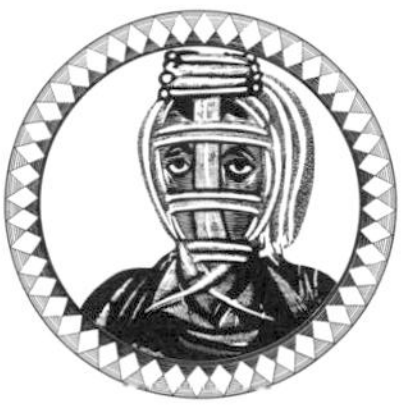

The Cornell Medical Center study indicated that 72 per cent of all people injured in automobile accidents sustain injuries to the face. Many of these are only soft tissue lesions, but an increasing number is associated with fractures of the bony structures. This kind of injury is becoming more common with the advent of speedier transportation. The incidence of extensive multiple fractures of ,the facial skeleton varies considerably in the series studied, but McCoy et al. (1962) reported that 40 per cent of all facial fractures in the Kansas City area were multiple facial fractures.

Multiple facial fractures usually are caused by automobile accidents. The head is thrown forward, and the face is struck against the instrument panel or against the rear of the front seat. The "guest passenger" injury described by Straith and the "facial smash" injury are those in which extensive fractures of the middle third of the face occur as the result of such an accident. The terminology "smash injury" occurs in the Smith Papyrus from ancient Egyptian times.

Many of these injuries involve only the middle third of the face, but some are complicated by coincident fractures of other facial bones (Fig. 288). McCoy et al. (1962) reported a series of 855 patients with fractures of the face. Forty per cent had fractures in the middle third of the face. Thirty-eight per cent had fractures of the mandible only. Twenty-two per cent had fractures of the nasal bones only. Of the 855 patients, 337 had fractures of the middle third of the face. Of these 337, 41 per cent also had fractures of the mandible and 28 per cent had associated nasal fractures.

Etiologic factors include severe crushing blows from the front or the side or even to both sides of the face simultaneously. Although most of such fractures are sustained in automobile accidents, they may have been sustained also in airplane, motorcycle, sports, and other accidents. As prophylactic measures, seat belts, shoulder harnesses, protective helmets, and the like are effective. It has been proved statistically by the Cornell study that such protective devices reduce materially the incidence of injuries to the face.

Injuries other than actual facial fracture may cause a delay in getting the patient under the care of the facial surgeon. In case of the severely injured patient, voluntary delay is advisable if the general condition of the patient contraindicates early treatment. Facial bone fractures usually are not acute surgical emergencies, and the patient's life should not be jeopardized by attempting definitive procedures if there is a question whether he can endure them. Yet even though immediate care of the fracture cannot be undertaken, helpful measures may

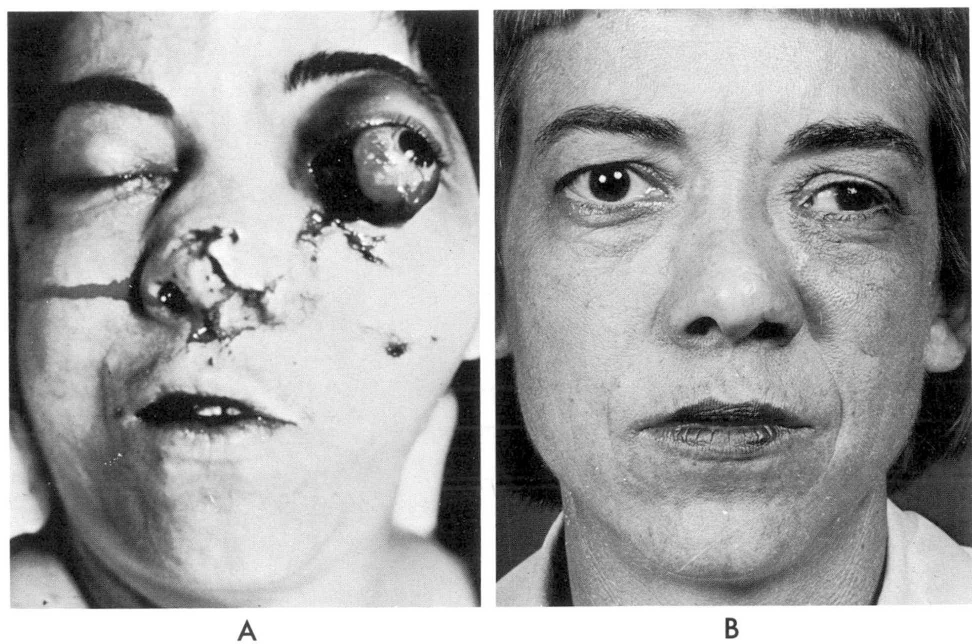

Figure 288. *A.* Severe fractures of the facial bones suffered in an automobile accident. The patient had fractures of the maxilla, nose, left zygoma, and mandible. The left eye was lost. She was treated by open reduction and direct wiring of multiple facial bones and enucleation of the eye. *B.* Postoperative view one year after treatment for multiple facial injuries. Patient has prosthesis in left orbit.

be carried out at the patient's bedside. Teeth, fragments of bone, blood clots, and soft tissue debris should be removed from the wound. Facial lacerations can be coapted with a few well-placed sutures, and a nasopharyngeal tube may be inserted to help keep open the patient's airway.

Elective tracheotomy is indicated in all patients with severe facial smash and intracranial injuries, and should be done early. Tracheotomy should be done even though the patient is not in extreme danger, for this facilitates his respiration. The tracheotomy makes it easier to keep the airway free from secretions if suction is used, and later the tracheal opening can be used as a preferred route for administration of anesthesia. As conditions improve, upper and lower arch bars may be applied at the bedside with little disturbance to the patient or danger to his well-being.

THE DIAGNOSIS OF MULTIPLE FACIAL FRACTURES

Upon admission it will be obvious by inspection that the patient has multiple facial injuries and probably many fractures of the facial skeleton. The clinical findings are those associated with individual fractures of the various facial bones. Edema usually is severe and may involve all the facial structures. Periorbital and perioral ecchymosis is a usual finding. Malocclusion due to fractures of the mandible and maxilla usually is quite severe, and mobility of fragments is elicited easily by digital manipulation. Edema, ecchymosis, and lacerations of the floor of the mouth and soft tissues of the palate may have occurred, and respiration will usually be labored because of partial obstruction of the airway.

Roentgenographic study should include a careful inspection of all the facial bones. The most useful roentgenographic approach to diagnosis of facial bone fractures is the chin-nose or Waters' view taken stereoscopically. Additional films are advisable to demonstrate the mandible, maxilla, and nasal bones in detail.

On palpation, irregularities may be noted over the nasal bony processes and about the margins of the orbit. Deformities of the mandible may be disclosed by intraoral palpation, and steplike deformities may be found along the lateral maxillary wall.

THE TREATMENT OF MULTIPLE FACIAL INJURIES

Methods of reduction and fixation have been described and discussed under the management of fractures of specific bones. These include open and closed methods of reduction with fixation by dental appliances and splints, interosseous wiring, internal wire suspension, suspension of fragments by outriggers on extraoral appliances, pin fixation, and metal plate fixation. Most multiple facial fractures can be managed with convenience, efficiency, and safety by using a combination of intermaxillary fixation and open reduction with internal wire fixation. The management of extensive facial fractures by interosseous and internal wire fixation was advocated by Adams (1942), and has been the basis for management for almost all facial fractures by the present authors since 1942. The principles of this management have been elaborated upon and their application to the edentulous patient discussed by Dingman and Alling (1954).

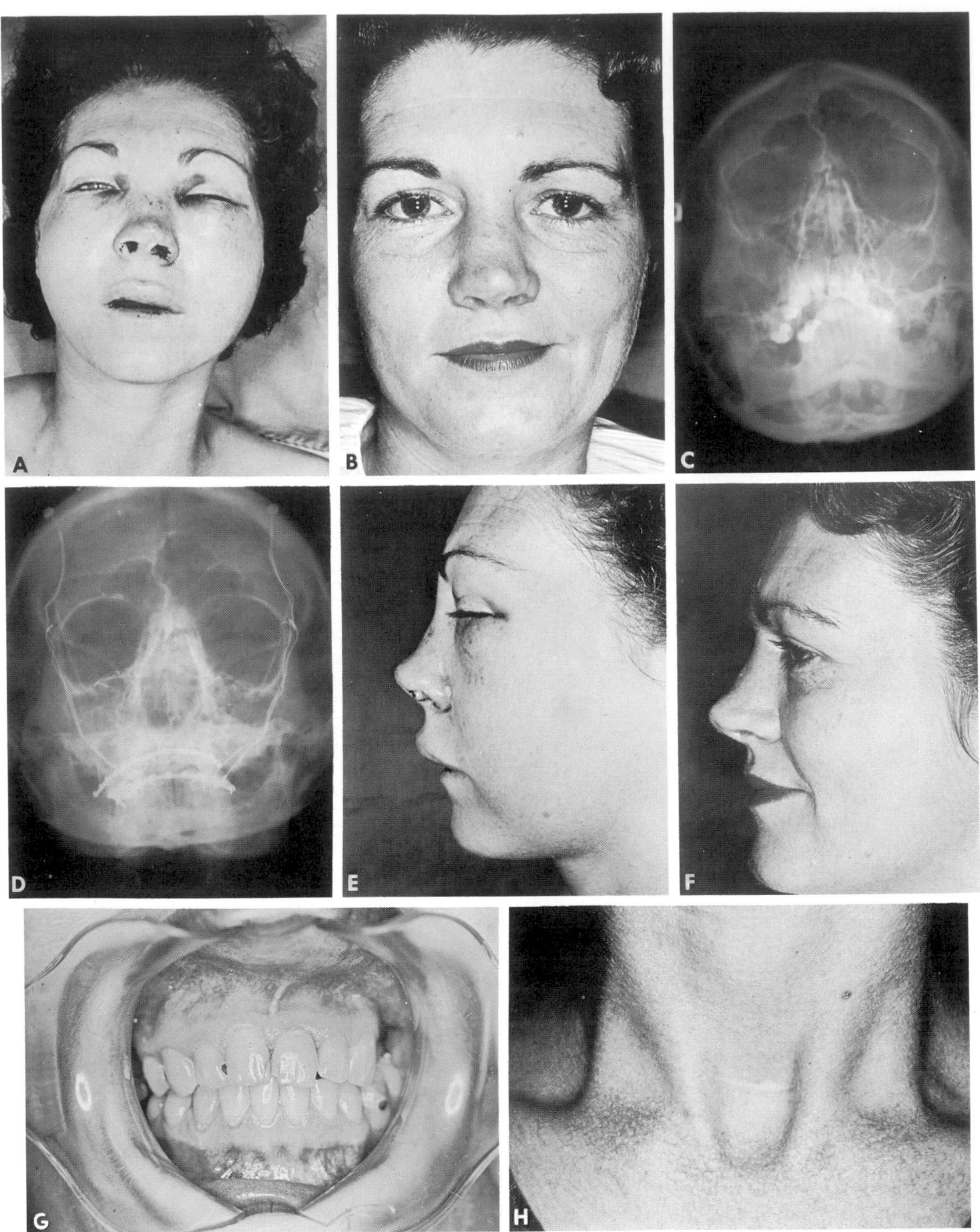

Figure 289. Craniofacial disjunction (Le Fort III) treated by interosseous wire fixation and craniofacial internal wire suspension. *A.* Appearance of the patient 24 hours after injury. *B.* Final result six months after treatment. *C.* Radiograph showing multiple facial fractures with loss of architectural detail of most of the facial bones. Note separation at the nasofrontal suture. *D.* Radiograph showing method of fixation of facial bones. *E.* Profile view on admission. *F.* Six months following treatment. *G.* Excellent postoperative occlusion. *H.* The anesthetic was administered through a tracheotomy. Note minimal postoperative scar.

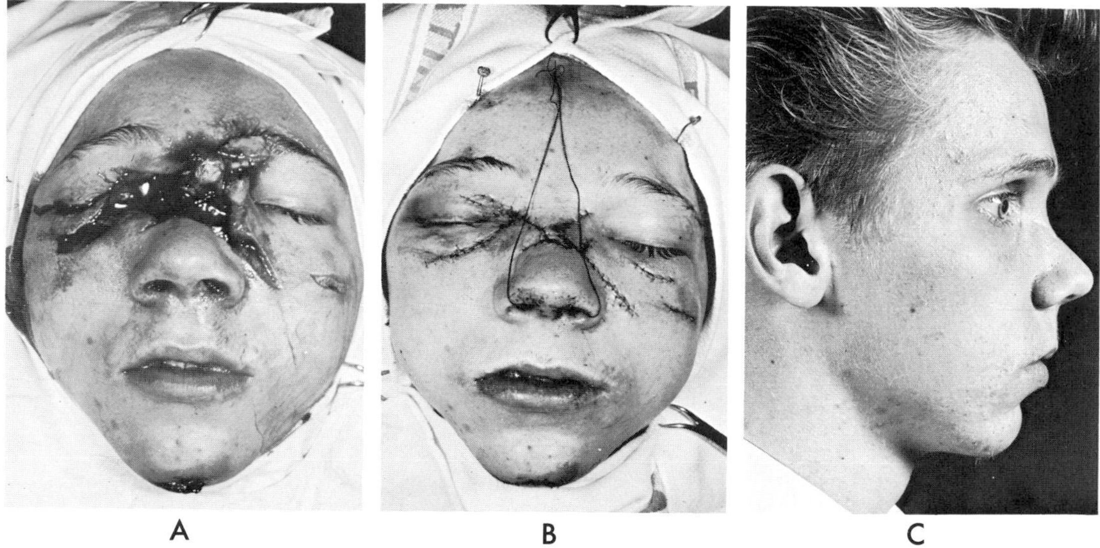

Figure 290. Compound fracture of facial skeleton with complete craniofacial disjunction. Extensive facial smash injury treated by craniofacial suspension and interosseous wire fixation. *A.* Appearance of the patient upon admission: open laceration into the nose, ethmoid area, cranial fossa, and right orbit. The right eye was lacerated beyond repair. *B.* Immediate postoperative appearance, after open reduction of multiple fractures through the lacerations and enucleation of the right eye. *C.* Appearance six months after operation with prosthesis in the right orbit.

General anesthesia with endotracheal intubation is the preferred method of preparing a patient for treatment of extensive facial injuries. An attempt to operate upon the severely injured patient under local anesthesia usually is unsatisfactory. The inflammatory reaction caused by the injury, the sensitivity of the tissues, the extensive force and manipulation necessary to reduce the fractures, all call for the use of general anesthesia. Elective tracheotomy, if not done immediately after the injury, should be performed preoperatively, for it facilitates the administration of the anesthetic and is especially indicated in the patient in whom the patency of the airway will be endangered by intermaxillary fixation and nasal packing. Endotracheal anesthesia, using the tracheotomy opening, makes it unnecessary for the anesthesiologist to be in the operative field, and the tracheotomy provides not only a satisfactory route for anesthesia but also a satisfactory postoperative airway.

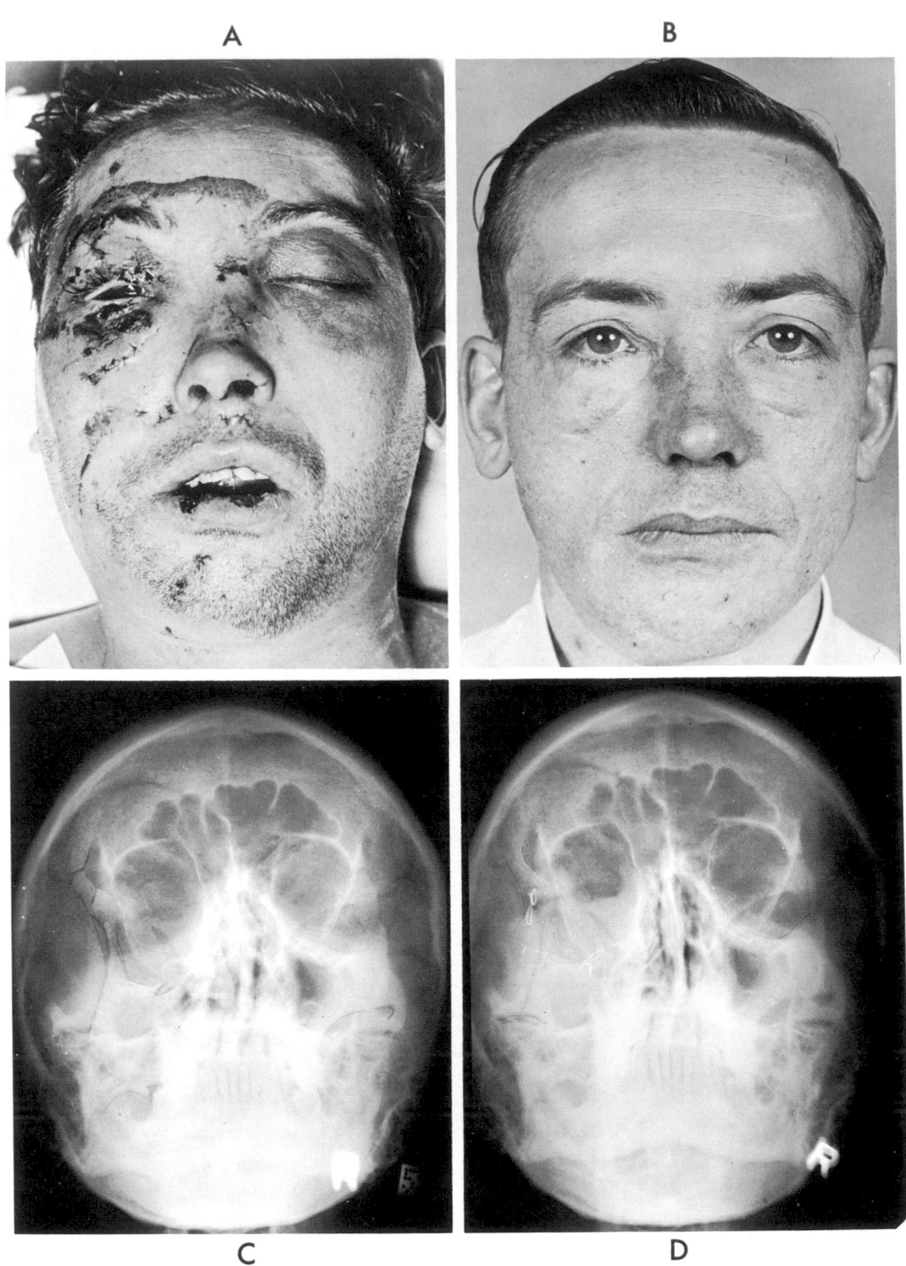

Figure 291. Typical guest-passenger facial injury. *A.* Appearance after injury. Note elongation of the face and depression of the nose and infraorbital areas. *B.* Appearance three months following operation. The patient was treated by interosseous wire fixation and craniofacial suspension. *C.* Radiograph demonstrating multiple fractures of the middle third of the face. *D.* Postoperative roentgenogram three months following treatment for multiple facial fractures.

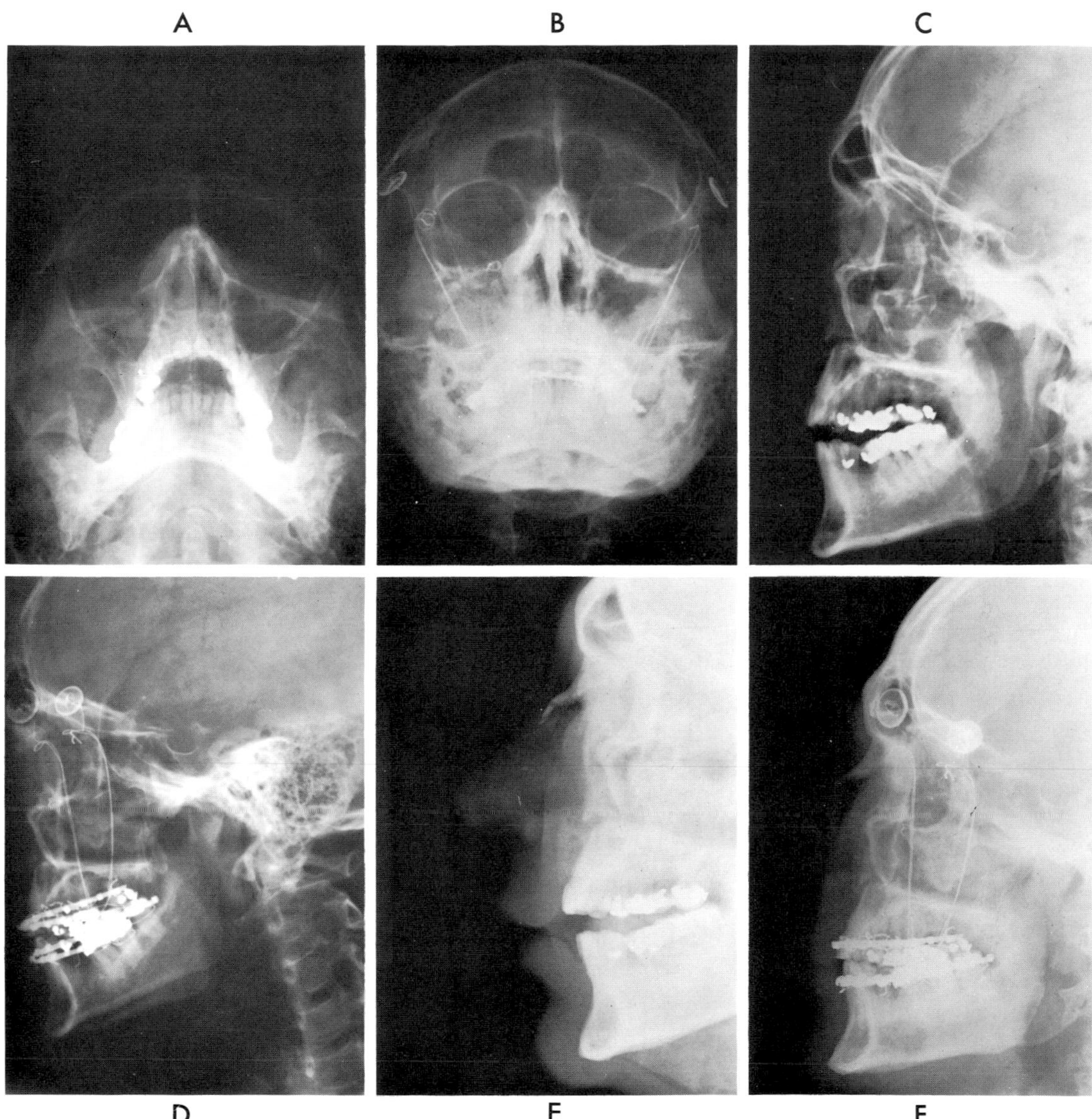

Figure 292. Radiographs of facial fractures sustained in an automobile accident in which the patient was thrown forward against the instrument panel. The injury resulted in multiple fractures of the middle third of the face. *A.* Preoperative radiograph (Waters' projection). *B.* Method of fixation following reduction. *C.* Lateral preoperative view showing malocclusion, posterior displacement of the maxilla, and separation at the nasofrontal suture line. *D.* Craniomaxillary fixation by means of arch bars and intermaxillary rubber band traction. *E.* Profile view showing fracture of the lower half of the nasal bones, open bite deformity, and fracture of the maxilla. *F.* Method of fixation following reduction of multiple facial fractures.

Multiple Fractures of the Middle Third of the Face Associated with Fractures of the Mandible

The following rules are useful in the management of multiple facial fractures that also involve the mandible:

1. The initial step is reduction of the mandibular fragments and their immobilization by the use of intraoral appliances, arch bars, or direct interosseous wiring. External pin fixation, although infrequently used, may be applicable in some cases.
2. The reconstructed mandible serves as a guide in assembling and reducing the maxillary fragments and determines the proper position of the maxilla at the time of fixation.
3. Fixation of the teeth in occlusion is attained by intermaxillary rubber band traction, direct wiring, or splints.
4. The mandibular-maxillary compound is forced into its proper position where it is held by internal wire suspension to the solid facial bone structures immediately above it. Fixation may be to the pyriform margin, the infraorbital ridges, the base of the zygoma, or the zygomatic processes of the frontal bone.

Concomitant reduction of nasal and zygomatic and maxillary fractures is carried out and fixation is attained by interosseous wiring to the frontal bone, the zygoma, and the maxilla. Associated nasal fractures are managed by direct wiring of the bone fragments, intranasal packing, and external splinting, or by through-and-through wires passed over metal plates on each side of the nose.

In an occasional case, support may be attained by means of a chin bandage suspended on each side by elastic traction from a head-cap. Suspension wires attached to upper arch bars and passed through the soft tissues of the cheek to a head-cap may be effective in some instances, but usually methods that are less cumbersome and more effective can be employed. The Kingsley splint and the Gunning type splint can be used only rarely in the modern management of fractures of the facial bones. The use of such appliances should be discouraged because of the probability of complications like nonunion or malunion.

A case history will illustrate the method of management of complicated multiple fractures of the facial bones:

Case Report

This 35-year-old male patient was seen the day following an automobile accident in which he sustained multiple facial injuries. He was driving a station wagon without a seat belt. His car was involved in a head-on collision with another automobile, and he thought that he was injured by being thrown against the steering wheel or against the instrument panel. He sustained lacerations with extensive contusions and abrasions of the face, fractures of the mandible, and multiple fractures of the bones of the middle third of the face. He was not unconscious following the accident and received treatment in the hospital emergency room for facial lacerations and severe bleeding from the nose.

The following day the patient was well oriented. His facial lacerations had been sutured, and his nose had been packed with petrolatum gauze. There was moderate ecchymosis of the lower lid on the right side and of the upper and lower lids on the left side. Extensive conjunctival and scleral chemosis was present on the left. There were palpable fractures of the nasal bones, and the left zygoma was obviously depressed. The maxilla was free-floating, easily movable, with movement at the root of the nose. The septum was deviated to the right side, and there was almost complete nasal blocking due to edema and hematoma of the septum. There was severe malocclusion of the teeth and anesthesia in the distribution of the left infraorbital nerve.

Palpation of the infraorbital regions revealed a steplike deformity at the zygomaticomaxillary and zygomaticofrontal suture lines on the left side. On the right there was minimal irregularity at the infraorbital margin at the junction with the frontal process of the maxilla. The nasal bones were loose and fractured and could be moved easily. On palpation of the anterior maxillary teeth, the entire middle third of the face could be moved up and down. There was noticeable movement at the bridge of the nose and about the orbits. The patient had no other injuries. Neurological examination was negative except for the anesthesia in the region of the distribution of the infraorbital nerve on the left. The patient had good vision in both eyes but diplopia in the inferior, superior, and lateral fields.

Roentgenographic examination confirmed the clinical impression of fracture of the left zygoma, pyramidal fracture of the maxilla, multiple fractures of the nasal bones, and fracture of the body of the mandible on the right side. Roentgenograms showed no fracture of the cervical spine.

Diagnosis: fracture of the left zygoma, pyramidal fracture of the maxilla, fracture of the nasal bones, and fracture of the body of the right mandible.

Treatment plan. The plan was to utilize closed reduction for the fracture of the mandible; open reduction and internal wire fixation for fractures of the maxilla and zygoma; and elevation, packing, and splinting of the nasal fractures.

Operation. In the operating room under infiltration and block anesthesia of the gingival mucosa with 1 per cent Xylocaine and 1:100,000 epinephrine, Erich bars were applied to the maxillary and mandibular arches. It was possible, under mandibular block anesthesia, to reduce manually the fracture of the body of the right mandible and to hold it in position by ligating the mandibular arch bar on both sides of the fracture. Ligatures were applied to all the available posterior teeth. After application of the arch bars, a tracheotomy was done under local anesthesia and a large tracheal tube inserted. The operation was continued under Fluothane anesthesia given through the tracheotomy. Incisions 1.5 cm. in length were made in the brow areas, and in the lower lids bilaterally, for exposure of the fractures. The zygoma was reduced by pressure with an elevator passed through the brow incision and carried down on the medial surface of the zygomatic arch.

Exploration of the orbital floor showed comminution with a depressed fracture and herniation of fat into the maxillary sinus. A thin section of preserved irradiated costal cartilage homograft was used to reconstruct the orbital floor. The fracture at the infraorbital margin on the left was wired and the right infraorbital margin was reduced and wired in the same manner. The fracture at the left zygomaticofrontal suture line was held by 25 gauge stainless steel wire passed through small drill holes on each side of the fracture site.

Internal wire fixation was done by passing 24 gauge stainless steel wire from the drill holes in the zygomatic process of the frontal bone downward on the medial surface of the zygomatic arch through a passing needle into the vestibule of the mouth opposite the premolar teeth. The teeth were brought into occlusion and held with intermaxillary rubber band traction. Upward pressure was applied on the mandible to force the maxilla into position where it was held by internal craniomandibular suspension with the wires tightly secured around the lower arch bar. The nasal fragments were reduced by upward and forward intranasal pressure with an Asch forceps. The septum was manipulated into position and held in the midline with intranasal packs of petrolatum. The intranasal splinting held the bones in position and a plaster splint was applied to the external nose. Rubber breathing tubes were used under the packs to permit equalization of air pressures in the nasopharynx.

Operation performed: open reduction for fractures of the zygoma and maxilla; reduction of fractures of the nasal bones and mandible; and tracheotomy.

The patient made an uneventful recovery. The tracheotomy tube was removed on the fourth day and the patient was able to breathe through his mouth and the nasal tubes. The intranasal supporting packs were removed on the seventh day, and on the eighth day the patient was discharged from the hospital.

The intermaxillary fixation and craniomandibular suspension wires were removed in the fifth week. Six months after operation the patient had excellent occlusion and minimal scarring at the operative sites; he had no complaints relative to his vision (Fig. 293 *A–F*).

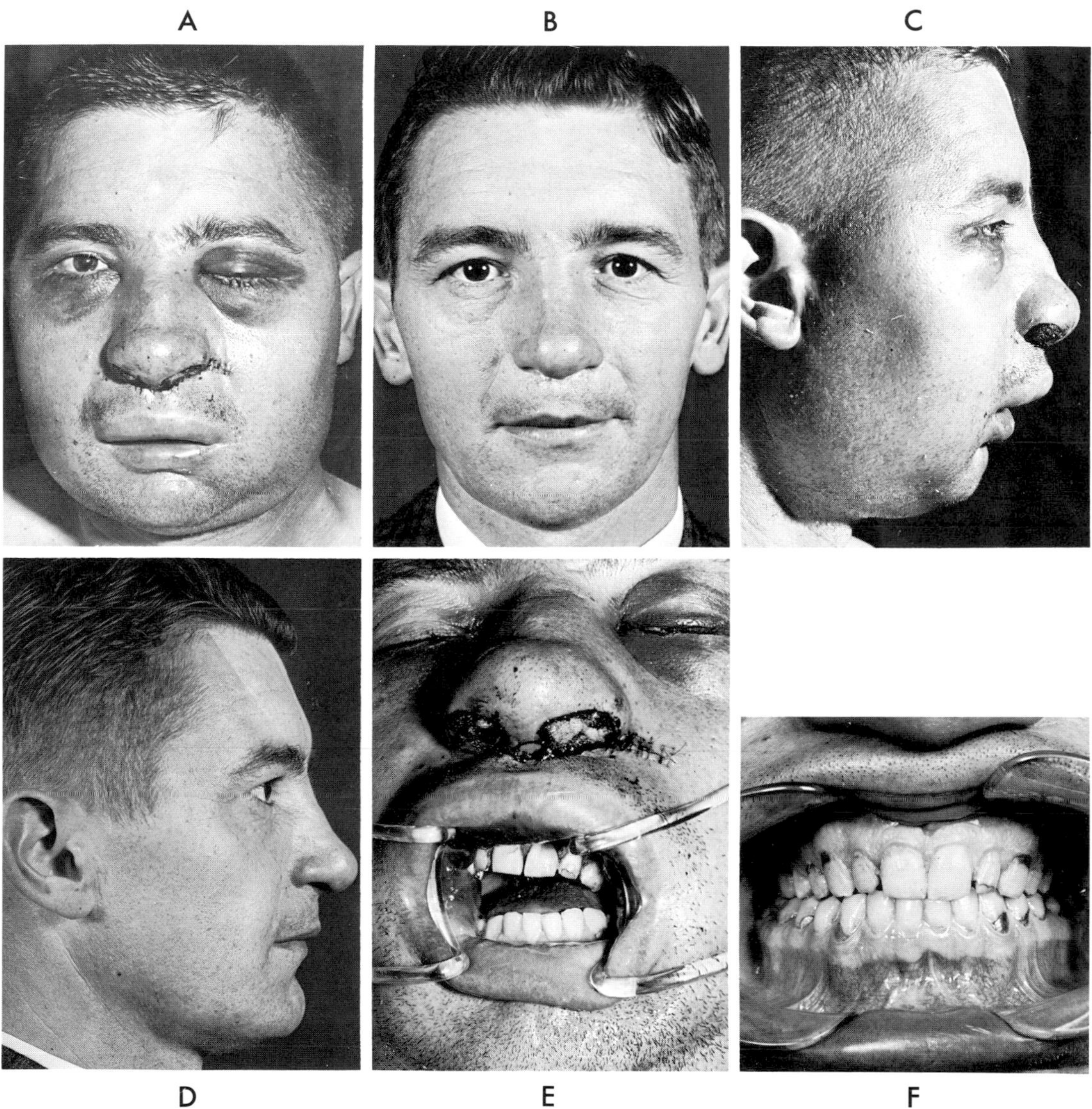

Figure 293. Multiple facial fractures, including the mandible, maxilla, zygoma, and nose, treated by interosseous wire fixation and craniofacial suspension with closed reduction of fracture of the mandible. *A*. Appearance of the patient a few hours after admission to the hospital and approximately eight hours following injury. *B*. Appearance one year after surgery. *C*. Profile view eight hours after injury. *D*. Profile view one year after treatment. *E*. Note severe malocclusion and edema of facial tissues eight hours after injury. *F*. Occlusion one year after treatment for multiple facial fractures.

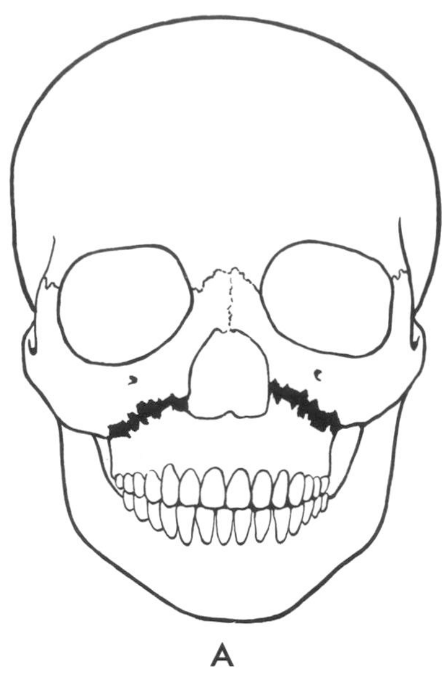

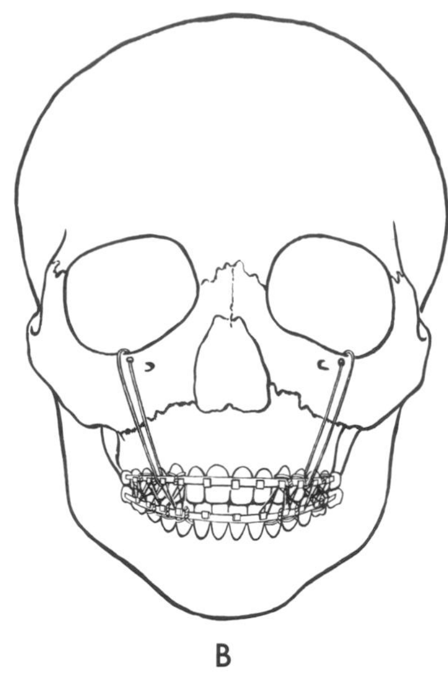

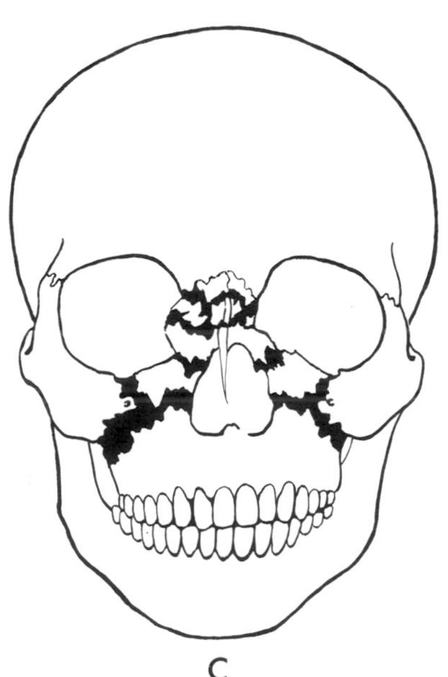

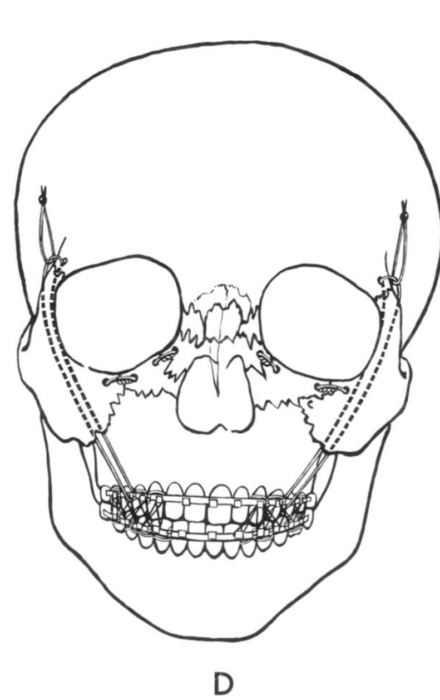

Figure 294. *A.* Transverse maxillary fracture (Le Fort I). *B.* Treatment by intermaxillary rubber band traction with arch bars and internal wire suspension from the infraorbital rim. *C.* Pyramidal type maxillary fracture (Le Fort II) associated with extensive comminution of the nasal, lacrimal, and ethmoid areas. *D.* Correction by intermaxillary fixation, craniomaxillary suspension, and interosseous wiring of fragments in the infraorbital region.

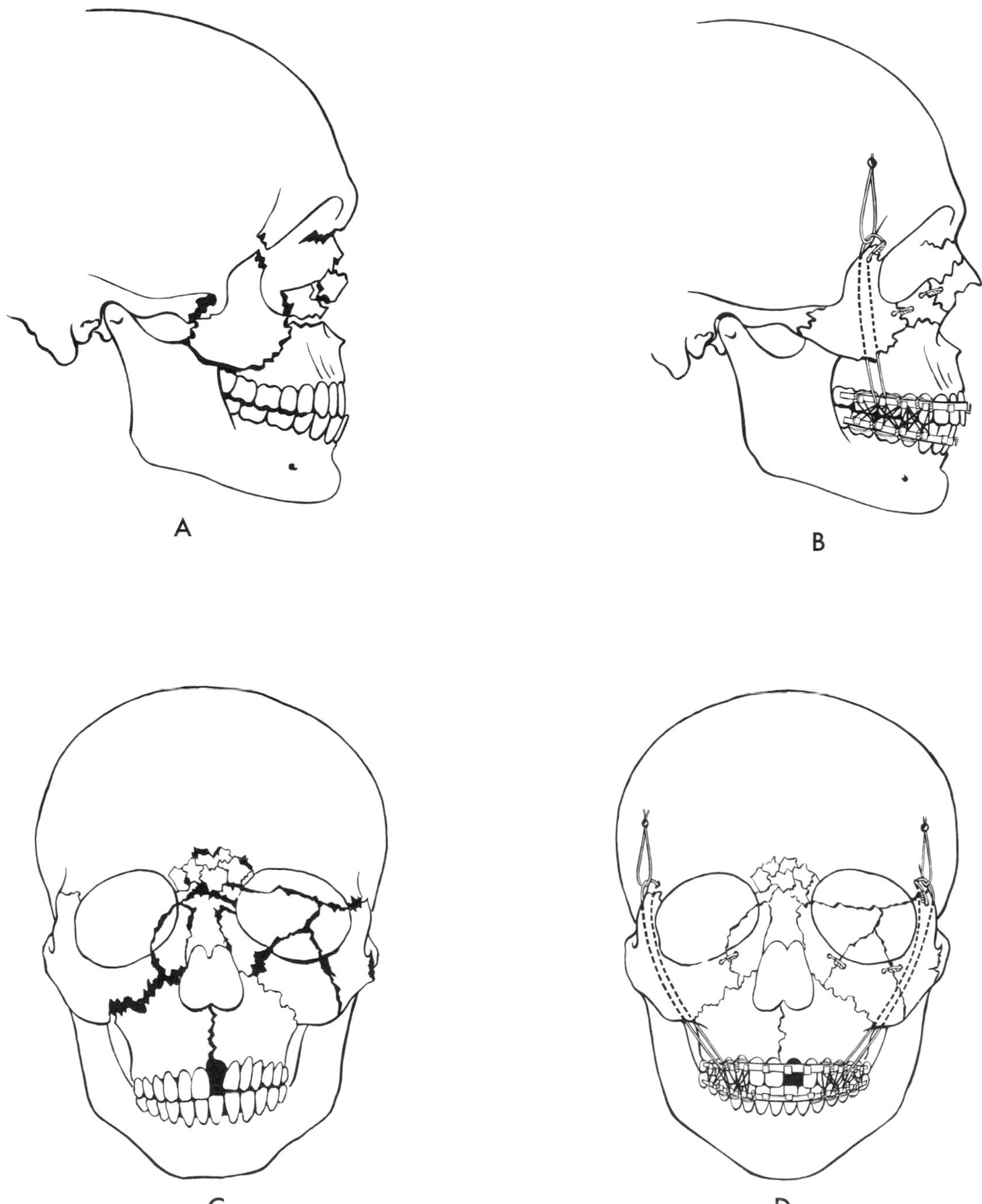

Figure 295. *A.* Fracture-dislocation of the upper portion of the facial skeleton. This kind of fracture is caused by a blow above the level of the nasal spine and results in compound comminuted fractures of the zygomatic, nasal, lacrimal, and ethmoid areas, with fracture of the maxilla. *B.* Reduction and interosseous wire fixation of multiple bone fragments, and craniomaxillary suspension with internal wire fixation. *C.* Diagram of multiple fractures of the middle third of the face, including maxilla, left zygoma, nasal, lacrimal, and ethmoid bones with involvement of the frontal sinus. *D.* Treatment by intermaxillary arch bar fixation, open reduction, and interosseous wire fixation of the fragments of the infraorbital bones, elevation of nasal and frontal bone fractures, fixation of fracture at the zygomaticofrontal suture line on left, and craniomaxillary internal wire suspension.

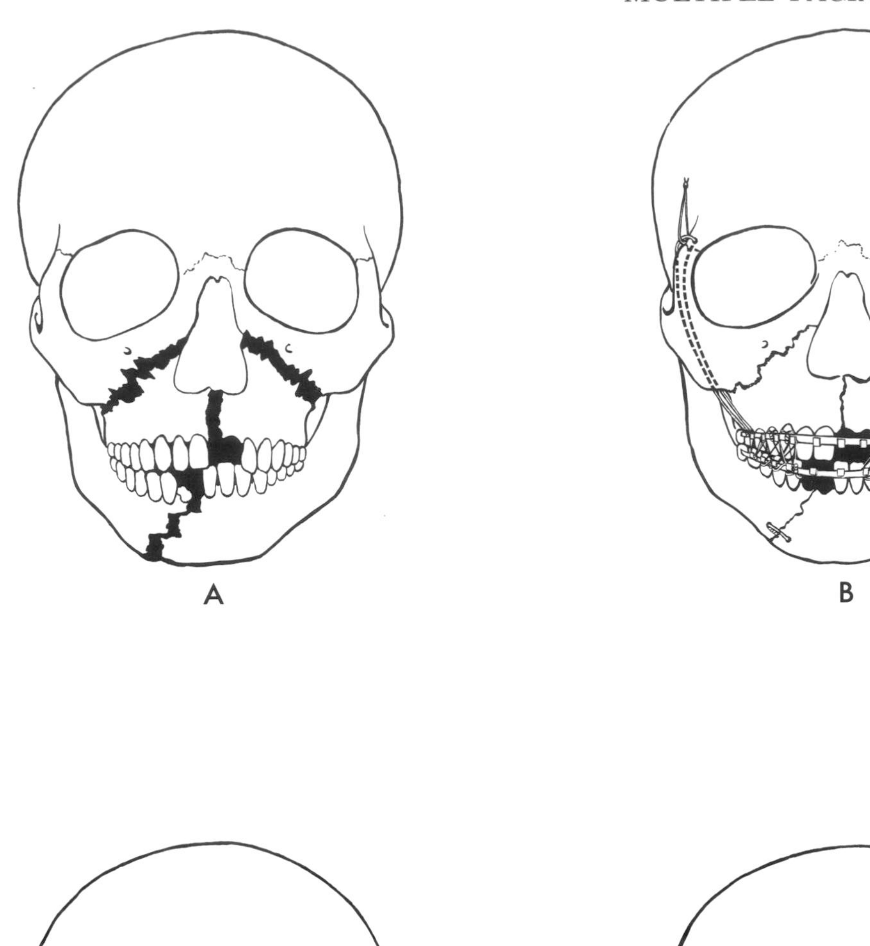

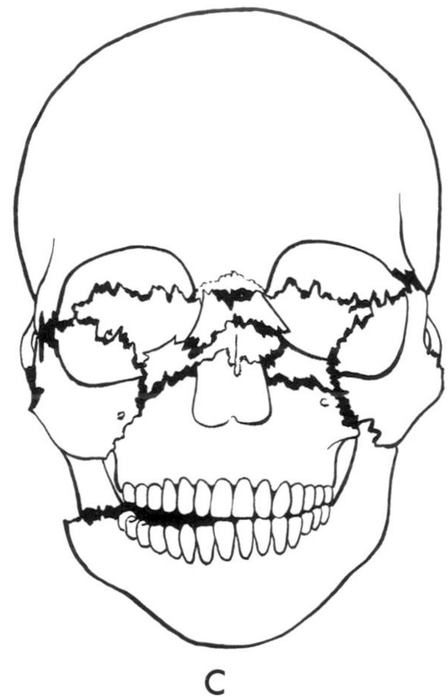

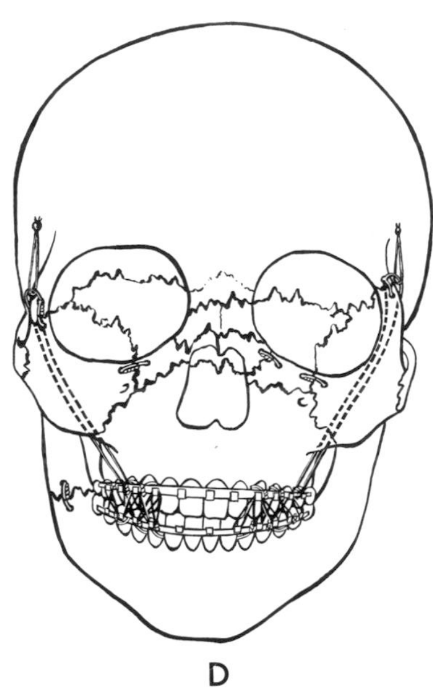

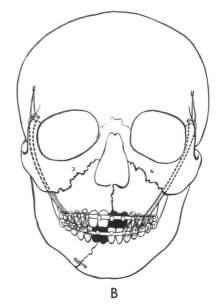

Figure 296. *A.* Pyramidal maxillary fracture with associated midline fracture of the maxilla and fracture in the region of the symphysis of the mandible. *B.* Treatment by open reduction and interosseous wiring of the mandibular fragments, intermaxillary fixation with arch bars and rubber band traction, and craniomaxillary fixation with internal suspension wires. *C.* Severe comminuted fractures of the middle third of the face with craniofacial disjunction and fracture of the mandible. *D.* Reconstruction of the mandible with open reduction, intermaxillary fixation, interosseous wiring at the zygomaticofrontal sutures, interosseous wiring of multiple fragments in the infraorbital regions, and craniomaxillary suspension.

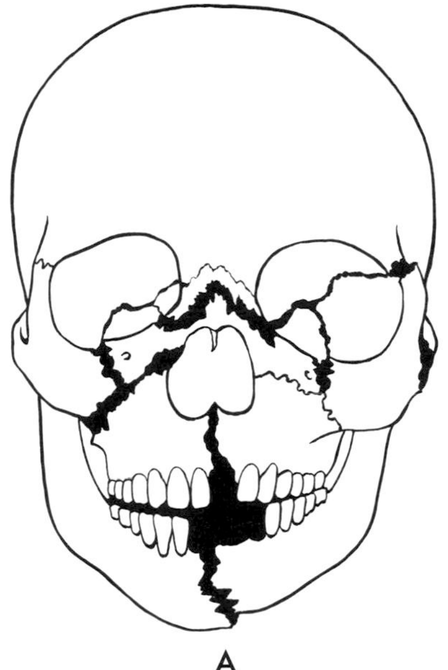

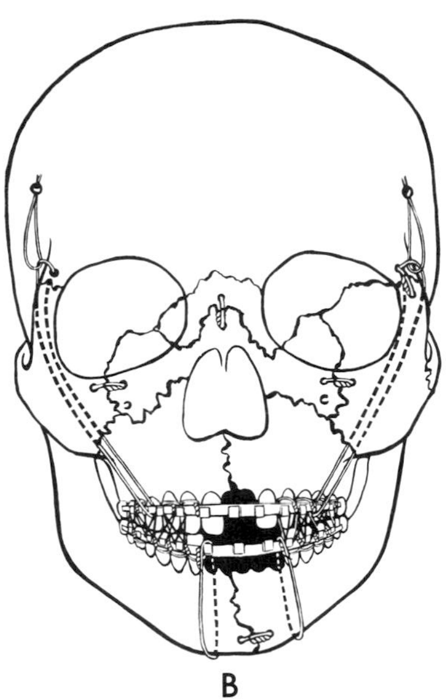

Figure 297. *A*. Multiple complex fractures of the maxilla, nasal bones, left zygoma, lacrimal, and ethmoid bones associated with fracture of the mandible. *B*. Treatment consists of reconstruction of the mandible by open reduction and interosseous wiring, application of upper and lower arch bars with supplemental circumferential fixation of the mandibular arch bar, intermaxillary rubber band fixation, and interosseous wire fixation of fractures of the left zygoma and nasal bones with craniomaxillary internal wire suspension.

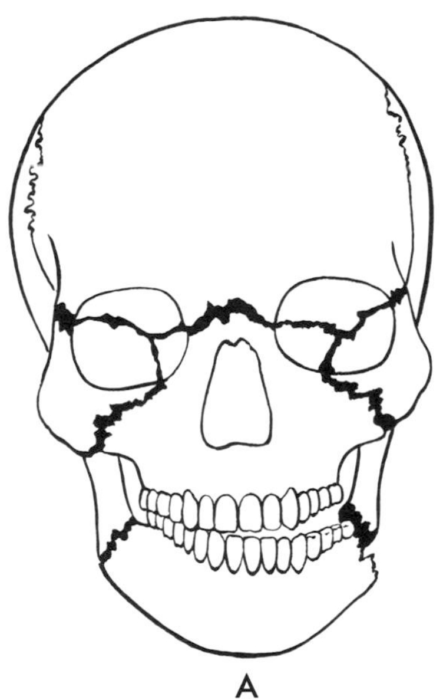

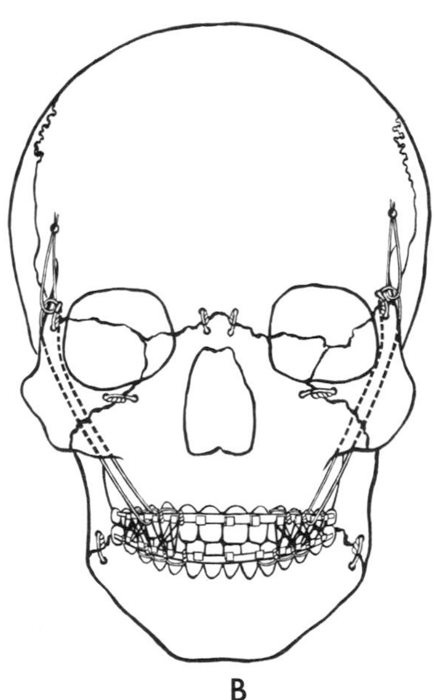

Figure 298. *A*. Multiple facial fractures including the maxilla, zygoma bilaterally, craniofacial disjunction, and bilateral fracture of the mandible. *B*. The primary step in the management of such fractures is reconstruction of the mandible by bilateral open reduction and interosseous wire fixation. Interosseous wire fixation is performed at the zygomaticofrontal suture, nasofrontal, and zygomaticomaxillary sutures. Intermaxillary rubber band fixation of the upper and lower jaws and craniomaxillary internal wire suspension fixation are also done.

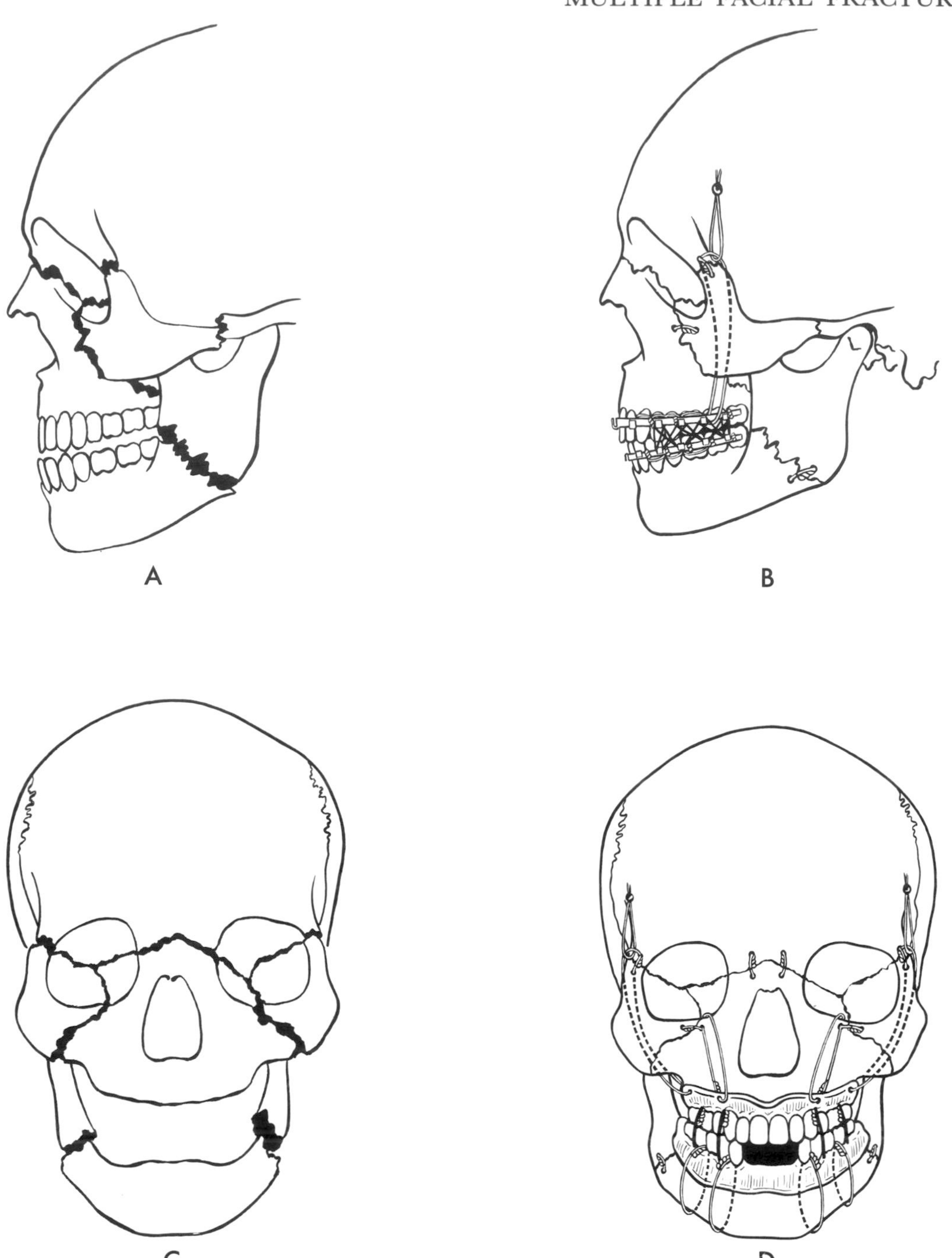

Figure 299. *A.* Profile view showing fracture of the middle third of the facial bones, open bite deformity, and fracture of the mandible. *B.* Method of fixation following reduction of multiple facial fractures. *C.* Multiple fractures of the middle third of the face, with bilateral mandibular fractures in the edentulous patient. *D.* The mandibular artificial denture is fixed with circumferential wires to the mandible. The maxillary artificial denture is used to suspend the maxilla and acts as a guide for placement of the maxillary fragments. Open reduction and interosseous wire fixation in conjunction with suspension of the upper denture from the infraorbital rims, and from the zygomatic processes of the frontal bone, provides excellent fixation for extensive fractures in the edentulous patient.

CHAPTER

11

FACIAL FRACTURES IN CHILDREN

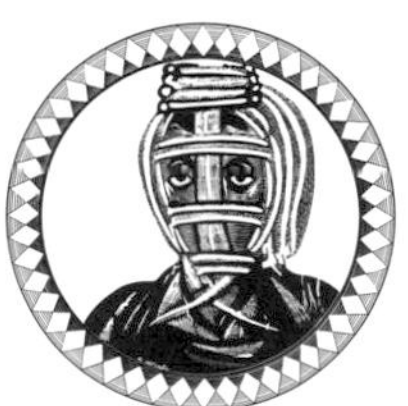

Facial bone fractures in children are relatively rare as compared with facial fractures in the adult. Reported series indicate that only from 1.4 per cent (Panagopoulos, 1957) to 10 per cent (Kazanjian and Converse, 1959) of all facial fractures occur in children. The etiological factors include falls, automobile accidents, playground accidents, sports events, and injuries from animals. The soft, resilient bony structure of the jaws in children is able to sustain a considerable impact without fracture, for bones are not so rigid as in older age periods. The resiliency of the child's facial skeleton predisposes to the development of greenstick fractures rather than complete separation at the site of fracture. Greenstick fractures are frequently seen in the region of the condyle of the mandible where there may be marked displacement of the condyle but a remaining attachment at the site of fracture.

Unerupted teeth in the line of fracture may result in loss or destruction of the developing tooth or maleruption and delayed eruption of the teeth. The method of reduction and fixation should take into account the developing tooth buds, and every effort should be made to avoid damage to them.

The bone heals rapidly and usually without complication. Fractures begin to heal immediately after the injury, and if reduction and fixation are not carried out within a few days, malunion may occur. It is advisable, therefore, to reduce fractures in children early in order to prevent complications.

The techniques of reduction and fixation used in adults may be used effectively in the management of children's fractures. The chief differences in the treatment of the child as against the adult patient concerns the size, shapes, and number of teeth available for application of appliances, the density of the bone, and the strong resistance to infection. During the period of mixed dentition, in which there are some permanent teeth and some deciduous teeth present, wiring of the teeth for fixation of the arch bars may present difficulties. Some problems arise because the anatomic development of the structures and the eruption of the teeth are incomplete, and the difficulty of reasoning with the child makes cooperation difficult in most cases. The greenstick fracture of the mandible is commonly seen in the younger child and most commonly occurs at the neck of the mandible. Fractures of the neck with medial displacement of the greenstick variety heal quickly with minimal treatment, and interference with the condylar growth centers occurs only rarely.

Severe fracture-dislocation of the condylar process in children results in complete separation of the process from the body of the mandible, and results in arrested development on the affected side with the typical facial deformity due to lack of growth, and asymmetry. The cartilaginous growth center may be destroyed, with cessation of growth of the mandible but without ankylosis (Fig. 335 *A–D*).

Diagnosis of fractures in children may be difficult because of the immature mentality, but most children are amenable to suggestion and the operator can do a reasonably thorough examination if he does not cause pain. The usual signs and symptoms of fractures seen in adult patients are present in facial bone fractures of children.

Radiography

It may be difficult for the roentgenologist to get satisfactory roentgenograms of the facial region because of lack of cooperation in the child. Sedation should be used if necessary, because radiographs in children must be taken very carefully in order to demonstrate the fractures. The jaws in children contain many developing and erupting teeth which may mask the fracture line.

Rate of Repair

Facial fractures in children unite rapidly and unless diagnosed and treated, early malunion occurs often, with disruption of the deciduous dental occlusion and deformity. Fractures of the mandible are movable for 10 days or two weeks, but fractures of the nose, the canthal region, and the maxilla become fixed after 7 to 10 days and are difficult to mobilize.

Sedation for the Child

If it is evident that cooperation cannot be obtained from the child because he is frightened or spoiled, then time should not be wasted and sedation should be used. The barbiturate drugs, chloral hydrate, or Demerol may be used safely in dosages estimated by the weight of the child. After a thorough physical examination has been carried out and the diagnosis has been established by clinical and x-ray examination, appropriate treatment should be instituted.

Principles of Management

The principles of management of facial fractures in children are not different from those employed in the management of the adult patient with similar injuries. In fact, facial fractures in children respond well to the usual methods of management used in adults. Differences in approach may be necessary because of the difficulty in getting complete cooperation from the small child. The simplest techniques that will result in proper reduction and good fixation should be used. Complicated forms of fixation should be avoided. Children may experiment or interfere with the fixation apparatus and by constant movement of the mandible may loosen or dislodge the wires and the appliances. Complications are more likely to occur in the child, and consideration of the effect of injury on the growth and development of the injured structures is important in the management of the injuries in children. Developmental deformities may result from injuries to the facial bones in children but may not be obvious until adolescence or young adult age.

Soft tissue injuries associated with fractures in children are managed in the usual manner. Resulting scars usually cause no disturbance of growth and development of the facial bones, but occasionally a dense, tight scar about the mouth or buccal vestibule results in developmental deformity of the mandible and malalignment of the teeth. If scar seems to be a factor in developmental deformity, it should be revised by appropriate reconstructive surgical procedures.

BIRTH INJURIES

Compression of soft tissues and damage to the facial bones by passage through the birth canal or by forceps delivery may result in permanent deformity. Fractures of the mandible and damage to the craniomandibular joint sometimes occur because of obstetrical maneuvers in which the obstetrician's finger is placed into the mouth of the child and forceful manipulation is used in delivery. J. Johnson (1962) treated a newborn baby who had complete separation of the mandible at the symphysis. The mother had been delivered by Smellie's maneuver, in which the body of the baby lies upon the forearm of the obstetrician and the aftercoming head is brought out by placing a finger in the infant's mouth and applying downward pressure. It is probable that ankylosis of the mandible seen in infants of 12 or 18 months is caused by birth injury.

Injury to the craniomandibular joint in children may result in developmental deformity owing to loss of the growth center in the mandibular condyle. The degree of malformation depends on the age of the infant when the injury destroyed the growth center. If growth ceases in infancy, gross deformity will result as the patient reaches adult life.

FRACTURES OF THE MANDIBLE

Although the management of fractures of the mandible in children is essentially the same as in the adult, the following differences may be mentioned.

1. The deciduous teeth may not provide good support for intermaxillary fixation. Between the ages of 6 and 12, children are in the stage of mixed dentition. The roots

of the temporary teeth are undergoing resorption and the teeth are exfoliating as the permanent teeth erupt to replace them. During the period of mixed dentition the teeth may be inadequate for the ligation of arch bars and for intermaxillary fixation.

2. Healing of fractures occurs early in children, and if treatment is not carried out within 5 or 7 days, malunion may occur. If a patient is seen later, it may be necessary to remove the callus in the fracture line in order to accomplish reduction.

3. General anesthesia is indicated in the management of children's fractures because fear and immature mentality result in lack of cooperation.

4. Fractures of the mandible are most likely to be greenstick in infancy. The cortical layer is thin and the inner cancellous portion is large and filled with developing tooth buds. These factors dispose to greenstick fracture rather than to the distinct break that occurs in the adult bone. In fractures of the condylar process there is usually some remaining contact between the bone segments. The fracture is of the greenstick type, which usually unites so that the condyle growth center continues to function. Fractures of the condylar process may result in complete separation of the growth center with interposition of soft tissue, muscle, and scar, which prevents union of the fragments. Ankylosis and deformity may result from loss of the growth center. In all fractures of the condylar process in children, the parents should be told of the possibility of damage to the growth center. Ankylosis may occur within six months to two years following injury to the mandibular condyle.

Mandibular fractures in children usually are compound and may be complicated by the presence of tooth buds in the line of fracture. Tooth buds do not interfere with reduction of the fracture, but delay of eruption may follow damage to a tooth bud.

Reduction and immobilization are the principles of management of fractures of the mandible in children and can be accomplished by manipulation and the usual methods of fixation. The methods of fixation

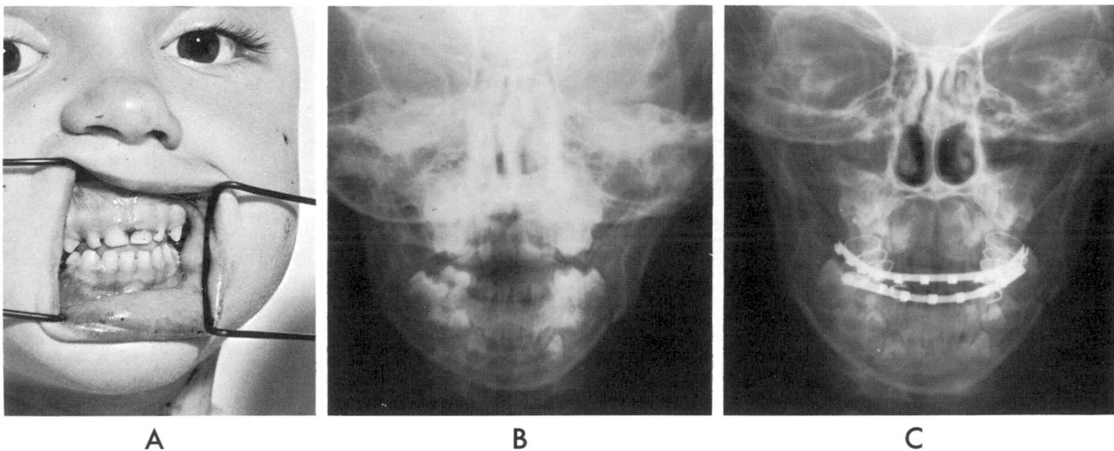

Figure 300. *A.* Malocclusion in a four-year-old child who suffered fracture of the left side of the mandible in an automobile accident. *B.* Preoperative radiograph showing fracture of the left side of the body of the mandible. *C.* Postoperative radiograph showing stabilization of the mandible with upper and lower arch bars and rubber band fixation.

may include the direct wiring method of Gilmer, the eyelet method of Ivy, or the cable wire method of fixation. Maxillary and mandibular arch bars may be applied effectively in children, but because of mixed dentition or small, short teeth, supplementary fixation by circumferential wires may be necessary. Open reduction with interosseous wiring is a safe, effective means of management of children's mandibular fractures when not enough teeth are present to permit occlusal fixation.

The mandible may be immobilized by passing one circumferential wire about the anterior region and another through the pyriform margin of the maxilla or the an-

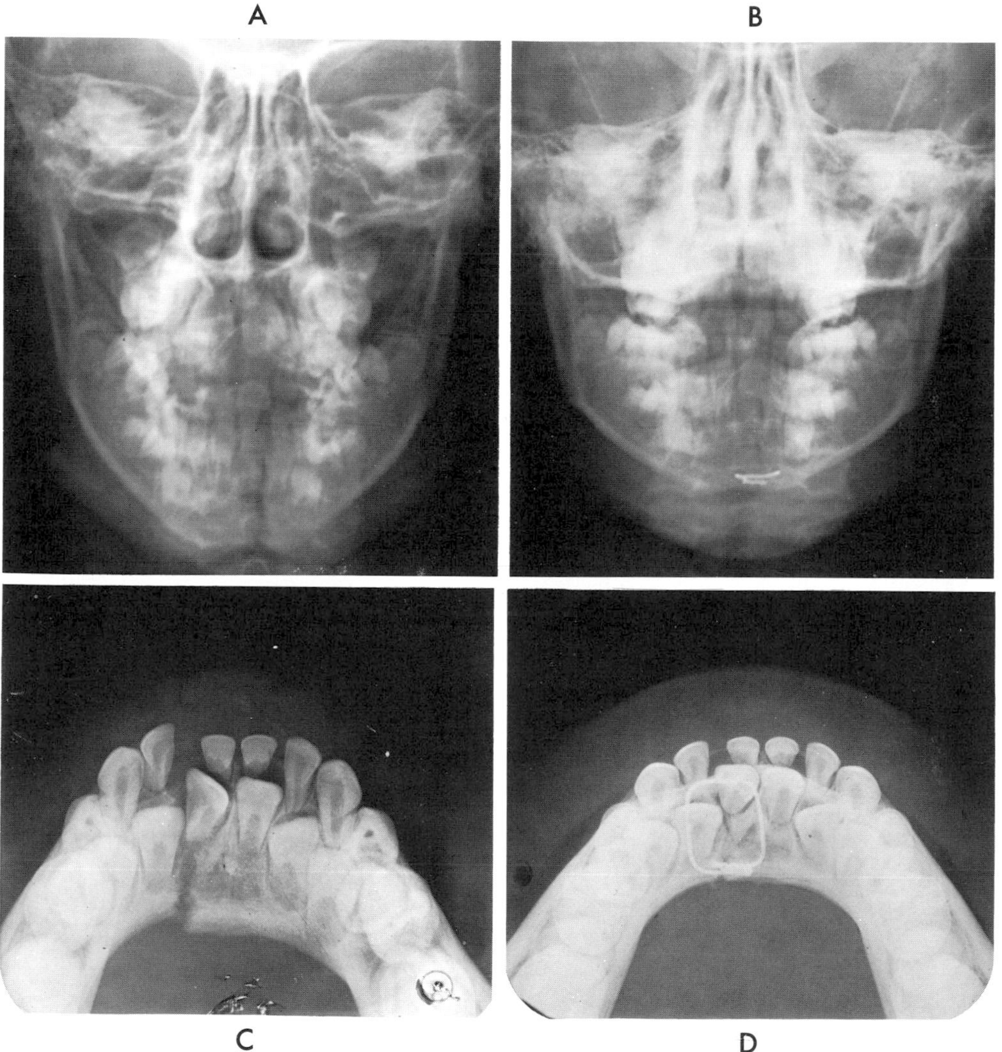

Figure 301. Fracture of the mandible in a four-year-old child, treated by open reduction and interosseous wire fixation. *A.* Radiograph of the mandible, showing fracture through the region of the symphysis. *B.* Postoperative view, showing interosseous fixation in the symphysial region. *C.* Occlusal film showing fracture of the symphysial region of the mandible. *D.* Occlusal film showing wire suture through the symphysial region.

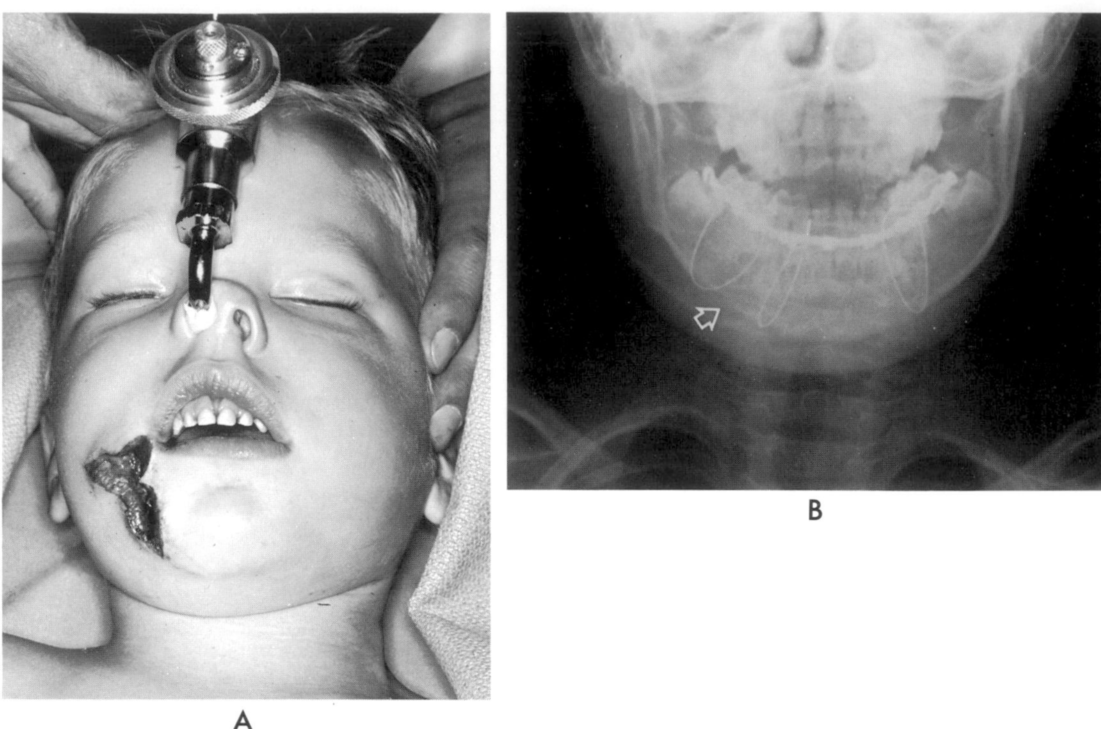

Figure 302. A. This two-year-old child was kicked in the face by a horse and suffered a severe laceration of the right cheek and fracture of the right mandible. *B.* The compound fracture was stabilized with a monomaxillary appliance consisting of an Erich arch bar ligated to the teeth and fixed by supplementary circumferential wiring.

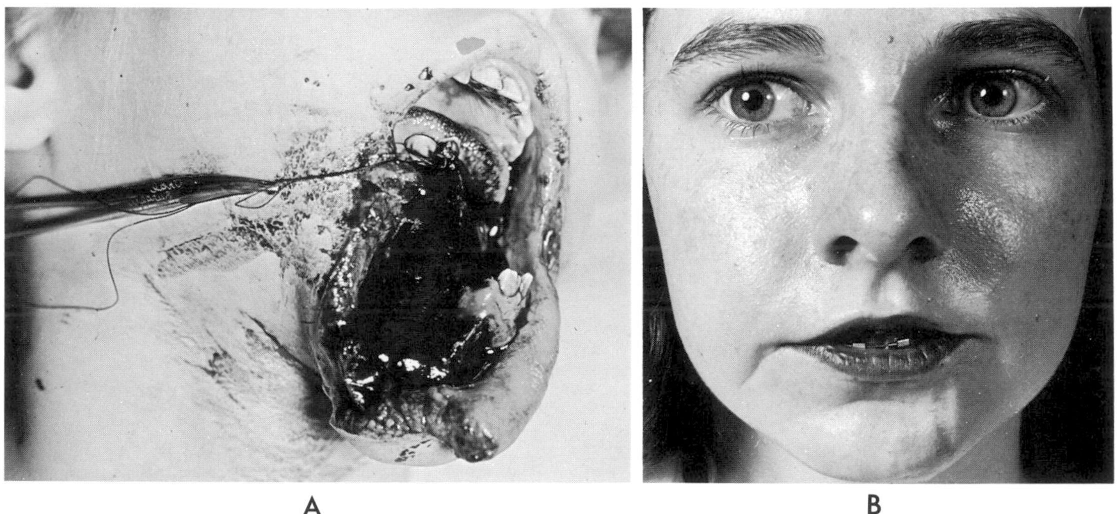

Figure 303. An eight-year-old girl with an extensive comminuted compound fracture of the anterior portion of the mandible from an automobile injury. *A.* The bone was shattered into pieces no larger than cornflakes. The mandible was reconstructed by wiring many of the small fragments together with fine stainless steel wire, careful closure of the soft tissues, placing the remaining teeth in occlusion, and fixation by direct wiring from the upper to the lower teeth. Multiple small bone fragments acted as a nidus for regeneration of the mandible. *B.* Patient five years after treatment has a solid, intact mandible. The lower teeth have been replaced by a prosthesis and function is excellent.

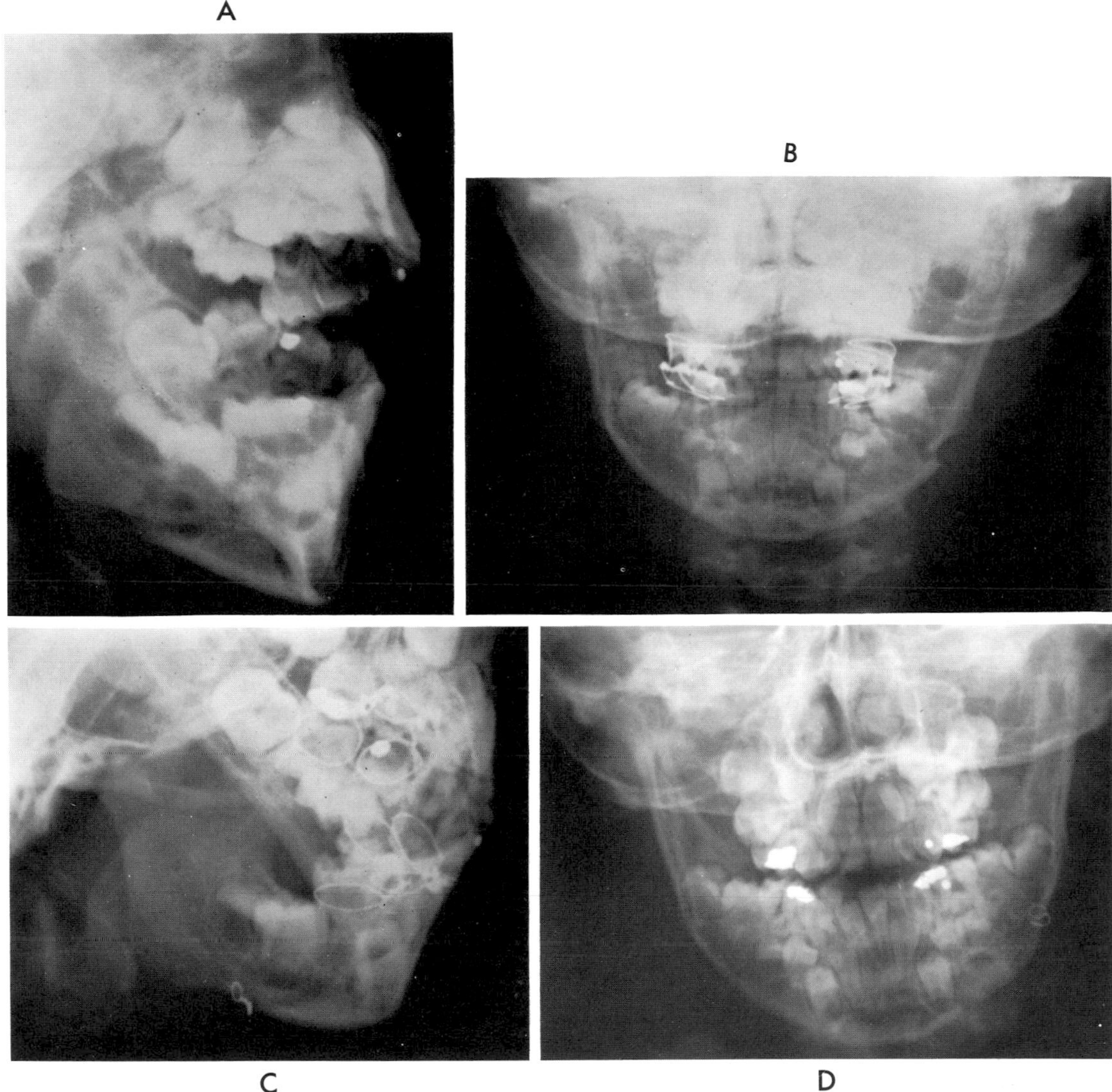

Figure 304. Fracture of the angle of the mandible on the left in a five-year-old child. *A*. Preoperative radiograph showing displacement and overriding. *B*. An attempt was made to treat this patient by intermaxillary wire fixation. Instability of the posterior segment necessitated open reduction. *C*. Lateral view showing fixation by interosseous wiring. *D*. Postoperative view three months following open reduction and direct wiring.

terior nasal spine. Each of these wires can be twisted into a loop and the two loops may be connected by rubber bands or wire fixation. Fractures in which there is minimal displacement may be treated by the use of a head-cap and chin traction for 7 to 10 days, during which time the segments will stabilize by rapid healing.

INJURIES TO THE TEETH AND ALVEOLAR PROCESS

Fractures of the teeth and alveolar process in children are relatively common results of falls or blows to the anterior part of the mouth. Teeth may be loosened or fractured with a segment of the alveolar bone, and every effort should be made to save them, especially in the anterior region where the permanent teeth erupt at an early age and loss is of great significance. Collateral circulation in the alveolar structures is excellent, the dental root canals are open, and the teeth and bone have an amazing ability to recover if properly supported and splinted for two or three weeks.

The anesthetized or unconscious child should be examined carefully for loose or dislodged teeth to avoid the possibility of aspiration. During the period of mixed dentition, the roots of the deciduous teeth undergo resorption and the teeth are easily dislodged.

Reimplantation of completely dislodged, partially developed permanent teeth in the child has resulted in success in many cases. But such success depends upon satisfactory splinting during the period of healing.

FRACTURES OF THE MAXILLA

Fractures of the maxilla are often associated with fractures of the zygoma in children. These are rare but result from violent forces rather than from falls or simple blows. Fractures are usually the result of automobile accidents, injuries from farm equipment, or kicks from animals. Treatment is the same as that for the adult patient. Many maxillary fractures respond to reduction and fixation with chin support or temporary head-cap appliances. Alveolar fractures in the maxilla can be supported by ligation of the teeth to an arch bar attached to the adjacent solidly fixed maxillary teeth. With craniofacial disjunction, open reduction and interosseous wire fixation or craniomaxillary suspension may be indicated, as described for the adult patient with a similar type of fracture. As in the adult, the mandible may be utilized as a guide for the proper positioning of the maxillary fragments.

The paranasal sinuses are small in children and need no practical consideration in the management of fractures of the maxilla. As the child becomes older, the sinuses become larger and in the teen-age patient they may be large enough to be involved in complications.

FRACTURES OF THE ZYGOMA

Fractures of the zygoma in children are relatively rare and are associated frequently with fractures of the maxilla. The violent forces that cause fractures of the zygoma usually result also in fractures of the orbital structures. Evaluation and cooperation with the ophthalmologist are important in cases of this kind. Inasmuch as many of the fractures are compound, it is advisable to reduce the fracture and fix it with direct wire sutures through the open wound as soon as possible after injury. The closed methods of reduction of the fractured zygoma in children may be effective, but the consequences of the inadequate reduction and fixation are such that open operation should be done if there is any question about the effectiveness of the reduction by closed methods.

FRACTURES OF THE NOSE

Nasal fractures in children are often missed or are untreated because they are consid-

(*Text continued on page 322.*)

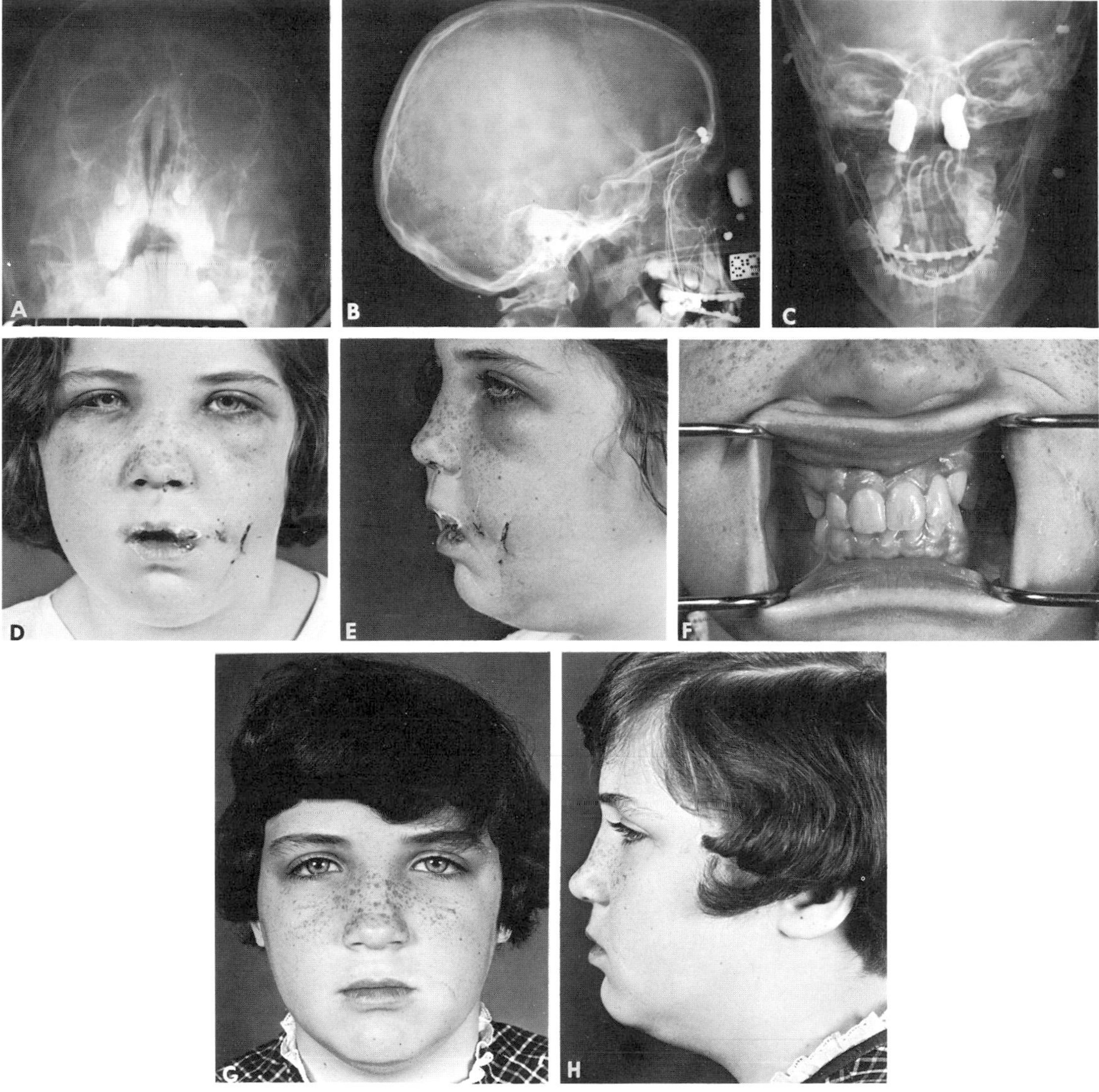

Figure 305. Extensive multiple fractures of middle third of the face, sustained in an automobile accident. *A*. Injuries included a pyramidal fracture of the maxilla, smash fractures of the nose, and bilateral infraorbital fractures. *B, C*. Treatment consisted of internal wire suspension of the facial bones with intermaxillary fixation by the use of arch bars and rubber band traction. A circumferential wire was placed around the anterior part of the mandible to supplement fixation of the lower arch bar. *D, E*. Appearance of patient two days after injury. Note flattening of the middle third of the face and loss of contour of the nose. *F, G, H*. One year after operation.

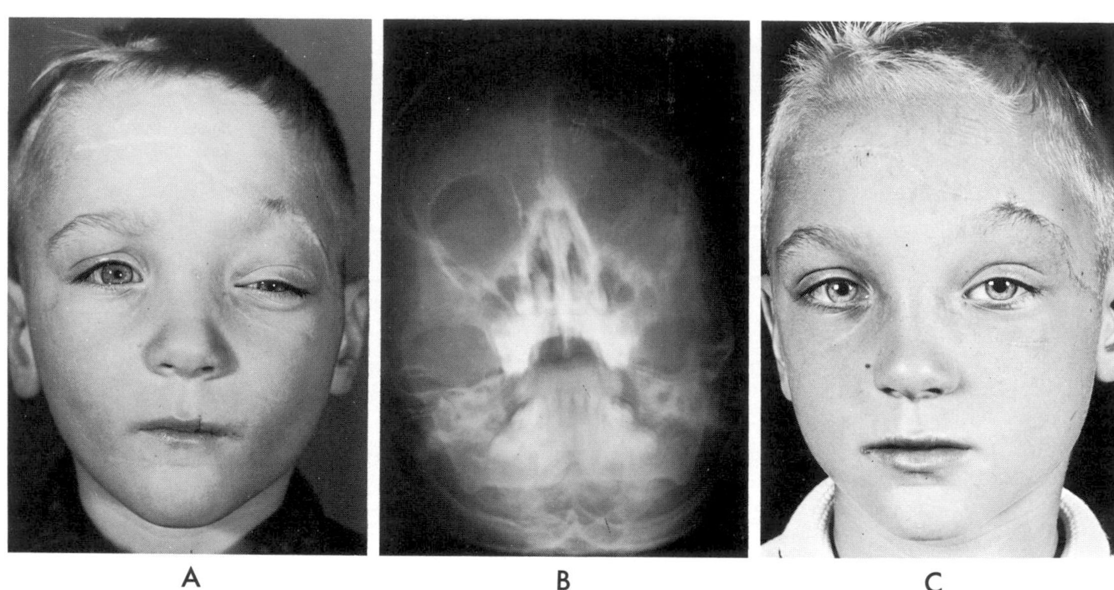

Figure 306. This three-year-old patient was knocked down and dragged by an automobile, and suffered fractures of the skull and left zygoma. The immediate treatment necessitated removal of the supraorbital ridge, another portion of the frontal bone, and the roof of the orbit. The depressed fracture of the zygoma was not treated immediately. Subsequently, open operation with osteotomy of the left zygoma was done, and a later procedure consisted of repair of the orbital floor by use of an autogenous iliac bone graft. *A*. Appearance of the patient nine months following injury. Note depression of the left eye and ptosis. *B*. Radiograph showing defects in the left orbit, supraorbital ridge, frontal bone, and roof of the orbit. *C*. Patient shown at age five years with result obtained by elevation of the left zygoma and reconstruction of the orbital floor with iliac bone grafts. No other operative procedure was performed to correct the ptosis.

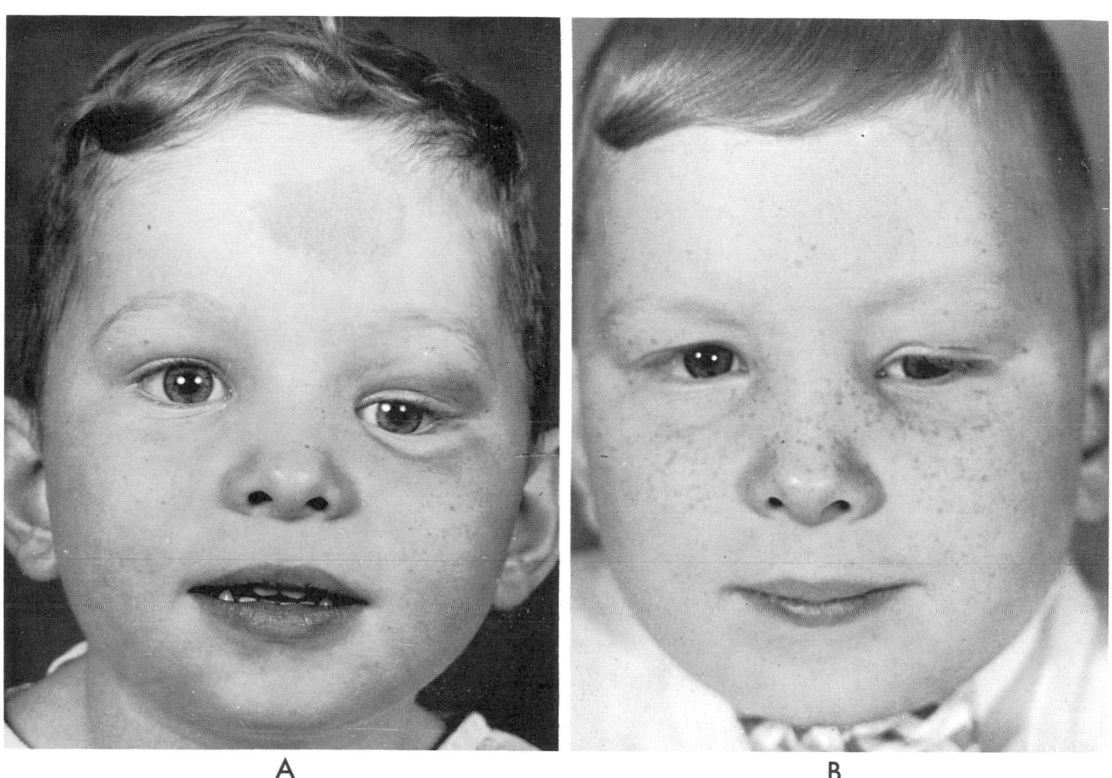

Figure 307. *A*. Two-year-old child with malunion fracture of the left zygoma and orbital floor. He was struck by an automobile and suffered extensive injury to the brain in addition to facial fractures. This photograph was taken six months after his injury. *B*. Postoperative result two years after reconstruction of the orbital floor with preserved irradiated costal cartilage homografts.

ered to be insignificant. Displacement of the bony and cartilaginous structures, although not great at the time of injury, may result in gross deformity as growth and development progress. Fractures of the septal cartilage and nasal bones are common in children.

The kind of fracture most frequently seen is the open-book type, with splaying outward of the fractured segments over the frontal process of the maxilla. These fractures are due to violent trauma from a direct frontal blow and may result in the displacement of the entire nasal bony bridge into the ethmoid region. The force of the nasal bones and frontal process of the maxilla striking against the lacrimal region may result in tearing of the medial palpebral ligament or displacement of the lacrimal bones, with flattening of the bony nose, increased separation between the medial canthi, and lateral displacement of the eyes with narrowing of the palpebral fissures. Fracture-dislocation of the cartilaginous septum, with telescoping or buckling of the cartilage, may result in nasal obstruction, which becomes progressively worse as the patient gets older.

Bleeding from the nose of a child who has been struck over the bony bridge suggests the presence of a fracture. The nasal bones, when displaced, act as secondary missiles which penetrate through the nasal mucoperichondrium or mucoperiosteum. Fractures in the child may be difficult to discover by means of roentgenograms, and the presence of edema and hematoma may make a clinical diagnosis difficult.

If a fracture is suspected it is advisable to place the child under anesthesia and to elevate and manipulate the nasal bones and carefully inspect the septum. Fractures or dislocations of the septum should be corrected by placing the tissues in position and supporting them with intranasal packs and splints if necessary. The structures usually will remain in position without fixation unless the comminution has been extensive and the lacerations of the soft tissues are severe. If indicated, the structures should be held in place by through-and-through wire fixation over soft metal plates, as has been described for the adult patient.

Fractures of the nose in children may not become evident until adolescent development results in gross nasal deformity.

The nasal tissues heal rapidly and, unless they are repositioned in a matter of two or three days, reduction may be difficult or impossible. When seen late, nasal deformities in children should not be corrected unless this can be done by a simple procedure. Extensive reconstructive procedures for deformity of the nose in children are inadvisable unless they become urgent for psychological reasons.

Chip fractures of the lower ends of the nasal bones depress the septum and result in subsequent twisting and deformity of the septum. A subsequent overgrowth may be productive of a severe deformity in adult life. Nasal obstruction from a deflection of the septum should be corrected if significant obstruction of the airway causes interference with the drainage of the sinuses. However, if the patient has a reasonably clear airway and is not embarrassed by his appearance, it is best to defer corrective procedures until he is 16 or 17 years of age. If the nasal defect is psychologically disturbing to the patient, the dorsum of the nose may be built up with grafts of bone or cartilage. Autogenous costal cartilage, rib, or iliac bone is satisfactory for building up the nasal dorsum. If the ilium is used as a source of graft material, the graft should be taken from the bony area of the ilium rather than from the crest, which usually is cartilaginous in children and does not provide substantial material for permanent grafts.

In one of our cases, traumatic nasal deformity in a 10-year-old child was disturbing psychologically to him and he refused to attend school. An acrylic implant was inserted subcutaneously through a midcolumellar incision. This was changed subsequently on two occasions for larger pieces during the developmental period, and finally, at the age of 18, a permanent iliac bone graft was inserted. The acrylic insert was useful in maintaining growth of the skin so that at the time of definitive surgery an adequate amount of tissue was present for final correction.

COMPLICATIONS OF FRACTURES IN CHILDREN

Early Complications

Early complications in children are rare. Infection may complicate compound fractures of the facial bones but is infrequent because of the excellent blood supply and the great resistance of the tissues. The use of antibiotic therapy in the management of facial injuries has decreased the number of infections and the cases of osteomyelitis. Obstruction of the airway and hemorrhage are managed by the usual methods. Malunion of fractures is an early complication in childhood injuries. The rapid healing of tissues may result in malunion, malocclusion, and facial deformity. This complication usually can be avoided by early reduction and fixation.

Late Complications

Late complications include malocclusion and delayed eruption or malformation of the teeth. Facial deformity may result from malunion or from interference with growth and development of the facial bones. Ankylosis of the mandible is a common complication of fracture of the neck with damage to the articulating surface of the head. This may occur unilaterally or bilaterally. It may be due to a compound fracture in the region of the condyle, but usually is due to aseptic necrosis of the articular surface of the condyle or to fracture with complete separation of the condyle from the ramus of the mandible. Trauma to the joint may cause aseptic necrosis without ankylosis. The dish-face deformity results from a fracture-displacement of the maxilla that is untreated or is permitted to heal in malposition.

Permanent diplopia due to fracture of the zygoma and orbital floor may occur. Sometimes correction can be accomplished by means of a graft of bone or cartilage with reconstruction of the orbital floor and zygomatic region. Saddle nose, or a flat nasal dorsum, may result from unreduced nasal bone fractures or from fracture-dislocation of the cartilaginous septum. Traumatic pseudohypertelorism may result from fractures with lateral displacement of the nasal and lacrimal bones and detachment of the palpebral ligaments (Fig. 308). Craniofacial disjunction may result in permanent, persistent cranionasal fistula with cerebrospinal rhinorrhea. Schneider and Thompson (1957) reported a number of cases in which acute meningitis occurred several years after facial injury, from untreated permanent fistula from the nose to the dura. Ankylosis may result in unilateral underdevelopment of the mandible with maldevelopment of the temporocranial region. The premature loss of teeth in the child results in the lack of normal development of the body and alveolar process of the maxillary and mandibular bones.

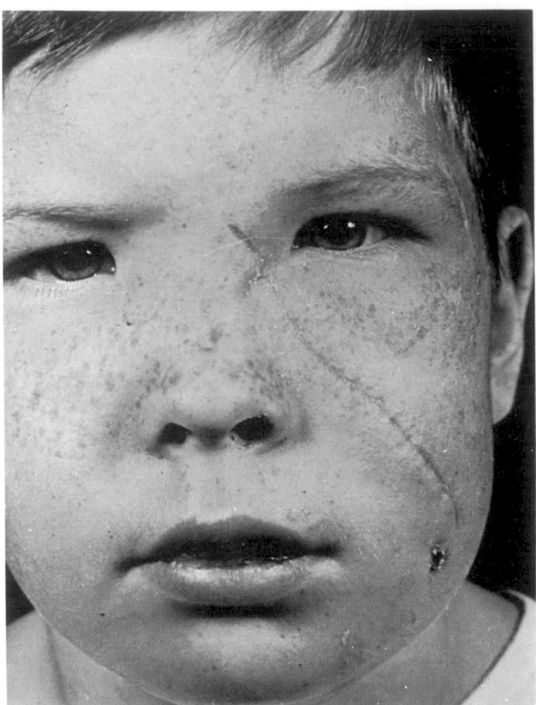

Figure 308. Pseudohypertelorism as a result of malunion fractures of the nasal bones and frontal processes of maxillae, lateral displacement of the lacrimal bones, and detachment of the palpebral ligaments. This is an extremely unfortunate complication of facial fractures, for it is nearly impossible to get a good final result in such a case. Early treatment may help prevent this deformity.

Case Report

A 6-year-old boy was transferred for treatment of facial fractures, having been treated initially in another hospital for shock following an automobile accident on the preceding day. On admission, his temperature was 100.2° F., pulse 144, blood pressure 124/85. Physical examination showed a sutured laceration over the right forehead, the nose out of alignment, and clotted blood filling the airway on both sides. The right upper and lower lids were edematous and ecchymotic. There was great deformity, with depression, over the right maxilla. The patient was unable to open his mouth more than 1.5 cm. The right maxilla was displaced downward and backward with the teeth still attached. There was tenderness upon palpation over the left side of the mandible, although no deformity was evident. There was clotted blood in the left ear, but both ear drums appeared normal. There were contusions and abrasions over the face and right wrist. Laboratory studies revealed 8 to 10 white blood cells in the urine, hemoglobin 13.5 gm. and white blood cell count 6200.

X-ray examination showed a right maxillary fracture with depression of the main portion of the maxilla inward and backward. The fracture line extended from the inferior anterolateral aspect of the right orbit, through the zygoma, and nearly parallel with the zygomatic arch. The medial fracture line was not identified radiographically but probably involved the medial inferior portion of the right orbit and extended down into the hard palate. There was a medially angulated condylar fracture of the mandible on the left. The preoperative diagnosis was fracture of the right maxilla with posteroinferior displacement, fracture of the left condylar process of the mandible, and facial lacerations and contusions.

Operation was performed under general anesthesia. With oral endotracheal intubation a tracheotomy was performed through a transverse incision. The trachea was entered through the third and fourth tracheal rings. A No. 4 tracheotomy tube was inserted. The oral tube was removed and the anesthesia was continued with cyclopropane and oxygen through the tracheotomy tube.

It was possible, after irrigating and cleansing the area, to assess more accurately the extent of the injuries. They involved the entire right maxilla, nose, and infraorbital margin with displacement posteriorly, inferiorly, and medially for about 2 cm.

The maxillary fragments were reduced by grasping the anterior portion of the maxilla with a towel clip and applying forward, upward, and lateral traction; no difficulty was encountered in the reduction. Erich bars were ligated with 25 gauge stainless steel wire to the upper and lower arches. A circumferential wire placed about the anterior part of the mandible was used to stabilize the lower arch bar, since the anterior deciduous teeth were short and did not offer adequate means for ligation of the bar around the necks of the teeth. Then upper and lower arch bars were joined with intermaxillary rubber bands, and in this way stable fixation of the loose maxillary fragment on the right was accomplished.

It was elected to investigate the fracture at the lateral margin of the lower orbital ridge. This was done through a small transverse incision parallel with and inferior to the orbital margin. The fracture site was exposed, and it was seen that adequate reduction had been achieved, leaving a separation of less than 2 mm. in the fracture. It was thought that no interosseous fixation was necessary, and the incisions were closed with 0000 catgut sutures in the subcutaneous tissues and 00000 nylon sutures in the skin. Then the nasal passages were examined and the fragments adjusted. Torn labial mucosa of the upper lip was seen, but it was not possible to approximate the mucosa accurately because of the loss of tissue and it was decided to allow this area to heal by granulation. The child tolerated the procedure well and was moved to the recovery room. Estimated blood loss: 100 cc.

Operation: tracheotomy, reduction of fracture of the right maxilla and nasal bones. The tracheotomy was maintained for six days. The postoperative course was uneventful and discharge from the hospital was possible on the tenth day. Fixation was maintained for five weeks. The appliances were removed under Demerol sedation and local application of topical xylocaine viscous to the gingival tissues. The final result was satisfactory from the standpoint of appearance and function (Figs. 309–316).

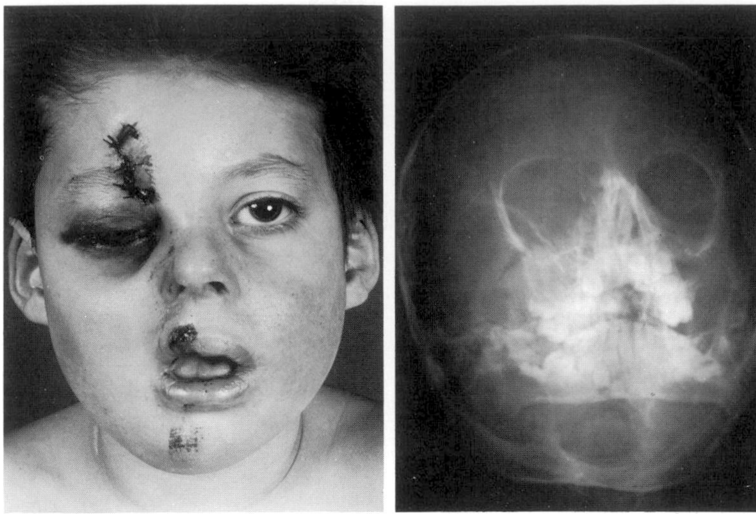

Fig. 309 Fig. 310

Figure 309. Unilateral depressed, displaced compound fracture of the right maxilla, zygoma, and nasal bone in six-year-old child 24 hours following injury in an automobile accident.

Figure 310. Radiograph (Waters' projection) showing right unilateral fracture and displacement of the maxilla, floor of the orbit, zygoma, and nasal bone. Note the normal maxillary sinus on the left and the clouded maxillary sinus on the right.

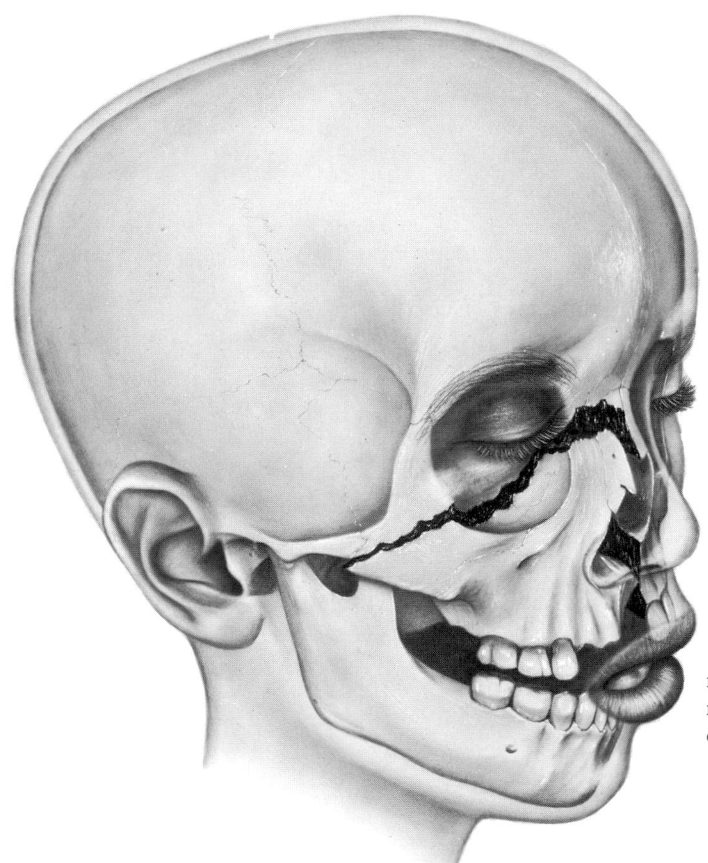

Figure 311. Extent of fracture of the right maxilla, zygoma, orbital floor, and nasal bone and extent of displacement of fracture.

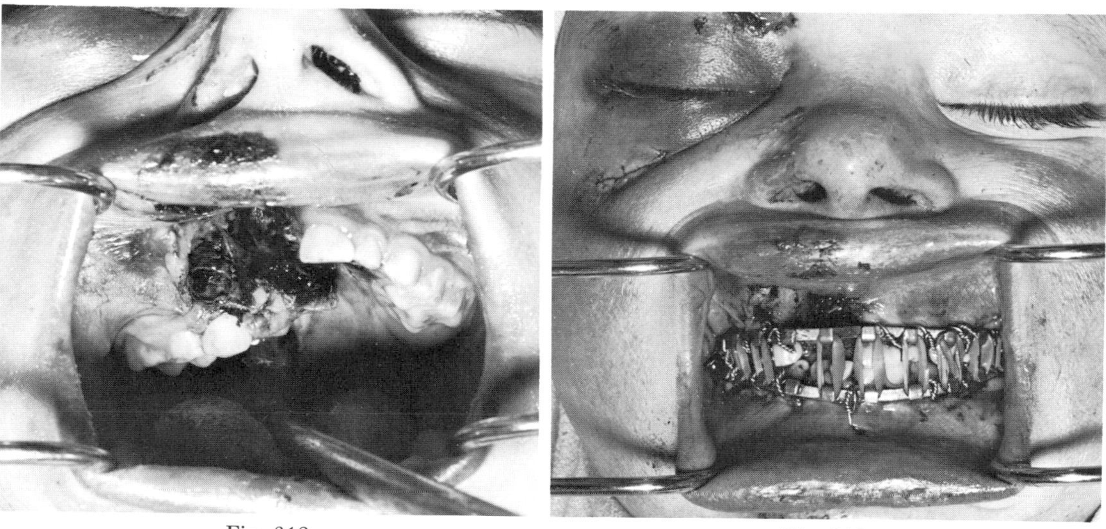

Fig. 312 Fig. 313

Figure 312. Intraoral view showing displacement of fracture.

Figure 313. Arch bars and intermaxillary rubber band traction utilized for fixation following reduction. Note circumferential wire passing around the mandible and the arch bar in the lower anterior region.

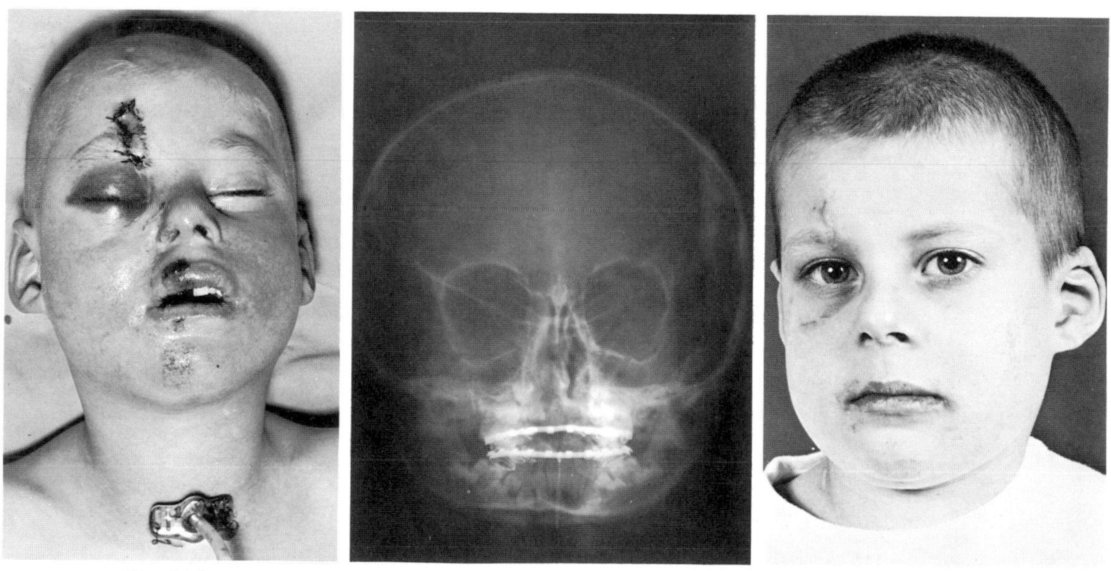

Fig. 314 Fig. 315 Fig. 316

Figure 314. Anesthetic being administered through tracheotomy.

Figure 315. Postoperative roentgenogram. Note excellent position of the reduced fragments, arch bars, and supplementary circumferential wire about the mandible for arch bar stabilization.

Figure 316. One month postoperative. Note restored facial contour and normal position of the right eye.

CHAPTER

12

COMPLICATED FRACTURES

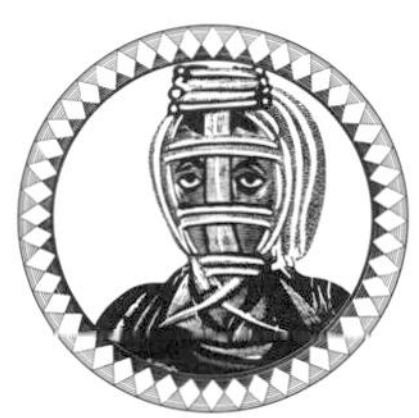

Most facial fractures are uncomplicated and involve only a single bone or possibly its immediate articulating bones. Some of these fractures, however, are complicated by associated soft tissue injuries, loss of bone structure, or extension into vital surrounding tissues. Some are complicated by local or general disease, such as cysts, malignant disease, or advanced constitutional disease, which interferes with the process of repair.

CRANIOFACIAL DISJUNCTION

Complete disjunction of the facial skeleton from the cranium may occur. The fractures extend through the zygomaticofrontal suture areas, the nasofrontal suture, the lateral and medial orbital walls, or the pterygoid process to result in complete separation of the skeletal structures composing the middle third of the face. Such fractures usually result from a direct frontal blow in the upper facial area and a shearing force which completely separates the facial bones from the skull. There is usually a multiplicity of injuries with comminution, but the maxilla may not be separated from the zygoma or from the nasal structures, and the entire middle-third bony structure may be completely detached from the base of the skull as a unit, and remain suspended only by the soft tissues. This injury is known as the Le Fort III fracture and is usually the result of the guest-passenger kind of injury in which the patient is thrown forward against the instrument panel, the back of the front seat, or the head of another passenger. Violent force sustained at a high level on the face usually results in a comminuted, separated, displaced fracture. Traumatic forces usually are directed from in front or from the side, but upward forces may result in displacement of fragments into the cranial fossa, laceration of the dura, and damage to the brain tissues. The entire maxilla may be driven upward and backward into the interorbital space or the pharynx.

Diagnosis is made on the basis of bleeding from the nose; periorbital, conjunctival, and scleral ecchymosis with facial edema; malocclusion of the teeth; and a dish-faced, long, or donkey-like appearance of the face. Controlled but forceful manipulation of the anterior maxillary region reveals movement of the facial bones. Palpation may reveal separation at the zygomaticofrontal and the nasofrontal sutures with a palpable space between the bony structures. Simultaneous bilateral bimanual palpation may reveal irregularities of the infraorbital margins from fractures of the zygoma and maxilla. Movement and crepitation of the nasal bones may reveal associated nasal fractures. Cerebrospinal rhinorrhea is noted if there is cranial extension with tearing of the dura.

Cerebrospinal rhinorrhea can result from the driving of displaced fractured segments of the maxilla or nose into the base of the skull with laceration of the dura. The crista galli may be fractured and driven into the brain. Clear fluid may be seen draining from the nostrils, from the open wound, or into the pharynx in fractures in which the cribriform plate or the floor of the anterior cranial fossa is damaged. Fragments of bone of the ethmoid-sphenoid-maxillary structures may be driven into the anterior cranial fossa and cause severe brain damage. Injury to the supraorbital ridge of the frontal bone may result in fractures that extend through the outer wall of the frontal sinus without fracture of the inner wall. Severe penetrating injuries may involve both the outer and inner walls of the frontal sinus with tears in the dura and leakage of cerebrospinal fluid into the wound or the nasal cavity.

CEREBROSPINAL RHINORRHEA

The large space between the medial orbital walls is known as the interorbital space and has been defined as the region made up primarily of the two ethmoidal labyrinths. The roof of the ethmoidal region on each side projects a few millimeters higher than the cribriform plate between the ethmoidal labyrinths. The roof of the space is formed by the cribriform plate in the midline and by the frontal bones near the ethmoid notch on each side. The floor of the space is on a horizontal plane between the lower borders of the ethmoidal labyrinths. Laterally the space is bounded by the medial walls of the orbit, which are formed by the laminae papyraceae of the ethmoid bone. Posteriorly the space is limited by the body of the sphenoid bone and anteriorly by the frontal process of the maxilla.

Cairns (1937) described three mechanisms by which cerebrospinal rhinorrhea might occur:

1. Fractures involving the posterior wall of the frontal sinus with penetration of fragments into the frontal lobe result in dural tear and brain damage. There may be a concomitant fracture extending into the cribriform plate.

2. Cerebrospinal rhinorrhea may occur from fracture of the nasal bones and frontal processes of the maxilla. Bone fragments are pushed into the ethmoidal labyrinth or into the interorbital space, with fracture of the roof of the ethmoid area and penetration of the dura. The cribriform plate may be involved by direct extension of a fracture or by telescoping fragments of the perpendicular plate of the ethmoid. Cerebrospinal rhinorrhea may result from tearing of the dural prolongations of the olfactory nerves which pass through the cribriform plate into the nasal area.

3. Cerebrospinal rhinorrhea may result from impaction and comminution of the interorbital space in high maxillary fractures with complete craniofacial disjunction. The mode of such injuries is similar to that described in the previous paragraph.

Cerebrospinal rhinorrhea may result from fractures involving the sphenoid, ethmoid, or frontal sinuses with tearing of the underlying or associated dura. Diagnosis is made by clinical and radiographic findings. Clinically, periods of unconsciousness following injury, conspicuous edema about the orbits, and ecchymosis of the lids and subconjunctival hemorrhage may be seen. Irritability and restlessness, with the patient thrashing purposelessly about the bed, suggest brain damage. There may be anesthesia of the supraorbital and infraorbital regions due to interference with the branches of the trigeminal nerve.

Evident deformity of the nasal dorsum and frontal structures may be present. The facial structures usually can be moved en bloc by forceful, controlled manipulation of the anterior maxillary region. Crepitation is not a reliable sign. In compound wounds the sinuses may be opened and can be brought into view through the wounds. Clear fluid escaping from the nostrils or from the wounds is most likely to be caused by cerebrospinal fluid leakage. In questionable cases the identity of the fluid may be ascertained by a simple laboratory test which demonstrates the presence of sugar but no mucin in the fluid and thus shows that it is actually cerebrospinal fluid; nasal secretions contain mucin but not sugar. Pulsation of the fluid at the nasal opening, or increase of fluid with the head in the dependent position, suggests that the fluid is cerebrospinal. The flow increases upon compression of both jugular veins. Disturbance of the sense of smell (dysosmia) is a helpful sign in establishing the diagnosis of dural tears. The patient may complain of a salty taste if cerebrospinal fluid drains into the mouth or nasopharynx.

Roentgenographic Examination

The situation and the severity of fractures in or near the cribriform plate are best seen in stereoscopic and laminographic films. Accumulation of air in the subdural, subarachnoid, and ventricular spaces suggests direct communication of these with the nasal cavity. The presence of air may not be evident for the first 24 hours, and repeat roentgenograms should be made if the patient continues to show increasing mental aberration. Displaced fragments of bone may be found near the cribriform plate, and buckling of the plate itself or displacement of the crista galli suggests the probability of lodgment of the fragments in the brain.

Radiographic examination is only an adjunct in arriving at a diagnosis of cerebrospinal rhinorrhea. The clinical findings are the most important.

Treatment of Cerebrospinal Rhinorrhea

Neurosurgical consultation is advisable in all cases of cerebrospinal rhinorrhea. The treatment depends upon the degree of the injury to the brain and the extent of penetration of fragments through the dural tears. The presence of cerebrospinal rhinorrhea is in itself not an indication for immediate surgical intervention. In most cases of severe facial injury the cerebrospinal drainage ceases after reduction and fixation of the fractured facial bones.

Some neurosurgeons are apprehensive about manipulation for the reduction of fractured facial bones in the presence of cerebrospinal rhinorrhea. Such manipulation should not be done if the patient is a poor surgical risk, but if one waits until all drainage subsides the best opportunity for reduction of the fractures will have passed. Reduction of these fractures becomes difficult after a week to 10 days and in many cases reduction is impossible after so long a wait. Schneider and Thompson (1957) noted that long-standing fistulas in the cribriform area eventually result in meningitis and sometimes in brain abscess and death.

Fistulae with bone fragments in the frontal lobe are indications for early surgical treatment. Excessive manipulation of the facial fractures should be avoided, and the patient should be prohibited from blowing his nose. Nasal packs which might prevent adequate drainage should not be used. Smoking should be prohibited. The head of the bed should be elevated to approximately 60 degrees from the horizontal. If suctioning of the nose is done, a sterile catheter should be used each time the suction is applied.

Surgical Repair for Cerebrospinal Rhinorrhea

The management of persistent cerebrospinal rhinorrhea is a neurosurgical problem, and if there is evidence of comminution, with fragments of bone in the frontal lobes, or if cerebrospinal rhinorrhea does not subside in a matter of three to five weeks, intracranial operation is indicated. Prophylactic antibiotics should be used to protect the patient from infection until the time of operation. Most surgeons feel that the intradural method of repair of cerebrospinal fluid fistulae has advantages over the extradural method. The elevation of a bone flap and the intradural approach facilitate placing of the graft and provide a better opportunity for effecting a tight closure. In some cases it is possible to close the dura without grafts. Bone spicules and necrotic brain tissue are removed by aspiration.

In some cases the intracranial procedure and facial fracture reduction may be done simultaneously. One operator reduces the fractures of the facial bones by manipulation, while the other observes the region of the cribriform plate to ascertain that no sharp spicules of bone are causing damage to the dura or the brain. Intermaxillary fixation and craniofacial suspension are proper. Operation should not be undertaken if the patient's general condition is serious or if there is respiratory obstruction, hemorrhage, or unconsciousness.

Elective tracheotomy should be done in cases of brain injury, and forceful manipulation of fragments is inadvisable. Slow reduction by intermaxillary rubber band traction may be helpful in preparing for the open operative procedure.

FRACTURES INVOLVING THE FRONTAL SINUSES

Violent injury to the supraorbital area may result in fractures of the outer or both walls of the frontal sinus. The more simple fractures involve only the outer wall and may result in a depressed fracture with deformity. Comminuted depressed fractures may be reduced through the open wound by using bone hooks or elevators. If the fragments do not appear to remain in good position after they have been pried up into position, direct interosseous wiring may be necessary.

Depressed outer wall fractures, if not compounded, may be elevated by a curved trocar passed through a frontal ethmoid approach into the floor of the frontal sinus. Patients with these fractures do not tend to have recurrent displacement because there is no musculature to force the reduced fragments out of position. With extensive comminution and lack of support for the fragments, the frontal sinus may be packed with rubber drains and the ends left protruding from the wound into the nasal cavity or through an anterior ethmoid opening. The packing may be removed through the nose after a week to 10 days, during which time consolidation of the fragments will have occurred.

There is a misconception among surgeons that compound depressed fractures of the anterior wall of the frontal sinus require radical excision of bone and obliteration of the sinus lining. This usually is unnecessary

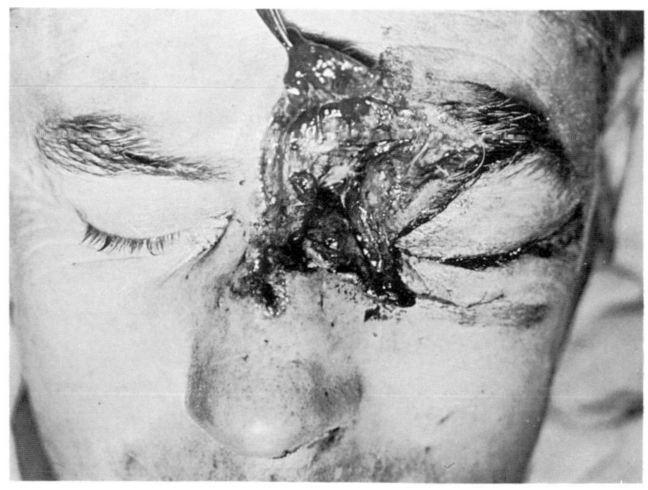

A

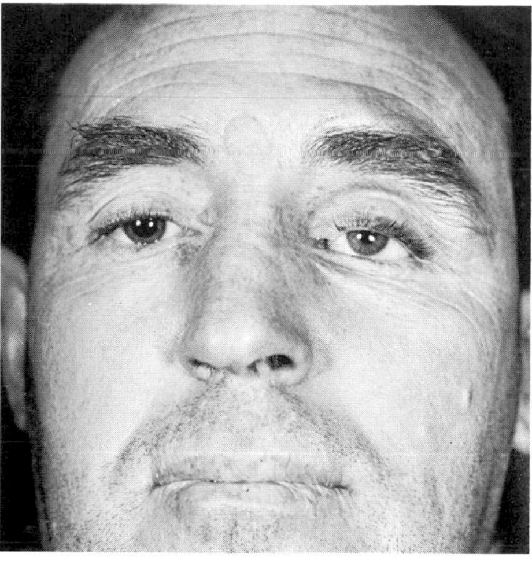

B

Figure 317. Complicated fractures of the nasal, lacrimal, ethmoid, and frontal bone, with puncture wound of the left eye sustained in an automobile accident. Treatment consisted of enucleation of the left eye, direct wiring of the bone fragments, and closure of the soft tissues. *A*. Appearance immediately after injury. *B*. Appearance one year after injury with prosthesis in the left orbit.

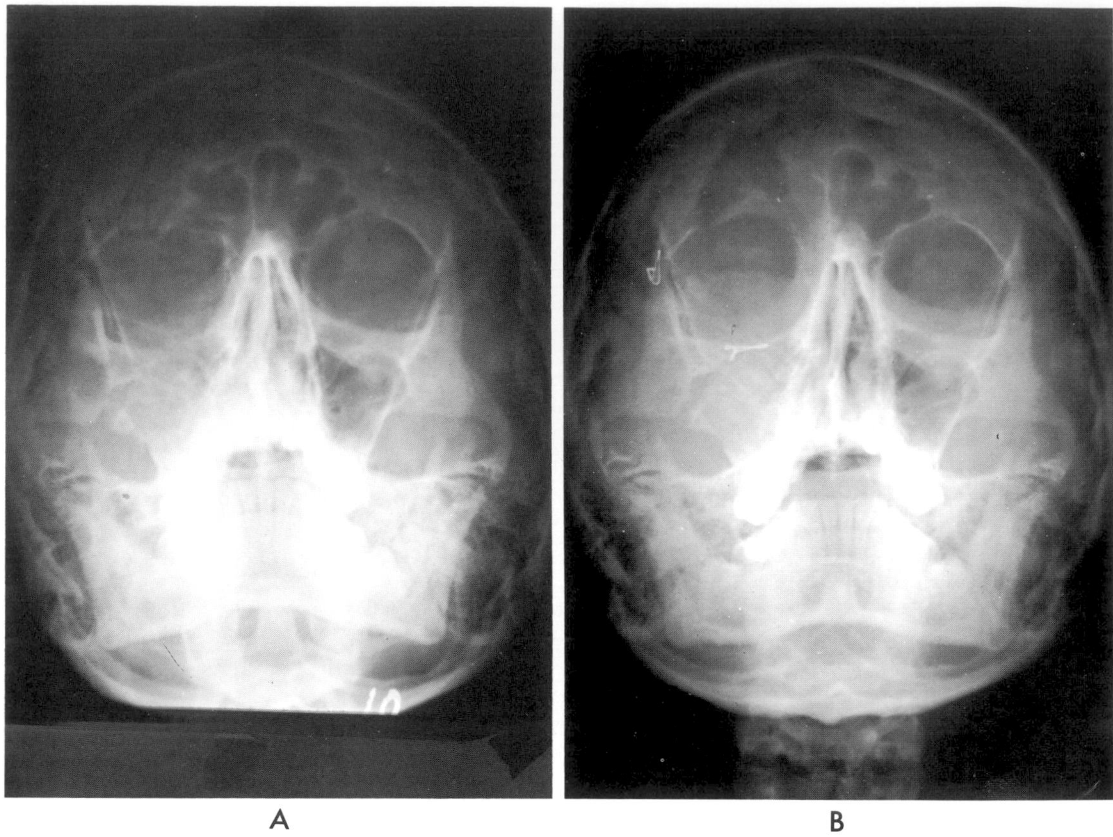

Figure 318. *A.* Compound fracture of the frontal bone on the right associated with fracture of the right zygoma. *B.* Roentgenogram following debridement of frontal bone and reduction of the fracture of the right zygoma.

surgery and results in severe deformity in many cases. There is no reason to suspect that the fragments will not heal in good position if they have soft tissue attachments, and even if detached, many of them will survive if they are covered adequately with soft tissues. More extensive fractures which involve the outer and inner walls of the sinus, with fragments of bone in the frontal lobes and lacerations of the dura and brain, require intracranial operation. Loose, displaced fragments should be removed, damaged brain tissue aspirated, and the dura repaired by approximation of the torn margins or by the use of grafts taken from the fascia lata.

Complications of Fractures of the Fronto-Ethmoid-Sphenoid Region

Complications of fractures in this region include damage to the brain and dura, meningitis, brain abscess, aerocele, orbital complications from splintered pieces of bone that have been driven into the orbital cavity or into the eye, injury to the optic nerve, damage to the extraocular muscles, injury to the lacrimal apparatus, hemorrhage from the ethmoidal vessels, detachment of the medial palpebral ligaments, dacryocystitis, pseudohypertelorism, and facial deformity. Unreduced or malunion fractures of the nasofrontal-ethmoidal region are found to result in depression of the upper part of the face. Widening of the distance between the medial canthi and lateral displacement of the eyes may occur. Detachment of the medial palpebral ligaments gives an ugly appearance with separation of the ligaments and an abnormally wide space between the eyes. Chronic ethmoidal and frontal sinusitis may result from obstruction of drainage from the upper part of the nose and from the anterior ethmoidal cells. Osteomyelitis of the frontal and ethmoidal bones is rare, but may be a complication of fractures of the nasofrontal-ethmoidal region.

FRACTURES COMPLICATED BY LOSS OF BONE STRUCTURE

Some fractures caused by penetrating injuries and gunshot wounds are complicated by the loss of large fragments of bone. This complication may occur in fracture of the mandible when large fragments are avulsed or so badly comminuted that they cannot maintain effectively the natural conformation of the mandible. Immediate use should be made of iliac bone grafts to bridge such defects if it is possible to get satisfactory closure of the soft tissues so that the graft will survive. But this procedure should not be attempted in the presence of gross contamination or in cases in which the blood supply of the soft tissues has been jeopardized to the point at which the graft cannot receive adequate nourishment. In questionable cases it is advisable to bridge the space by plates fixed with wires or screws, or simply to close the soft tissues, or to secure the fragments by intermaxillary fixation.

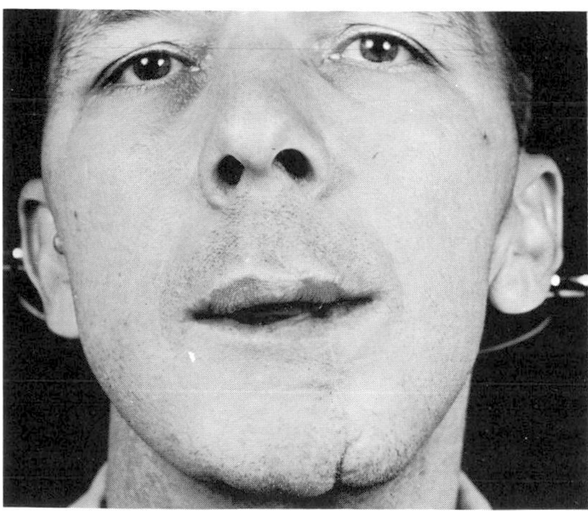

A

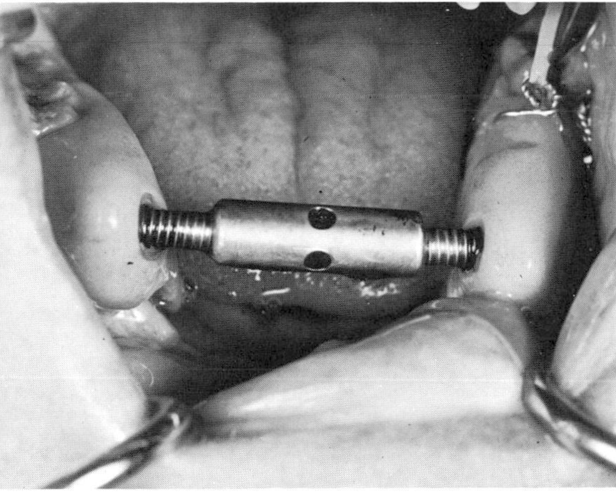

B

Figure 319. *A*. Appearance of patient with loss of the anterior part of the mandible from gunshot injury. Bone from the canine region to the opposite canine region was lost. Scar tissue contracture had pulled the two halves of the mandible almost together in the midline. Reconstruction called for iliac bone graft to the anterior part of the mandible. *B*. A jackscrew appliance was utilized to spread the two halves of the mandible and to reposition them so that a bone graft could be inserted for reconstruction of the anterior part of the mandible.

FRACTURES COMPLICATED BY LOSS OF SOFT TISSUE AND BONE

If large portions of soft tissue and bone have been avulsed completely, as may happen in gunshot wounds or in other violent injury, definitive care should not be attempted. Careful debridement of the tissues should be performed and all structures that can possibly be saved should be retained. In addition, sharp, jagged edges of bones that might interfere with healing should be trimmed with rongeurs, and the bone ends should be covered by adjacent soft tissues or by rotation of muscle or skin flaps from a nearby area. Exposed bone is highly susceptible to infection and may be lost because of inadequate blood supply.

Primary closure of the wound usually can be obtained by suturing mucosa to skin over the exposed bone, or by the use of split skin graft dressings, so that early closure of the wound can be obtained (Fig. 321 *A–F*). Early closure of the wound greatly decreases the incidence of infection, reduces the necessity for frequent changes of dressings, and tends to prevent the formation of excessive scar tissue, which may be troublesome later during the stages of definitive repair. The principles involved in the management of such wounds are the prevention of infection, the stabilization of the fragments, the covering of all exposed bone surfaces, the conservation of tissues, early primary wound closure, the prevention of scar contractures, and the retention of viable bone segments.

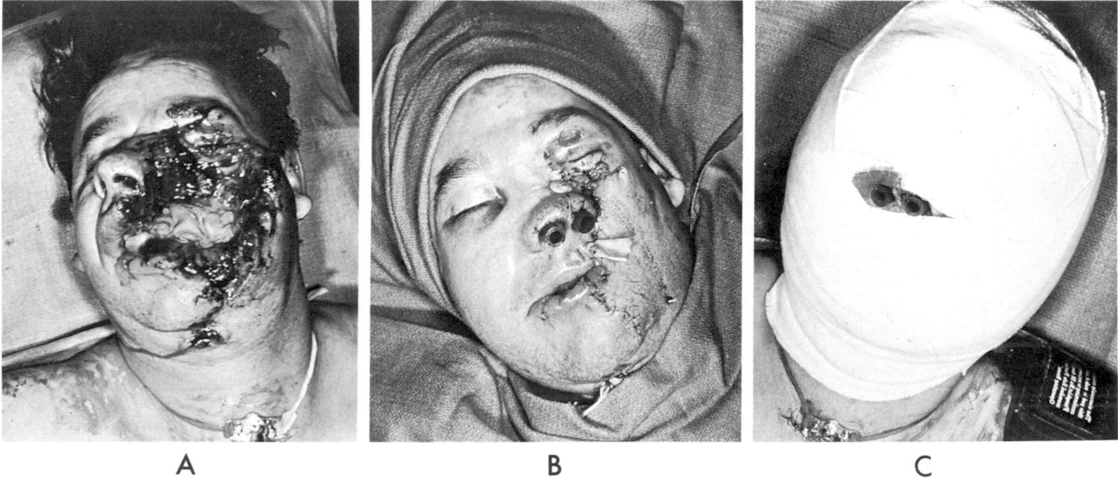

Figure 320. Gunshot wound of face. This patient attempted suicide by placing a shotgun under his chin. *A*. Note the small wound of entry and the large wound of exit with loss of bone and soft tissues. The pack is placed in the maxillary region to control hemorrhage. *B*. The principles of careful, conservative debridement and primary closure of the wound have been well followed. Nasopharyngeal airways help support the tissues and permit early removal of the trachetomy tube. *C*. A firm, large head dressing was used to support the bone and soft tissues of the face.

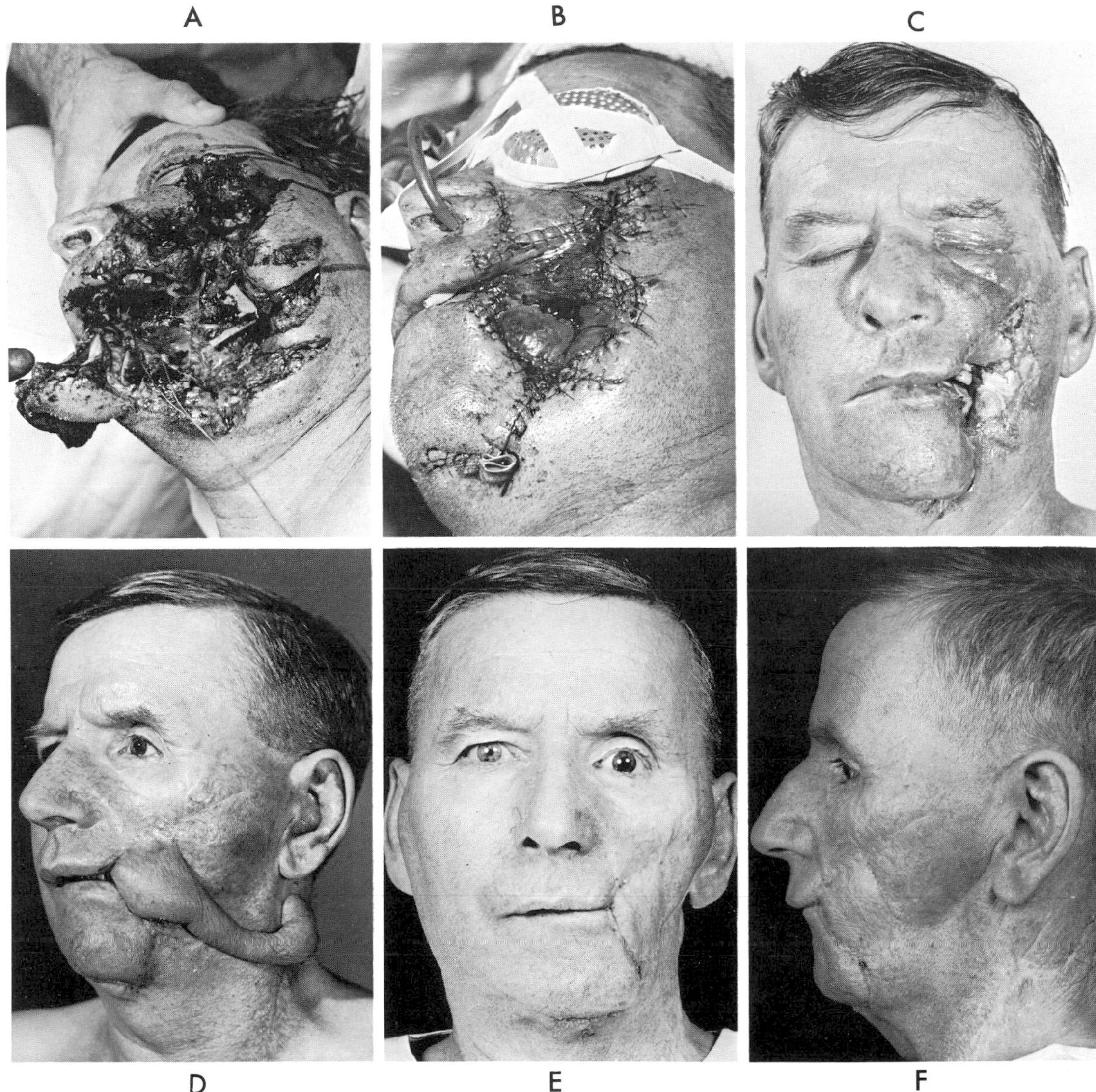

Figure 321. Shotgun wound of the left side of the face with extensive loss of soft tissue and bone, including the lining of the mouth and skin overlying the mandible. Reconstruction consisted of replacement of the covering and lining of the floor of the mouth, the lip and the cheek, with reconstruction of the mandible by use of bone grafts. *A*. Appearance of patient three hours after injury. *B*. The immediate repair. The mucous membrane was sutured to the skin margins to provide a closed wound to minimize infection and prevent excessive scar tissue formation. *C*. One month after initial treatment. The left eye was lost as a result of the injury. *D*. Tube pedicle flap from the neck, with a skin graft lining of the flap for reconstruction of the cheek. *E*. Following cutting and return of tube pedicle to the neck. *F*. Lateral view following soft tissue reconstruction of the face.

CHAPTER

13

POSTOPERATIVE CARE AND COMPLICATIONS

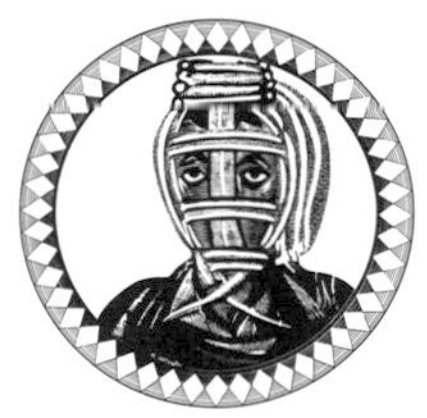

In the postoperative management of patients with facial injuries, certain general considerations are important for the well-being, comfort, and happiness of the patient and for ensuring an orderly and uninterrupted process of repair. Adequate fluid replacement and maintenancc of fluid balance are primary considerations in all patients who have suffered loss of fluid and electrolytes through perspiration, vomiting, drainage from the wound, diarrhea, and shock. The patient's condition should be evaluated carefully and electrolyte balance should be reestablished at the earliest moment possible. Severe loss of blood from facial injuries or other injuries in other regions may have reduced the blood volume to unphysiologic levels. Associated injuries and shock may have resulted in the loss of large amounts of blood and tissue fluids in local regions or in the thoracic and abdominal cavities, with serious decrease in volume of the circulating blood. Hemoglobin, hematocrit, and blood volume studies should be performed when they are indicated and deficiencies corrected promptly. Persistent bleeding from the oral and nasal cavities is uncommon in facial injuries, but if continued may be a source of loss of blood, fluid, and electrolytes. Repeated laboratory studies should be carried out as they become advisable; laboratory findings change rapidly in the postoperative period and should be ascertained at reasonable intervals to detect deficiencies of physiologic importance.

MANAGEMENT OF THE SEVERELY INJURED PATIENT

Although necessarily under the direction of a specialist who should formulate the program and make the decisions in the event of differences of opinion, management of the severely injured patient sometimes is better carried out by coordinated team effort. Consultation with the appropriate medical and surgical specialists should be sought freely.

Damage to the orbit and its contents is not uncommon in cases of extensive multiple facial fractures, and may require the highly specialized skill and care of an ophthalmologist. Subdural hematoma, extradural hematoma, and cerebral hemorrhage are ever-present dangers and should be suspected if changes of personality, lack of orientation, or changes in the state of consciousness occur. Neurosurgical consultation is imperative in such cases and also in all patients with a history of concussion and loss of consciousness at the time of injury. Cerebrospinal rhinorrhea also requires the attention of the neurosurgical consultant. Fractures of the cervical spine, damage to the structures of the middle ear, or thoracic and abdominal and extremity injuries may require the services of other surgical specialists. Cardiac difficulties, diabetes, liver disease, and other medical conditions should have the attention of a consultant trained to handle such problems.

DIETARY CONSIDERATIONS

Immediately following injury and in the early postoperative period, the patient, because of obstruction to the alimentary passages or because of unconsciousness which renders him unable to take adequate fluid and other dietary substances, may require transnasal gastric gavage. This is done best through a small polyethylene gastric tube. The patient's requirements should be estimated and a formula made up that contains the 24-hour food, fluid and vitamin requirements.

The Barron food pump, which delivers a continuous flow of liquid food mixture, may be helpful, especially in patients who have had severe injuries and who do not regain consciousness within the first few days. A small, flexible polyethylene tube is easy to insert and causes very little irritation to the mucosa of the nose, pharynx, and esophagus. The tube should be exchanged at three- or four-day intervals and put through the opposite nostril to avoid irritation. Instillation of food into the stomach in controlled, small amounts permits the gastrointestinal tract to absorb the food adequately, thereby eliminating the complications of acute gastric dilatation, distention, and nausea and vomiting.

Special diets may be arranged in consultation with the dietitian, but the standard diet may be liquefied in a food blender and fed into the Barron pump. One of our patients, who remained unconscious for more than six months, was maintained in an excellent state of nutrition and hydration by this technique. Three times daily the food from a regular diet tray was liquefied in the food blender, and this provided all the elements needed to keep him in excellent physical condition. The patient succumbed at last from injuries to the brain stem, which he had sustained in falling from a great height during the construction of a building.

If it is expected that tube feeding will be only a few days, feeding at regular intervals, by passing the liquefied formula into the gavage tube with an Asepto syringe, usually is satisfactory. To provide an adequate dietary intake, as much as two quarts of liquid may be necessary to carry the quantities of proteins, carbohydrates, and fats required during a 24-hour period. The diet must be delicately balanced in order to obviate diarrhea, which is a common complication of an unbalanced liquid diet. Patients on an inadequate diet, or those who will not cooperate, may lose as much as 20 pounds during the month or six weeks during which intraoral fixation is maintained. This loss of weight may be significant in that it may interfere with healing and thus may result in nonunion or delayed union of the fracture.

Most patients are able to maintain an adequate intake without tube feeding if the state of consciousness is satisfactory. A liquid diet can be taken by mouth even in the presence of complete fixation of the dentition with the teeth wired in occlusion. There is enough room between the teeth and the retromolar region to permit adequate intake of fluid and food. It is unnecessary to extract teeth to facilitate feeding when the teeth are fixed in occlusion.

In addition to the usual breakfast, luncheon, and dinner feeding, the patient should have supplementary feedings in the midmorning, mid-afternoon, and before sleeping at night. Patients who are employed and busy during the day should be encouraged to take supplementary feedings at these times. These supplements may be milk containing eggs and other food additives, or concentrated food substances which will complement the liquid diet. Adequate vitamin intake should be assured by the daily use of a concentrated multivitamin liquid. The quantity necessary should be calibrated, and the patient should be advised to place the vitamin drops directly into the

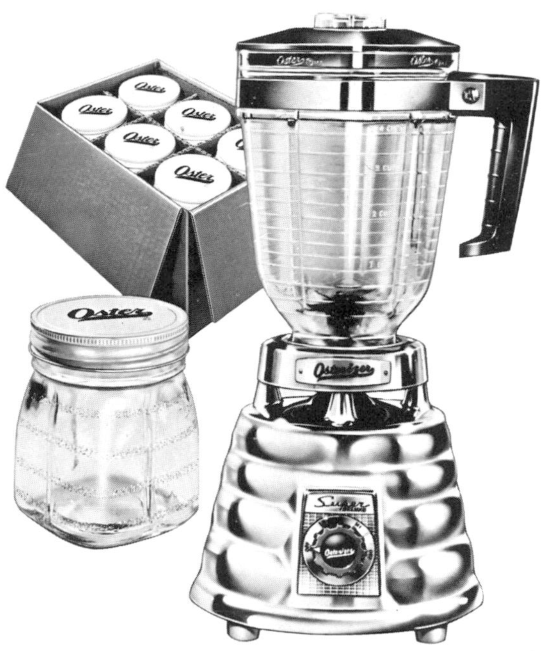

Figure 322. An electric food blender is indispensable in preparing an adequate, tasty, liquid diet for the patient whose teeth are fixed by intermaxillary appliances. The sharp cutting blades of the blender liquefy foods instantaneously.

mouth and not to attempt to mix them into a formula. Vitamins in an oil vehicle tend to separate from the liquid and accumulate on the side of the container, and most of them are lost if mixed into the formula. A liquid diet usually is more palatable if it is cold, and so the formula should be kept under refrigeration. Some patients prefer hot foods such as soups and heated beverages.

The patient should be encouraged to keep a weight record from day to day, and if there is persistent weight loss the diet should be changed. Most patients lose some weight, but this should not be over 3 to 5 pounds in the average adult during the course of a month or six weeks. Most patients can return to their usual activities a week or 10 days after reduction of fractures unless there is a complication. Patients who are engaged in work requiring light physical effort, or those in sedentary occupations, may return to full activity, but heavy manual work should not be attempted during the convalescent period.

When the patient leaves the hospital, he should be instructed in regard to his dietary intake and should be given suggestions concerning the care of his mouth and his local wound, if this seems pertinent. We have found it desirable to give the patient a list of printed instructions, for most patients are overwhelmed by lengthy verbal instructions at the time of discharge. Unless the details are written, the patient may not recall some of them. A small booklet that outlines the details of dietary management and contains suggestions for variations in the diet is helpful to the patient (Dingman, 1957). The manual we have used also contains suggestions covering the recording of weight, the care of the mouth, and other facts which we think are important for the patient to understand during his postoperative period.

LOCAL CONSIDERATIONS

Care of the Wound and the Affected Part

The local wound should receive meticulous care daily to prevent the accumulation of dried blood, serum, and crusts on the suture line and food about the intraoral appliances. Accumulation of crusts predisposes to infection about the sutures and may result in permanent marking along the wound margin. Increasing redness and swelling during the immediate postoperative period, with tenderness and increased tissue temperature, suggests the possibility of localized infection. If these signs are noted, a few sutures should be removed and the wound probed and drained. Drainage and local application of moist compresses usually will bring infection under control within a short time. Drains placed in the wound at the time of the operation will have attained the purpose for which they were inserted within 48 hours; however, if redness, tenderness, and drainage persist, drains should be left in the wound longer.

Although infection following operations about the face and jaws is not a common complication, one should remember that the operations are done in a potentially contaminated area and that infection can occur. Wound infection should be recognized early and appropriate measures taken for its control. Cultures of pus for the determination of the identity of the organisms and tests for sensitivity are necessary for prescribing the proper antibiotics.

Strict hygienic measures should be taken in order to maintain adequate oral hygiene. A clean mouth promotes the patient's comfort and reduces the possibility of local oral wound infection or of pulmonary infection due to aspiration. Frequent washing of the mouth with antiseptic solutions is helpful. The most useful are weak solutions of hydrogen peroxide, dilute solutions of essence of Caroid, and the vigorous use of a small toothbrush with toothpaste or hydrogen peroxide to loosen plaques of food and mucus that accumulate about the teeth and appliances. Frequent suctioning of excess saliva and mucus from the mouth with a small rubber catheter or suction tip will add immeasurably to the patient's comfort. The patient himself can be trained to pass a small rubber tube into the nose to remove secretions from the posterior pharyngeal area. The unconscious or disoriented patient must have help in this, and the nursing staff should be instructed in the techniques of the daily care of the mouth with small brushes or swabs and suction. Immediately after the operative procedure, cracking, fissuring, and abrasion of thc lips may produce severe discomfort. Frequent application to the lips of petrolatum from a tube kept at the bedside for use by the patient himself will keep the tissues free of crusts and will promote early healing.

Suture Removal and Wound Splinting

If facial lacerations and surgical wounds have been closed carefully, the subcutaneous sutures usually make it unnecessary to providc prolonged fixation of the wound with surface sutures. To avoid scarring from the sutures along the wound margin, absolute cleanliness from day to day is imperative and early removal of the sutures is advisable. Sutures in the face are removed on the second or the third day. In this short period it is obvious that the wound will not be well healed and will need additional support. This support can be obtained by strips stuck to the skin with collodion or by commercially available tape or paper strips. To get the best possible result from wound closures, it is advisable to splint the wound by this method for two or three weeks. This will prevent stretching and separation of the wound margins and will lessen the final scarring.

PERIOD OF FIXATION FOR TREATMENT OF FACIAL FRACTURES

The fixation appliances must be maintained for a period adequate to ensure reasonable stability during wound healing. The length of time necessary depends upon the extent of the injury, the amount and degree of comminution, the age and general condition of the patient, and the presence or absence of complications. In children, fixation of facial bone fragments for two or three weeks is adequate. Healing takes place rapidly and support no longer is necessary after that time. Fixation for four weeks usually is adequate in the 20- to 30-year age group, whereas in older individuals fixation for four to eight weeks may be necessary before the bone will have healed well enough to maintain stability without appliances. Fixation should be prolonged in cases in which infection of the local wound has occurred or the patient has suffered from a general reaction incident to the injury. Single fractures heal more readily than multiple fractures and require a shorter time of fixation. Our estimates are average and the judgment of the surgeon must be exercised.

If intermaxillary fixation has been used,

rubber bands or vertical fixation wires between the arch bars can be removed at the usual time and the site of fracture tested for stability by manual manipulation. If the site of fracture is springy or appears to be delayed in healing, or if there is nonunion, the intermaxillary fixation should be re-established for a period of two or three weeks. The wound can be tested again after this period. The appliances should not be removed until it is evident that stability has been attained. In most cases it is advisable to remove the intermaxillary fixation when healing seems satisfactory but to leave the arch bars in place and permit the patient to have use of his jaws during the day and wear rubber bands at night. To be certain that the appliances are no longer necessary, in some cases the patient may be permitted full use of his jaws with the arch bars still in place for about a week. If there has been no shifting during a period of 7 to 10 days, the arch bars and all the appliances may be removed.

After prolonged fixation, temporary trismus, or difficulty in opening the mouth, will be found following the release of the intermaxillary traction. If the patient is permitted to use the jaws for a week, the removal of the arch bars will be facilitated considerably by his ability to open his mouth. In the immediate postoperative period, he should be advised to continue a soft diet and not to attempt to eat hard foods. Tenderness and discomfort in the temporomandibular joints will occur and the muscles will tire easily, but these soon disappear and usually in a week or two function will be normal.

The removal of the wires and appliances is not difficult. In small children a general anesthetic may be necessary for removal of the wires and arch bars. In the adult this usually can be done as an office or outpatient procedure. To minimize the discomfort associated with the removal of the wires the patient should be given light sedation if indicated, and local anesthesia may be used. Before removing the craniofacial internal wire suspension, the mouth should be prepared by detergents and antiseptic solutions in order to reduce the bacterial flora to a minimum. Although infection following removal of wires is uncommon, it is possible to infect the deep structures by pulling the wires from the mouth up through the temporal region. Craniofacial suspension wires are easily removed by cutting the wires in the mouth, so that the ends are free, and applying traction to the pull-out wire in the temporal region. Occasionally, if a heavy wire has been used for suspension, difficulty is encountered in pulling the wire loose and disengaging it from the drill hole in the zygomatic portion of the frontal bone. If difficulty is encountered, a local anesthetic is injected into the skin in the brow region, the wound is opened, and the wire will be identified quickly. The wire can be removed easily with a wire-twisting forceps or a heavy hook. The edges of the wound are reapproximated easily with a few small sutures.

Care of the Mouth Following Removal of Appliances

After removal of the arch bars or wires, the gingiva and soft tissues may appear to be damaged or irritated and highly inflamed. Stains may be left on the teeth by the wires or by the accumulation of food about the arch bars. Such sequelae disappear after a few days if usual oral hygiene is instituted. Dental prophylaxis will remove stains and calculus that has accumulated about the teeth. Some of the teeth may feel slightly loose to the patient, but they will tighten in a few weeks unless they are involved directly in the line of fracture. Teeth of questionable viability that are retained require extraction. If it is obvious that they will not be useful teeth, they should be extracted. It is advisable to defer extraction of teeth for several months after healing to avoid refracture as a complication of the extraction.

The small interosseous wire ligatures utilized to affix small bone fragments in the infraorbital region, frontal process, or near or in the zygomaticofrontal suture cause little, if any, irritation and need not be removed. Occasionally in a thin individual, a wire at the inferior border of the mandible can be felt under the skin. This may be noted by the patient when he shaves over the area and, if annoying, the wire should be removed. Occasionally, a foreign body reaction about the site of a wire may necessitate its removal.

At the end of the period of fixation the bones may seem to be reasonably stable; nevertheless, complete bony regeneration may not have occurred. For all practical purposes the patient has a satisfactory clinical union. Roentgenograms taken within the first few months will still show the fracture, usually with the evidence of callus formation. Complete obliteration of the fracture by healing may not occur for a year or a year and a half. A final postoperative roentgenogram should be obtained in order to determine the status of the tissues at the site of the healed fracture. In patients who have sustained small losses of bone bridged by plates or pins, partial regeneration may be expected if the periosteum has been retained. Sometimes such regeneration is satisfactory for function without the necessity for bone grafts.

PERSISTENT ANESTHESIA

Anesthesia of the lower lip, the infraorbital or nasal areas, or areas of the forehead usually is transient, and complete recovery of sensation can be expected in a matter of 12 to 18 months. Such recovery depends, of course, upon the extent of damage to the nerve. The crushed nerve usually regenerates faster than the nerve that has been severed. Regeneration is dependent upon the degree of alignment of the nerve following reduction of the fracture. If large sections of the maxilla or the mandible have been avulsed completely together with parts of nerves, regeneration cannot be expected. Patients adjust quite well to such anesthesia, however, and sometimes sensory and motor nerve regeneration does occur from anastomosis with other nerve systems or fibers in the area. Nerve regeneration usually is complete, but sometimes the nerve never is regenerated. If nerve regeneration fails and is considered to be due to obstruction in the nerve pathway, exploration may discover the cause of the obstruction, and elimination of it may permit nerve regeneration. Some cases may be complicated by neuroma or troublesome postoperative paresthesias; these, however, require special consideration.

CHAPTER

14

REPAIR OF RESIDUAL DEFORMITIES

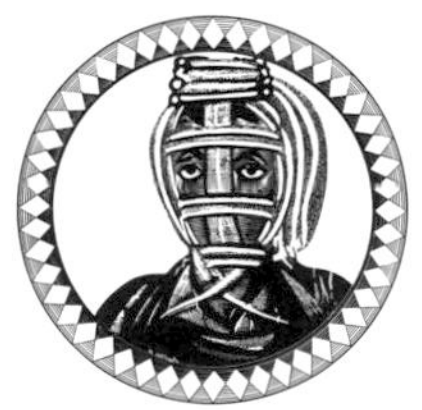

Residual deformity following traumatic injury to the facial bones may be of significance from the standpoint of the appearance of the patient or malfunction of the organs involved. Defacement that remains may cause psychological disturbance or social and economic problems of great concern to the patient. Disturbances of function may interfere with the ability to speak, swallow, breathe, or see satisfactorily.

Deformities of the facial skeleton may be divided into those without and those with loss of tissue. When there is no loss of tissue but simply displacement of parts, deformities result from failure to diagnose the original condition correctly during the acute phase, or from failure to correct impaction or to replace all the injured tissues into proper position.

A critical evaluation of the displacement

(Text continued on page 350.)

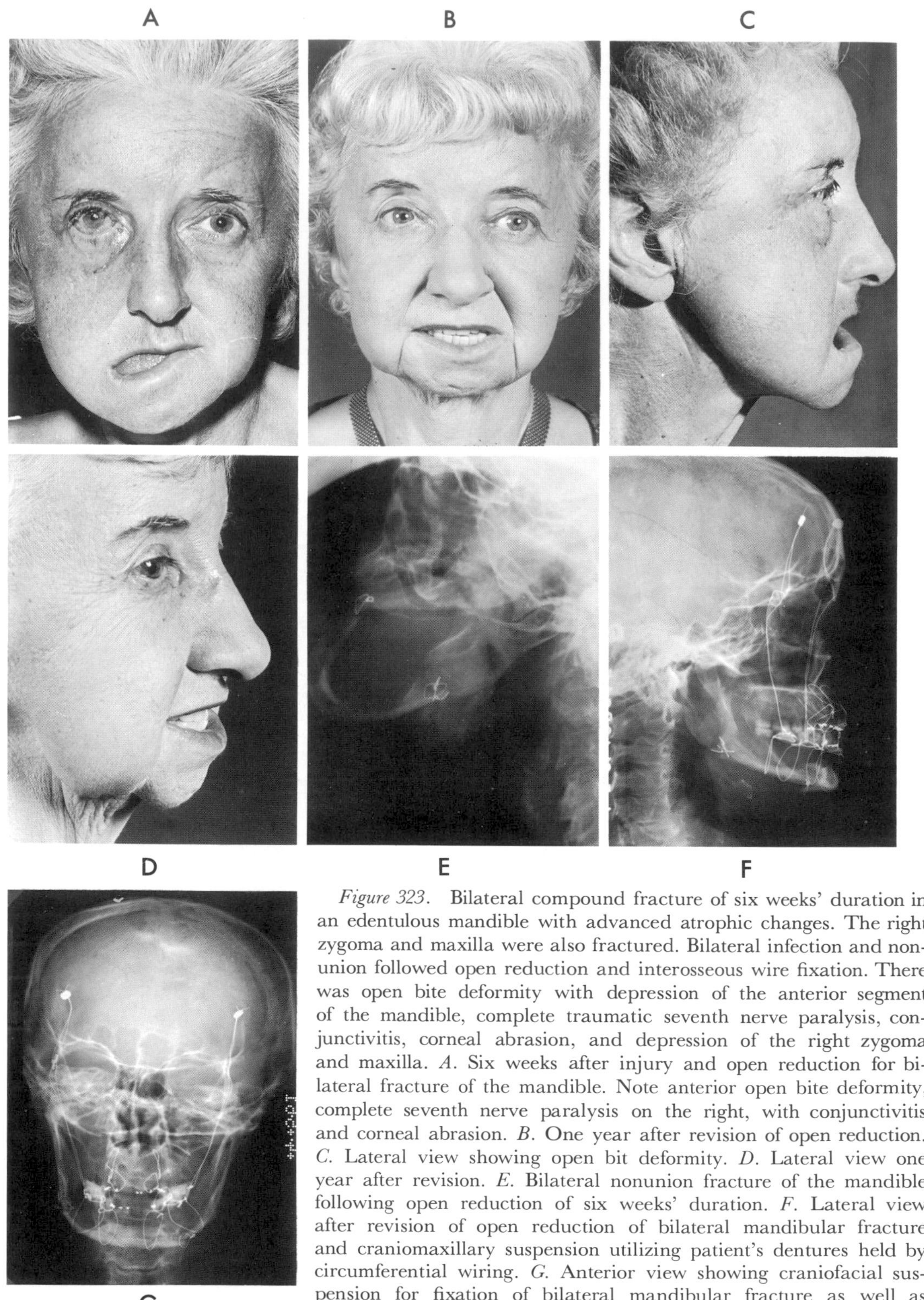

Figure 323. Bilateral compound fracture of six weeks' duration in an edentulous mandible with advanced atrophic changes. The right zygoma and maxilla were also fractured. Bilateral infection and nonunion followed open reduction and interosseous wire fixation. There was open bite deformity with depression of the anterior segment of the mandible, complete traumatic seventh nerve paralysis, conjunctivitis, corneal abrasion, and depression of the right zygoma and maxilla. *A.* Six weeks after injury and open reduction for bilateral fracture of the mandible. Note anterior open bite deformity, complete seventh nerve paralysis on the right, with conjunctivitis and corneal abrasion. *B.* One year after revision of open reduction. *C.* Lateral view showing open bit deformity. *D.* Lateral view one year after revision. *E.* Bilateral nonunion fracture of the mandible following open reduction of six weeks' duration. *F.* Lateral view after revision of open reduction of bilateral mandibular fracture and craniomaxillary suspension utilizing patient's dentures held by circumferential wiring. *G.* Anterior view showing craniofacial suspension for fixation of bilateral mandibular fracture as well as fracture of the zygoma.

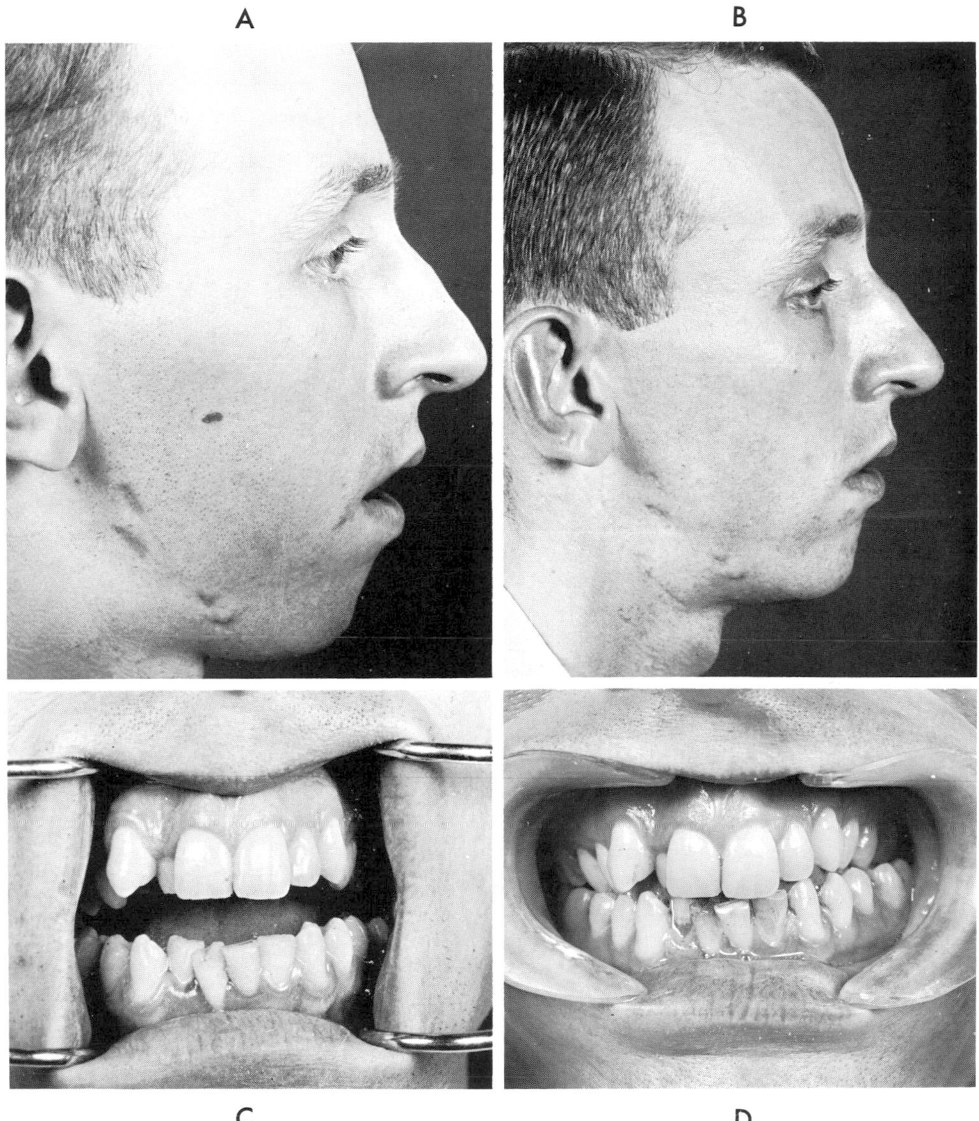

Figure 324. *A*. Bilateral open bite deformity due to telescoping and malunion of the segments of bilateral mandibular subcondylar fractures. The patient was seen six months after injury with occlusal contact on the molar teeth only. *B*. Six months following bilateral osteotomy of the mandible. *C*. Preoperative view showing open bite deformity due to shortening of the ramus of the mandible bilaterally. *D*. Occlusion six months after bilateral osteotomy of the mandible.

and its degree must be made before correction can be carried out. In cases of loss of bone and soft tissue due to destruction from the primary injury, the quantity and the quality of the material lost must be known and replacement must be based upon this knowledge. Obvious external deformity usually will suggest the location and extent of the fracture lines, since the fragments will carry with them large portions of attached soft tissues, or their abnormal position may fail to give support to the soft tissues. Elongation of the face suggests that unreduced fractures remain in the midfacial skeleton. Flatness of the cheek suggests underlying fracture-dislocation of the zygoma, and a depressed eye suggests fracture of the orbital floor. Deviation of the tip of the nose suggests fracture-dislocation of the cartilaginous septal structures, and a flat, saddle-type nose may be the result of residual nasal deformities from fractures. The dish-faced appearance of the patient indicates imperfectly united fractures of the middle third of the face. Malocclusion and open bite deformity indicate malunion of mandibular or maxillary fractures (Fig. 324 *A–D*).

Residual deformities may be corrected by refracture and repositioning of the bones, by use of onlay or inlay grafts, or by the use of prosthetic appliances. Disimpaction, refracture, replacement, and efficient retention of the new fragments is the method of choice in reconstruction when there is malposition but no loss of tissue. In some less significant deformities, bone or cartilage grafts may give a satisfactory result.

In cases of extensive loss of soft tissue and bone structures, clinical evaluation of the loss will indicate or dictate the type of procedure necessary for repair of the deformity.

DEFORMITIES OF THE FRONTAL BONE

Defects in this area usually have no subjective importance as they cover a relatively silent area of the brain. Deformities of the forehead may be due to malunion of depressed fractures or to traumatic loss of bone. Fractures healed in malposition are very difficult to dislodge by osteotomy, and it usually is better to camouflage the defect than to attempt elevation of the healed depressed fractures. Improvement may be obtained by the use of dermal fat grafts, bone or cartilage grafts, or acrylic or other nonbiologic materials.

The result obtained by the use of dermal fat grafts is unpredictable because it is impossible to determine the amount of shrinkage that will take place. Generally, dermal-fat grafts should be overcorrected by at least 25 per cent. We prefer fresh, autogenous iliac cancellous bone or cartilage grafts for correction of frontal bone defects. Quick-setting synthetic acrylic material may be used for correction of bony defects of the forehead. This material is convenient to use and is contoured easily at the operating table, and, although nonbiologic, it does serve to give satisfactory contour in many cases. Approach to the defect is gained through scars in the region of the deformity, through the eyebrows, or through an incision above the hairline.

RESIDUAL DEFORMITIES OF THE NASAL BONES AND CARTILAGES

The nasal bones are fractured more often than any of the other facial bones. Residual deformity may result from failure to recognize displacement of tissues or from neglect of the acute injury. Fractures of the nose in childhood with minimal displacement may become significant deformities as the facial structures grow and develop.

The defect may involve both bony and cartilaginous structures or the cartilaginous

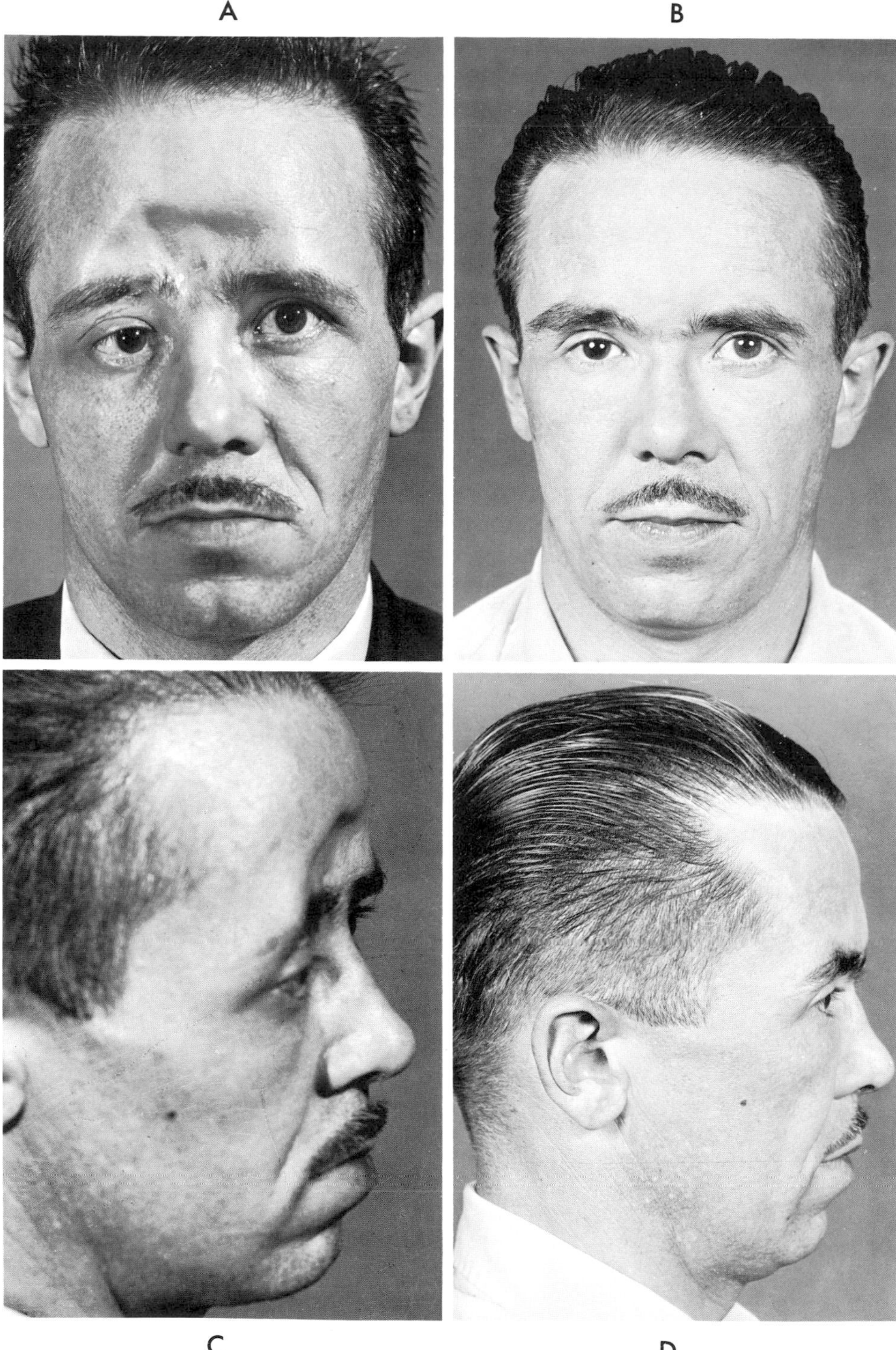

Figure 325. Malunion fracture of the right zygomatic compound and traumatic defect of the forehead. *A.* Preoperative frontal view. *B.* Four months after correction by osteotomy, open reduction, wire fixation of the right zygoma, and bone graft to the floor of the orbit and frontal bone. Dr. Bruce Fralick performed an extraocular muscle procedure upon the right eye because of a paretic right lateral rectus muscle. *C.* Preoperative profile view. *D.* Postoperative profile view. (From Dingman, R. O.: Symposium: malunited fractures of zygoma; repair of deformity. Tr. Am. Acad. Ophth., *57:*889–896, Nov.–Dec., 1953.)

structures only. Usually a defect of the bone is associated with defects of the lower cartilaginous tissues of the nasal dorsum. The deflected or bowed nose and the broad, flat, saddle nose are the deformities most commonly seen. The bowed nose is usually the result of a lateral force fracture with displacement of the bones and septum in the direction of the force. The most gratifying results from correction of this kind of deformity occur with nasal osteotomy and septal reconstruction. In most such cases the bony arch has a long side and a shortened side. To correct the defect, a wedge osteotomy or partial bone removal should be done on the long side, and a simple osteotomy on the short side, in conjunction with a septal reconstruction. The excess bone is removed on the long side, and at the same time the dorsal hump in reduced by sawing the bone a little lower on the long side of the nose. If the deformity is not long standing, the septum may spring back to the midline at the time the osteotomy is done. But in most cases it is necessary to carry out septal reconstruction by placing submucosal cuts in thc cartilage to relieve the spring, and to resect the posterior deviated septum. Septal reconstruction gives very gratifying results in the correction of post-traumatic septal deformities (Steffensen, 1947; Dingman, 1961).

The depressed nasal bridge is repaired best by a supportive graft. The authors prefer a block of contoured cancellous iliac bone, but cartilage grafts may give satisfactory results. Grafts may be inserted through midcolumellar incisions or through an intranasal intercartilaginous incision about 1 cm. above the lower border of the nostril between the upper lateral and alar cartilages. The skin of the nose along the dorsum is undermined by blunt dissection to the lower edges of the nasal bones where the periosteum is incised and reflected from the midline. The residual nasal bone is freshened by an osteotome or bone bur, and a small slot is prepared in the glabellar area of the frontal bone with the chisel or bone bur for the reception of the graft.

Some grafts remain securely seated in the prepared bed, but, if insecure, they may be fixed by wiring directly to the nasal bones with a 25 gauge stainless steel wire. This wire is placed by drilling a hole through the nasal bone near the crest of the ridge. A wire is passed through the hole and brought subcutaneously over the bone graft and back through the stab wound of entry. The wire is then twisted securely over the top of the graft. This gives positive fixation against the nasal bone and prevents tipping of the lower end of the graft by the pressure of the nasal tip. If the skin pressure at the tip seems to be greater than can be tolerated, a columellar strut should be placed to give support to the lower end of the bone graft; the strut is carried from the undersurface of the dorsal graft to the anterior nasal spine.

MALUNION FRACTURE OF THE ZYGOMATICOMAXILLARY COMPOUND

Unrecognized or inadequately replaced fractures of the zygomatic compound result in malunion fractures. Fibrosis occurs early and manipulation a few weeks after the injury is difficult; it may be impossible to get satisfactory position of the fragments. Mobilization of the fragments is possible by open operation and may be accomplished months or even years following the injury. Through a small, well-placed incision in the brow and the infraorbital region, the fracture lines can be re-established by the use of osteotomes for elevation of the depressed fracture.

It may be necessary to refracture the bone

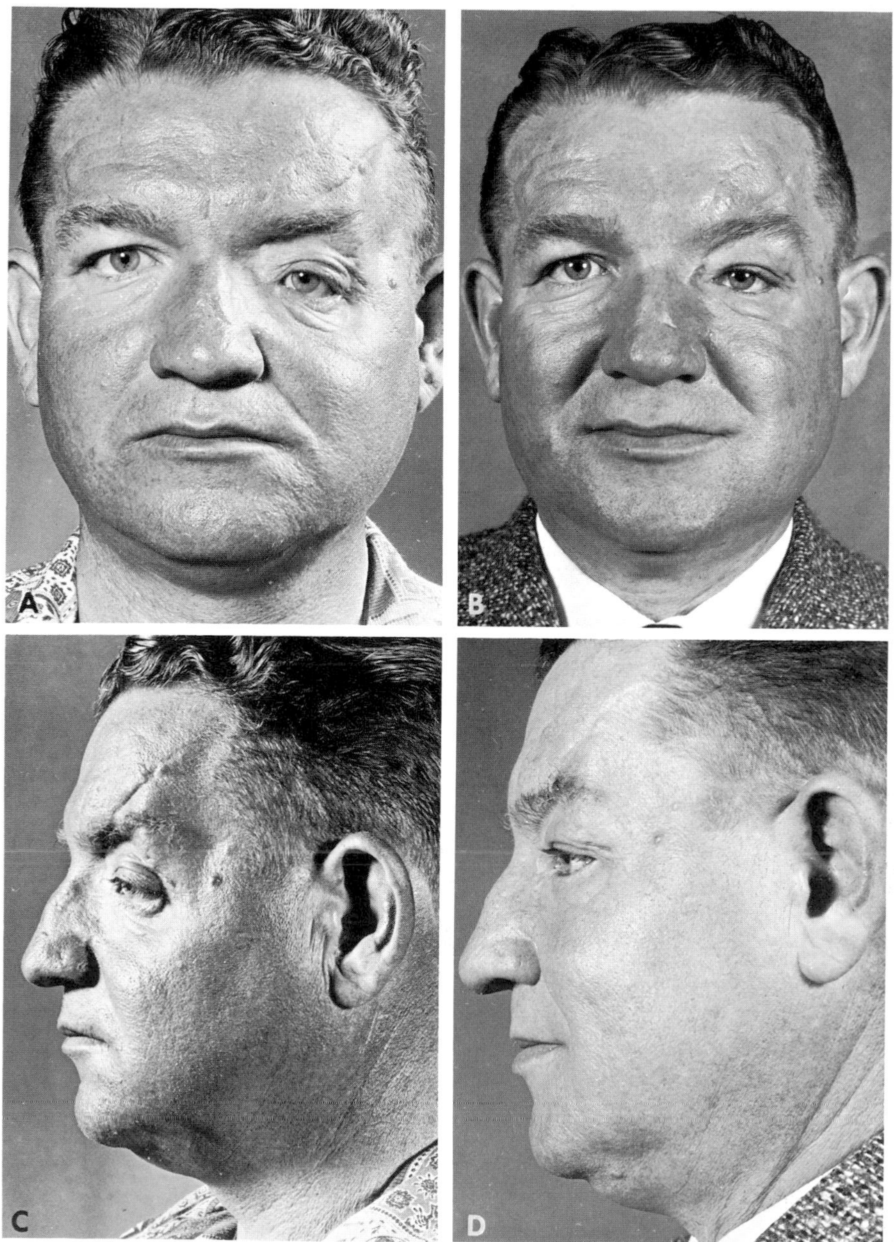

Figure 326. Malunion fracture of the left zygoma. *A.* Patient four years after fracture-dislocation of the left zygomaticomaxillary compound. *B.* One year after open osteotomy, repositioning of the zygoma, and application of preserved irradiated costal cartilage homograft to the orbital floor. *C.* Lateral view four years after primary injury. *D.* Lateral view one year following osteotomy, repositioning of the zygoma, and cartilage graft to the orbital floor.

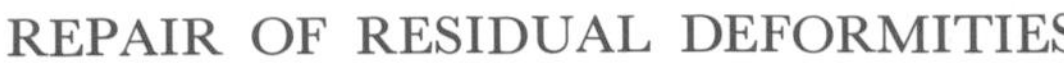

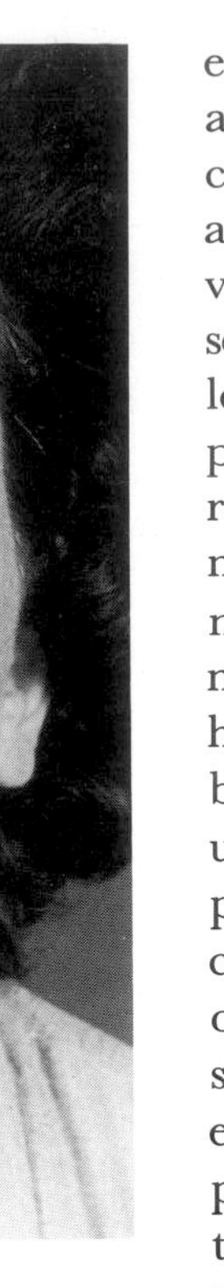

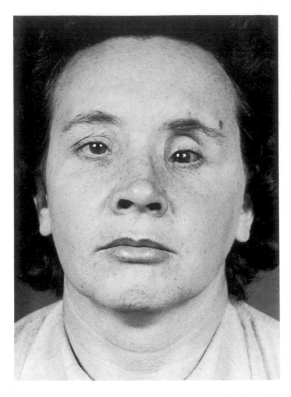

Figure 327. Malunion fracture of the left zygoma with depression of the orbital floor and depression of the left eye with enophthalmos and diplopia. Note that the patient puts her head in a posterior position in an attempt to obtain binocular vision without diplopia.

at the zygomaticomaxillary and the zygomaticofrontal suture lines and along the lateral orbital wall. The lower part of the zygomaticomaxillary suture is exposed subperiosteally through an intraoral approach. After satisfactorily immobilizing the fragments, they are replaced in normal position where they are held by direct interosseous wiring after the method of Adams.

Severe injury, with healing in malposition, may result in derangement or loss of the infraorbital rim and the orbital floor. The usual deformity consists of flatness of the cheek and depression of the globe with enophthalmos and diplopia. The disturbance in vision is usually of greater significance to the patient than the cosmetic disability. In an attempt to overcome double vision, the patient may turn or tilt his head so that the eyes can function on the same level. Attempts to overcome the diplopia by prisms are generally unsatisfactory. To correct the deformity an attempt should be made to place the bone fragments in as nearly normal a position as possible. If a few months have passed since the injury, the healing at the fracture sites may take place by soft tissue union which can be broken up with elevators. The fracture lines are approached through brow and infraorbital incisions and, if necessary, through an incision over the zygomatic arch. The orbital floor should be inspected, and the bone should be elevated and secured with interosseous wires passed through small holes on either side of the fracture site. If satisfactory elevation of the orbital floor cannot be obtained by this method, iliac bone or preserved irradiated costal cartilage grafts may be placed in the orbital floor to obtain additional elevation of the eye.

When the deformity is due to malunion and the healing of a conglomerate mass of small fragments, it is inadvisable to attempt osteotomy.

RESIDUAL DEFORMITY IN FRACTURES OF THE MAXILLA

Impacted or incompletely reduced fractures of the maxilla become fixed early by fibrous tissue, but bony union occurs later than does bony union in the mandible area. Horizontal fractures of the maxilla of three or four weeks' standing still can be reduced by traction. If it is impossible to obtain appreciable movement by digital manipula-

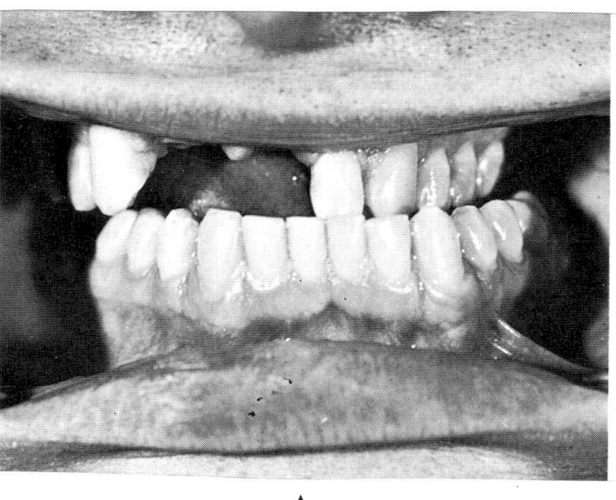

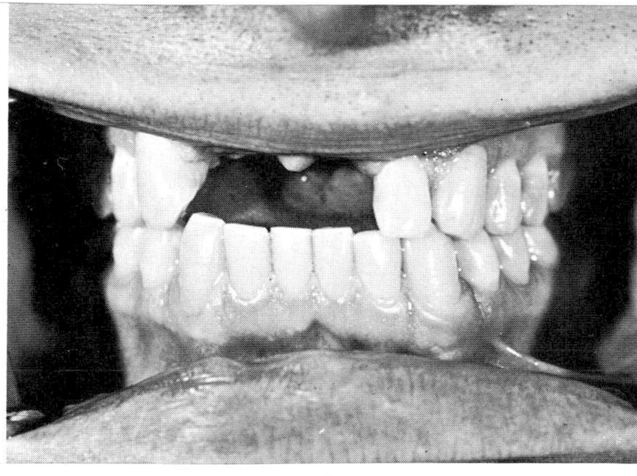

Figure 328. Malunion fracture of the maxilla with malocclusion, treated six weeks after injury by refracture, manipulation, and repositioning of the maxilla. *A.* Malunion with malocclusion six weeks following injury. *B.* Occlusion two months following repositioning.

tion, continuous traction by weight and pulley may effect reduction, but this requires considerable effort in preparing metal cap splints and also requires hospitalization of the patient. Forward traction can be obtained by applying an arch bar attachment to the upper jaw and providing the traction by the use of rubber bands attached to an outrigger on a head-cap. Appliances of this type are annoying and unsightly and may result in pressure sores on the forehead. In some cases the fracture lines can be re-established by forceful manipulation of the maxilla under anesthesia.

The use of an upper impression tray containing impression compound may be helpful in getting control of the maxillary fragment. While soft, the compound with the tray is forced up over the teeth to the sulcus in a fashion similar to taking a dental compound impression. The tray with its compound is left in position and chilled with cold water to cause hardening of the compound. Pressure applied to the handle of the tray permits movement in any desired direction so that the fibrous union at the fracture sites may be broken up. Usually the maxilla can be mobilized by this method and brought forward into normal position with the mandibular teeth where it can be fixed in occlusion by intermaxillary rubber band traction and secured by suspension to the infraorbital ridges or to the zygomatic process of the frontal bone. Such fixation will permit healing in normal position. For unilateral fracture of the maxilla, this same procedure is followed with a smaller bridge tray. If greater force is needed, refracture can be accomplished by osteotomy.

Malunion Fractures of Several Months' Duration

Cases that have progressed to bony malunion require osteotomy in order to establish normal anatomic relations. Under endotracheal anesthesia the operation is done through an incision made on the undersurface of the upper lip to expose the floor of the nose. The mucoperiosteum is elevated until the floor of the nasal cavity is identified. The dissection is carried posteriorly along the floor of the nose and the lower

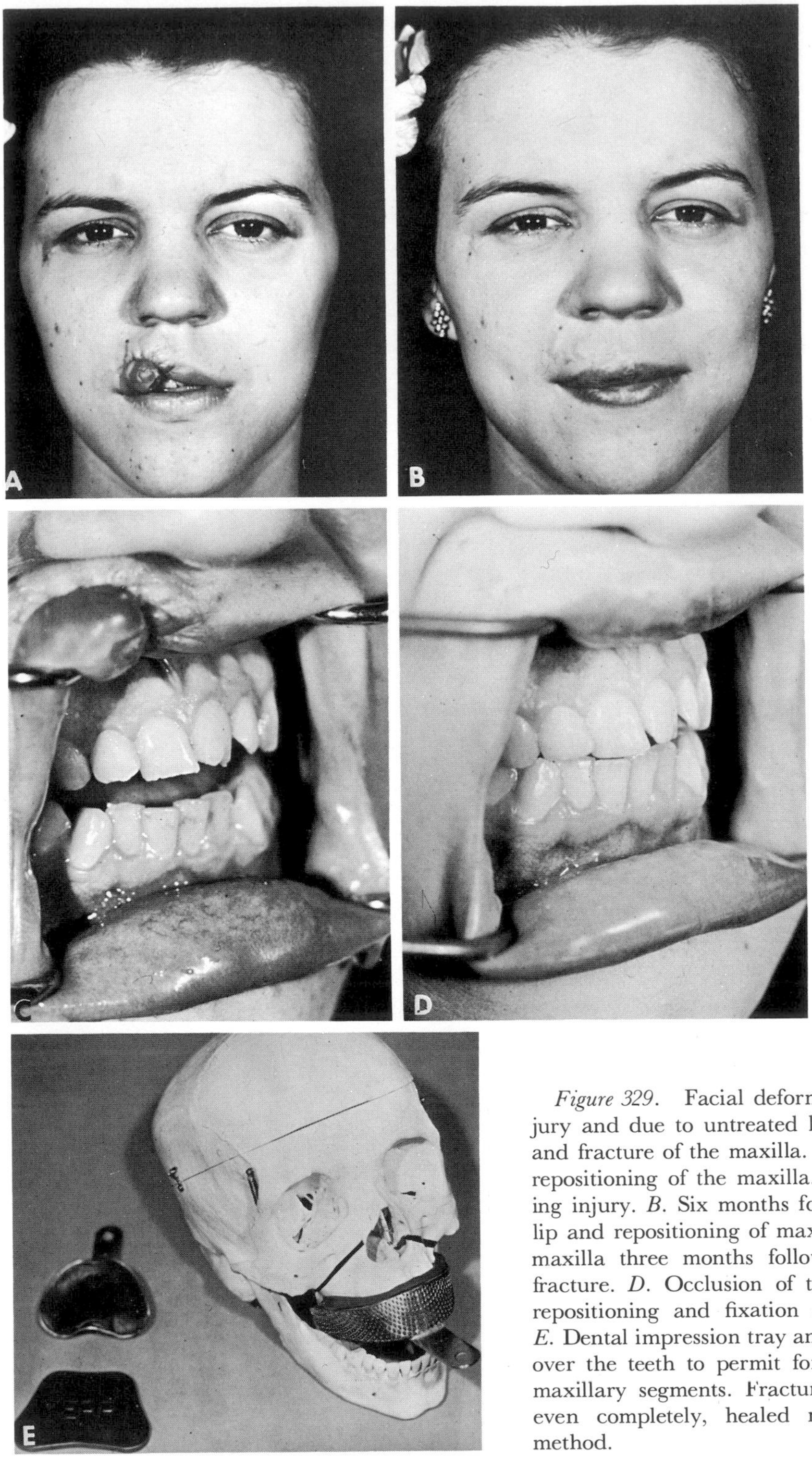

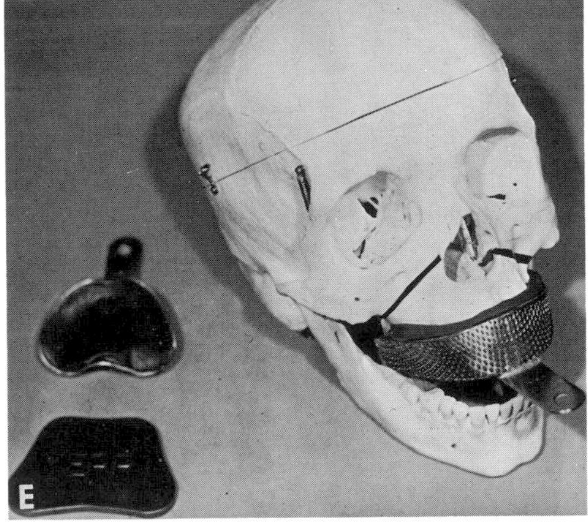

Figure 329. Facial deformity three months after injury and due to untreated laceration of the upper lip and fracture of the maxilla. Treated by refracture and repositioning of the maxilla. *A.* Three months following injury. *B.* Six months following revision of scar of lip and repositioning of maxilla. *C.* Malposition of the maxilla three months following transverse maxillary fracture. *D.* Occlusion of teeth six months following repositioning and fixation of the maxillary fracture. *E.* Dental impression tray and dental compound placed over the teeth to permit forceful manipulation of the maxillary segments. Fractures that have partially, or even completely, healed may be reduced by this method.

part of the septum on both sides, exposing the floor and the lateral nasal wall, and the lower part of the septum. Dissection is continued on the lateral surface of the bone from the premolar region to the tuberosity region without disengaging the gingival attachments. In most cases it is impossible to identify the original fracture site.

A thin osteotome is driven along the floor of the nose to separate the nasal septum. Then the osteotome is used on each lateral wall and on the lateral wall of the maxilla up to the region of the tuberosity. The plane of the osteotomy is parallel to the alveolar process and level with the nasal floor. Usually it is possible to obtain completely free movement of the fractured bone, but fibrous union in the region of the pterygoid plates may make mobilization difficult. Usually the maxilla can be disimpacted forcibly, and forward traction will bring the maxilla into a position where occlusion of the teeth can be established (Fig. 330 *A–F*).

Craniofacial Disjunction with Malunion

The deformity associated with this injury may vary from slight open-bite and minor nasal derangement to the extreme dish-face deformity. It is possible to mobilize the Le Fort III fracture of the nasomaxillary structures after several weeks by the impression tray technique or by the use of a large disimpaction forceps. Complete freedom may not be obtained, but the fibrous union in unsatisfactory position will be disrupted enough so that anterior traction on an arch bar attached by a strong rubber band to a head-cap-outrigger appliance will reduce the deformity rapidly. Then intermaxillary traction is performed, but the forward pull exercised by the outrigger is continued for 10 days to prevent a recurrence of the dislocation or contracture from intact fibrous tissue, which might dislocate the maxilla upward and backward and result in an open-bite deformity with occlusion of the teeth only in the molar region.

One must be sure that the occlusal relations of the teeth are correct and also that the relation of the incisal edge of the maxillary anterior teeth to the upper lip is satisfactory. It is possible to have elongation of the anterior portion of the face and still have the teeth in occlusion.

Recurring cerebrospinal rhinorrhea usually does not occur following refracture, even though such rhinorrhea may have occurred with the initial injury. It is possible that new leakage may occur, however, so that medication with antibiotics is advisable.

Well-healed multiple facial fractures present the most difficult problems and, in most cases, are treated by methods of reconstruction which include grafts and prostheses. Most of these measures, however, give inadequate and disappointing results. Nasal deformity may be corrected by osteotomy, by using grafts of bone or cartilage.

Cases of this type may not be treated completely by osteotomy, but the contour of the face may be improved considerably to facilitate the final reconstructive procedures. The operation consists simply of a combination of multiple osteotomies, as for individual fractures. It may be necessary to do bilateral nasal, zygomatic, maxillary, and pterygoid osteotomies. The procedure to be used is determined by careful evaluation of the deformity. Effective mobilization of the fractured facial bones is best achieved by attacking the problem in exactly the same sequence as the impact that caused the fracture originally. When there has been no treatment for several months, the fracture lines still may be identified through carefully selected incisions, and may be mobi-

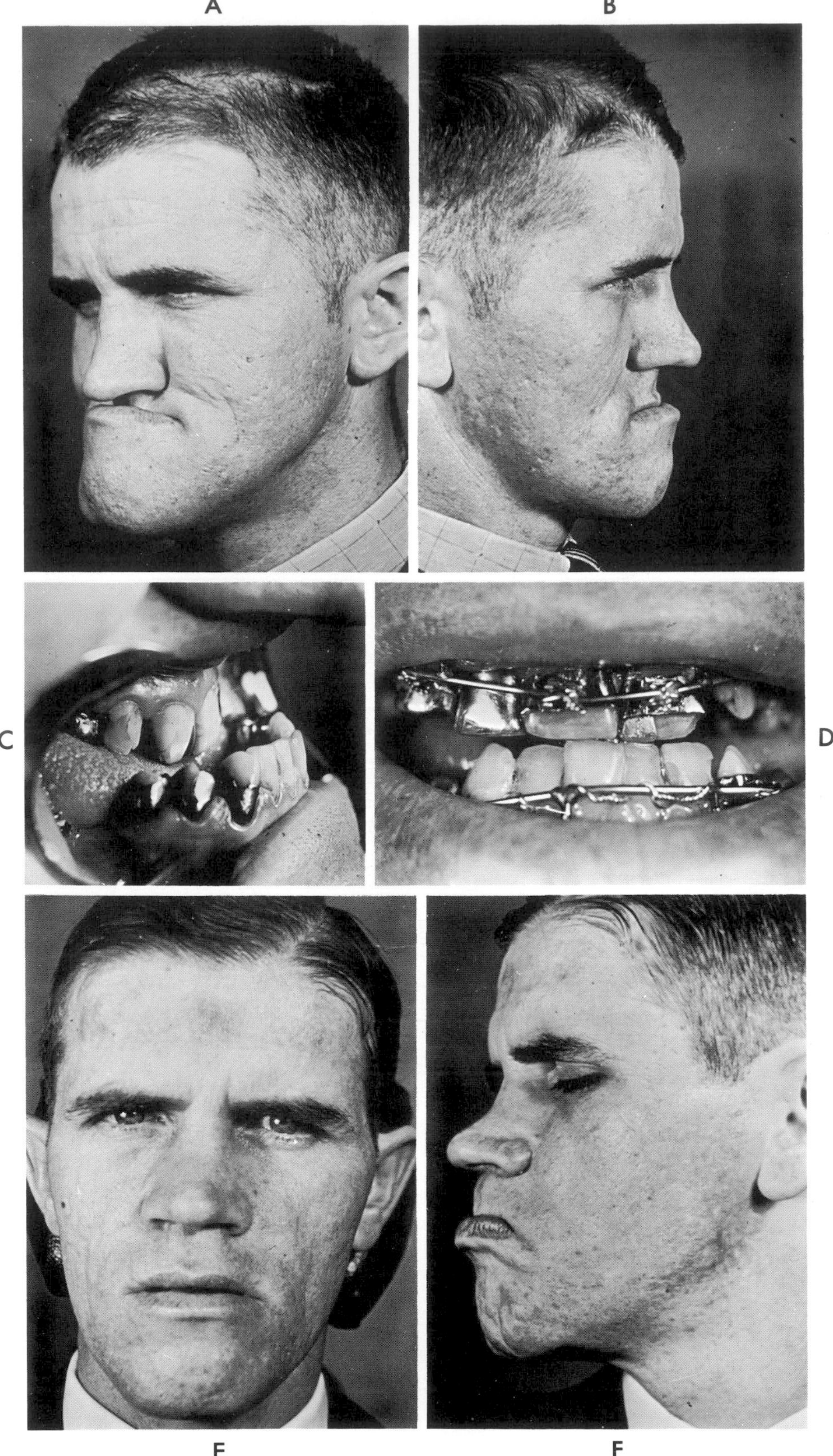
A
B
C
D
E
F

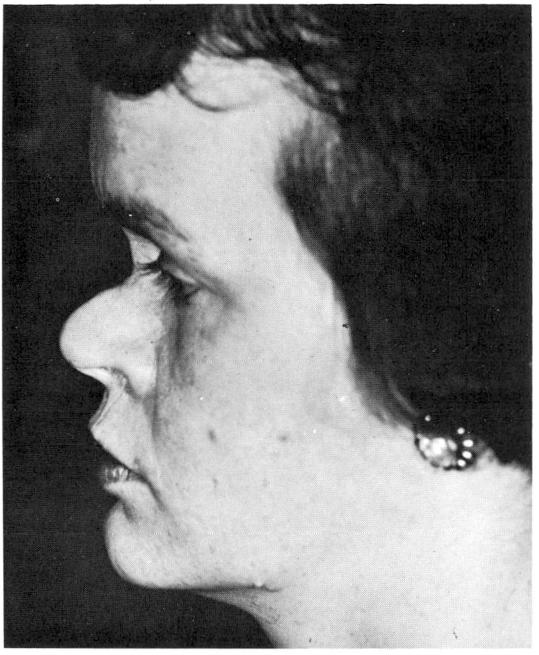

Figure 331. Facial deformity that resulted because craniofacial disjunction was not recognized. Three years after injury.

Figure 330. Deformity due to healed fracture-dislocation of the maxilla. *A–C.* Fifteen months after injury. The fractured maxilla was treated with a Kingsley splint, which does not permit evaluation of the occlusal relations. The deformity was noted after the appliance was removed. *D–F.* Result obtained by osteotomy of the maxilla and by forward traction and fixation. (From Dingman, R. O., and Harding, R. L.: The treatment of malunion fractures of the facial bones. Plast. & Reconstruct. Surg., *7:*505–519, June, 1951.)

lized by breaking up the fibrous unions with osteotomes and elevators.

Malunion fractures of long standing require the application of bold but carefully controlled forces through areas that are impossible to visualize completely if one wishes to get adequate mobilization. The procedures are daring and heroic, but the end results justify their use in well-selected patients who are impossible to treat by other means. Fixation of the bones after osteotomy and reduction depends upon the extent of the procedure, and may include any of the methods and appliances ordinarily applied in the management of acute fractures.

Case Report

A 28-year-old white male was seen in October 1949. At the age of 17 he suffered multiple facial fractures in an automobile accident. He was not expected to live and no treatment was given for the facial injuries. After recovery, his remaining teeth were removed. There was no other treatment.

He was seen 11 years after his injury with a typical dish-face deformity due to posterior displacement of the entire zygomaticomaxillary, nasal, lacrimal, and ethmoid compound. All the bones were solidly fixed in malposition and dislocated posteriorly. The relation of the maxilla to the mandible was such that there was no possibility of wearing artificial dentures. Rebuilding of the face with bone or cartilage alone appeared to be impractical. After careful consideration, the following plan was agreed upon by the staff and the patient: (1) osteotomy of the facial bones with replacement in normal position if possible; (2) replacement of lost nasal skin by median forehead flap; (3) reconstruction of any residual bony deformity with iliac bone grafts; (4) replacement of the medial palpebral ligaments; and (5) mouth rehabilitation with artificial dentures.

The operation was done under oral endotracheal anesthesia. Through appropriate incisions, osteotomy with sharp osteotomes under carefully controlled force was carried out along the lines of articulation of the various bones, as shown in Figure 332. The blood loss in this procedure was enough to warrant replacement transfusion at the time of operation. After mobilization, the bones were pulled forward manually and maintained by attachment with rubber band traction to a modified Erich appliance by means of stainless steel wires passed through drill holes in the maxilla and zygomatic bones. The nasal bones were supported by intranasal rubber-covered Erich appliances. Figure 332 *D* shows the patient three weeks after surgery. Following the removal of the appliances the bones remained in excellent position.

CARE OF OTHER RESIDUAL DEFECTS

Some patients have residual defects due to extensive loss of bone and soft tissue. Before planning the reconstruction an exact evaluation of the lost structures must be undertaken in order to determine accurately the quality and quantity of tissue necessary for repair. The lost tissues may include the external skin, the lining of the vestibule of the lip, bone for support of the jaw, and the lining for the floor of the mouth and cheek. After assessment of the lost structures, a plan is outlined for repair.

Figure 333 *A–G* illustrates a patient in whom there was extensive loss of the skin of the neck and submandibular area, the lower lip, the mandible, the floor of the mouth, the anterior portion of the tongue, and a portion of the upper lip on the left side.

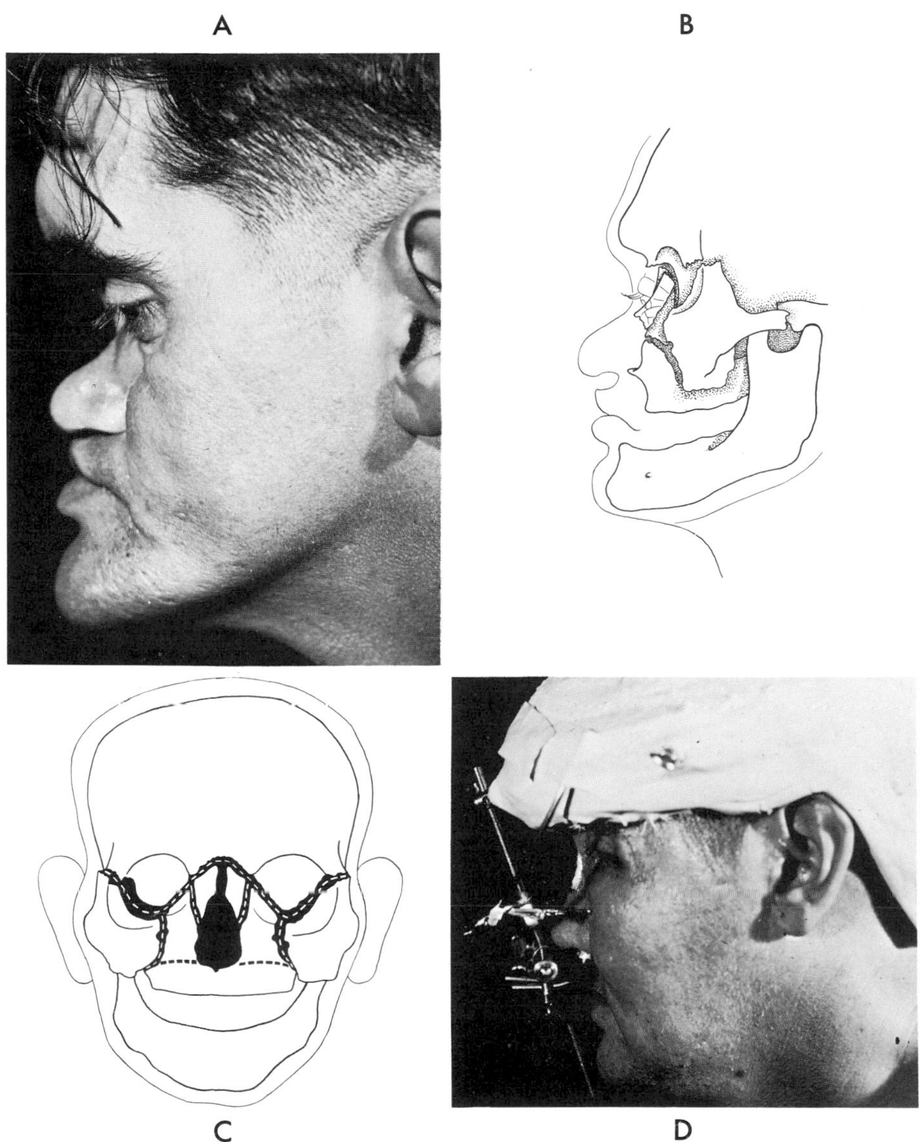

Figure 332. Malunion fracture of the facial bones. *A.* Dish-face deformity of 11 years' duration following multiple facial bone fractures. *B–C.* Artist's illustration of fractures drawn from study of the radiographs. *D.* Three weeks after osteotomy for correction of dish-face deformity. (From Dingman, R. O., and Harding, R. L.: The treatment of malunion fractures of the facial bones. Plast. & Reconstruct. Surg., *7:*505–519, June, 1951.)

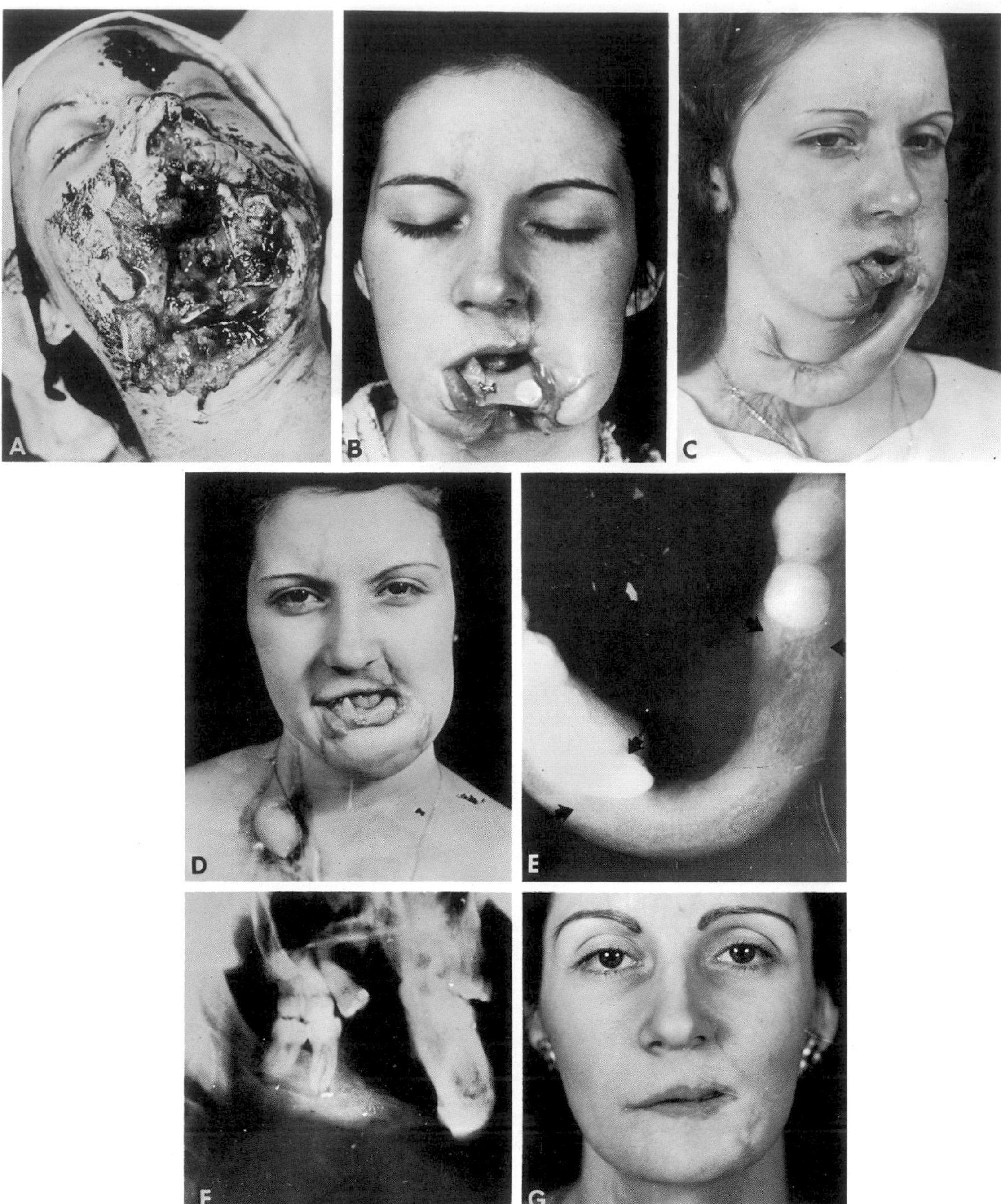

Figure 333. Self-inflicted gunshot wound of the face with extensive loss of bone and soft tissue. *A.* Six hours following gunshot wound. *B.* One month following injury. The mandible on each side is supported with an acrylic splint held to the mandible by means of circumferential wires. *C.* Tube pedicle flap based on the neck and transferred to the left side of the face. *D.* Tube cut and attached to the right side of the face. Six months later bone graft was employed for mandibular reconstruction. *E.* Iliac bone graft for reconstruction of the mandible. *F.* Lateral view of iliac bone graft. *G.* The final appearance after reconstruction consisting of replacement of the covering and lining of the lip and the lining of the floor of the mouth, resurfacing of neck, and reconstruction of the mandible with an iliac bone graft.

REPAIR OF RESIDUAL DEFORMITIES

Before reconstruction of the bone, adequate soft tissue with a good blood supply must be available for nourishment and support of the bone graft. In some cases, local tissues can be shifted into the defect to provide a covering of soft tissue. In cases of extensive loss, pedicle flaps from the neck, chest, or back may be necessary. The best color match can be obtained with skin from the immediately adjacent area. In some cases, however, it may be inadvisable to produce extensive scarring of the neck or chest, especially in women, in order to get a flap for reconstruction of the face. Skin brought from a distance by using the arm as a carrier may give satisfactory tissue for reconstruction. If taken from a distance, it has the disadvantage of poor color matching and the texture may not be the same as that of the skin of the face. In women, cosmetics will compensate for poor color match.

Thc mandible may be reconstructed with fresh autogenous bone grafts from the iliac crest. Grafts from the ilium are excellent when there is a question of contour. The desired contour for reconstruction of almost any of the facial bones can be obtained from grafts from the ilium, for this bone has a combination of curves and broad surfaces that provide grafts of almost any size and shape needed for facial bone reconstruction. The ilium is also desirable for graft material because of the great abundance of bone. The bone has sufficient stability to permit its use in areas where strength is required and is soft enough to permit it to be worked easily into the proper form. The cancellous iliac bone provides grafts that are most likely to "take" in the recipient area; it vascularizes early.

Bone grafts also may be obtained from the tibia or from the ribs. The choice of the donor region depends upon the experience and desires of the surgeon and the requirements for the use of the bone. Tibial bone is dense and will withstand great force. It is harder to contour because of its density, and especially in women it is undesirable as a source of graft material because a scar on the anterior medial aspect of the leg may be emotionally disturbing.

Rib grafts are useful in children. The grafts are easy to obtain and the rib will regenerate within a few months if the periosteum is left intact and carefully closed. This is a desirable source of grafts for repair of large defects, since grafts can be taken repeatedly from the same area. The disadvantage of the rib grafts is their small size, but when smaller segments of bone suffice, the ribs offer an excellent source of supply.

Late reconstruction of maxillary and nasal defects may be accomplished by means of bone or cartilage grafts. Depressed areas in the infraorbital and anterior maxillary region may be reconstructed by bone or cartilage overlays on the anterior maxillary wall and the infraorbital ridge.

The use of synthetic sponges is gaining some favor among American surgeons. Their use is controversial, and many feel that they produce foreign body reactions that subsequently result in loss of the sponges. It is a sound principle to use fresh autogenous biologic materials for reconstruction in the facial area whenever possible. Synthetic materials and metals frequently cause foreign body reactions and loss of the prosthesis. Foreign body reaction and infection usually cause rejection of the implant. The nonbiologic implants do very poorly in areas with thin coverage, such as the infraorbital, lateral orbital, and frontal areas.

In conclusion, it should be stressed that the majority of secondary or late residual deformities without loss of tissue are largely avoidable. Too much emphasis cannot be placed upon the vital importance of complete and unequivocal disimpaction in order that the fundamental principle of replacing normal tissues into their normal position and retaining them there can be realized. "In other words: Unravel—Disimpact—Reset—Resuture" (Gillies, 1955).

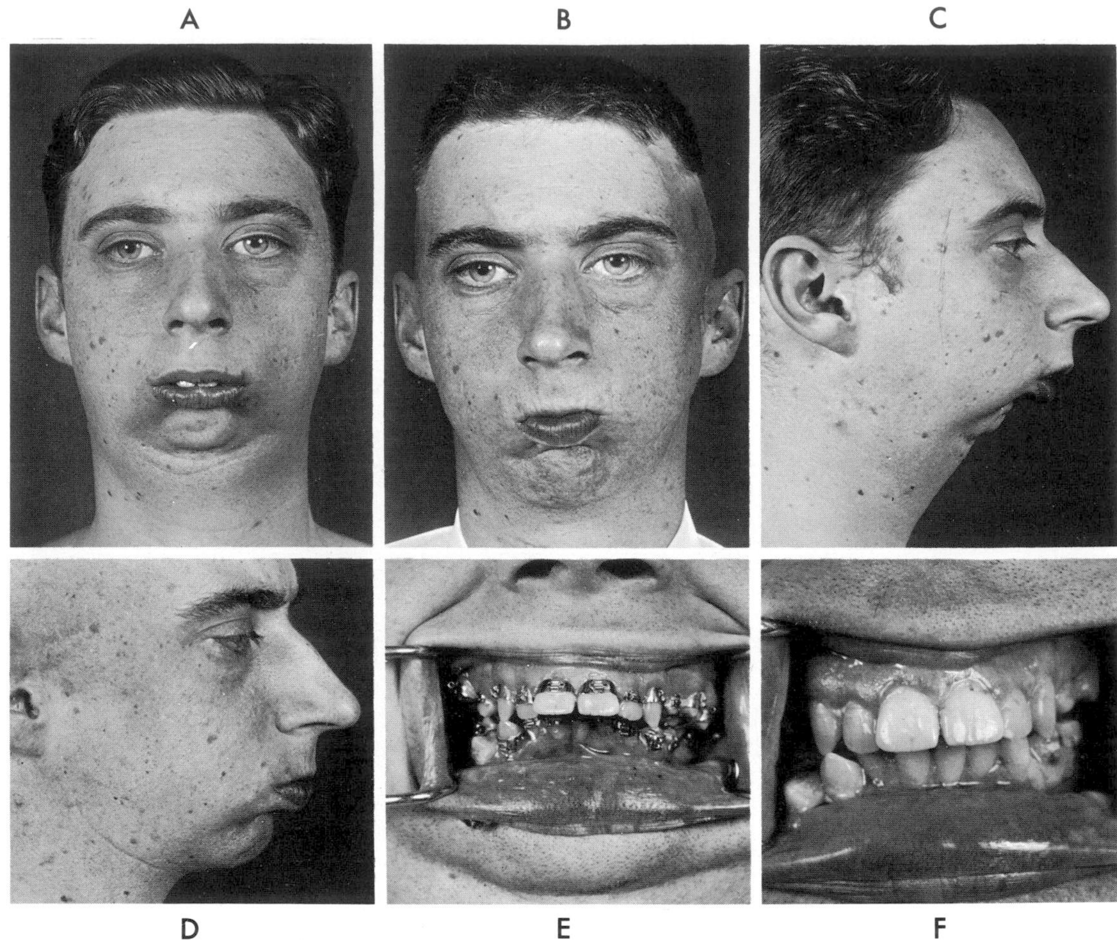

Figure 334. Facial deformity incidental to traumatic destruction of the growth centers of the mandibular condyles bilaterally. The patient injured his mandible in a fall at the age of two years, at which time the mandible ceased to develop normally. Improvement was obtained by bilateral arthroplasty of the temporomandibular joints, osteoplastic step operation for advancement of the mandible, and iliac bone graft to the anterior mandible. The patient died of a brain tumor before the total reconstruction was completed. *A.* Preoperative view showing underdevelopment of the mandible. *B.* Appearance following sliding osteotomy of the mandible and bone graft to the symphysial region. *C.* Profile view showing marked developmental deformity of the mandible. *D.* Profile view following surgery. *E.* Patient was unable to open his mouth more than 1 or 2 mm. for the intake of food. *F.* Occlusion following bilateral arthroplasty of the temporomandibular joints and sliding osteotomy of the mandible. Opening of 3.5 cm. was possible after arthroplasty.

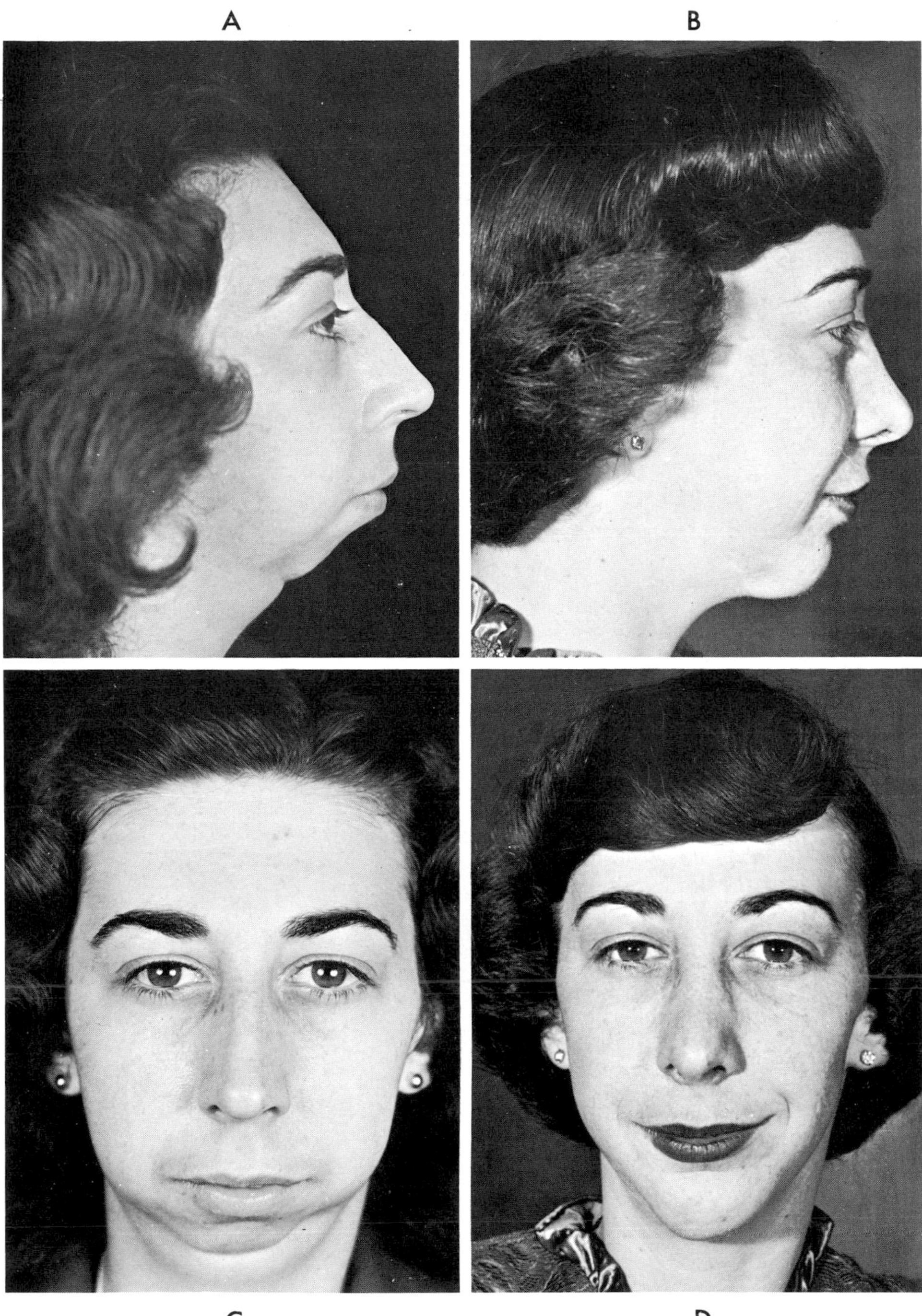

Figure 335. A 20-year-old woman with developmental deformity of the mandible without ankylosis, incident to injury at 10 years of age. Reconstruction was performed by means of sliding osteotomy of the mandible and iliac bone graft to the symphysial region. *A.* Profile view showing developmental deformity due to bilateral destruction of condyle growth centers. This patient had no ankylosis. She was able to open her mouth normally. *B.* Profile view following sliding osteotomy, iliac bone graft, and rhinoplasty. *C.* Frontal view before operation, showing underdevelopment of the mandible. *D.* Result following sliding osteotomy of the mandible and iliac bone graft to build up the contour of the chin. This case is interesting in that the patient had severe developmental deformity without ankylosis.

EPILOGUE

Is there another part of the body which is more nearly one's self than is the face? For it is the origin of respiration and of nutrition. Its senses are the wonderful means by which one discovers the uniqueness of one's being in the great universe. The configuration of its features, which has evoked so urgently the incomparable creations of sculptors and painters and poets, is that which distinguishes one from all others.

The incredibly complex arrangements of its parts, from the microscopic to the most massive, have given to man alone among terrestrial beings the power of intelligible speech and the great gift of his ability to make music. The ceaselessly mobile lines of the countenance conceal or reveal the recondite workings of the spirit. The eyes have been named the windows of the soul.

Is there another part of the body which is more nearly one's self?

G. KASTEN TALLMADGE

REFERENCES

Adams, W. M.: Internal wiring fixation of facial fractures. Surgery *12:* 523–540, (Oct.) 1942.

Adams, W. M., and Adams, L. H.: Internal wire fixation of facial fractures; 15-year follow-up report. Am. J. Surg. *92:* 12–17, (July) 1956.

Anderson, R.: Ambulatory method of treating fractures of shaft of femur. Surg. Gynec. & Obst. *62:* 865–873, (May) 1936.

Angle, E. H.: Classification of malocclusion. Dental Cosmos *41:* 248–264, 1899.

Apollonius von Kitium: Illustrierter Kommentar zur der Hippokratischen Schrift περι ἄρθρων, hrsg. von H. Schöne. Leipzig, 1896.

Babbitt, D. P.: Personal communication.

Barsky, A. J.: *Principles and Practice of Plastic Surgery.* Baltimore, Williams & Wilkins Co., 1950.

Baudens, J. B.: Fracture de la mâchoire inférieure. Bull. Acad. de méd., Paris, *5:* 341–342, 1840.

Berg, A.: Ein Fall einer veralteten, doppelseitigen Unterkieferverrekung. Ztschr. f. Stomatol. *24:* 876–887, 1926.

Bettmann, O. L.: *A Pictorial History of Medicine.* Springfield, Ill., Charles C Thomas, 1956.

Bouisson: Über die Reduktion einer veralteten Luxation des Unterkiefers. Der Zahnarzt *8:* 91–96, 1853.

Braunstein, P. W.: Medical aspects of automotive crash injury research. J.A.M.A. *163:* 249–255, (Jan.) 1957.

Breasted, J. H.: *The Edwin Smith Surgical Papyrus* (published in facsimile and hieroglyphic transliteration with translation and commentary). Chicago, University of Chicago Press, 1930, 2 v.

Brown, J. B., Fryer, M. P., and McDowell, F.: Internal wire-pin immobilization of jaw fractures. Plast. & Reconstruct. Surg. *4:* 30–35, (Jan.) 1949.

Brown, J. B., Fryer, M. P., and McDowell, F.: Internal wire-pin fixation for fractures of upper jaw, orbit, zygoma and severe facial crushes. Plast. & Reconstruct. Surg. *9:* 276–283, (March) 1952.

Brown, J. B., and McDowell, F.: Internal wire fixation for fractures of jaw: preliminary report. Surg. Gynec. & Obst. *74:* 227–230, (Feb.) 1942.

Brown, J. B., and McDowell, F.: *Plastic Surgery of the Nose.* St. Louis, C. V. Mosby Co., 1951.

Brunschwig, H.: *Das Buch der Cirurgia des Hieronymus Brunschwig.* Strassburg, Johann Grüninger, 1497.

Buck, G., Jr.: Fracture of the lower jaw, with displacement and interlocking of the fragments. Annalist, N. Y., *1:* 245–246, 1846–1847.

Cairns, H.: Injuries of frontal and ethmoidal sinuses with special reference to cerebrospinal rhinorrhea and aeroceles. J. Laryng. & Otol. *52:* 589–623, (Sept.) 1937.

Campbell, D. A.: Discussion. *In* Glas, W. W., King, O. J., Jr., and Lui, A.: Complications of tracheostomy. Arch. Surg. *85:* 62, (July) 1962.

Castiglioni, A.: *A History of Medicine* (Krumbhaar tr.). Ed. 2. New York, Alfred A. Knopf, Inc., 1947.

Celsus, A. C.: Cornelii Celsi de medicina liber incipit. Florentiae, Nicolaus, 1478.

Chalmers J. Lyons Club: Fractures involving the mandibular condyle; post-treatment survey of 120 cases. J. Oral Surg. *5:* 45–73, (Jan.) 1947.

Chopart, F., and Desault, P. J.: Traité des maladies chirurgicales, et des opérations qui leur conviennent. Paris, Villier, 1797, 2 v.

Converse, J. M.: Personal communication. The use of collagen film, electron beam sterilized for reconstruction of the orbital floor, 1962.

Converse, J. M., and Smith, B.: Reconstruction of the

floor of the orbit by bone grafts. Arch. Ophth. *44:* 1–21, (July) 1950.

Cornell University Automotive Crash Injury Research: The injury-producing accident: a primer of facts and figures. New York, (Aug.) 1961.

Daremberg, C. V. (ed.): Glossulae quatuor magistrorum super chirurgiam Rogerii et Rolandi. Neapoli et Parisiis, J. B. Baillière, 1854.

Darnall, W. L.: The use of the modified Baker anchorage in the naval dental service. U.S. Nav. M. Bull. *19:* 42–45, (July) 1923.

Desault, P. J.: Oeuvres chirurgicales. Publié par Xav. Bichat. Paris, C. Ve Desault, an VI (1798).

DesPrez, J. D., and Kiehn, C. L.: Methods of reconstruction following resection of anterior oral cavity and mandible for malignancy. Plast. & Reconstruct. Surg. *24:* 238–249, (Sept.) 1959.

Devine, J. C.: Personal communication.

Dingman, R. O.: Use of rubber bands in treatment of fractures of bones of face and jaws. J. Am. Dent. A. *26:* 173–183, (Feb.) 1939.

Dingman, R. O.: Symposium: malunited fractures of zygoma; repair of deformity. Tr. Am. Acad. Ophth. *57:* 889–896, (Nov.-Dec.) 1953.

Dingman, R. O.: *You Can Still Eat.* Ann Arbor, Mich., Caduceus Press, 1957.

Dingman, R. O.: Local anesthesia for rhinoplasty; and the nasal septum in rhinoplastic surgery. Plast. & Reconstruct. Surg. *28:* 251–260, (Sept.) 1961.

Dingman, R. O., and Alling, C. C.: Open reduction and internal wire fixation of maxillofacial fractures. J. Oral Surg. *12:* 140–156, (April) 1954.

Dingman, R. O., and Grabb, W. C.: Surgical anatomy of the mandibular ramus of the facial nerve based on the dissection of 100 facial halves. Plast. & Reconstruct. Surg. *29:* 266–272, (March) 1962.

Dingman, R. O., and Grabb, W. C.: Mandibular laterognathism. Plast. & Reconstruct. Surg. *31:* 563–575, (June) 1963.

Dingman, R. O., and Harding, R. L.: The treatment of malunion fractures of the facial bones. Plast. & Reconstruct. Surg. *7:* 505–519, (June) 1951.

Dingman, R. O., and Moorman, W. C.: Menisectomy in the treatment of lesions of the temporomandibular joint. J. Oral Surg. *9:* 214–224, (July) 1951.

Duverney, J. G.: Traité des maladies des os. (De la fracture de l'apophyse zygomatique. *1:* 182), Paris, De Bure l'aîné, 1751, 2 v.

Erich, J. B.: Fractures of the facial bones. Mil. Surgeon *88:* 637–639, (June) 1941.

Erich, J. B.: Treatment of fractures of the upper jaw. J. Am. Dent. A. *29:* 783–793, (May) 1942.

Erich, J. B.: Treatment of bilateral fractures of the edentulous mandible. Plast. & Reconstruct. Surg. *9:* 33–41, (Jan.) 1952.

Erich, J. B., and Austin, L. T.: *Traumatic Injuries of the Facial Bones: An Atlas of Treatment.* Philadelphia, W. B. Saunders Company, 1944.

Federspiel, M. N.: Jaw fractures; the value of orthodontic appliances to immobilize. Wisconsin M. J. *26:* 300–304, (June) 1927.

Federspiel, M. N.: Maxillo-facial injuries. Wisconsin M. J. *33:* 561–568, (Aug.) 1934.

Franzen, I. G.: Personal communication as quoted by *Patterns of Disease,* a publication of Parke, Davis & Company, (July) 1962, p. 4.

Freeman, B. S.: The direct approach to acute fractures of the zygomatic-maxillary complex and immediate prosthetic replacement of the orbital floor. Plast. & Reconstruct. Surg. *29:* 587–595, (May) 1962.

Fry, W. K., Shepherd, P. R., McLeod, A. C., and Parfitt, G. J.: *The Dental Treatment of Maxillofacial Injuries.* Oxford, Blackwell Scientific Publications, 1943.

Garrison, F. H.: *An Introduction to the History of Medicine.* 4th ed. Philadelphia, W. B. Saunders Co., 1929.

Georgiade, N. G.: Personal communication.

Gerrie, J. W., and Lindsay, W. K.: Fracture of maxillary-zygomatic compound with atypical involvement of orbit. Plast. & Reconstruct. Surg. *11:* 341–347, (May) 1953.

Gillies, H. D.: The diagnosis and treatment of residual traumatic deformities of the facial skeleton. *In* Rowe, N. L. and Killey, H. C.: *Fractures of the Facial Skeleton.* Baltimore, Williams & Wilkins Co., 1955, Ch. 26.

Gillies, H. D., Kilner, T. P., and Stone, D.: Fractures of the malar-zygomatic compound, with a description of new X-ray position. Brit. J. Surg. *14:* 651–656, (April) 1927.

Gilmer, T. L.: Fractures of the inferior maxilla. Ill. S. Den. Soc. Trans.: 67–104, 1881; Disc. 104–106.

Gilmer, T. L.: A case of fracture of the lower jaw with remarks on treatment. Arch. Dent. *4:* 388–390, (Sept.) 1887.

Ginestet, G., Desorthes, and Houessou: Luxation irréductible de la mâchoire suivie d'ankylose. Revue de Stomatologie *49:* 655–656, (Oct.) 1948.

Glas, W. W., King, O. J., Jr., and Lui, A.: Complications of tracheostomy. Arch. Surg. *85:* 56–63, (July) 1962.

Gorens, S. W.: Personal communication.

Gottlieb, O.: Long-standing dislocation of the jaw. J. Oral Surg. *10:* 28–32, (Jan.) 1952.

Graefe, C. F.: J. der Chir. u. Augenheilk. *IV:* 583–593, 1823.

Graham, G. G., and Peltier, J. R.: The management of mandibular fractures in children. J. Oral Surg. *18:* 416–423, (Sept.) 1960.

Gregory, T. G.: Personal communication, 1957. Quoted by Kazanjian, V. H., and Converse, J. M.: *The Surgical Treatment of Facial Injuries.* 2d ed. Baltimore, Williams & Wilkins Co., 1959, p. 164.

Gunning, T. B.: The treatment of fracture of the lower jaw by inter-dental splints. New York M. J. *3:* 433–448 (Sept.) and *4:* 11–29 (Oct.) 1866; *4:* 274–277 (Jan.) 1867.

Hagan, E. H., and Huelke, D. F.: An analysis of 319 case reports of mandibular fractures. J. Oral Surg. *19:* 93–104, (March) 1961.

Hayward, J. R.: Treatment methods for jaw fractures. J. Oral Surg. *20:* 273–280, (July) 1962.

Hendrix, J. H., Jr., Sanders, S. G., and Green, B.: Open reduction of mandibular condyle. Plast. & Reconstruct. Surg. *23:* 283–287, (March) 1959.

Holmes, W. N.: Personal communication.

Ivy, R. H.: Observations of fractures of the mandible. J.A.M.A. *79:* 295–297, (July 22) 1922.

Ivy, R. H.: Personal communication.

Johnson, J. B.: Personal communication.

Johnson, W. B.: New method for reduction of acute dislocation of the temporomandibular articulations. J. Oral Surg. *16:* 501–504, (Nov.) 1958.

Johnston, G. B.: Multiple severe automotive injuries. Evaluation and management. N. Carolina Med. J. *22:* 335–338, (Aug.) 1961.

Jolly, M.: Condylectomy in the rat. An investigation of the ensuing repair in the region of the temporomandibular articulation. Austral. D. J. *6:* 243–256, (Oct.) 1961.

Kazanjian, V. H.: Treatment of automobile injuries of the face and jaws. J.A.D.A. *20:* 757–773, (May) 1933.

Kazanjian, V. H., and Converse, J. M.: *The Surgical Treatment of Facial Injuries.* 2d ed. Baltimore, Williams & Wilkins Co., 1959.

Keen, W. W. (ed.): *Surgery, Its Principles and Practice.* Philadelphia, W. B. Saunders Co., 1906–1921, 8 v.

King, J. M.: Personal communication.

Kingsley, N. W.: *A Treatise on Oral Deformities as a Branch of Mechanical Surgery.* New York, D. Appleton & Co., 1880.

Kinloch, R. A.: Rare form of fracture of the lower jaw, successfully treated by suture of the fragments. Am. J. M. Sc., n.s., *38:* 67–70, 1859.

Kissling, A. C., Jr.: Personal communication.

Knight, J. S., and North, J. F.: The classification of malar fractures: an analysis of displacement as a guide to treatment. Brit. J. Plast. Surg. *13:* 325–339, (Jan.) 1961.

Laignel-Lavastine, P. M. M.: Histoire Générale De La Médecine, de l'art dentaire et de l'art vétérinaire. Paris, Michel, 1936–1949, vol. 2.

Lambotte, A.: *Chirurgie Opératoire Des Fractures.* Paris, Masson & Cie., 1913.

Lang, W.: Traumatic enophthalmos with retention of perfect acuity of vision. Trans. Ophth. Soc. U. Kingdom *9:* 41–45, 1889.

Laurentian Manuscript, LXXIV, 7, Laurentian Library, Florence, Italy.

Le Fort, R.: Fractures de la mâchoire supérieure. Cong. internat. de méd. C.-r., Paris, 1900, sect. de chir gén., pp. 275–278.

Le Fort, R.: Étude expérimentale sur les fractures de la mâchoire supérieure. Rev. de chir., Paris, *23:* 208, 360, 479, 1901.

Lenormant, C., and Darcissac, M.: Le procédé des "anses métalliques transosseuses" pour la contention des branches montantes, dans les fractures du maxillaire inférieur; son application dans un cas de fracture double retrodentaire de la mâchoire inférieure. Bull. et mem. Soc. nat. de chir. *53:* 503–507, (April 2) 1927.

Lillie, R. H.: Personal communication.

Litzow, T. J., and Royer, R. Q.: Treatment of long-standing dislocation of the mandible: report of case. Proc. Staff Meetings Mayo Clinic *37:* 399–403, (July 18) 1962.

Lothrop, H. A.: Fractures of the superior maxillary bone, caused by direct blows over the malar bone. A method for the treatment of such fractures. Boston Med. & Surg. J. *154:* 8–11, (January 4) 1906.

MacKinney, L.: Personal communication.

Manwaring, J. G. R.: Replacing depressed fractures of the malar bone. J.A.M.A. *60:* 278–279, (Jan. 25) 1913.

Marks, J. L.: Personal communication.

Matas, R.: Fracture of the zygomatic arch: a simple method of reduction and fixation, with remarks on the prevalence, symptomatology and treatment of this fracture. N. Orl. M. & S. J. *49:* 139–157, (Sept.) 1896.

McCoy, F. J., Chandler, R. A., Magnan, C. G., Jr., Moore, J. R., and Siemsen, G.: An analysis of facial fractures and their complications. Plast. & Reconstruct. Surg. *29:* 381–391, (April) 1962.

Meade, J. W.: Tracheotomy—its complications and their management. A study of 212 cases. New Eng. J. Med. *265:* 519–523, (Sept. 14) 1961.

Merrill, V.: *Atlas of Roentgenographic Positions.* St. Louis, C. V. Mosby Co., 1949, v. 2.

Meschan, I.: *An Atlas of Normal Radiographic Anatomy.* 2d ed. Philadelphia, W. B. Saunders Co., 1959.

Mörch, E. T.: Tracheostomy and mechanical hyperventilation. Armamentarium (V. Mueller & Co., Chicago) *3:*(6):4–7, 1960.

Müller, G. M.: Long-standing dislocation of the mandible: manual reduction. Brit. M. J. *1:* 572, (Apr. 13) 1946.

Musselman, M. M.: In discussion of paper by Glas, W. W., King, O. J., Jr., and Lui, A.: Complications of tracheostomy. Arch. Surg. *85:* 63, (July) 1962. (Death rate corrected to 3 per cent by personal communication.)

National Education Association: Summary of results of studies evaluating driver education. Washington, D.C., National Commission on Safety Education, 1961.

National Safety Council: *Accident Facts, 1961.* Chicago, 1961.

Natvig, P., and Dingman, R. O.: Osteomyelitis of the jaws in infants. Am. J. Surg. *94:* 873–876, (Dec.) 1957.

Oliver, R. T.: A method of treating mandibular fractures. J.A.M.A. *54:* 1187–1191, (April 9) 1910.

Olmstead, E. G.: Personal communication.

Panagopoulos, A. P.: Management of fractures of the jaws in children. J. Internat. Coll. Surgeons *28:* 806–815, (Dec.) 1957.

Panagopoulos, A. P., and Dietrich, W. C.: Anesthesia in operative procedures on fractures of children's jaws. Dental Items of Interest *75:* 655–662, (Aug.) 1953.

Parke, Davis & Company: Automobile accidents: special report. *Patterns of Disease,* (July) 1962.

Parker, S.: Personal communication.

Peacock, E. E., Jr.: Management of facial fractures in unconscious patients. Am. Surgeon *24:* 639–646, (Sept.) 1958.

Pfeiffer, R. L.: Roentgenography of exophthalmos with notes on roentgen ray in ophthalmology. Am. J. Ophth. *26:* 724, (July); 816 (Aug.); 928 (Sept.) 1943.

Pfeiffer, R. L.: Traumatic enophthalmos. Arch. Ophth. *30:* 718–726, (Dec.) 1943.

Pifteau, P.: Chirurgie de Guillaume de Salicet. Toulouse, 1898.

Priscianus, T.: *Octavii Horatiani rerum medicarum lib. quatour* . . . Argentorati, apud. J. Schottum, 1532.

Reiche, C. F. G.: De maxillae superioris fractura. Berol., 1822.

Risdon, F. E.: Treatment of nonunion of fractures of the mandible by free autogenous bone grafts. J.A.M.A. *79:* 297–299, (July 22) 1922.

Risdon, F. E.: Arthroplasty of the temporomaxillary joint. J.A.M.A. *85:* 2011–2013, (Dec. 26) 1925.

Risdon, F. E.: Ankylosis of the temporomaxillary joint. J.A.D.A. *21:* 1933–1937, (Nov.) 1934.

Robert, C. A.: Nouveau procédé de traitement des fractures de la portion alvéolaire de la mâchoire inférieure. Bull. gén. de thérap. méd. et chirurg. *42:* 22–25, 1852.

Roland of Parma [surnamed Capellati]: Libellus de cyrurgia editus sive compilatus a magistro Rolando feliciter incipit. *In:* Guy de Chauliac. Cyrurgia Guidonis de Cauliaco . . . Bruni, Theodorici, Rolandi, Rogerii, Lanfranci, Bentapaliae . . . Venetiis, Andrea Torresanus de Asula, 1499, pp. 135–146 ff.

Rowe, N. L., and Killey, H. C.: *Fractures of the Facial Skeleton.* Baltimore, Williams & Wilkins Co., 1955.

Ruetenick, F. G.: Dis. de fractura mandibulae, Berol., 1823.

Ryff, W. H.: *Die gross Chirurgei, oder volkommene Wundtartzenei.* Frankfurt am Main, C. Egenolph, 1545.

Safian, J.: *Corrective Rhinoplastic Surgery.* New York, Paul B. Hoeber, Inc., 1935.

Schelble, J. A.: Personal communication.

Schlomovitz, H. H.: Personal communication.

Schneider, R. C., and Thompson, J. M.: Chronic and delayed traumatic rhinorrhea as a source of recurrent attacks of meningitis. Ann. Surg. *145:* 517–529, (April) 1957.

Schullian, D. M.: Personal communication.

Sicher, H.: Structural and functional basis for disorders of the temporomandibular articulation. J. Oral Surg. *13:* 275–279, 1955.

Sicher, H.: *Oral Anatomy.* 3d ed., St. Louis, C. V. Mosby Co., 1960.

Sicher, H.: Personal communication.

Sicher, H., and Tandler, J.: *Anatomie für Zahnärzte.* Wien and Berlin, J. Springer, 1928.

Späth, J.: Komplicirte Fraktur des Unterkiefers. Med. Cor. Bl. d. Württemb. ärztl. Ver., Stuttgart, *6:* 276–277, 1836.

Spencer, W. G. (trans.): Celsus' *De medicina.* London, W. Heinemann, 1935.

Spencer, W. G.: *"De Medicina" of Celsus.* London, W. Heinemann, 1938.

Stader, O.: A preliminary announcement of a new method of treating fractures. North Am. Vet. *18:* 37–38, (Jan.) 1937.

Steffensen, W. H.: Reconstruction of the nasal septum. Plast. & Reconstruct. Surg. *2:* 66–71, (Jan.) 1947.

Stener, R. D.: Treatment of fractures of the lower maxilla. Brit. J. Dent. Sci. *20:* 658–661, 1877.

Stevenson, R. L.: *A Child's Garden of Verses* (Good and Bad Children). New York, Grosset & Dunlap, 1957.

Straith, C. L.: Guest passenger injuries. J.A.M.A. *137:* 348–351, (May 22) 1948.

Tallmadge, G. K.: Personal communication.

Tandler, J.: *Topographische Anatomie dringlicher Operationen.* Berlin, J. Springer, 1916.

Thoma, K. H.: The history and treatment of jaw fractures from World War I to World War II; collective review. Surg. Gynec. & Obst., Int. Abst. Surg. *78:* 281–312, (April) 1944.

Topetzes, N. J.: Personal communication.

Vicq d'Azyr, F.: Œuvres, recueillies et publiées avec des notes, et un discours sur sa vie et ses ouvrages, par Jacq. L. Moreau. 6 v., 8°; atlas, 39 pl., 4°. Paris, L. Duprat-Duverger, 1805.

Williamson, G. C.: *The History of Portrait Miniatures,* "Carolus II Mag. Brit. Regi Archichirurgus." London, George Bell & Sons, 1904.

Winter, L.: The use of the modified Baker anchorage in the early treatment of fractures of the mandible and maxilla. Dental Cosmos *62:* 91–93, 1920.

REFERENCES

Winter, L., Jr.: Personal communication.

Wiseman, R.: *Several chirurgical treatises.* London, R. Royston, 1676.

Wiseman, R.: *Eight chirurgical treatises.* 3d ed. London, B. Tooke & L. Meredith, 1696.

Withington, E. T. (tr.): (with notes by Tallmadge, G. K.). Corpus Hippocraticum.

Withington, E. T., and Jones, W. H. S. (eds.): Hippocrates' Works (with English translation). London, W. Heinemann, 1923–1931, 4 v.

INDEX

Page numbers in *italic* type refer to illustrations.

χρυσίῳ, ἔστ' ἂν κρατυνθῇ τὸ ὀστέοι
ίνῳ· ἔπειτα ἐπιδεῖν κηρωτῇ καὶ σπλήν
καὶ ὀθονίοισιν ὀλίγοισι, μὴ ἄ
α, ἀλλὰ χαλαροῖσιν. εὖ γὰρ εἰδ
ι ἐπίδεσις ὀθονίων γνάθῳ κατεαγεί
μὲν ἂν ὠφελέοι, εἰ χρηστῶς ἐπιδέο
δ' ἂν βλάπτοι, εἰ κακῶς ἐπιδέο
δὲ παρὰ τὴν γλῶσσαν ἐσματεῖσθαι
λὺν χρόνον ἀντέχειν τοῖσι δακτύλ
οῦντα τοῦ ὀστέου τὸ ἐκκλιθέν· ἄριο
εἰ δύναιτο· ἀλλ' οὐχ οἷόν τε.

Ἢν δὲ ἀποκαυλισθῇ παντάπα
ον—ὀλιγάκις δὲ τοῦτο γίνεται—κατορθ
τὸ ὀστέον οὕτω, καθάπερ εἴρηται. ὁ
ορθώσῃς, τοὺς ὀδόντας χρὴ ζευγνύναι,
ν εἴρηται· μέγα γὰρ ἂν συλλαμβάνο
οεμίνην, προσέτι καὶ εἴ τις ὀρθῶς ζε
χρή, τὰς ἀρχὰς ῥάψας. ἀλλὰ γὰρ
ἐν γραφῇ χειρουργίην πᾶσαν διηγεῖσ
καὶ αὐτὸν ὑποτοπεῖσθαι χρὴ ἐκ
μένων. ἔπειτα χρὴ δέρματος Καρ
ἢν μὲν νηπιώτερος ᾖ ὁ τρωθείς, ἀ
τῷ χρῆσθαι, ἢν δὲ τελειότερος ᾖ, α